Spinal
Reconstruction

Spinal Reconstruction

Clinical Examples of Applied Basic Science, Biomechanics and Engineering

edited by

Kai-Uwe Lewandrowski
University of Arizona
and
Center for Advanced Spinal Surgery
Tucson, Arizona, U.S.A.

Michael J. Yaszemski
Mayo Clinic College of Medicine
Rochester, Minnesota, U.S.A.

Iain H. Kalfas
Cleveland Clinic Foundation
Spine Institute
Cleveland, Ohio, U.S.A.

Paul Park
University of Michigan Health System
Ann Arbor, Michigan, U.S.A.

Robert F. McLain
Cleveland Clinic Foundation
Spine Institute
Cleveland, Ohio, U.S.A.

Debra J. Trantolo
A.G.E., LLC
Princeton, Massachusetts, U.S.A.

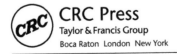

CRC Press
Taylor & Francis Group
Boca Raton London New York

CRC Press is an imprint of the
Taylor & Francis Group, an **informa** business

CRC Press
Taylor & Francis Group
6000 Broken Sound Parkway NW, Suite 300
Boca Raton, FL 33487-2742

First issued in paperback 2019

© 2010 by Taylor & Francis Group, LLC
CRC Press is an imprint of Taylor & Francis Group, an Informa business

No claim to original U.S. Government works

ISBN-13: 978-0-8493-9815-5 (hbk)
ISBN-13: 978-0-367-38949-9 (pbk)

This book contains information obtained from authentic and highly regarded sources. While all reasonable efforts have been made to publish reliable data and information, neither the author[s] nor the publisher can accept any legal responsibility or liability for any errors or omissions that may be made. The publishers wish to make clear that any views or opinions expressed in this book by individual editors, authors or contributors are personal to them and do not necessarily reflect the views/opinions of the publishers. The information or guidance contained in this book is intended for use by medical, scientific or health-care professionals and is provided strictly as a supplement to the medical or other professional's own judgement, their knowledge of the patient's medical history, relevant manufacturer's instructions and the appropriate best practice guidelines. Because of the rapid advances in medical science, any information or advice on dosages, procedures or diagnoses should be independently verified. The reader is strongly urged to consult the relevant national drug formulary and the drug companies' and device or material manufacturers' printed instructions, and their websites, before administering or utilizing any of the drugs, devices or materials mentioned in this book. This book does not indicate whether a particular treatment is appropriate or suitable for a particular individual. Ultimately it is the sole responsibility of the medical professional to make his or her own professional judgements, so as to advise and treat patients appropriately. The authors and publishers have also attempted to trace the copyright holders of all material reproduced in this publication and apologize to copyright holders if permission to publish in this form has not been obtained. If any copyright material has not been acknowledged please write and let us know so we may rectify in any future reprint.

Except as permitted under U.S. Copyright Law, no part of this book may be reprinted, reproduced, transmitted, or utilized in any form by any electronic, mechanical, or other means, now known or hereafter invented, including photocopying, microfilming, and recording, or in any information storage or retrieval system, without written permission from the publishers.

For permission to photocopy or use material electronically from this work, please access www.copyright.com (http://www.copyright.com/) or contact the Copyright Clearance Center, Inc. (CCC), 222 Rosewood Drive, Danvers, MA 01923, 978-750-8400. CCC is a not-for-profit organization that provides licenses and registration for a variety of users. For organizations that have been granted a photocopy license by the CCC, a separate system of payment has been arranged.

Trademark Notice: Product or corporate names may be trademarks or registered trademarks, and are used only for identification and explanation without intent to infringe.

A CIP record for this book is available from the British Library.

Library of Congress Cataloging-in-Publication Data available on application

Visit the Taylor & Francis Web site at
http://www.taylorandfrancis.com

and the CRC Press Web site at
http://www.crcpress.com

Preface

Spinal fusion remains at the center of many reconstructive procedures of the spine. However, several new concepts have recently emerged, which led many spine surgeons to rethink traditional approaches to common clinical problems. Examples of these new trends include use of artificial disc replacements for reconstruction of degenerated spinal segments instead of interbody fusion devices, percutaneous pedicle screw fixation systems instead of open screw placement, and minimal invasive decompressions through small percutaneously placed tubes instead of open, wide laminectomy procedures through large incisions. Minimally invasive techniques are now aided by computerized navigation systems; substitute, and expander materials are increasingly employed as adjuncts to autologous bone grafts; and growth factors, such as BMP-2, are now strongly considered as a replacement material for iliac crest bone grafts.

With the ongoing expansion and aggressive marketing of novel spinal device and implant systems, judging many of the newer developments presents a growing challenge to clinicians as it is not clear whether all of these innovative concepts represent true improvements over established clinical standards of care. Extensive work is currently underway to study the healing success and decrease in morbidity with less rigid implant systems, more bioactive and mechanically sound bone graft substitutes, and growth factor applications to establish clinical outcomes and rates of failure.

The illustrative description of the development of a new generation of materials and devices capable of specific biological interactions to improve reconstruction of the spine and to enhance reconstitution of diseased spinal segments are at the heart of this new reference text: *Spinal Reconstruction: Clinical Examples of Applied Basic Science, Biomechanics and Engineering*. Improvement of these materials and devices is in a constant state of activity, with the challenge of replacing older technologies with those that allow better exploitation of advances in a number of technologies; for example, motion preservation; navigation; less rigid, biologically active, and/or biodegradable implants that exert less stress to adjacent levels; drug delivery; recombinant DNA techniques; bioreactors; stem cell isolation and transfection; cell encapsulation and immobilization; and 3D scaffolds for cells. The chapters within this text deal with issues in the selection of proper technologies that address biocompatibility, biostability, and structure/function relationships with respect to specific clinical problem scenarios. Other chapters also focus on the use of specific biomaterials based on their physiochemical and mechanical characterizations. Integral to these chapters are discussions of standards in analytical methodology and quality control.

The readers of *Spinal Reconstruction: Clinical Examples of Applied Basic Science, Biomechanics and Engineering* will find it derived from a broad base of backgrounds ranging from the basic sciences (e.g., polymer chemistry and biochemistry) to more applied disciplines (e.g., mechanical/chemical engineering, orthopedics, and pharmaceutics). To meet varied needs, each chapter provides clear and fully detailed discussions. This in-depth but practical coverage should also assist recent inductees to the circle of spinal surgery and biomaterials. The editors trust that this reference textbook conveys the intensity of this fast-moving field in an enthusiastic presentation.

Kai-Uwe Lewandrowski

Contents

Contributors

Frank L. Acosta, Jr. Department of Neurological Surgery, University of California, San Francisco, California, U.S.A.

Michael Alapatt Boston University School of Medicine, Boston, Massachusetts, U.S.A.

Matías Alfonso Department of Orthopaedics, University Clinic of Navarra, Pamplona, Spain

Christopher P. Ames Department of Neurological Surgery, University of California, San Francisco, California, U.S.A.

Yasuchika Aoki Department of Orthopedic Surgery, Graduate School of Medicine, Chiba University, Chiba City, and Chiba Rosai Hospital Ichihara, Chiba, Japan

Henry E. Aryan Department of Neurological Surgery, University of California, San Francisco, California, U.S.A.

Thomas W. Bauer Department of Anatomic Pathology and Orthopaedic Surgery and The Spine Institute, The Cleveland Clinic Foundation, Cleveland, Ohio, U.S.A.

Stephanie Beeler Department of Neurosurgery, University of Iowa, Carver College of Medicine, Iowa City, Iowa, U.S.A.

Jose Luis Beguiristain Department of Orthopaedics, University Clinic of Navarra, Pamplona, Spain

Edward Benzel The Cleveland Clinic Foundation, Cleveland, Ohio, U.S.A.

Debdut Biswas Department of Orthopaedics and Rehabilitation, Yale University, New Haven, Connecticut, U.S.A.

Ashok Biyani Department of Bioengineering and Orthopedic Surgery, University of Toledo, Toledo, Ohio, U.S.A.

Ciaran Bolger Department of Neurosurgery, Beaumont Hospital, Dublin, Ireland

Christopher M. Bono Department of Orthopaedic Surgery, Harvard Medical School, Brigham and Women's Hospital, Boston, Massachusetts, U.S.A.

Joseph C. Cauthen III Neurosurgical and Spine Associates PA, Gainesville, Florida, U.S.A.

Robert H. Chamberlain Barrow Neurological Institute, Phoenix, Arizona, U.S.A.

Boyle C. Cheng Department of Neurological Surgery, UPMC Health System, University of Pittsburgh School of Medicine, Pittsburgh, Pennsylvania, U.S.A.

Susan Chubinskaya Department of Biochemistry and Section of Rheumatology, Rush University Medical Center, Chicago, Illinois, U.S.A.

Neil R. Crawford Barrow Neurological Institute, Phoenix, Arizona, U.S.A.

Lieven A. Danneels   Department of Rehabilitation Sciences and Physiotherapy, Ghent University, Ghent, Belgium

Reginald Davis   Greater Baltimore Neurosurgical Associates PA, Baltimore, Maryland, U.S.A.

Hugo J. De Cuyper   Hospital Jan Palfijn—Campus Gallifort, Antwerp, Belgium

Rick B. Delamarter   Spine Research Foundation, The Spine Institute, Santa Monica, California, U.S.A.

Michael J. DePalma   Department of Physical Medicine and Rehabilitation, Virginia Commonwealth University, Richmond, Virginia, U.S.A.

Nabil Ebraheim   Spine Research Center, University of Toledo and Medical University of Ohio, Toledo, Ohio, U.S.A.

Ahamed Faizan   Department of Bioengineering and Orthopedic Surgery, University of Toledo, Toledo, Ohio, U.S.A.

Leonora Felon   Department of Bioengineering and Orthopedic Surgery, University of Toledo, Toledo, Ohio, U.S.A.

Mark R. Foster   Department of Orthopaedic Surgery, University of Pittsburgh School of Medicine, Pittsburgh, Pennsylvania, U.S.A.

Takeshi Fuji   Department of Orthopaedic Surgery, Osaka Koseinenkin Hospital, Osaka, Japan

Peter C. Gerszten   Department of Neurological Surgery, UPMC Health System, University of Pittsburgh School of Medicine, Pittsburgh, Pennsylvania, U.S.A.

Vijay K. Goel   Department of Bioengineering and Orthopedic Surgery, University of Toledo, Toledo, Ohio, U.S.A.

Jonathan N. Grauer   Department of Orthopaedics and Rehabilitation, Yale University, New Haven, Connecticut, U.S.A.

Steven Griffith   Anulex Technologies Inc., Minnetonka, Minnesota, U.S.A.

Mats Grönblad   Division of Physical Medicine and Rehabilitation, University Central Hospital, Helsinki, Finland

Mark R. Grubb   Northeast Ohio Spine Center, Akron/Canton, Ohio, U.S.A.

Helen E. Gruber   Carolinas Healthcare System, Charlotte, North Carolina, U.S.A.

Edward N. Hanley, Jr.   Carolinas Healthcare System, Charlotte, North Carolina, U.S.A.

Hiroshi Hashizume   Department of Orthopaedic Surgery, Wakayama Medical University, Wakayama City, Wakayama, Japan

Kyoji Hayashi   Department of Orthopaedic Surgery, Graduate School of Medical and Dental Sciences, Kagoshima University, Kagoshima, Japan

Hwan Tak Hee   Department of Orthopaedic Surgery, National University of Singapore, Singapore

David D. Hile   Stryker Biotech, Hopkinton, Massachusetts, U.S.A.

Patrick W. Hitchon   Department of Neurosurgery, University of Iowa, Carver College of Medicine, Iowa City, Iowa, U.S.A.

Frank S. Hodges   University of Alabama at Birmingham, Birmingham, Alabama, U.S.A.

Scott J. Hollister   Department of Biomedical Engineering, University of Michigan, Ann Arbor, Michigan, U.S.A.

Michio Hongo   Department of Orthopedic Surgery, Akita University School of Medicine, Akita, Japan

Noboru Hosono   Department of Orthopaedic Surgery, Osaka Koseinenkin Hospital, Osaka, Japan

Tadashi Inaba   Department of Mechanical Engineering, Mie University, Tsu, Mie, Japan

Aditya V. Ingalhalikar   Department of Neurosurgery, University of Iowa, Iowa City, Iowa, U.S.A.

Adrian P. Jackson   Premier Spine Care, Overland Park, Kansas, U.S.A.

Masahiko Kanamori   Department of Orthopaedic Surgery, University of Toyama, Toyama, Japan

Yuichi Kasai   Department of Orthopaedic Surgery, Mie University Graduate School of Medicine, Tsu, Mie, Japan

Takaya Kato   Department of Mechanical Engineering, Mie University, Tsu, Mie, Japan

Yasuji Kato   Department of Orthopaedic Surgery, Toyonaka Municipal Hospital, Toyonaka, Japan

Mamoru Kawakami   Department of Orthopaedic Surgery, Wakayama Medical University, Wakayama City, Wakayama, Japan

Michael O. Kelleher   Department of Neurosurgery, Beaumont Hospital, Dublin, Ireland

Naomi Kobayashi   Department of Anatomic Pathology and Orthopaedic Surgery, The Cleveland Clinic Foundation, Cleveland, Ohio, U.S.A.

Setsuro Komiya   Department of Orthopaedic Surgery, Graduate School of Medical and Dental Sciences, Kagoshima University, Kagoshima, Japan

Leslie L. Korbee   Cincinnati Orthopaedic Research Institute, Cincinnati, Ohio, U.S.A.

Paul H. Krebsbach   Department of Biologic and Materials Sciences, University of Michigan, Ann Arbor, Michigan, U.S.A.

Donald W. Kucharzyk   The Orthopaedic, Pediatric and Spine Institute, Crown Point, Indiana, U.S.A.

Koichi Kuribayashi   Department of Immunology and Pathology, Kansai College of Oriental Medicine, Kumatori-Cho, Osaka, Japan

Frank La Marca   Department of Neurosurgery, University of Michigan, Ann Arbor, Michigan, U.S.A.

Adolfo Espinoza Larios   Barrow Neurological Institute, Phoenix, Arizona, U.S.A.

James P. Lawrence   Department of Orthopaedics and Rehabilitation, Yale University, New Haven, Connecticut, U.S.A.

Carlos J. Ledezma   Department of Neurological Surgery, University of Southern California, Los Angeles, California, U.S.A.

Kai-Uwe Lewandrowski   University of Arizona and Center for Advanced Spinal Surgery, Tucson, Arizona, U.S.A.

Isador H. Lieberman   The Cleveland Clinic Foundation, Cleveland, Ohio, U.S.A.

Tae-Hong Lim   Department of Biomedical Engineering, University of Iowa, Iowa City, Iowa, U.S.A.

Chia-Ying Lin   Department of Neurosurgery, University of Michigan, Ann Arbor, Michigan, U.S.A.

Timothy Lindley   Department of Neurosurgery, University of Iowa, Carver College of Medicine, Iowa City, Iowa, U.S.A.

Takuji Matsumoto   Department of Orthopaedic Surgery, Wakayama Medical University, Wakayama City, Wakayama, Japan

Shunji Matsunaga   Department of Orthopaedic Surgery, Imakiire General Hospital, Kagoshima, Japan

James Maxwell   Scottsdale Spine Care, Scottsdale, Arizona, U.S.A.

Linda McEvoy   Department of Neurosurgery, Beaumont Hospital, Dublin, Ireland

Dennis McGowan   Spine and Orthopedic Surgery Associates, Kearney, Nebraska, U.S.A.

Adam G. Miller   Cincinnati Orthopaedic Research Institute, Cincinnati, Ohio, U.S.A.

Thomas J. Milroy   The Orthopaedic, Pediatric and Spine Institute, Crown Point, Indiana, U.S.A.

Naohisa Miyakoshi   Department of Orthopedic Surgery, Akita University School of Medicine, Akita, Japan

Hideshige Moriya   Department of Orthopedic Surgery, Graduate School of Medicine, Chiba University, Chiba City, Chiba, Japan

Yoshimi Nagatomo   Department of Orthopaedic Surgery, Graduate School of Medical and Dental Sciences, Kagoshima University, Kagoshima, Japan

Kazuo Ohmori   Department of Orthopaedic Surgery, Nippon-Kokan Hospital, Kanagawa, Japan

Seiji Ohtori   Department of Orthopedic Surgery, Graduate School of Medicine, Chiba University, Chiba City, Chiba, Japan

Walter Peppelman, Jr.   Pennsylvania Spine Institute, Harrisburg, Pennsylvania, U.S.A.

Joseph H. Perra   Twin Cities Spine Center, Minneapolis, Minnesota, U.S.A.

Ben B. Pradhan   Spine Research Foundation, The Spine Institute, Santa Monica, California, U.S.A.

Gary W. Procop   Clinical Microbiology, The Cleveland Clinic Foundation, Cleveland, Ohio, U.S.A.

E Raymond S. Ross   Hope Hospital, Eccles Old Salford, U.K.

Koichi Sairyo   Department of Orthopedics, University of Tokushima, Tokushima, Japan

Hiroshige Sakai   Department of Anatomic Pathology and Orthopaedic Surgery, The Cleveland Clinic Foundation, Cleveland, Ohio, U.S.A.

Toshinori Sakai   Department of Orthopedics, University of Tokushima, Tokushima, Japan

Hassan Serhan   DePuy Spine, Raynham, Massachusetts, U.S.A.

John Sherman   Orthopedic Consultants PA, Edina, Minnesota, U.S.A.

Yoichi Shimada   Department of Orthopedic Surgery, Akita University School of Medicine, Akita, Japan

Chelsey Simmons Harvard University, Cambridge, Massachusetts, U.S.A.

Ghassan Skaf American University of Beirut, Beirut, Lebanon

Curtis W. Slipman Department of Rehabilitation Medicine, The Penn Spine Center, Hospital of the University of Pennsylvania, Philadelphia, Pennsylvania, U.S.A.

Michael L. Swank Cincinnati Orthopaedic Research Institute, Cincinnati, Ohio, U.S.A.

Kazuhisa Takahashi Department of Orthopedic Surgery, Graduate School of Medicine, Chiba University, Chiba City, Chiba, Japan

Steven M. Theiss University of Alabama at Birmingham, Birmingham, Alabama, U.S.A.

Daisuke Togawa Department of Anatomic Pathology and Orthopaedic Surgery and The Spine Institute, The Cleveland Clinic Foundation, Cleveland, Ohio, U.S.A.

Masataka Tokuda Department of Mechanical Engineering, Mie University, Tsu, Mie, Japan

Jukka Tolonen Department of Internal Medicine, University Central Hospital, Helsinki, Finland

Debra J. Trantolo A.G.E., LLC, Princeton, Massachusetts, U.S.A.

Atsumasa Uchida Department of Orthopaedic Surgery, Mie University Graduate School of Medicine, Tsu, Mie, Japan

Guy G. Vanderstraeten Department of Rehabilitation Sciences and Physiotherapy, Ghent University, Ghent, Belgium

Carlos Villas Department of Orthopaedics, University Clinic of Navarra, Pamplona, Spain

Brian Walsh University of Wisconsin, Madison, Wisconsin, U.S.A.

Shih-Tien Wang Department of Orthopedics and Traumatology, Taipei, Taiwan

William C. Welch Department of Neurological Surgery, UPMC Health System, University of Pittsburgh School of Medicine, Pittsburgh, Pennsylvania, U.S.A.

Andrew P. White Department of Orthopaedic and Neurological Surgery, Thomas Jefferson University Hospital, Philadelphia, Pennsylvania, U.S.A.

Takuya Yamamoto Department of Orthopaedic Surgery, Graduate School of Medical and Dental Sciences, Kagoshima University, Kagoshima, Japan

Kazunori Yone Department of Orthopaedic Surgery, Graduate School of Medical and Dental Sciences, Kagoshima University, Kagoshima, Japan

Kenneth Yonemura Department of Neurosurgery, University of Utah, Salt Lake City, Utah, U.S.A.

Munehito Yoshida Department of Orthopaedic Surgery, Wakayama Medical University, Wakayama City, Wakayama, Japan

1 The Role of Minimally Invasive Surgery in Instrumented Lumbar Fusion

Donald W. Kucharzyk and Thomas J. Milroy
The Orthopaedic, Pediatric and Spine Institute, Crown Point, Indiana, U.S.A.

Over the years, we have seen the new and innovative techniques that have allowed the surgeon to minimize exposure to potentially maximize the patient's outcome. Minimally invasive surgical approaches and treatment have become the standard in many surgical specialties. When we look at this evolution, we are drawn to the use in the surgical procedure for a cholecystectomy (1). The minimally invasive approach via laparoscopy has now replaced the traditional open approach, and the results have shown less morbidity and movement of this procedure to an ambulatory outpatient procedure. In orthopedics, this has been seen with the advent of the arthroscope, where an open procedure was the standard and the only option. Now, one can treat many joints, especially the knee and shoulder, with a minimally invasive approach through the arthroscope.

This concept of minimally invasive surgery has now become evident in all aspects of orthopedics—especially, most recently, with total hip and total knee replacement surgery with the main driving force for minimally invasive surgery being sooner and quicker recovery. The results from this approach to the hip and knee have shown promise. Spine surgery has also had its evolution from the classic open laminectomy and discectomy to microdiscectomy, which has evolved into, and in many centers, is now an ambulatory outpatient procedure. The reason for this transition and the success has been based on the premise of less bone disruption, less bleeding, less paraspinal muscle damage than that which was seen with the classic approach (2–4). Concerns have existed with any procedure in the lumbar spine, open or via microdiscectomy, as to the degree of soft-tissue dissection and stripping of the paraspinal muscles and damage during muscle retraction. Problems have been identified from these, which include elevated creatinine phosphokinase MM (5), a high incidence of low back pain (6), and an increased incidence in the development of failed back syndrome (7).

As a result, any approach that minimizes these problems and can improve surgical outcomes and rehabilitation time would be met with support from the spinal community.

In the advent of the progression to a minimally invasive approach to the spine for decompression and discectomy, we have seen the evolution from the open approach, where good clinical results have been seen to the micro-approach, which has also evolved into a small incision ambulatory procedure with good surgical and clinical outcomes (8).

If we believe our concerns about muscle damage and their effects, and a new approach, such as minimally invasive or minimal access were developed, then it should provide access channels to the spinal anatomy and bony structures with minimal muscle stripping and damage. The first system to address this was METRx^{TM} (Medtronic Sofamor Danek) (Fig. 1), which involved a tubular retraction system that allowed direct visualization, minimal muscle stripping and damage, and the ability to perform a decompression and discectomy. Foley (9) and Hilton (10) have reported their results, showing a reduction in hospital stay, improved clinical outcomes, and quicker return to work with the METRx system.

Additional systems have now been developed to provide access to the spine and provide results similar to that reported. Such systems include the DePuy Pipeline^{TM} (which provides access through a retractor system that allows it to be expanded to the size and length needed), NuVasive MaXcess^{TM} (which is similar to the others with distracters that provide access to any length of the spinal exposure needed) (Fig. 2), Endius (which is different from the others in that it utilizes an arthroscopic camera system to visualize the operative field

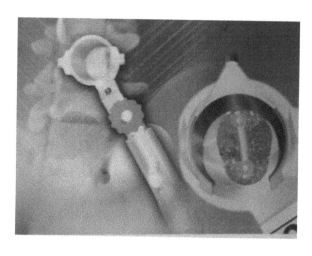

FIGURE 1 Medtronic METRx™ minimally invasive system with next generation X-tube modification for screw and rod insertion. *Source*: Courtesy of Medtronic Sofamor Danek, Memphis, Tennessee.

and visualize the spine), and EBI VuePass Tubular (which uses a radiolucent tubular system that provides ease with accessing radiographs for placement of the retractors and identifying the levels, and moreover is free of metal interference on X-rays) (Fig. 3). In addition, with the ability to perform a decompression and discectomy through this approach, these systems allow the surgeon to perform an interbody fusion as well.

With proper positioning and placement of the initial guide wires, and paying attention to the angle for the type of procedure desired, followed by proper placement of the retractors, one can approach the interspace and perform a posterior lumbar interbody fusion (PLIF) or transforaminal interbody fusion (TLIF).

The technique begins by identifying the proper landmarks for the skin incision (Fig. 8) and then under C-arm visualization guide wires at the specific levels. Proper positioning involves the placement of the guide wires 3 to 5 cm from the midline (Fig. 4) and at the specific level and angle based on the approach. If performing a PLIF, then a more direct approach is used (Fig. 5), and for a TLIF, a more angled position is utilized for the insertion point (Fig. 6). The radiographs shown in Figure 7 can be used to ascertain proper position and placement. Subsequently, through dilators and a small fascial incision (Fig. 8), the muscle fibers are split and separated along the muscle plane, so as to prevent muscle damage and injury. Permanent retractors are then inserted for the specific system used, and the standard procedure that would be done open can be performed. A decompression, facetectomy, discectomy can be easily performed and an interbody fusion can be completed (Fig. 9).

Preliminary studies have shown that in this approach and technique, fewer complications have been reported; no graft or implant failure have been seen; decreased blood loss;

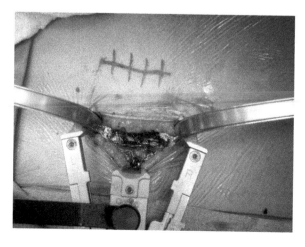

FIGURE 2 The NuVasive MaXcess™ system (Nuvasive, San Diego, California) for insertion of pedicular screws and rods with direct view of facets and landmarks for screw placement and decompression for interbody fusion.

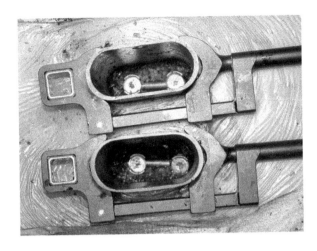

FIGURE 3 EBI VuePass™ (EBI, L.P., Parsippany, New Jersey) minimally invasive system showing ability to perform bilateral access to the spine for instrumented fusion with ease of graft insertion in posterolateral gutter.

shorter hospital stays; and good clinical outcomes are reported (11,12). However, with this technology, we were unable to stabilize the spine posteriorly with instrumentation, and could only provide anterior column support via interbody fusion after a decompression in the initial systems that were developed. As technology has continued to evolve and strove to identify a process to instrument the spine posteriorly, a percutaneous system, through a minimally invasive approach, would be ideal (13,14). This minimally invasive concept has now given rise to a truly percutaneous system, the Sextant System.

The Sextant System™ (Medtronic Sofamor Danek) allows one to insert pedicle screws percutaneously with the aid of radiographic C-arm. The technique involves the insertion of percutaneous guide wires first, followed by dilators over the guide wires. The pedicles are then prepared and screws inserted. With the screws inserted, extenders are attached to the screw heads and aligned and interlocked.

This allows the screw heads to be aligned appropriately and the arc-shaped rod awl is driven through to engage each screw head, and then the arc-rod insertor is utilized to pass the rod into the screws, and locking nuts are applied. This system lends itself well as a supplement for an anterior approach, but can also be applied to posterior decompression with or without interbody fusion, using a Wiltse approach, with insertion of the screws through this incision and percutaneous screw insertion on the opposite side. The Sextant System allows one to perform a single-level instrumented fusion in its initial design, and currently, multiple-level instrumented fusions with the next-generation Sextant System. This system does have its limitations in its use, especially with severe deformities of the spine, patients with increased lumbar lordosis, and if considering instrumentation at the L5-S1 level or if a posterolateral fusion is to be performed. As with any

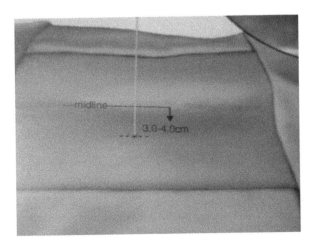

FIGURE 4 Initial placement of skin marking and guide pin insertion point. *Source*: Courtesy of Medtronic Sofamor Danek, Memphis, Tennessee.

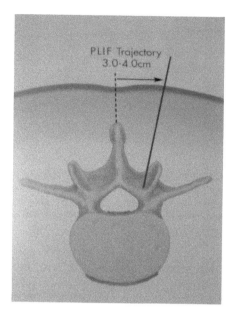

FIGURE 5 Guide pin angle for insertion for a minimally invasive approach for performing a posterior lumbar interbody fusion. *Source*: Courtesy of Medtronic Sofamor Danek, Memphis, Tennessee.

evolving technology, modification and refinement will occur and move to a still minimally invasive access approach with more visualization of the spine and greater flexibility in the performance of additional procedures, such as an instrumented fusion with posterolateral fusion, which is limited in the percutaneous system.

Systems that have evolved and which allow the insertion of pedicular screws through a minimally invasive approach and incision, coupled with the ability to perform a posterolateral fusion, include the Medtronic X-Tube™ (Fig. 1), Spinal Concepts Pathfinder, DePuy Aperture, DePuy Viper, NuVasive SpherRx™ and SpherRxDBR™, and Endius.

These systems utilize a Wiltse approach (15) to provide an intramuscular plane to the spine, between the multifdus and longisimus. Guide wires are placed, and taps and screws are inserted. Rods are then inserted through both direct visualization and placement or with the aid of slotted connectors that align the screw heads for placement of the rods, and then locking screws are guided into place (Fig. 11). Advantages include less blood loss, less

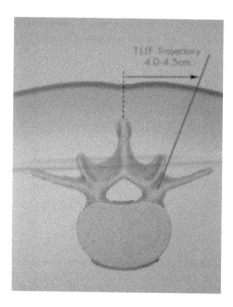

FIGURE 6 Placement and angle for direction of system for a transforaminal interbody fusion approach. *Source*: Courtesy of Medtronic Sofamor Danek, Memphis, Tennessee.

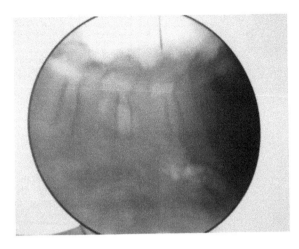

FIGURE 7 Radiographic image of proper placement and angle on lateral radiograph for the appropriate level.

muscle damage, the ability for reduction of a spondylolisthesis, compression and distraction across a spinal segment, and use in multilevel instrumented fusions. Disadvantages include limitations in the ability to decompress the spine, visualization of the neural structures for discectomy, and the ability to perform an interbody fusion.

The ability to perform all aspects of a fusion through a minimally invasive approach have taken all that was previously developed and evolved it, so as to include decompression, interbody fusion, and instrumentation through a single simple approach. Systems that have been developed include the Medtronic Quadrant System (Fig. 10), NuVasive MaXcess (Fig. 2), Endius ATAVI, and the EBI VuePass System (Fig. 3). These systems allow one to have direct visualization of the spine, potentially less muscle damage, limited dissection of the soft tissues and preservation of the tissues, the ability to perform a decompression, perform a PLIF or TLIF, and insert pedicular screws and instrumentation. These systems are all applicable for either single- or multi-level fusions. Advantages are similar in all these systems, with the exception of the EBI VuePass System that allows one to utilize C-arm easily as the retractor system is radiolucent, and allows the surgeon to perform the surgery his way with little change in his technique.

The advantages of the EBI VuePass System include the ability to span a multi-level segment for instrumented fusion; the ability to insert bilateral tubes for simultaneous work on both sides of the spinal column; the ability to use any spinal instrumentation system or interbody fusion device that one desires; and ease to perform a posterolateral fusion with minimal movement of the retractor system (Figs. 3 and 11). This system encompasses all these and has been shown to have reproducibility, and as a result offers distinct advantages over any of the current available systems.

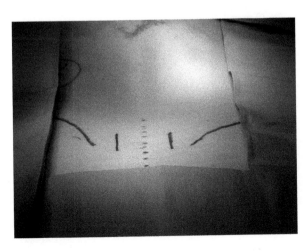

FIGURE 8 Landmarks and placement of skin incision for minimal access and minimally invasive approach to the lumbar spine.

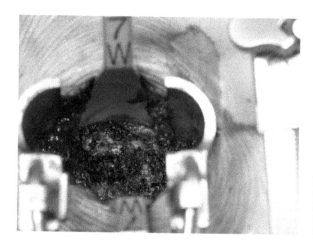

FIGURE 9 Direct visualization of anatomic structures of the lumbar spine through the Medtronic Quadrant System with visualization of facets and landmarks for screw insertion and decompression.

Nevertheless, the influx of all these systems and the interest in minimally invasive spine surgery, the premise at the advent of these technologies, was to decrease surgical morbidity, decrease hospitalization days, decrease pain, cause less muscle damage, offer a quicker return to functional activity, and most importantly offer reproducibility.

We have seen that through minimally invasive surgery, we can decrease our overall blood loss; decrease the surgical morbidity associated with these procedures; and offer less pain with less muscle damage, as seen with many microdiscectomy procedures, now being performed as an outpatient.

To see the overall effect of minimally invasive fusion surgery in terms of hospital stay, complications, operative time, and rehabilitation, the authors undertook a study comparing a matched group of 12 patients in each group, with one receiving minimally invasive fusion versus a standard open approach in the other. The results revealed that the overall operative time was only lengthened by 20 minutes (105 minutes in the open vs. 125 minutes in the minimally invasive); blood loss was reduced by 50% in the minimally invasive group (75 cc) compared with the open group (150 cc); hospitalization was reduced by 1.25 days (1.75 days in the minimally invasive group with two patients discharged in 23 hours compared with three days in the open group), and no additional complications were reported.

With reference to rehabilitation potential, the results were dramatic with those patients in the minimally invasive group into physical therapy (PT) one day sooner, 50% ahead in terms of

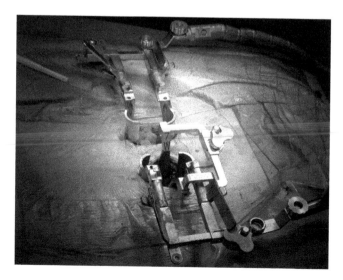

FIGURE 10 Medtronic Quadrant™ System for minimally invasive surgery with bilateral simultaneous access retractor placement.

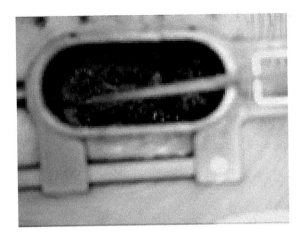

FIGURE 11   Direct visualization via EBI VuePass™ (EBI, L.P., Parsippany, New Jersey) of landmarks and anatomy for screw insertion and decompression.

aerobic activities as well as strengthening and conditioning when compared with those in the open group at one month. At two months, over again, the minimally invasive group was 60% ahead of the open group in terms of overall strength and endurance, and 80% were ready to return to work compared with 45% in the open group.

At three months, 95% of the patients in the minimally invasive group returned to work compared with 65% in the open group, and all patients were accessed via Functional Capacity Evaluations, and matched to job requirements, before these patients returned to work. This study concludes that minimally invasive spine surgery and fusion does offer distinct advantages in terms of overall ability to improve rehabilitation, improve strength and endurance, and return patients to functional activities and work at a sooner time frame than with the standard open fusion.

Interest in minimally invasive surgery and fusion continues to expand as it has a potential to deliver benefits to the patient, surgeon, and the hospital. As the technology is enhanced, and our understanding of the indications continues to grow, and with proper patient selection and proper system selection, greater patient satisfaction can be potentially achieved.

Preliminary study has shown the efficacy of this technology, and most importantly that with the right system, the surgeon does not have to alter his technique and can perform the surgery his way and not be governed by the system or the technology. This technology has the potential to continue to decrease surgical morbidity and offer quicker recovery time and return to functional activities, including work, than with the standard open approaches.

REFERENCES

1. Topcu O, Karakayali F, Kuzu MA, et al. Comparison of long-term quality of life after laparoscopic and open cholecystectomy. Surg Endosc 2003; 17(2):291–295.
2. Regan JJ, Guyer RD. Endoscopic techniques in spinal surgery. Clin Orthop 1997; 335:122–139.
3. Foley KT, Smith MM. Microendoscopic discectomy. Tech Neurosurg 1997; 3:301–307.
4. Roh SW, Kim DH, Cardoso AC, Fessler RG. Endoscopic foraminotomy using MED system in cadaveric specimens. Spine 2000; 25(2):260–264.
5. Kawaguchi Y, Matsui H, Tsuji H. Back muscle injury after posterior lumbar spine fusion. A histologic and enzymatic analysis. Spine 1996; 21:941–944.
6. Gejo R, Matsui H, Kawaguchi Y, et al. Serial changes in trunk muscle performance after posterior lumbar fusion. Spine 1999; 24:1023–1128.
7. Sihvonen T, Herno A, Palijiarvi L, et al. Local denervation atrophy of paraspinal muscles in postoperative failed back syndrome. Spine 1993; 18:575–581.
8. Findlay GF, Hall BI, Musa BS, Oliveira MD, Fear SC. A 10-year followup of the outcome of lumbar microdiscectomy. Spine 1998; 23(10):1168–1171.

9. Foley KT, Smith MM, Rampersaud YR. Microendoscopic discectomy. In: Schmidek HH, ed. Operative Neurosurgical Techniques: Indications, Methods, and Results. 4th ed. Philadelphia, PA: W.B. Saunders, 2000.
10. Hilton DL. Microdiscectomy with a minimally invasive tubular retractor. In: Perez-Cruet, Fessler RG, eds. Outpatient Spinal Surgery. St. Louis, MO: Quality Medical Publishing, Inc, 2002:159–170.
11. Foley KT, Lefkowitz MA. Advances in minimally invasive spine surgery. Clin Neurosurg 2002; 49:499–517.
12. Foley KT, Holly LT, Schwender JD. Minimally invasive lumbar fusion. Spine 2003; 28:26–35.
13. Foley KT, Gupta SK, Justis JR, Sherman MC. Percutaneous pedicle screw fixation of the lumbar spine. Neurosurg Focus 2001; 10:1–8.
14. Lowery GL, Kulkarni SS. Posterior percutaneous spine instrumentation. Euro Spine J 2000; 9(suppl):S211–S216.
15. Wiltse LL. The paraspinal sacrospinalis-splitting approach to the lumbarspine. Clin Orthop 1973; 91:48–57.

2 | Minimally Invasive Transforaminal Lumbar Interbody Fusion

Mark R. Grubb
Northeast Ohio Spine Center, Akron/Canton, Ohio, U.S.A.

INTRODUCTION

An increasingly popular method for lumbar arthrodesis is transforaminal lumbar interbody fusion (TLIF) (1–5). In a manner similar to posterior lumbar interbody fusion (PLIF) (6,7), TLIF provides for a 360° spinal fusion. Traditional posterolateral onlay techniques have been reported to have lower arthrodesis rates than interbody lumbar fusion techniques (8–12).

Transforaminal lumbar interbody fusion and PLIF offer a number of potential benefits over conventional posterolateral intertransverse arthrodesis, including increased fusion surface area; copious fusion blood supply via cancellous vertebral body bone; complete access for medial and lateral decompression; and restoration of intervertebral body height (8). Unfortunately, with PLIF, retraction and manipulation of the neural elements are required for disc space access. This has linked PLIF with a significant rate of neurologic injury (13–17).

As a more lateral approach, TLIF provides access to the disc space without the need for significant retraction of the nerve roots or thecal sac. Transforaminal lumbar interbody fusion is a unilateral procedure, and therefore avoids the need for bilateral dissection within the epidural space. It also makes revision surgeries less challenging, as there is less need to mobilize the nerve roots away from scar tissue. Finally, important midline supporting bony and ligamentous structures are preserved with TLIF.

Conventional posterior lumbar surgery, regardless of the fusion technique, is associated with significant soft-tissue morbidity that can adversely affect patient outcomes (18–23). Reduction in the iatrogenic soft tissue injury that occurs with muscle stripping and retraction during routine spinal exposure is the rationale of minimally invasive posterior lumbar fusion techniques (24–26). In this Chapter, we will outline the indications, surgical technique, results, and complications of performing the TLIF procedure using a minimally invasive approach.

Iatrogenic soft tissue and muscle injury that occurs during routine surgical exposure accounts for most of the significant morbidity of open instrumented lumbar fusion procedures. The deleterious effects of extensive muscle stripping and retraction have been well documented in the medical literature (18–23,27). These negative effects of lumbar surgery occur so commonly that the term fusion disease has been used to describe their occurrence. The effects of retractor blade pressure on the paraspinous muscles during surgery have been evaluated by Kawaguchi et al. (18,19) and Styf et al. (23). They found that elevated serum level of creatine phosphokinase MM isoenzyme, a direct marker of muscle injury, is related to the retraction duration and pressure. The beneficial effects of surgery can be negated by the long-term problems of this iatrogenic muscle injury. Rantanen et al. (21) concluded that patients who had poor outcomes after lumbar surgery were more likely to have persistent pathologic changes in their paraspinous muscles. It has been shown that patients who had undergone fusion procedures had significantly weaker trunk muscle strength than discectomy patients (20).

Minimally invasive spinal surgery with a less traumatic approach aims to achieve the same objectives as open surgery. However, reducing the approach-related morbidity must be accomplished without reducing procedure efficacy.

Surgical Technique

Following the induction of general endotracheal anesthesia, the patients were positioned prone on a Jackson (OSI) table. The patients were prepped and draped in the usual sterile manner. Lateral and anteroposterior (AP) C-arm fluoroscopic images were obtained. With the use of fluoroscopic guidance and an 18-gauge spinal needle, a 2.5-cm incision was centered on the interspace of interest approximately 5.0-cm lateral to the midline. The TLIF approach was carried out on the side ipsilateral to the worst radiculopathy. Contralateral Pathfinder (Abbott Spine, Austin, Texas, U.S.A.) pedicle screws and rod were placed through a separate 2.5-cm, mirror-image incision centered over the interspace. Through this incision, one can distract the interspace using the Pathfinder distracter, and then provisionally tighten the screw–rod connections in the distracted position. On the TLIF side, electrocautery was used to incise the fascia, after which serial dilators were used to create a muscle-sparing surgical corridor, as originally described for the microendoscopic discectomy (MED) procedure (28–31). An appropriate-length 22 diameter METRx (Medtronic Sofamor Danek, Memphis, Tennessee, U.S.A.) tubular retractor was docked on the facet joint complex (Fig. 1). The remainder of the procedure can be performed with the operative microscope or with loupe magnification, depending on surgeon preference. A total facetectomy was carried out using a high-speed drill. The removed bone was denuded of all soft tissue, morselized, and then later used for interbody graft material. The lateral margin of the ligamentum flavum was resected to expose the ipsilateral exiting and traversing nerve roots. Typically, only the most lateral margin of the traversing root was exposed so that it could be identified, protected, and decompressed as necessary. If needed, though, the tubular retractor could be wanded (angled) medially so that a more extensive decompression could be carried out (including decompression of central canal stenosis) (Fig. 2).

A discectomy was next performed through the ipsilateral tubular retractor. Epidural veins were controlled with bipolar cautery and thrombin-soaked Gelfoam was used for additional hemostasis, as necessary. At this point, distraction was performed, which allowed better access to the interspace, improved visualization of the annulus, and further, protected the nerve roots. Intervertebral distraction was performed in a bilateral and simultaneous manner by using the interbody paddles inserted into the disc space through the ipsilateral METRx tube, and applying the Pathfinder distracter to the contralateral pedicle screws (Fig. 3). This distraction was maintained via provisional tightening of the contralateral Pathfinder construct. However, if anterolisthesis was present and reduction was warranted, it could be accomplished using the Pathfinder reduction instruments (Fig. 4). The distracted position allowed improved access to the contralateral side of the interspace to complete the discectomy and prepare the endplates for fusion. Typically, cartilaginous materials were removed from the endplates, but their cortical portions were retained. Structural allograft bone, cages, bone morphogenetic protein (BMP), various bone graft expanders, and/or local autologous bone graft can be placed into the interspace, depending on surgeon preference. The local autograft

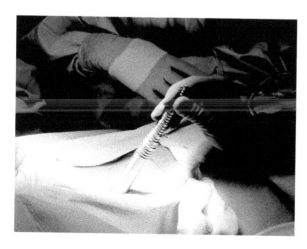

FIGURE 1 Dilation up to 22 mm using serial dilators, approximately 4 to 5 cm from midline with oblique orientation.

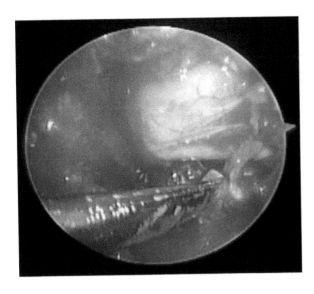

FIGURE 2 View through tubular retractor. The port has been wanded to allow a more extensive decompression of the thecal sac.

(combined with a BMP-soaked collagen sponge or other bone graft expander) was placed anteriorly and contralateral to the annulotomy within the interbody space (Fig. 5).

Additional autograft bone was placed into the interspace after insertion of the structural graft, if space allowed. Once the interbody fusion had been carried out, the contralateral pedicle screw construct was compressed using the Pathfinder Compressor. The tubular retractor was removed and an ipsilateral Pathfinder pedicle screw–rod construct was

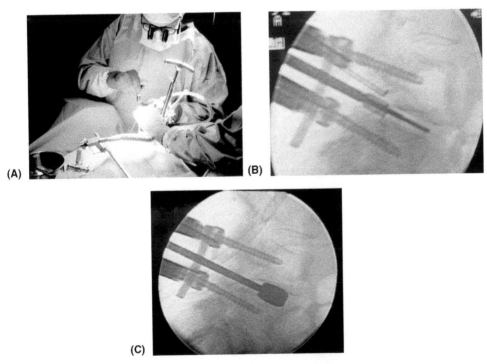

FIGURE 3 **(A)** Distraction using intervertebral paddle distracter (in hand) and Pathfinder distracter applied to contralateral pedicle screws. **(B)** Lateral fluoroscopic view of paddle distracter inserted into disc space and Pathfinder distracter placed on contralateral pedicle screws: predistraction. **(C)** Lateral fluoroscopic view following simultaneous application of Pathfinder distracter and rotation of intradiscal paddle distracter. Note the significant change in disc space height.

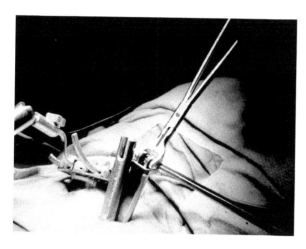

FIGURE 4 Spondylolisthesis reduction instrumentation.

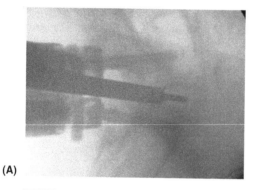

(A)

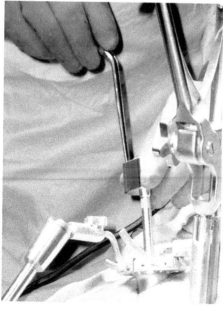

(B)

FIGURE 5 (**A**) Lateral fluoroscopic image showing
placement of implant spacer within the disc space. (**B**)
Placement of morselized autograft into disc space via funnel.

placed through the same incision. Bilateral compression was applied to the construct prior to final tightening, providing compression of the bone graft within the middle column and recreating lordosis.

Clinical Study

A nonrandomized, prospective study was carried out on patients treated with a uniform surgical technique by a single surgeon. The patient group consisted of 31 patients with mean age of 54.2 years. All patients were taking narcotic medications prior to surgery. Slightly over half of the patients were working preoperatively.

All interbody procedures were performed via unilateral TLIF procedure. The TLIF component was performed through a 22-mm tubular retractor. Exposure of the disc space through the foramen followed facetectomy. Subtotal discectomy allowed for the interbody cage and bone graft to be placed in an oblique fashion. Bilateral percutaneous pedicle-screw instrumentation was then completed. Percutaneous pedicle-screw instrumentation was accomplished under electromyogram (EMG) and fluoroscopic control. Patients were assessed radiographically and clinically preoperatively and at 3, 6, 12, and 24 months.

All surgeries were for one-level disease, primarily spondylolisthesis. All of the devices were implanted via unilateral TLIF. The average surgical data: EBL-estimated blood loss: 125 cc, 211- minute surgical time, hospital stay of 2.2 days. There were five complications: one CSF-cerebral spinal fluid leak (unrelated to pedicle-screw insertion), one ileus, one right leg numbness (resolved), one superficial wound infection and one interbody graft retropulsion (required re-operation). Mean Oswestry scores were preoperation, 31.2; 12 months, 19.9; and 24 months, 18.1. Mean back pain scores were preoperation, 8.8; 12 months, 3.2; and 24 months, 2.8. Two-thirds of the patients were working at two years postoperation. Six of the 31 patients retired at two years postoperation, and four were on disability at two years. Nearly, 96.8% patients demonstrate rigid fusion on flexion–extension films at two years post-operation. The reoperation rate was 3%. At 24 months, 19% of patients were taking narcotic medications. Ninety-seven percent of patients were satisfied with the outcome of the surgery.

DISCUSSION

In this chapter, we have discussed the minimally invasive TLIF (MITLIF) procedure. Special-ized instruments, such as a tubular retractor system and the Pathfinder system have made the TLIF procedure feasible. Serial dilation of the paraspinous operative corridor allows the surgeon to dissect through the muscle and fascia with minimal tissue trauma. Percutaneous pedicle screws can be placed through the same incisions.

The creation of a working channel between the muscle fibers permits access to the bony anatomy without the need for muscle stripping, unlike the open TLIF procedure. As a result, the estimated blood loss in our experience averaged only 125 mL, including pedicle-screw placement. Blood loss during conventional lumbar fusion surgery can be quite significant; in fact, patients commonly donate autologous blood preoperatively or a cell saver is used during the surgery. None of our patients required a blood transfusion. Compared with similar open procedures, patients had less postoperative pain following the MITLIF. Narcotic use was significantly reduced postoperatively. In addition, the hospital stay was at a relatively short average of 2.2 days.

We have outlined the many potential benefits of the MITLIF procedure. Minimally invasive transforaminal lumbar interbody fusion does have its drawbacks and limitations. A learning curve that must be surmounted before technical proficiency can be achieved is not insignificant. Standard landmarks that are visualized during open procedures may be unex-posed during minimally invasive procedures, and lead to anatomic disorientation. Minimally invasive transforaminal lumbar interbody fusion is more technically demanding than open TLIF. This is attributed to a number of factors, including working in a smaller area and the need for longer and bayoneted surgical instruments. Additionally, placement of percutaneous pedicle screws requires the surgeon to be able to accurately interpret AP and lateral fluoro-scopic images to safely insert these devices. Screw misplacement can be minimized by attention to anatomic detail. Use of intraoperative electromyography is also helpful in avoiding this potential complication. Image guidance systems would possibly further reduce screw placement error.

When severe neural compression is present on the side contralateral to the TLIF approach, consideration should be given to direct decompression of the neural structures on that side. This can be accomplished by inserting a tubular retractor through the contralateral incision, prior to contralateral percutaneous pedicle-screw placement.

SUMMARY

To summarize, this chapter has briefed on the rationale, suggested benefits, and techniques of MITLIF. Although the efficacy and outcomes of open spinal decompression and fusion procedures have been validated in numerous longitudinal studies, these surgeries typically involve significant soft-tissue dissection and muscle retraction. The MITLIF techniques aim to minimize iatrogenic damage to the soft tissues around the lumbar spine, while allowing the surgeon to perform effective decompression and fusion. As with all new surgical techniques, MITLIF has a learning curve in addition to its associated disadvantages.

CONCLUSION

Minimally invasive transforaminal lumbar interbody fusion offers a number of potential advantages over traditional open lumbar fusion techniques. It is a technically demanding procedure. It is a feasible option for many patients, and can be performed with a relatively low complication rate.

REFERENCES

1. Harms JG, Jeszenszky D. The unilateral transforaminal approach for posterior lumbar interbody fusion. Orthop Traumatol 1998; 6:88–99.
2. Harms JG, Rollinger H. A one-stage procedure in operative treatment of spondylolisthesis: dorsal traction-reposition and anterior fusion. Z Orthop Ihre Grenzeb 1982; 120:343–437.
3. Lowe TG, Tahernia AD, O'Brien MF, et al. Unilateral transforaminal posterior lumbar interbody fusion (TLIF): indications, technique, and 2-year results. J Spinal Disord 2002; 15:31–38.
4. Moskowitz A. Transforaminal lumbar interbody fusion. Orthop Clin North Am 2002; 33:359–366.
5. Rosenberg WS, Mummaneni PV. Transforaminal lumbar interbody fusion: technique, complications, and early results. Neurosurgery 2001; 48:569–575.
6. Cloward RB. Spondylolisthesis: treatment by laminectomy and posterior interbody fusion. Clin Orthop Relat Res 1981; 154:74–82.
7. Cloward RB. The treatment of ruptured lumbar intervertebral discs by vertebral body fusion. I. Indications, operative technique, after care. J Neurosurg 1953; 10:154–168.
8. Hacker RJ. Comparison of interbody fusion approaches for disabling low back pain. Spine 1997; 22:660–666.
9. Fraser RD. Interbody, posterior, and combined lumbar fusions. Spine 1995; 20:S167–S177.
10. Branch CL. The case for posterior lumbar interbody fusion. Clin Neurosurg 2000; 47:252–267.
11. Branch CL, Branch CL Jr. Posterior lumbar interbody fusion: the keystone technique. In: Lin PM, Gill K, eds. Lumbar Interbody Fusion. Rockville, MD: Aspen, 1989:211–219.
12. McLaughlin MR, Haid RW, Rodts GE, et al. Posterior lumbar interbody fusion: indications, techniques, and results. Clin Neurosurg 2000; 47:514–527.
13. Fraser RD. Interbody, posterior, and combined lumbar fusions. Spine 1995; 20:S167–S177.
14. Elias WJ, Simmons NE, Kaptain GJ, Chadduck JB, Whitehill R. Complications of posterior lumbar interbody fusion when using a titanium-threaded cage device. J Neurosurg (Spine 1) 2000; 93:45–52.
15. Ray CD. Threaded titanium cages for lumbar interbody fusions. Spine 1997; 22:667–680.
16. Stonecipher T, Wright S. Posterior lumbar interbody fusion with facet-screw fixation. Spine 1989; 14:468–471.
17. Lin PM. Posterior lumbar interbody fusion technique: complications and pitfalls. Clin Orthop Relat Res 1985; 193:90–102.
18. Kawaguchi Y, Matsui H, Tsuji H. Back muscle injury after posterior lumbar spine surgery. A histologic and enzymatic analysis. Spine 1996; 21:941–944.
19. Kawaguchi Y, Matsui H, Tsuji H. Back muscle injury after posterior lumbar spine surgery. Part 2: histologic and histochemical analyses in humans. Spine 1994; 19:2598–2602.

20. Mayer TG, Vanharanta H, Gatchel RJ. Comparison of CT scan muscle measurements and isokinetic trunk strength in postoperative patients. Spine 1989; 14:33–36.
21. Rantanen J, Hurme M, Falck B, et al. The lumbar multifidus muscle five years after surgery for a lumbar intervertebral disc herniation. Spine 1993; 18:568–574.
22. Sihvonen T, Herno A, Paljiarvi L, et al. Local denervation atrophy of paraspinal muscles in postoperative failed back syndrome. Spine 1993; 18:575–581.
23. Styf JR, Willen J. The effects of external compression by three different retractors on pressure in the erector spine muscles during and after posterior lumbar spine surgery in humans. Spine 1998; 23:354–358.
24. Foley KT, Lefkowitz MA. Advances in minimally invasive spine surgery. Clin Neurosurg 2002; 49:499–517.
25. Khoo LT, Palmer S, Laich DT, Fessler RG. Minimally invasive percutaneous posterior lumbar interbody fusion. Neurosurgery 2002; 51:S166–S181.
26. Foley KT, Holly LT, Schwender JD. Minimally invasive lumbar fusion. Spine 2003; 28:S26–S35.
27. Gejo R, Matsui H, Kawaguchi Y, et al. Serial changes in trunk muscle performance after posterior lumbar surgery. Spine 1999; 24:1023–1028.
28. Foley KT, Smith MM. Microendoscopic discectomy. Tech Neurosurg 1997; 3:301–307.
29. Perez-Cruet MJ, Foley KT, Isaacs RE, et al. Microendoscopic lumbar discectomy: technical note. Neurosurgery 2002; 51:S129–S136.
30. Fessler RG, Khoo LT. Minimally invasive cervical microendoscopic foraminotomy: an initial clinical experience. Neurosurgery 2002; 51:S37–S45.
31. Guiot BH, Khoo LT, Fessler RG. A minimally invasive technique for decompression of the lumbar spine. Spine 2002; 27:432–438.

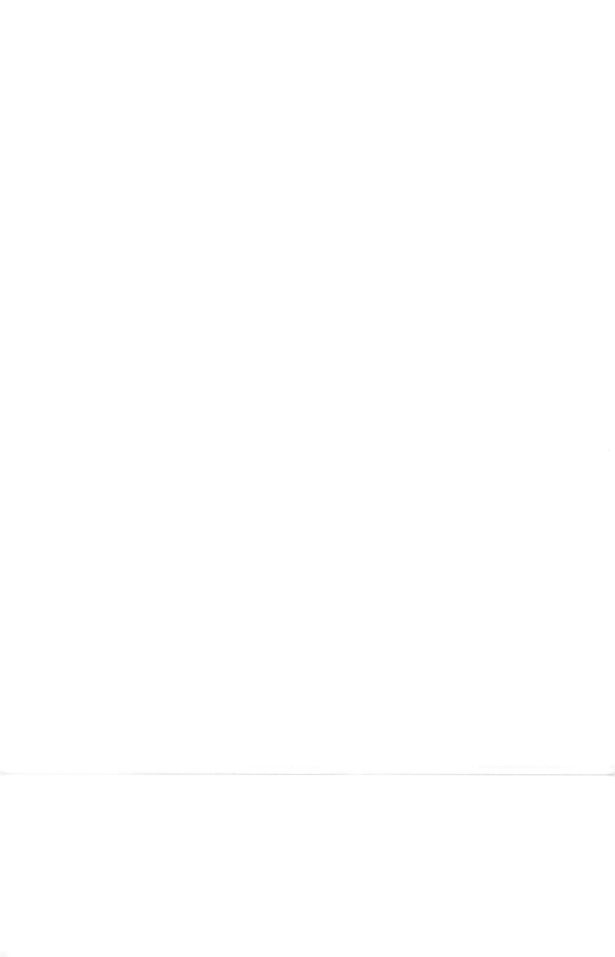

3 | Nonendoscopic Percutaneous Disc Decompression as Treatment of Discogenic Radiculopathy

Michael J. DePalma
Department of Physical Medicine and Rehabilitation,
Virginia Commonwealth University, Richmond, Virginia, U.S.A.

Curtis W. Slipman
Department of Rehabilitation Medicine, The Penn Spine Center, Hospital of the University of Pennsylvania,
Philadelphia, Pennsylvania, U.S.A.

INTRODUCTION

Lumbar pain and sciatica are responsible for a significant portion of health care expenditure afflicting approximately 10 million individuals at an estimated cost of several billion dollars in diagnosis, treatment, and lost wages (1,2). A variety of spinal structures can serve as the source of incapacitating lumbar pain. However, the lumbar intervertebral disc has been demonstrated to be the most common cause of chronic low back pain (3). Lower limb pain in the presence of lumbar pain may be somatically referred from deep spinal structures (4) or may be the manifestation of nerve root insult (5). Intervertebral disc herniation has long been recognized as a common source of neural injury (6,7), and can present as lower limb pain with or without motor or sensory deficits (8). Radicular signs and symptoms are addressed in a therapeutically different fashion than axial discogenic symptomatology. These treatment measures have been molded by the prevailing theory of spinal pathophysiology.

Cervical spine disorders have been estimated to affect 9% to 12% of the general population, and rival their lumbar counterpart as a common presenting complaint to the health care practitioner (9). Cervical intervertebral disc herniation was first discovered in the 1920s after presenting as myelopathy, and was believed to be because of spinal cord tumors (10,11). In 1936, Hanflig first ascribed upper limb radicular pain to cervical arthritis-induced cervical nerve root inflammation (12). Shortly thereafter, Semmes and Murphey (13), followed by Spurling and Scoville (14), and Michelson and Mixter (15), correlated cervical nerve root irritation with cervical intervertebral disc herniation in the absence of cord compression. Succeeding studies established the relationship between cervical radiculopathy and radicular pain, and cervical intervertebral disc protrusions (16–18). Subsequent clinical studies established the most common etiologies of cervical radiculopathy as cervical intervertebral disc herniation (19) followed by cervical spondylosis (20).

The implicit premise founded by these early works (6,13) has been that biomechanical compression of neural elements was the sole etiologic factor leading to the manifestation of signs and symptoms. However, there is evidence that mechanical influence is not the sole etiologic factor (21–30). There is little correlation between the severity of radiculopathy and the size of disc herniation (22,25,26,31). Resolution of symptoms after conservative treatment has been observed without a concurrent reduction in disc herniation volume (25,26). Mixter and Ayers, a year after Mixter and Barr's hallmark paper, demonstrated that radicular pain could occur without significant disc herniation (27). However, it was not conclusive if this "radicular pain" was nerve root-mediated or somatically referred from another spinal structure. It is probable that, in most instances, biomechanical injury is not the singular cause for the expression of lumbar radicular symptoms related to lumbar intervertebral disc herniation.

Early observations by Haberman and later Lindahl (29) in 1949 established the presence of pathologic changes including inflammatory cells in nerve roots of patients suffering from sciatica. Subsequent animal studies have demonstrated autoimmune and inflammatory reactions to autogenous nucleus pulposus (32,33). The human intervertebral disc has been shown to be a potent source of phospholipase A$_2$ (PLA$_2$) (28), a regulator of the inflammatory cascade which causes perineural inflammation, conduction block, axonal injury (34), and dorsal root demyelination and mechanically induced ectopic discharges in the rat animal model (35). Herniated cervical (36,37) and lumbar (37,38) intervertebral discs have been observed to spontaneously produce increased amounts of other potentially neurotoxic inflammatory mediators (37,39). A rapid transport route may exist bridging the epidural space and intraneural capillaries, providing quick access for this nuclear material to spinal nerve axons (40).

In stark contrast to the peripheral nerve, the nerve root lacks a perineurium, which provides tensile strength and a diffusion barrier (41,42). Consequently, the nerve root possesses less resilience to tension forces and chemical irritants (42). Furthermore, the epineurium, which provides mechanical cushion to resist compression, is less abundant or developed, in the nerve root (42). Within the nerve root itself the fasciculi do not branch to form a plexiform pattern; instead, they run in parallel loosely held together by connective tissue (41,42). Hence, the nerve root is not as well suited to withstand either mechanical or chemical insult as compared with a peripheral nerve. Furthermore, once the inflammatory cascade is initiated, the nerve root lymphatic system is poorly equipped to adequately clear the inflammatory mediators (42). An inflamed nerve root is thus predisposed to a chronic inflammatory reaction with invasion by fibroblast with eventual development of intraneural fibrosis (42).

Cadaveric studies have discovered a functional tethering of the nerve root to the intervertebral foramen (42,43). When an intervertebral disc herniates in a posterior or posteriolateral fashion, the exiting nerve root is placed under tension and not always compressed (42). The ensuing inflammatory response sensitizes the involved nerve root, decreasing its resilience to biomechanical influences. An inflamed nerve will fire repetitively with just minor perturbations; whereas, a nonirritated nerve will tolerate more vigorous manipulation without prolonged firing patterns (41,44). The length to which a nerve root must be stretched for it to incur neurophysiologic dysfunction is believed to be 10% to 15% of resting length (45,46). Clinically, nerve root irritability can be appreciated by elevating the involved lower limb with the knee extended, straight leg raising (SLR). Goddard et al. (43) demonstrated stretch without displacement of the nerve root upon raising the affected limb 20–30 to 70°. As no nerve root motion is occurring, the radicular pain elicited by this maneuver is a consequence of nerve root tension (43). In asymptomatic patients, this movement is nonpainful despite the same amount of tension placed on the neural elements. Provocative SLR has been demonstrated to be indicative of elevated prostaglandin E2 levels at the disc herniation–nerve root interface (47). Hence, dural tension signs are markers of nerve root inflammation and do not necessarily imply nerve root compression.

The natural history of radiculopathy because of a herniated intervertebral disc treated conservatively including spinal injections is marked by gradual improvement over a period of a few weeks to three to five months (48–55). Over this time period, 50% to 60% of these herniations will resolve to a variable degree (25,26,52,56). Asymptomatic disc herniations have been documented to occur in both the cervical (57–59), and lumbar (21,23,24,60) spines. Thus, the extension of nuclear material through a rent in the annular fibers presumably represents a reversible anatomical abnormality responsible for limb pain owing to nerve root insult. Such an injury results in both biochemical and biomechanical harassment of the spinal nerve root. Over a period of time, both or either of the biomechanical and biochemical insults will abate allowing for resolution of signs and symptoms of nerve root injury. In this sense, a component of the disc herniation pathophysiology will effectively reverse. Whether or not the associated nerve root injury reverses depends on the level of nerve injury (neurapraxia versus axontmesis) (61). If symptoms persist despite physical therapy, oral anti-inflammatory medications, and a tincture of time, fluoroscopically guided transforaminal epidural corticosteroid (TFESIs) or selective nerve root injections (SNRIs) are the appropriate successive steps in the treatment algorithm (49,50,52,53). The majority of the patients' symptoms will improve with one to four injections (55,62–68) as the inflammatory response of the herniation is rendered inert. The remaining one-fourth to one-third of patients who do not respond to conservative care and do not appreciate a steroid benefit from TFESIs and/or SNRIs may require mechanical decompression of the offended nerve root(s) in order to alleviate the neural compression and the source of inflammation (50–53).

Open surgical discectomy has traditionally been the standard of care for persistent radicular limb pain owing to a herniated intervertebral disc (6). Although surgical results have been quite successful (69,70), open surgery is not without risks (71–73). Prospective trials have observed a major complication rate of 1.6% to 13% (71,72) ranging from major neurologic injury (71) and nerve injury (72), discitis (72), to intraoperative death (71,72). Advent of the microdiscectomy technique has not decreased surgical complication rate. Pappas et al. observed a rate of complication of 10.8% including two vascular injuries, one fatal, and a major injury in 654 cases (73). Reoperation rates for recurrent disc herniation range from 5% to 21% (74–78). Primary protrusions without an anular defect are more likely to require revision surgery than extruded or sequestered disc fragments (74,78). Despite the favorable natural history of discogenic radiculopathy (50–52), a protracted conservative regimen addressing severe radicular symptoms should be avoided to maximize odds for a successful outcome (79). Treatment for a contained herniation-induced radiculopathy unresponsive to physical therapy, oral anti-inflammatory medications, and spinal injections might best be achieved by one of a variety of percutaneous disc decompressive techniques (80–124). Disc decompression via the percutaneous approach was pursued as a means by which to decompress a reversible anatomical defect alleviating neural injury with less morbidity and mortality than the open surgical approach.

The predominant indication for decompression remains limb pain owing to a reversible anatomic source (80–83,88,89,98,106,108,110,119–124). Some studies fail to differentiate these two symptomatically distinct groups (90,94,97,104,109,117,118); in these studies, meaningful conclusions regarding treatment efficacy are difficult to formulate. Consequently, the use of percutaneous disc decompressive procedures to treat solely axial pain remains speculative with less structured support than similar treatment of discogenic radiculopathy. Because of such difficulties, this Chapter will *not* attempt to discuss the efficacy of nonendoscopic percutaneous decompressive techniques for axial pain, but will focus primarily on efficacy and safety for limb pain.

DISCOGENIC BEHAVIOR AND PATHOPHYSIOLOGY

In a healthy adult intervertebral disc, the nucleus pulposus behaves as a semi-fluid mucoid mass. Under loads, the nucleus will deform owing to an applied pressure while maintaining an incompressible volume. Consequently, once the nucleus incurs pressure from any angle it will attempt to deform and effectively transmit the applied pressure in multiple directions (7). The nucleus is comprised of 70% to 90% of water largely contained within the chemical domains of large molecular proteoglycans (125). This immense volume of hydration provides the nucleus with its fluidity. Type II collagen fibrils (126), small elastic fibers, and other noncollagenous proteins (127) are interspersed throughout the proteoglycan network. These proteinaceous nuclear components provide a viscous stiffness facilitating transmission of pressure (7). Chondrocytes are embedded in the proteoglycan meshwork located near the vertebral endplate where they manufacture the proteoglycan and collagen constituents of the nucleus (128).

Surrounding the nucleus circumferentially is the annulus fibrosus composed of proteoglycans imbibing water (128), and both type I and II collagen fibers, with type I predominating (129), intermixed with elastic fibers (130). The collagen fibers are concentrically arranged into parallel sheets of lamellae (131). Fibers within each lamellar sheet run at an angle of 65° to 70° vertically and alternately in direction from one lamellae to the next (132). A binding proteoglycan gel helps maintain a linear cohesion between adjacent lamellae (128). Although the lamellae circumscribe the nucleus, the posterior portion of the annulus fibrosus is relatively thinner than its anterior and lateral counterparts (133), and the lamellae in the posterolateral region of the disc are structurally incomplete (134).

The construction of tightly packed lamellae endows the annulus fibrosus with an element of stiffness to withstand axial compressive loads transmitting weight from one vertebra to the next (135,136). However, without a nucleus the annulus will deform under a constant load causing buckling of the collagenous lamellae (7), and may be less resilient to translatory and

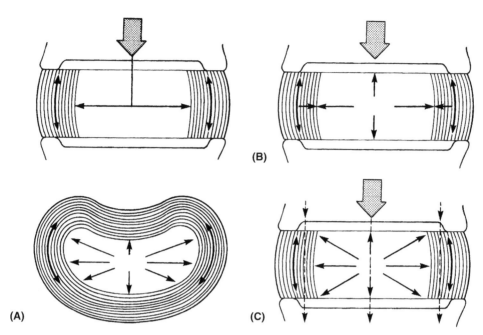

FIGURE 1   The mechanism of weight transmission in an intervertebral disc. (**A**) Compression raises the pressure in the nucleus pulposus. This is exerted radially onto the anulus fibrosus and the tension in the anulus rises. (**B**) The tension in the anulus is exerted on the nucleus preventing it from expanding radially. Nuclear pressure is then exerted on the vertical end-plates. (**C**) Weight is borne, in part, by the anulus fibrosus and by the nucleus pulposus. The radial pressure in the nucleus braces the anulus, and the pressure on the end-plates transmits the load from one vertebra to the next.

torsional strains. When presented with a vertical load, the nucleus will deform but not compress. As the nuclear height is reduced under a load, the nucleus exerts counterpressure both outward against the annulus and vertically against adjacent endplates (7). An equilibrium is established whereby radial nuclear expansion is balanced by annular resistance owing to the tensile strength of the annular fibers. Consequently, load is transmitted from one vertebra to the next as pressure is transferred by the nucleus to the verterbral endplates lessening the load placed on the annulus. Yet, the pressure imposed on the annulus by the nucleus effectively prevents annular buckling augmenting the annular capacity to bear weight (Fig. 1) (7). Conceptualizing the nucleus of the intervertebral disc as a contained semi-fluid, incompressible tissue will allow one to then realize how a breach in containment of the nuclear contents triggers a progressive degenerative cascade that can eventually lead to herniation of nuclear material.

Relative to the intervertebral disc, both intrinsic and extrinsic factors interact accomplishing the herniation of nuclear material. Internal derangement or internal disc disruption has been vastly studied to better delineate the sequence of events culminating in disc injury (137–151). The vertebral endplate can be damaged under sustained (139) or repetitive loads (138), which can be related to forceful muscle contraction (140). A damaged vertebral endplate deforms more when placed under a load (139) allowing for either more space for the nuclear contents to occupy or passage of the nucleus through the endplate resulting in a drop in intradiscal pressure (141). Consequently, this relatively decompressed nucleus is less resilient to withstand an applied axial load placing greater forces on the adjacent annular fibers (142). Delamination of the annular lamellae ensues as high stress gradients disrupting the proteoglycan glue and forcing the inner annulus inward and outer annulus outward (142,143). Reduction in the nuclear intradiscal pressure inhibits nuclear chondrocytes from producing more proteoglycans (144,152) interfering with water retention and ultimately restoration of nuclear volume effectively promoting a catabolic state in the disc (7,142). Elevated annular peak stresses impair disc cell metabolism and interfere with reparative efforts of the collagen network (142,144). Endplate injury might additionally interfere with metabolite transport into the nucleus from the vertebral body vasculature (145,148), or by instigating an inflammatory (146,147) or auto-immune reaction (7) in the intervertebral disc. Circumstantial evidence exists suggesting an integral role of endplate damage in disc herniation as Schmorl's nodes have been associated with lower lumbar disc herniation on magnetic resonance imaging (MRI) (149). Other factors have been deemed to be associated with degenerative disc changes and structural changes themselves should not be viewed as simply markers of the aging disc (142,153,154). Cigarette smoking increases the incidence of disc degeneration (150), and a genetic predisposition may also exist contributing to disc degeneration (151,155,156).

A critical degree of disc degeneration may not be a prerequisite to herniation of nuclear tissue. The incidence of disc herniation in the adolescent population has been observed to be consistently less than 15% (157) and perhaps less than 5% (158,159). Seventy-three percent of 63 adolescent disc herniation cases retrospectively reviewed had sustained a single precipitat-ing traumatic event. None of these cases revealed evidence of vertebral endplate fracture intraoperatively (156). Although inconclusive, the cumulative findings from these studies would suggest that congenially weakened annular fibers were integral in herniation of nuclear material. The fact that 27% of these adolescent herniations were not traumatically induced and no structural endplate abnormality was observed supports the notion that intervertebral disc herniation in the adolescent may be related to a congenially weakened annular fiber.

Extrinsic variables also play a contributory role in disc injury, one of which, cigarette smoking, was previously mentioned (51). Additionally, various spinal movements will expose the intervertebral disc to injurious forces. Flexion and extension in the sagittal plane and torsion in the axial plane impose different stresses on the disc. As the spine flexes, the anterior annulus is compressed and will tend to buckle (137) as the nucleus is deformed poster-iorly and is not able to fortify the annular fibers (7). As the long extensor musculature of the spine contracts to control flexion, intradiscal pressure increases owing to this applied load by the muscle contraction (7). Consequently, an increased pressure is exerted on an already stretched posterior annulus as the vertebral bodies separate. Concurrently, a flexed spine will incur greater anterior shear force owing to a relative decrease in posterior shear force gen-eration by the spinal long extensor musculature (160). Rotation in the axial plane with a center of rotation within the geometric center of the vertebral body prestresses annular fibers. As further rotation occurs, the axis of rotation shifts posteriorly to the zygapophyseal joints sub-jecting the disc to additional lateral shear forces (Fig. 2) (7). Combined flexion and rotation greatly increases the risk of injury as annular fibers are maximally prestressed in flexion when additional rotation strains the involved annular fibers beyond their normal strain limit (161). The combination of lateral shear and torsion strain results in circumferential tears in the outer annulus (162) typically located in the posterolateral annular region (163) where annular strain is high (164). These circumferential tears can coalesce to form radial extensions providing a channel through which nuclear contents may extrude. The posterior annular fiber's capability to withstand both tension and pressure is inherently compromised owing its structural attenuation (134) in this region of the disc. Furthermore, any previous injury or degeneration will have weakened the lamellae in that area of the intervertebral disc increasing the responsibility of the remaining intact lamellae in supporting the applied load (7). Conse-quently, the pressure exerted by the nucleus may herniate nuclear content through a newly developed rent in the annular fibers.

Repetitive movements in the sagittal plane with or without superimposed axial rotation will repetitively tax the intact intervertebral discs which may lead to nuclear degeneration and annular disruption. Damage to the vertebral endplate reduces intranuclear pressure in adjacent discs by up to 57%, and doubles the amount of compressive stress in the posterolateral annular fibers (140). Similar effects occur consequent to other structural changes such as radial fissures and posterior herniation that create more space available for the nucleus (154). Consequently, greater force is transmitted to the annulus. Bogduk has previously described this scenario (7). If one-third of a disc's annular fibers are injured and rendered dysfunctional, the remaining fibers would have to contend with the same load and thus increase their individual stress by 43%. Disruption of two-thirds of the annular fibers would increase the stress on the remaining one-third by three times their normal strain. These structural alterations may manifest

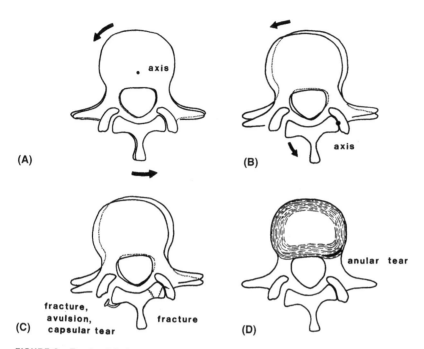

FIGURE 2 Torsion injuries to a lumbar intervertebral joint. (**A**) Rotation initially occurs about an axis through the posterior third of the intervertebral disc, but is limited by impaction of a zygapophysical joint. (**B**) Further rotation occurs about a new axis through the impacted joint. The opposite joint rotates backwards while the disc undergoes lateral shear. (**C**) The impacted joint may suffer fractures of its articular processes, its subchondral bone or the parts interarticularis. The opposite joint may suffer capsular injuries. (**D**) Subjected to torsion and lateral shear, the annulus fibrosus suffers circumferential tears.

clinically as intermittent or fluctuant axial lumbar pain that may progress to constant symptomatology or acutely progress to nuclear herniation resulting in radiculopathy. Such a patient may report explosive onset of lower limb pain with concurrent reduction in the midline axial lumbar pain. The new lower limb syptomatology is related to insult of a nerve root from frank herniation of nuclear material instigating an inflammatory reaction and increasing nerve root tension and perhaps compression. In this instance, both biochemical and biomechanical alterations are responsible for radicular signs and symptoms. Successful outcome may be achieved without significantly addressing the mechanical effects of the herniation. However, in the minority of patients, the mechanical influence will prevail after initial therapeutic interventions warranting more aggressive treatment.

EFFICACY OF NONENDOSCOPIC PERCUTANEOUS DISC DECOMPRESSION BY TECHNOLOGY
Enzymatic Degradation—Chymopapain

Chymopapain is a protease derived from the latex of the papaya tree and was first isolated by Jansen and Balls 65 years ago (165). The enzyme acts exclusively on the nuclear noncollagen ground substance producing loss of glycosaminoglycans and water resulting in volume reduction (166). The efficacy of intradiscal chymopapain in treating lumbar radiculopathy because of herniated intervertebral discs was first reported by Lyman Smith in 1964 who coined the term chemonucleolysis (167). Since this initial investigation, intranuclear injection of chymopapain has become the most extensively evaluated and regulated minimally invasive intervention for radicular pain recalcitrant to conservative treatment (168). More recently, collagenase has been investigated and compared with chymopapain (169,170). Despite 42 years of clinical and basic science research, chemonucleolysis remains a controversial treatment for discogenic radiculopathy (168).

Smith observed in an uncontrolled study, improvement of sciatica in 10 patients treated with intradiscal chymopapain. Each patient was suffering from intractable symptomatology despite other treatments, demonstrated signs of nerve root injury, and had been deemed "operative cases." Seven patients experienced complete relief of their lower limb symptoms, and three had gradual improvement. One patient eventually experienced recurrent contralateral lower limb symptoms necessitating open surgical discectomy. Nine patients had two discs injected after the performance of discography indicating an "abnormal" disc. Follow-up correspondence was short, however, occurring at or within two months (167).

The first prospective, randomized, controlled trial was orchestrated by Schwetschenau et al. and published in 1976 (171). Sixty-eight of 130 appropriate patients were randomized to 1 ml of 20 mg chymopapain/5 ml of saline or 1 ml of 20 mg sodium iothalamate/5 ml of saline placebo solution. Each patient demonstrated one or more signs of lumbosacral radiculopathy corroborated by myelographic evidence of a correlative disc abnormality that did not respond to three weeks of conservative care. Each subject was evaluated by history and physical examination at six weeks, three months, six months, and one year. Outcome was categorized as completely asymptomatic, greatly improved, and moderately improved. Two of the initial 68 patients were lost to follow-up. Of the 66 enrolled patients, 35 had been randomized to receive placebo and 31 received chymopapain. No statistically significant difference was observed between the groups. However, mutiple methodologic flaws preclude the formulation of any conclusion. Among the concerns are that the investigators used a potentially therapeutic, active placebo agent; chose a therapeutically inadequate chymopapain dose; were admittedly inexperienced leading to improper needle placement; and committed improper timing of code break (80,81).

Javid et al. engineered a much more sound study in which 55 patients were randomized to receive 3 ml of chymopapain (3000 units/1.5 ml) while 53 patients were randomized to 3 ml of pyrogen-free saline (80). Each patient had persistent lumbosacral radicular pain despite six weeks of conservative care with reproduction of this pain with SLR, and either myotomal weakness, dermatomal sensory abnormality, or a diminished muscle stretch reflex. Myelography revealed a correlative, single-level disc abnormality, and discography confirmed internal injury of this disc. Outcomes were measure primarily at six weeks and six months by assessing improvement in radicular signs and symptoms, and subjective improvement as deemed by the patient and physician. Three patients were lost to follow-up. Eighty-two percent of the chymopapain patients had a successful clinical course with 91% of the successful cases attributable to the chymopapain intervention. In contrast, just 41% of the placebo arm achieved successful outcome attributable to the placebo intervention. The remaining 59% crossed over to the chymopapain arm and 91% of these cases were then successfully treated. Although six months is a short follow-up interval, this investigation proved that chemonucleolysis is clearly superior to placebo in treating patients with lumbosacral radiculopathy because of disc herniation, and is a safe procedure when performed by orthopedic specialists (80).

Fraser published two-year data after randomizing 30 patients to receive 2 ml (8 mg) of intradiscal chymopapain and 30 patients to receive 2 ml of intradiscal saline (82). Each patient had not responded to 6 to 24 weeks of conservative care including physical therapy. Myelography demonstrated a corroborative posterolateral disc herniation affecting the clinically suspected nerve root. All patients reported radicular pain on SLR to 50° or less. Outcomes were measured by pain rating and the patient's subjective report of the treatment assessed at six months and again at two years while maintaining blinding of both the investigator and the patients. All 60 initial patients were evaluated at both follow-up intervals. Seventy-three percent of the chymopapain group versus 47% of the control group felt the treatment was successful at two years. Fifty-three percent of the treatment group was pain-free at two years compared with 23% in the saline group. At the time of follow-up, 40% of the saline group and just 20% of the chymopapain group had required laminectomy. Fraser's work provided the first prospective, controlled long-term follow-up data demonstrating a sustained therapeutic benefit of chymopapain to treat lumbosacral radiculopathy because of disc herniation.

Three years later, Dabezies et al. published the largest prospective, randomized, controlled trial of 173 patients suffering from lower limb radicular pain recalcitrant to at least two weeks of conservative care (81). Myelography and/or computed axial tomography revealed a soft disc herniation offending the involved nerve root, and each patient's physical examination included an associated diminished muscle stretch reflex, sensory abnormality, myotomal weakness, or dural tension signs. Eighty-seven patients received 2 ml (8 mg) of chymopapain, and 86 received an equivalent volume of cysteine-edetate-iothalamate in a randomized fashion. Patients were assessed at six weeks, three months, and six months after intervention and improvement was defined by subjective improvement in pain, normalization of neurologic findings, and a return to previous level of occupation. This study contained an inordinately large number of code breaks as patients requested to become unblinded in order to pursue chymopapain treatment once the sponsor announced it would afford all patients in the placebo arm the opportunity to travel out of the country for treatment. Including the results after the code breaks revealed successful outcome in 71% in the treatment arm compared with 45% in the control group at six months. These numbers changed to 67% and 44%, respectively when the code-break patients were excluded from data analysis. These findings are commensurate with previously published studies (80,82).

Gogan and Fraser published 10-year data of their 60 patients initially studied at six months and two years (83). Their protocol has previously been described. All the patients had remained blinded to identity of their intervention and were assessed by an independent observer who was unaware of the original therapy. Each patient answered the question of whether or not their treatment was successful. Each patient was then evaluated by the investigator and determined to be pain-free, moderately improved, unimproved, or worse. Eighty percent of the chymopapain patients compared with 34% of the saline group found their treatment successful. Of the chymopapain group, 53 percent were completely pain-free at 10 years in contrast to 23% of the saline group at 10 years. Six of the 30 chymopapain patients eventually underwent open surgical discectomy at the treated level but none of these cases occurred two years after treatment. In short, 77% of the chymopapain patients and 38% of the saline patients achieved a good result at 10 years.

This study provided definitive evidence that chymopapain treatment of discogenic lumbosacral radiculopathy can achieve therapeutic benefit in properly selected patients not responding to conservative care. There is a distinct increase in the number of patients relieved of limb pain and a faster rate of improvement in patients treated with chymopapain compared with saline. The laminectomy rate did not reach statistical significance at two years but did by 10 years (83).

Cervical chemonucleolysis has not been studied as intently as in the lumbar region. Gomez-Castresana published an initial series of 40 patients treated for 44 cervical herniated intervertebral discs (172). Eighty-five percent were successfully treated at a mean follow-up of 21.4 months (172). These results have been stable and expanded to a successful treatment of 90% of 147 patients treated for 171 cervical intervertebral disc herniations (173). All patients were available at a mean follow-up of 101 months (2–103 months), and 72% of repeat MRIs demonstrated a reduction in the size of the disc herniation (172).

Efficacy of chemonucleolysis compares well with that of open surgical discectomy (84,85). Outcomes at one year were not significantly different between patients treated with chemonucleolysis versus open surgical discectomy in a randomized, prospective, controlled trial (85). However, this trial did show a statistically significant difference at six weeks and three months in favor of the surgical group (85). In Nordby's experience, good to excellent results occurred at six weeks in 80% of 100 patients treated with chemonucleolysis. Eighty-five percent of their 100 surgical counterparts experienced good to excellent results at six weeks. Although open surgical discectomy was statistically superior ($P = 0.13$) than chemonucleolysis at six weeks, no statistical difference was measured at six months or one year (168). In a retrospective review 10 years after treatment, Tregonning et al. observed minimal difference in efficacy between 145 patients treated with chymopapain and 91 patients treated surgically (86). Overall, mean success rates of chemonucleolysis in trials comparing it with open surgical discectomy have been calculated to be 66% compared with 77% for open surgery (84). Taking into account similar efficacy between chemonucleolysis and open surgical discectomy, the former may be more cost-effective than the latter in treating discogenic lumbosacral radiculopathy because of the lower associated costs (87).

Enzyme Degradation—Collagenase

The potential risk of allergic reactions and other complications such as central nervous system damage have led to the development of colllagenase as an alternate enzyme to effect intervertebral disc herniation (170). In a double blind study, collagenase produced successful outcomes in 80% of the treated patients compared with 30% in the placebo group (169). However, collagenase may not be as effective as chymopapain. Wittenberg et al. observed good and excellent results in 72% of the patients treated with chymopapain compared with 52% of the patients treated with collagenase (170). Eight-eight percent of the chymopapain group and 80% of the collagenase group were available at follow-up at five years. However, the collagenase group experienced an increased rate of neurologic injury which is discussed later in the Chapter.

Mechanical Decompression—Automated Percutaneous Discectomy

Although chemonucleolysis has been well studied providing strong evidence attesting to its efficacy, its use has fallen out of favor because of concerns over catastrophic complications. By 1994, most centers in the United States had discarded chemonucleolysis as a means to decompress a herniated intervertebral disc because it was perceived as less effective than standard open discectomy, and the associated complication rates were higher than could be accepted on the basis of this efficacy (174). Consequently, in late 1999, Boots Pharmaceuticals (Lincolnshire, IL, U.S.A) halted the manufacturing and distribution of its chymopapain product (93). Alternative means to achieve mechanical decompression of the herniated disc percutaneously were pursued. Pioneering investigations of mechanical percutaneous disc decompression initiated in the mid-1970s (91) incorporated large canulas with an associated risk of nerve injury, and required the involvement of modified pituitary forceps which proved to be cumbersome and time-consuming (91,92). In 1984, Onik first introduced an automated percutaneous device by which to mechanically remove herniated nuclear material in order to decompress the affected nerve root (90). Using this technique, a 2-mm, 8-inch long blunted closed-tip probe containing a side port with a reciprocating blade is placed within the nucleus. Suction is applied through the inner cannula pulling nuclear material into the port. The sharpened end of the inner cannula is pneumatically driven across the port severing the aspirated nuclear material from the parent source. The removed nuclear material is then aspirated into a collection container (90).

Following Onik's initial case report of immediate resolution of lower limb radicular pain in a 33-year-old male after automated percutaneous lumbar discectomy (APLD) was performed on a L4-5 intervertebral disc protrusion (90), Maroon and Onik published their initial results of the first 20 patients treated with APLD (175). Eighty percent of the treated patients experienced good to excellent improvement at a six-month follow-up interval. Four patients did not improve and eventually required microsurgical excision of sequestered disc fragments. Findings of a multicenter prospective trial by these investigators and others revealed a reported 75% success rate at follow-up at least one year after the procedure in 327 patients treated by APLD. Patients who experienced persistent lower limb greater than axial lumbar pain, provocative SLR, and two out of four signs of radiculopathy despite at least six weeks (mean duration of 11.6 months) of conservative care (94) were enrolled. However, objective data such as visual analog scale (VAS) scores and disability assessment were not reported, findings prior to one year were not revealed, and 18% of the discectomies involved two levels which clouds statistical assessment of the intervention's efficacy.

A subsequent prospective study of 518 patients by Davis and Onik (95) with similar inclusion criteria demonstrated a success rate of 85% at a minimum follow-up of one year after removing a mean of 2.1 g of nuclear material. Patients were evaluated at three-month intervals up to two years after the procedure. However, data from evaluations prior to one year were not presented in the article; yet, the authors did comment that 70% of successfully treated patients returned to work within two weeks (95). Davis and Onik confirmed the absence of intervertebral disc extrusion but did not clarify the size of the herniation volume. The absence of the postprocedure data at three-month intervals prevents an assessment of the rate of improvement which might allow commentary regarding the efficacy of the intervention relative to the natural history of the condition. A regression toward the mean analysis might have proven helpful to demonstrate a plateau of the patients' signs and symptoms prior to treatment because no control group was available for comparison. Fiume et al. found similar results in 64% of the 84 treated patients with small to medium disc protrusions at a mean follow-up of 22 months. The investigators removed a mean of 2.3 g of nuclear material, and reported pain relief and return to work at 24 and 21 days, respectively (96).

In a large prospective study of 1525 patients, Teng et al. found a success rate of 83%, 56% of patients became pain-free, and 26% of patients greatly improved, at a mean follow up of 18.3 months with 51 patients lost to follow-up (176). Using a device with a revolving blade rotating 400 cycles per minute, the authors treated 1289 patients who presented with sciatica and 185 patients presenting with complaints of primarily low back pain. These diagnostic categories were not separated prior to data analysis. Patients had persistent symptoms after a minimum of two months of conservative care and demonstrated a corroborative disc herniation on MRI or computed tomography (CT).

In a prospective assessment of over 1350 patients treated with APLD, Bonaldi observed successful outcomes in 67.5% patients at six months. He found favorable results in certain subgroups (97). Almost 80% of 83 elderly patients who are 70 years or older, experienced good or excellent results, and 78% of 108 postsurgical patients suffering a recurrent disc herniation at the previously treated level appreciated good or excellent results (97). His technique included the injection of 80 mg of methylprednisolone and 1 ml of 0.5% bupivicaine into the nucleus upon completion of the discectomy. In patients with radicular complaints, he injected 40 mg of methylprednisolone and 1 ml of bupivicaine around the offended nerve root. All patients demonstrated a corroborative protruded disc on MRI or CT or postdiscography CT (97). Bonaldi's data suggests that the addition of corticosteroid and anesthetic does not significantly alter the effect of APLD on clinical outcome. However, his patient cohort was not pure and contained patients with both purely axial and radicular pain, thus preventing the assessment of the effect of corticosteroid on clinical signs and symptoms. Yet, his work is the largest investigation of postsurgical patients with recurrent disc herniation. Seventy-eight percent success rate in this subgroup approaches findings in earlier work (95). However, a 9.6% rate of loss to follow-up, short follow-up interval, and outcomes measured largely by postal questionnaires were flaws of the study.

In a prospective audit of 30 patients presenting with radicular signs and symptoms owing to a contained disc herniation, Ramberg and Sahlstrand recorded immediate improvement in radicular pain and improved SLR at one week after APLD in 20 patients (98). A mean of 0.9 g of nuclear material was aspirated from the herniated discs (range 0–2.1). Four patients were lost to follow-up but were included in the initial assessments. Ten patients eventually required open surgical intervention. The remaining 16 patients demonstrated gradual improvement over the ensuing five weeks with gradually less improvement between six weeks and final follow-up at two to five years (98). Disability as measured by the Oswestry Disability Scale improved most dramatically from six weeks to follow-up at two to five years.

In a prospective, randomized trial, Revel et al. compared APLD with chemonucleolysis in 141 patients with lumbosacral radiculopathy unresponsive to 30 days of conservative medical treatment (99). Each patient had a corroborative disc herniation at a single level as detected by MRI, CT, or myelography. Seventy-two patients underwent chemonucleolysis in which 2 ml (4000 U) of chymopapain was administered intradiscally into each treated disc. Sixty-nine patients underwent APLD but the volume of the nuclear tissue removed was not reported. Thirty-two patients did not complete the study and were treated as failures. At six months follow-up, 61% of the chemonucleolysis group and 44% of the APLD group considered the treatment outcome to be successful. The patient had to consider his or her improvement better than "moderate" to be categorized as a treatment success. In contrast, the investigators judged 77% of the chemonucleolysis group and 83% of the APLD group as successfully treated. At one year, 83% of the chemonucleolysis patients felt their outcome was successful while 61% of their APLD counterparts held the same conviction. The authors did not attribute the low rate of success for APLD to a particularly low rate of loss to follow up (3%).

Chatterjee et al. randomized 31 patients to APLD and 40 patients to microdiscectomy as treatment for lumbosacral radiculopathy owing to a small disc protrusion unresponsive to six weeks of conservative care (100). At six months, 29% of the APLD group, after removal of a mean of 2.1 g of nuclear content, and 80% of the microdiscectomy group experienced good or excellent results. Twenty of the 22 failed APLD cases elected to undergo microdiscectomy and 13 (65%) achieved good or excellent results, which is less than the 80% success rate of the microdiscectomy group. This calculation may underestimate the failure of microdiscectomy in this subgroup of patients if all 22 had undergone surgery with just 13 successful outcomes leading to a 59% success rate. Furthermore, the 80% success rate observed in the surgical group is less than the 93% success rate in initial microdiscectomy cases encountered in an independent trial pursued by the investigators (93).

Grevitt et al. enrolled 137 patients into a prospective study utilizing VAS, Oswestry Back Disability form, and Short Form 36 as outcome measurement tools to assess improvement in radicular signs and symptoms after APLD (177). Each patient did not improve despite conservative care of physical therapy and epidural steroid injections, and the mean duration of preprocedure symptoms was 16 months (3–26 months). Twenty-two patients were lost to follow-up, and 17 patients eventually required surgical intervention. At a mean follow-up period of 55 months, 52% of patients were successfully treated with APLD. If the 22 patients lost to follow-up had been successfully treated, successful outcome may have been achieved in 64% of the patients. Two of the surgical cases had persistent radicular pain because of sequestered disc material at the index level. The majority of patients eventually undergoing late surgery were being treated for persistent and progressive axial lumbar pain. The authors did not report any results of further diagnostic evaluation, such as provocative discography or diagnostic facet joint blocks, to verify the source of persistent lumbar pain.

Few data have been collected regarding the role of automated percutaneous cervical discectomy. Bonaldi reported his experience in treating 84 patients over a 13-year time period. Sixty percent of cervical radicular patients experienced complete regression of pain and 20% appreciated a satisfactory, partial regression of pain (178). These data were communicated as an oral presentation, and the investigator did not report the duration of preprocedure symptoms, length of conservative care, or follow-up interval.

Thermal Decompression—Laser

The poor performance of APLD compared with conventional open discectomy interfered with its momentum as a minimally invasive percutaneous decompressive technology. In 1986, Choy and Ascher employed thermal technology to remove nuclear contents effectively decompressing the intervertebral disc (179). The term *laser* is an acronym for light amplification by stimulated emission of radiation (180). The laser–tissue interaction in biological tissues is determined by the physical properties of the laser (wavelength, pulse-length, energy density), and the optical, biomechanical, and biochemical properties (absorption, heat conduction, scattering, reflection) of the targeted tissue. The absorption spectrum of the nucleus pulposus is comparable with other water-containing tissues (180). Therefore, ablating nuclear tissue by energy absorption will best be achieved by utilizing a laser with wavelength matched to the known absorption bands of water—the visible and infrared regions (115). Choy and Ascher reported their experimental findings of reducing intradiscal pressure in human cadaveric lumbar discs using the laser wavelengths emitted by neodymium embedded in an Yttrium-Aluminum-Garnet crystal, Nd:YAG (103). The Nd:YAG laser is the most widely used medical laser system and produces a distribution of the applied energy within the nuclear tissue (180).

Choy communicated his initial clinical experience with percutaneous laser disc decompression (PLDD) in 12 patients suffering from "symptomatic lumbar disc herniation." Each patient was treated using a Nd:YAG laser via a 400-μm optical fiber. Nine of these 12 patients experienced improvement during the two-minute procedure after not improving with conservative care of an undisclosed period of time. Five of these initial nine patients subsequently underwent repeat surgery for recurrent symptoms, while four out of the initial 12 remained symptom-free at 7–16-month follow-up (179). However, despite all 12 patients demonstrating a symptomatic disc herniation, the report did not reveal if all 12 patients complained of radicular or axial lumbar pain. The period of preprocedure conservative care may not have been long enough to allow natural improvement in a certain number of cases. Technical details consequent to the novelty of the new procedure may have interfered with adequate nuclear absorption, hence decompression.

Choy later reported his findings after treating 333 patients who had persistent radicular symptoms despite three months of conservative care because of a contained lumbosacral disc herniation by MRI or CT (103). Patients demonstrating spondylolisthesis, central or lateral canal stenosis, or advanced disc degeneration were excluded. At a mean follow-up of 26 months, 78.4% of 333 patients were assessed as having good to fair results as defined by the Macnab criteria. Sixty-four percent of 261 good to fair patients experienced relief during the procedure, 21% experienced gradual and progressive relief starting three to four days after the procedure, and 24% reported partial recurrence on postprocedure day one with gradual improvement over the ensuing two to three weeks. Each patient was treated using the Nd:YAG laser connected to a 400-μm optical fiber for three to four minutes. The authors did not differentiate the proportions of fair or good responses which might represent two different clinical outcomes despite being grouped together in the same category. Although the Macnab criteria for a fair result includes no signs of radiculopathy, patients in this group may be functionally nonproductive and might still require certain medications because of intermittent episodes of mild lumbar or radicular pain. Choy has published his subsequent experiences (104,105) with inhomogenous patient populations complaining of either radicular or axial pain, undergoing treatment of multiple levels, again relying on loosely defined outcome criteria at long-term follow-up.

McMillan et al. found the short-term improvement of PLDD beneficial, primarily in patients suffering from lumbosacral radicular symptoms rather than axial lumbar pain (106). Each patient underwent PLDD with the Nd:YAG laser in a similar fashion to Choy's description. Of 30 patients with primarily radicular pain at baseline, 24 (80%) demonstrated improvement as measured by the American Academy of Orthopedic Surgeons Pain Assessment Questionnaire, and the mean scores improved by 68% between baseline and follow-up. Assessment was completed at follow-up evaluations at three months, and each patient underwent treatment of one segmental level after MRI evidence of a corroborative disc herniation with less than 50% reduction in disc height (106). Although flawed by a short follow-up period, McMillan utilized an objective measurement tool to document improvement in an endpoint.

Relying on the modified Macnab criteria for assessment, Casper et al. treated 222 patients who presented with signs and symptoms of lumbosacral radiculopathy (107). Each patient did not respond to six weeks of conservative care including physical therapy, anti-inflammatory medications, selective nerve root blocks, and epidural steroid injections (107). Patients who were deemed to be symptomatic because of central or lateral canal stenosis or disc herniation sequestration were excluded. Each patient underwent PLDD using Holmium:YAG (Ho:YAG) laser with a Sidefire fiber containing a 550-μm optical fiber (107). Good and excellent results were deemed successful while fair or poor were unsuccessful. Eighty-four percent of treated patients were successfully treated at a follow-up of one year. Of these, 62.5% experienced excellent results and 37.4% experienced good results. Only one patient was lost to follow-up because of nonprocedure-related death. Of the 35 failures, 10 underwent open surgery for sequestered disc fragment, lateral stenosis, or suspected discitis, 12 underwent a second PLDD at the index level, and 13 experienced fair or poor outcomes. Although the modified Macnab criteria more stringently evaluate postprocedure outcomes that were impressive, the absence of a control group precludes conclusion that PLDD was solely responsible for the measured improvement. However, the mean duration of preprocedural symptoms was 24.8 months, which presumably would have allowed for natural regression toward the mean.

In a prospective study of 50 patients, Nerubay et al. performed PLDD using carbon dioxide laser (108). The range of preprocedure symptom duration was four months to 10 years with a mean of 33 months. Each patient had complaints of axial and radicular pain accompanying advanced imaging evidence of a corroborative disc herniation despite three months of conservative care. Patients whose imaging revealed spinal stenosis, spondylolisthesis, or large disc herniation were excluded. Sixty percent of patients had excellent results using Macnab's criteria, 14% had good results, and no improvement or worsening symptoms were observed in 26%. Follow-up was carried out up to two to five years with a mean of 2.8 years. This was a small study of 50 patients but with adequate preprocedure conservative care.

Percutaneous laser disc decompression has been applied to the cervical spine with success (109,110). In a prospective study of 105 patients with cervical and/or upper limb radicular pain, Knight et al. observed a good or excellent outcome in 51%. Eight patients were lost to follow-up and the mean follow-up was 43 months. Another 25% of the patients experienced functional improvement. Each patient failed to improve with at least six months of conservative care and demonstrated a corroborative disc abnormality on MRI. Provocative discography was performed to verify the painful level in patients with multilevel involvement. Eighty milligrams of depo-medrol was injected intradiscally in addition to laser treatment. The study cohort enrolled in Knight's work was not homogenous as patients had either axial or radicular pain.

In a more pure patient population, Choy evaluated 93 patients after treating cervical radicular symptoms due to MRI-documented disc herniations unresponsive to three months of conservative care (110). Just 58 patients were available at an undisclosed follow-up evaluation conducted by a telephone interview. Ninety percent of these patients were reportedly improved by the Macnab criteria. However, if the remaining 35 patients were considered failures in addition to the other six (10% of 58), the success rate would decrease to 56% at an undisclosed follow-up interval.

Twenty-eight out of 31 prospectively studied patients treated with Ho:YAG laser using a 400-nm-wide probe tip demonstrated objective and subjective improvement in their cervical radicular complaints at six weeks follow-up (111). In this study, Siebert enrolled patients after an undisclosed duration of conservative care and symptoms. Yet, the follow-up interval was short and the outcome measures were not stringent. In a smaller study, Harada prospectively evaluated seven patients with cervical radiculopathy and corroborative MRI findings of disc herniation at one week and then again at three to six months (112). Each patient had not improved with six weeks of conservative care while the length of symptoms preprocedure was not reported. The authors treated the herniated cervical discs using the Nd:YAG laser and reported a good result defined by Macnab criteria in all patients and improvement in the Japan Orthopedic Association (JOA) score for cervical radiculopathy. The number of treated patients was low and the authors did not perform statistical analysis on the change in the mean JOA scores from baseline to each time point.

Nonthermal Decompression—Nucleoplasty

Radiofrequency ablation (RFA) of tissue is the process of applying directed radiofrequency energy to targeted tissue to destroy or modify that tissue. RFA has been applied to various tissues including tonsillar and pharyngeal tissues (181), cardiac muscle and nervous tissue (182), and peripheral nerves (183). Radiofrequency ablation was pursued in the orthopedic arena to shape and remove articular tissue (184). Anecdotal evidence has been generated attesting to more rapid healing of cartilaginous soft tissue with less scarring with RFA as compared with lasers and electrocautery (185). In contrast to its laster counterpart, RF heating causes less tissue destruction without a similar amount of inadvertent thermal damage to adjacent tissue. Application of RFA to the intervertebral disc was a logical extension of this new technology.

Nucleoplasty is the percutaneous decompression of an intervertebral disc by the application of patented Coblation™ (Arthrocare, Sunnyvale, California, U.S.A.) technology in which RF energy is applied to a conductive medium causing a focused plasma field to form around the energized electrodes. This plasma field contains highly ionized particles of sufficient energy to cleave organic molecular bonds within the tissue forming a channel (186). The by-products of this nonheat-driven process are the elementary molecules and low molecular weight inert gases which escape via the introducer needle (186,187). As the RF probe is withdrawn, the newly created channel is thermally treated producing a zone of thermal coagulation. Thus, nucleoplasty combines coagulation and tissue ablation to form channels within the nucleus and decompress an intervertebral disc herniation (188).

Initial data regarding the efficacy of nucleoplasty were presented in 2001. Singh reported improvement in both axial and radicular pain in a small cohort of patients evaluated postprocedurally at three months (188). However, patients with complaints of either axial lumbar pain or radicular pain were enrolled in the study. A year later, Sharps and Isaac published their findings again in a cohort of patients with mixed complaints of axial lumbar and radicular lower limb pain (117). The authors initially enrolled 49 patients and reported a 79% success rate at three months in 41 patients. A successful outcome was defined as a greater than 2-point reduction in visual analogue scale (VAS) score, patient satisfaction, absence of narcotic use, and return to work. The authors additionally reported a decrease in the mean VAS score of 3.3 points among the 13 patients who were assessed at 12 months after the procedure. The authors, however, did not report the narcotic utilization, return to work, or patient satisfaction data (117). Later in 2002, Singh et al. prospectively studied 80 patients with either lumbar or radicular pain (118). Sixty-nine patients were available for follow-up evaluation at 12 months by either telephone interview or clinical encounter. Seventy-five percent of these 69 patients reported a reduction in their pain scores which were statistically significant with 54% of patients reporting relief of 50% or more. Compared with baseline, nearly half of the patients reported statistically significant improvement in their sitting, standing, and walking capabilities (118). However, this was an uncontrolled study and assessment of improvement can only be suggested to be attributable to the intervention, and different diagnostic categories, axial versus radicular, were evaluated similarly.

In the largest clinical trial investigating nucleoplasty in the lumbar spine, Alexandre et al. studied 1390 patients presenting with either axial or radicular pain because of a contained disc herniation demonstrated by advanced imaging studies (119). The symptoms had been ongoing for a minimum of three months despite appropriate conservative care. At 12 months, 55.8% of the treated patients achieved excellent (total resolution of symptoms, full return of function) results and 24.9% good (fairly total symptom resolution, good quality of life) results. However, the authors did not confirm how many subjects were available at follow-up. No prospective, controlled trials investigating nucleoplasty's utility in treating specifically lumbosacral radiculopathy have been published. A multicenter trial is underway assessing nucleoplasty's efficacy versus therapeutic selective nerve root injections for lumbar radicular pain because of contained disc herniations.

Application of nucleoplasty in the cervical spine has been studied (120–122). Slipman and DePalma reported successful outcome in 91% of 21 patients at six months in an uncontrolled study (120). The investigators employed a two-pronged approach by injecting corticosteroid and anesthetic around the affected nerve root directly after completion of the nucleoplasty procedure (120). Each patient demonstrated a corroborative disc herniation of ≤5 mm. Also, in each instance, there had to be an objective correlating finding indicative of root involvement: myotomal deficit, or positive electrodiagnostic evaluation, or positive diagnostic selective nerve root block. The average VAS score decreased from a preoperative level of 6.9 to 1.3 at six months, and eight patients were without pain at six months. Their findings were sustained at 12 months in that 19 of 21 patients experienced successful outcome (121). The average VAS rating at 12 months was 1.4. The average duration of preprocedure symptoms was 10 months, and each patient had been deemed an appropriate operative candidate by a fellowship-trained spine surgeon (121). Nardi et al. prospectively evaluated 50 consecutive patients with cervical radiculopathy because of a contained disc herniation (122). The authors incorporated a randomized control group of 20 patients and demonstrated a complete resolution of symptoms in 80% of the treatment arm at a follow-up of 60 days (122). No patients in the control group reported complete relief at 60 days, and approximately 75% reported no change in their symptoms. Nardi, however treated patients with a contained herniation ≤3 mm, and enrolled patients with axial or radicular pain (122).

Mechanical Decompression—Dekompressor Probe™

In January 2001, the Food and Drug Administration (FDA) approved the clinical use of a new 1.5-mm percutaneous lumbar discectomy probe, the Dekompressor Probe™ (Stryker, Kalamazoo, Michigan, U.S.A.), for the treatment of contained intervertebral disc protrusions (123). This device is a disposable hand-held instrument driven by a battery-powered subminiature DC motor connected to an implant grade precision ground titanium probe with a helical auger as its distal tip (189). A 17-gauge outer cannula provides access to the disc via an extrapedicular approach. When activated, the auger tip rotates at 12,000 rotations per minute creating localized suction removing nuclear material and aspirating it through the cannula into a collection chamber using an Archimedes pump principle (123,124,189). The thixotropic nature of the nucleus in which nuclear material becomes less viscous when in motion provides an ideal application for the Archimedes pump mechanism employed by the Dekompressor Probe (189). The helical auger tip is relatively inactive when engaged in the more fibrous annular tissue (189).

The first human application was reported in 2003 in an open forum describing the successful treatment of a 36-year-old male suffering from contained 4.5-mm herniation at L4-5 and 9.5-mm herniation at L5-S1. Alo et al. then pursued a prospective study of 50 consecutive patients with stringent inclusion and exclusion criteria (123). Each patient presented with lumbosacral radicular signs and symptoms of at least six-month duration because of a corroborative contained disc herniation ≤6 mm in size. Conservative care including physical therapy, oral analgesic and anti-inflammatory medications, and transforaminal epidural corticosteroid and anesthetic injection did not provide lasting relief. Subsequent to these failed therapeutic injections each patient underwent confirmatory diagnostic selective nerve root blocks with 0.5–1.5 cc of anesthetic with a positive response defined as >80% reduction in the preblock radicular pain level for the duration of the pharmacologic effect of the anesthetic. Twelve patients underwent percutaneous decompression at two levels, and outcomes were assessed at six months regarding VAS rating, analgesic usage, patient satisfaction, and functional improvement. Patient satisfaction and functional improvement were assessed subjectively by asking each patient if these parameters had improved. During decompression, 0.75 to 2.0 cc of nuclear material was removed. At follow-up, 74% of the patients had reduced their analgesic intake, 90% reported improvement in their functional status, 80% reported an overall satisfaction with their treatment, and the reduction in the mean VAS rating was 60.25%, which was significant ($P < 0.001$). Six patients experienced zero radicular pain at six months. No remark was made regarding surgical intervention of any of the treatment failures, and objective, validated outcome measurement tools for patient satisfaction and function were not utilized, and the follow-up interval was short.

In a subsequent study reported by Amoretti et al., 10 patients were retrospectively reviewed at a range of 6 to 10 months after percutaneous disc decompression using the Dekompressor Probe (124). Each patient had a history of recalcitrant "sciatica" related to a corroborative contained intervertebral disc herniation on MRI that did not improve despite CT-guided periradicular "infiltration," and any medical therapy. The authors did not reveal the volume of tissue removed, and assessed outcome by VAS ratings and analgesic usage. At a mean follow-up of 8.6 months (6–10), eight patients (80%) were satisfactorily treated with a decrease in VAS rating of more than 70% and complete elimination of medical therapy. The two failed cases initially experienced improvement with one undergoing open discectomy for an extrusion that may have been misinterpreted on initial MRI evaluation, and the second responded to medical treatment. This was a small retrospective study without validated outcome measures other than VAS ratings that suggests improvements may be stable beyond six months. Although no other clinical trials have been published, our experience using Dekompressor to treat lumbar radiculopathy because of contained disc herniations after no prolonged benefit from transforaminal epidural steroid injections or therapeutic selective nerve root injections mirrors the results of Alo (123) and Amoretti (124).

SAFETY OF NONENDOSCOPIC PERCUTANEOUS DISC DECOMPRESSION BY TECHNOLOGY
Enzymatic Degradation

The overall complication rate of chemonucleolysis has been calculated as 3.7% with a rate of severe complications of 0.45% (190). However, this calculation may be an overestimate. Data reported to the FDA revealed 121 adverse reactions in approximately 135,000 patients (191). Of the 121 adverse events reported to the FDA (191), seven cases were of fatal anaphylaxis, 24 cases of infection, 32 cases of hemorrhage, 32 cases of neurologic deficits (such as paraplegia, paraparesis, hemiparesis, and foot drop), and 15 miscellanous cases of cardiac and respiratory complications. The overall mortality rate was 0.019% (191). The most common side effect is backache and stiffness ranging from 15% (80) to 100% (167). Lumbar muscle spasm or guarding has been observed in 36% to 41% of patients treated with chymopapain (80). Discitis (82,83), lower limb deep venous thrombosis (83), anaphylactic shock and death (90), acute transverse myelitis (90) [a causal relationship between chymopapain and central nervous system (CNS) could not be substantiated (192)], and cerebral hemorrhage (193) have been rarely reported. Anaphylaxis was recognized in one of 87 patients receiving chymopapain in Dabezies' 1987 study (81). However, since then the incidence of anaphylactic reactions has decreased to 0.25% because of sensitivity testing and antihistamine administration preinjection (168). Males have lower incidence of an anaphylactic reaction than do females, 0.3% versus 0.9%, respectively. African-American women, however, are at an increased risk with a reported incidence of 2% (84). No epidural or intraneural fibrosis has been observed (81). Although the incidence of anaphylaxis may be less with collagenase, neurologic deficit may be increased (170).

Loss of disc height does occur after chymopapain administration (82,167,194,195). Fraser demonstrated no difference in disc height loss between discs treated with chymopapain and saline but did not assess for a change relative to baseline in each group (82). Liesveth et al. observed an average disc height loss of 15.8% at 31 to 124 months after treating intervertebral discs with chymopapain (194). However, reconstitution of disc height was achieved over this same time period in discs treated with a lower dose of chymopapain (194). Maintenance of disc height loss in the discs treated with higher dose of chymopapain had an impact on the success of the intervention (194) and will be discussed under mechanism of action. However, these investigations used serial plain radiography which requires accurate placement of the central ray of the X-ray beam which can be difficult (195). Using digital lateral radiographs and CT, Mall et al. documented an invariable loss of disc height in 16 out of 17 patients treated with chemonucleolysis (only 16 were evaluated by digital radiography). However, the authors did not differentiate change in disc height relative to successful versus nonsuccessful cases (195).

Chemonucleolysis has been compared with open surgical discectomy regarding complication rates. A meta-analysis performed by Bouillet revealed an overall complication rate of 3.7% and rate of serious complications of 0.45% in 43,662 chemonucleolysis patients compared with 26% and 4.2%, respectively in 2051 surgery patients (190). No mortalities were reported in the chemonucleolysis group compared with three deaths reported in the surgical group (190). In a separate meta-analysis, Nordby and Wright found 15 times more infections, six times more neurological and vascular problems, and an overall mortality three times greater in laminectomy patients than chemonucleolysis patients (191). Brown performed a third literature analysis and concluded that chemonucleolysis is 3 to 20 times safer than surgery for the treatment of lumbosacral radiculopathy as a result of disc herniation (196).

Automated Percutaneous Discectomy

After treatment with APLD, most patients will experience mild paravertebral lumbar muscle spasm or guarding lasting a few days. Rarely, these spasms are severe (94), and appear to require analgesic medications less frequently than after chemonucleolysis (42% vs. 10%) (99). Discitis occurs with similar frequency as in provocative discography with an observed incidence of 0.06% to 0.2% (94,97,176). Rare cases of psoas muscle hematoma have been reported (94,97). The overall complication rate as observed in large trials has fallen between 0.06% (176) and 0.95% (97). Permanent injury to neural elements, dura, urinary tract, gastrointestinal system, or major blood vessels is extremely rare and has not been encountered in large trials (94,95,97,176). However, two isolated cases of cauda equina injury have been documented as a result of probe misplacement (159,197). Disc height loss of greater than 50% occurred less frequently in levels treated by APLD compared with chemonucleolysis (99).

Laser

The most common side effect of PLDD is postprocedure paraspinal muscle spasm or guarding which occurs in 10% of the cases (113). These symptoms can vary from mild stiffness to disabling pain with the patient listing toward the side of tightness (113). Typically, the lumbar pain dissipates over three to four days and can be addressed with oral muscle relaxers (113). Although not reported in most trials (102–108), Choy and Knight have remarked in personal communications about postprocedure sacroilitis occurring in 2% of lumbar cases and speculate that this may be because of an unlocking of the sacroiliac joint leading to overused "friction" related sacroilitis (113). Infectious and aseptic discitis each occur with an incidence of 0.3% per treated disc (105), and in Choy's experience infectious discitis has not occurred since the implementation of routine preprocedure intravenous antibiotics (105). In Choy's initial experience with 47 treated cervical intervertebral discs, one retroesophageal abscess had been encountered for a complication rate of 2% (105). However, this rate has decreased to 0.6% after treating 178 total discs in 93 patients (113), and is in accordance with Casper's findings of a 0.4% incidence of aseptic discitis per disc level treated (107). Thermal injury of nervous tissue has been observed with an incidence varying from 0% to 0.8% (105–107), or as high as 8% in one study (108) and is likely related to incorrect fiber placement (113). Most cases are transient and resolve over one to five months (107,108) but permanent injury can occur (108). Isolated cases of intestinal injury, sympathetic chain irritation (114), introducer needle heating (113), and dislodgement of needle tips have been reported (113). Thermal endplate necrosis has been reported (98) but has not been encountered by experienced physicians (103–107). Its occurrence appears to be operator-related and due to rotation of the side-firing probe in a cephalad and/or caudad direction thus directing the laser beam toward an endplate (113). Data regarding changes in disc height have not been tabulated.

Nucleoplasty

The most common side effect of lumbar nucleoplasty is localized soreness at the procedure site which was observed at 24 hours in 48% of the 150 patients treated at The Penn Spine Center (Philadelphia, PA, U.S.A.) (198). Axial lumbar pain can be a complaint in 5% of patients for up to 10 to 14 days (198). Less commonly at 24 hours, 9% of patients reported new areas of inconsequential leg pain and 8% new areas of lumbar pain. No permanent neurologic, vascular, or orthopedic injury has been observed (117–122). Intradiscal temperatures have been measured exceeding 60°C within 3 to 4 mm of the nucleoplasty probe tip (199). However, histologic studies have not found gross or microanatomical evidence of extreme tissue damage (200,201). Within the nucleus, a small 1.0-mm channel is created surrounded by intact fibrocartilage cells and collagen matrix. No alteration of the proteoglycan or collagen structure, or endplate damage has been observed to occur (200,201). Furthermore, no damage of the neural elements has been documented (117–122,200,201). If the applicator is maintained at a distance of 3 to 4 mm from any critical structure, unintentional thermal damage may be avoided (120).

Dekompressor Probe[TM]

Of the 60 published Dekompressor cases, no complications have been reported (123,124). Complications were not specifically reported by Alo et al. (123), but Amoretti (124) remarked that no complications were encountered at any point in the postprocedure period. Nuclear tissue removed in Alo's study reportedly did not reveal evidence of tissue injury in any of the samples (123). Direct and intentional operation of the device against annular fibers did not visually affect or remove annular tissue in lamb cadavers (189). In our experience, a minority of patients will report localized soreness at the insertion site that eventually resolves over five to seven days. Equally common, patients may experience mild, transient paresthesias in the distribution of the previously affected nerve root around seven days after the procedure that eventually resolve over the ensuing seven to ten days. The first author has encountered one case in which a patient developed severe radicular pain 24 to 28 hours after the decompressive procedure that was subsequently abolished within 24 hours of the completion of a transforaminal epidural steroid injection at the index level. Of all the cases we published and performed, we are not aware of any infections, vascular injury, viscous injury, or injury of neural elements. Presumably, risk of infection would be similar as with discography.

MECHANISM OF ACTION OF NONENDOSCOPIC PERCUTANEOUS DISC DECOMPRESSION BY TECHNOLOGY
Enzymatic Degradation

Chymopapain is a potent proteolytic enzyme that rapidly degrades the proteoglycan core protein and releases fragments containing a few glycosaminoglycan chains (166). Consequently, the intranuclear viscosity and molecular weight, and water-imbibing capacity are reduced or lost lowering disc volume, intradiscal pressure, and disc space height (166,167,195,202,203). It has been postulated that this enzymatic degradation and resultant remodeling of the disc architecture causes an "internal decompression" of the nerve root under influence by the disc herniation alleviating symptomatology (195,204,205). However, radiologic studies have not always confirmed a concurrent reduction in disc herniation volume after chemonucleolysis upon the initial reduction in clinical signs and symptoms (205–210). An additional mechanism of action has been substantiated as integral in symptom reduction and may be more active within the acute to subacute time period after treatment (203,205,207,209).

Studies using serial contrast-enhanced CT have documented that regression of the herniated mass did not occur until six weeks to six months after administration of intradiscal chymopapain, despite partial or complete resolution of symptoms in a fraction of the time (210,211). Similar serial studies utilizing MRI have documented that the size and signal characteristics of the intervertebral disc and herniation are not altered within an initial time frame of 6 to 12 weeks after chemonucleolysis (206,207,209,212). The consistency of the herniated disc material may be altered perhaps explaining a subtle decompression of the nerve root without gross changes in the herniation volume. McCulloch and Macnab hypothesized that the integrity of the disc herniation was changed from that of a "golf ball" to that more of a "cotton ball" of collagen fibers (213). However, McCulloch and Macnab did not render experimental evidence in support of their contention which has been challenged by experimental evidence demonstrating a lack of change in the physical properties of the herniated disc material within two weeks after chymopapain injection (214). Suguro provided histologic evidence explaining failure of chemonucleolysis in a relatively collagenous disc fragment lacking an abundance of proteoglycans (215). Disc desiccation induced by chemonucleolysis of nuclear proteoglycans can be detected by the loss of the nuclear tau 2 (T2) weight signal on MRI around two weeks after chymopapain treatment before which clinical improvement has already occurred (206). A detectable reduction in herniation volume may not be seen until four weeks after treatment but progresses beyond one year after chemonucleolysis (206). Hence, chymopapain's efficacy may very well be partially related to its ability to induce a cicatricial process marked by fibrocartilaginous remodeling that eventually matures the herniated fragment. In fact, posterolateral and far lateral soft disc herniations presenting with primarily limb pain have correlated well in a cohort of 3000 patients with successful outcome after chemonucleolysis of that disc (88). Chemonucleolysis may achieve a more rapid, but no more complete, resolution of the disc herniation that eventually occurs spontaneously (212).

Anti-inflammatory properties of chymopapain may account for early and rapid clinical improvement that cannot be entirely explained by morphologic changes on advanced imaging studies. Saal postulated that chemonucleolysis may degrade nuclear PLA_2 whose presence has been documented in acute disc herniation (28). Such conjecture provides an attractive explanation for the efficacy of chemonucleolysis. The time course of early clinical improvement after intradiscal chymopapain administration mirrors that after performance of transforaminal epidural steroid/anesthetic injections, which modify solely an inflammatory condition and not structural abnormalities (62,216). Transforaminal epidural steroid injections (62,216) and intradiscal chymopapain injection (80–83) provide immediate and lasting relief despite little change in disc herniation morphology (206–212). Using an experimental inflammatory neuropathy rat animal model, Sawin et al. demonstrated that perineural deposition of chymopapain or betamethasone (but not saline) significantly reduced both PLA_2 activity and neuropathic behavioral changes (205). Equally as important, Sawin et al. did not observe histologic evidence of neurotoxicity after direct topical administration of chymopapain to the rat sciatic nerve segments (205). Watts in his review of 13,000 chemonculeolysis cases did not discover report of damage to extradural nervous tissue (203). Chymopapain injected into the nucleus may extrude into annular defects and eventually enter the anterior epidural space and contact adjacent neural elements (217). Intranuclear chymopapain may exert two biochemical effects by extension into the epidural space thereby directly reducing the activity of inflammatory cytokines offending the affected nerve root (205,217), and/or or by inactivating intradiscal proinflammatory and inflammatory cytokines. Herniated discs produce increased levels of metalloproteinases, nitric oxide, interleukin-6 (IL-6), prostaglandin E2 (36–38), and tumor necrosis factor-alpha (TNF-α) has been documented in both, more so in the latter, nuclear and annular material of herniated human intervertebral discs (39,218). Perhaps, these cytokines provide a proteinaceous substrate for chymopapain leading to their proteolysis or disruption of their synthesis. An extensive literature review failed to produce a systematic study of the effect of chymopapain on inflammatory cytokines or their production.

The mechanism of action of chemonucleolysis most likely involves both biochemical and biomechanical effects. Immediate reduction in intradiscal pressure (219) and disc height reduces tension on the affected nerve root (220). Within 24 hours, anti-PLA$_2$ effects and disruption of intradiscal cytokine production relax inflammatory insults of the nerve root. Improvement gradually progresses as further desiccation occurs and nuclear remodeling is completed (206,212) leading to a variable and gradual reduction in herniation size (212) and presumably more inert disc herniation.

Automated Percutaneous Discectomy

Inspection of the clinical response after APLD from the available data reveals a trend for quickest improvement within two to four weeks after treatment (98,99,101). Ramberg observed a 26% improvement in the median VAS rating at 24 hours after APLD. This improvement increased to 66% by one week (98). Concurrently, SLR significantly improved with the fastest rate of improvement by one week after APLD (98). These findings are supported by Revel's data whereby the greatest improvement in lower limb VAS ratings and SLR occurred by the time of discharge presumably within 24 hours after completion of the procedure (99). In Revel's study, greater improvement occurred in SLR after APLD than chemonucleolysis ($P < 0.02$). In a prospective study of 57 patients with lumbosacral radiculopathy, Shapiro observed at two weeks a reduction in lower limb radicular pain in 88%, and return to work in all patients working prior to APLD. Thirty-four percent of these patients eventually experienced recurrent symptoms over a 2.5-year follow-up period. However, it was not clear in the manuscript how many of these recurrences were attributable to a subsequently new herniation (101). It appears that radicular symptoms treated by APLD improve quickly within one to seven days with the quickest rate of improvement within the first two weeks (90,96,98,99,101). Yet, these clinical changes cannot be explained solely by reduction in volume of the disc herniation as appreciated by MRI (221,222). No reduction in the size of disc herniation was detected immediately and at six weeks after APLD (221). These findings seem stable over longer follow-up with 80% of cases demonstrating no change in disc morphology at a mean of 14 months (222). Thus, volume reduction does not appear to contribute to clinical improvement after APLD.

Alternatively, a reduction in intradiscal pressure has been measured after APLD which may account more readily for postoperative clinical improvement (223–225). In intervertebral discs with disupted outer annular fibers, annular pressure increases proportionally with increase in intranuclear pressure, and the nuclear pressure is higher than the annular pressure despite greater transfer from the nucleus to the annulus (226). No correlation has been established between the absolute amount of nuclear material removed and the clinical success of the APLD procedure (90,227). Simply piercing the annulus alone may sufficiently decompress the intervertebral disc (225,228,229). Radial bulging increases by an average of 0.22 mm per gram removed by APLD (223) but may increase to as much as 0.45 mm upon removal of 4.6 gm. Under 1000 N load, radial bulge averages 0.3 mm per gram of nucleus removed (231), and others have observed radial bulging only after conventional surgical discectomy and not after percutaneous discectomy (225). Disc height is reduced by an average of 1.43 mm after removal of 4.6 g of nucleus during 45 minutes of APLD (224). However, after removal of just 1 g, disc height is reduced by 0.8 mm (230). Interestingly, when intact discs are subjected to an 800 N compressive load the posterolateral disc margin bulges 0.3 to 0.4 mm (231), and does not change significantly after APLD (225). However, disc biomechanics after APLD have not been investigated under flexion and axial rotation movements while bearing an axial load, nor have biomechanical parameters been investigated after APLD in herniated discs with disrupted annular fibers.

Once nuclear material breaches the inner annular fibers reaching the outer annular fibers resulting in a contained disc herniation there is a consequential attrition of the annular fibers opposing the extruding nuclear material. Consequently, nuclear contents will transgress toward the annular defect resulting in approximation of inflammatory markers to the adjacent nerve root, and a focal increase in annular pressure (228). Puncture of the annulus will decompress the disc dissipating a portion of the intradiscal pressure away from the herniated region. A drop in intradiscal pressure after APLD will help reduce annular pressure, thus less contact force will be transduced to the nerve root. Similarly, a reduction in disc height will reduce nerve root tension by reducing contact force on the nerve root by the disc protrusion (220,232). Although a specific biochemical effect of APLD has not been well delineated, the decompressive effect on the nerve root may remove the impetus for production of inflammatory markers consequent to nerve root compression (233). Furthermore, removal of a portion of nuclear material may actually remove a portion of the source of the inflammatory markers (39). Immediate improvement in radicular limb pain within 24 hours, therefore, is likely due to a local decompression of and reduction of tension on an inflamed nerve root. Subsequent further improvement within the next one to two weeks is likely related to any anti-inflammatory effects from a relative reduction in the machinery producing these inflamogens. An inflamed nerve root will not tolerate minor perturbations, whereas an uninflamed nerve root will tolerate manipulation (41,42). Hence, immediate improvement after APLD is likely a manifestation of less mechanical influence on an inflamed nerve root. Unlike chemonucleolysis, APLD does not disrupt the proteoglycan nuclear matrix as the histology is recognizable (228). Consequently, the intervertebral disc does not enter a similar degree of remodeling as it would after chemonucleolysis. Therefore, the primary mechanism of action for APLD involves internal decompression of the disc alleviating a degree of nerve root tension thus improving periradicular blood flow, and mechanically removing some of the source of inflammatory cytokines. Despite a lack of experimental evidence, it is a possibility that the mere interrogation of the annular and nuclear tissue triggers a healing state within the disc (234).

Laser

The mechanism of action of PLDD has been presumed to be related to a reduction in intradiscal pressure (113). Choy constructed a closed system to investigate intervertebral disc pressure changes in human cadaveric spines. After preloading the disc with an axial load and maintaining the elevated intradiscal pressure, a Nd:YAG laser was applied to the loaded disc. A reduction of 55.6% of the mean intradiscal pressure was documented compared with a 15% reduction in the mean reduction of control discs. The investigators did not statistically analyze baseline differences between the two groups, and standard deviations were not reported to allow a calculation of effect size. The mean baseline intradiscal pressure in the treated group was 2350 mm Hg compared with an approximate mean of 2100 mm Hg in the control group. However, the range was much greater in the treated group with the highest pressure reaching approximately 3400 mm Hg compared with a maximum value in the control group of approximately 2300 mm Hg. The higher pressures in the treated group may have been a consequence of longer loading time (31 minutes) than in the control group (10 minutes). Furthermore, the elapsed time since the initiation of lasing was 33 minutes in the treatment group before final intradiscal pressure measurement. In contrast, the control group values were measured 20 minutes after final loading. Yet, Choy subsequently measured in vivo a drop in intradiscal pressure from a mean of 300 mm Hg to a mean of 154 mm Hg after PLDD in eight patients. However, others have corroborated an in vitro reduction of intradiscal pressure after treatment with Nd:YAG laser (235). Yet, a reduction in nuclear hydration, prostaglandin content, and collagen meshwork was not maintained in an animal model between days 1 and 60 after Nd:YAG laser discectomy (236).

Alternatively, Quigley et al. evaluated the change in elastance of porcine lumbar intervertebral discs after treatment with Nd:YAG and Ho:YAG lasers, and APLD (115). After treatment with the Nd:YAG laser, a 12.7% reduction in mean elastance, or the disc's recoil behavior, was observed which was statistically significant. The investigators did not interrogate a control disc to evaluate for any change in the porcine disc's elastance consequent to just piercing the annulus. Quigley et al. did remark that their study involved discs with intact annular fibers devoid of degenerative changes. The authors admitted to assuming that the comparative mass and volume data would be similar in both intact and degenerative discs (115). However, if annular disruption is present, intranuclear pressure is less than that in an intact disc (226). Therefore, the removal of a minute volume of nuclear material similar to Quigley's study, may not achieve a similar reduction in intranuclear pressure. Until interverterbral discs with injured annular fibers containing herniated nuclear material are studied, a conclusion cannot be rendered regarding whether the herniation will tend to recoil less toward the nerve root versus toward the nucleus. Perhaps, this reduction in recoil might be explained by a more even distribution of pressure, hence load, across the annular fibers due to a decrease in annular stiffness in discs treated by laser discectomy (237,238).

In order to better detect any morphologic change in intervertebral disc herniation volume, Hellinger et al. evaluated the density of disc herniations before and afer PLDD (239). Without clearly delineating an explanation for their measurement protocol, Hellinger et al. assessed the intervertebral discs using Houndsfield units after CT scanning. After treating 21 patients for radiculopathy due to a single-level corroborative disc herniation, the density of the index disc herniation was reduced by a mean of 20% (239). Vaporization of nuclear material (235) by absorption of the laser produces gases that extend into the outer annular fibers permeating its defects and the herniation itself. Consequently, the density of the protrusion decreases and its consistency softens (239). Kutschera's observation of decreased annular stiffness might be somewhat explained by a reduction in herniation density. This suggestion is solely speculative without experimental support. However, MRI myelography has demonstrated improvement in intradural cerebrospinal flow at the segmental level of the disc herniation after laser discectomy supporting the presence of a reduction in intraspinal pressure (240). Such an improvement may alleviate radicular venous congestion and counteract vascular insult of the nerve root in addition to reducing minor perturbations of an inflamed nerve root.

Nucleoplasty

The mechanism of action of nucleoplasty has been presumed to be related to its ability to reduce intradiscal pressure (241). In an in vitro study of three fresh human cadaver spines, Chen et al. documented 100% reduction in intradiscal pressure after creation of six channels, almost complete reduction after first two channels, with Coblation technology in healthy intervertebral discs of a 54-year-old cadaver body. In contrast, two older cadaver spines, 77 and 81 years of age, demonstrated a 3.7% and 5.8% drop in intradiscal pressure, respectively (241). A total of 19 discs were treated with each spine contributing both the control and treatment discs. A greater range in intradiscal pressure was observed in the healthy control discs compared with the degenerative control discs. In addition to the 17-gauge Coblation probe, a 25-gauge spinal needle was placed intradiscally to monitor pressure change. Each disc was pressurized by injecting saline through the 25-gauge needle. The authors did not explain how they accounted for potential intradiscal decompression after the saline loading because of dislodgement of the Coblation probe or 25-gauge spinal needle. Perhaps, the wide range of intradiscal pressures measured in the healthy cadaver discs was a manifestation of the recoil of the contained disc after fluid loading by forcing some fluid out via one or both of the trans-annular conduits, hence reducing intradiscal pressure. Inspection of the degenerative disc data reveals less variability in the control group intradiscal pressure which might be explained by a stiffer annular perimeter. If annular defects were present in the degenerative discs, intradiscal pressure would not increase upon saline injection until 45 psi was reached (226), a value the investigators fell short of by injecting up to 30 psi (241). Chen et al. suggest that the desiccated discs are less decompressible because of a higher fibrotic nature on the nuclear material (241). The healthy discs with more nuclear hydration may allow greater exposure of the proteoglycans to the bond-breaking effects of the Coblation plasma field. Although speculative, percutaneous disc decompression with Coblation technology may be more efficacious at treating younger herniated discs with less disc dessication (241).

In vitro study has been published documenting a biochemical affect of plasma decompression on intervertebral discs (234). Using a minipig model, O'Neill et al. measured the changes in inflammatory cytokines, proteoglycan content, and biochemical parameters in Coblation-treated intervertebral discs. The treated discs demonstrated significantly higher ($P < 0.01$) mean concentration of interleukin (IL)-8 levels, and significantly lower mean levels ($P = 0.05$) of IL-1 (235) six weeks after percutaneous discectomy. However, no differences were noted between groups for IL-6 ($P > 0.15$) and tumor necrosis factor (TNF)-α concentrations ($P > 0.25$). Histologically, the treated discs demonstrated a larger proportion of degenerative discs than controls. Biomechanically, the treated discs demonstrated a trend ($P > 0.4$) showing decreased stiffness. A stab incision model was employed as part of the control arm to establish degenerative changes within the intervertebral disc. A threefold increase in mean IL-8 concentrations and complete reduction in IL-1 concentration was noted between the treated group and the stab-induced degenerate model. Although the experiment lacked a true control group in which the intervertebral discs were interrogated by the 19-gauge Coblation probe without initiation of the plasma field, it appears that the changes in the biochemical milieu of the discs were attributable to the plasma field discectomy.

The ramifications of O'Neill's contributions are that an overall anabolic state is induced in the disc after treatment with Coblation technology (234). IL-1 is neurotoxic, induces nerve hypersensitivity (242,243), and its effects are prostaglandin-mediated (234) providing a mechanism for involvement in radicular pain (242,243) due to disc herniation (244). In contrast, IL-8 is neuroprotective (245) and relies on sympathomimetic amines to render its effects (246). Thus, it seems most probable that IL-1 is a key pathophysiologic factor in the generation of radicular pain consequent to an intervertebral disc herniation (234). The instigating factor triggering these alterations can only be suggested. Although IL-1 and TNF are potent stimulators of IL-8 expression, neither was elevated in the treated discs. Cellular stimulation may enhance IL-8 expression (247), and it is possible that the stress imposed on the disc during plasma discectomy accomplished this enhancement (234). A by-product of plasma discectomy is the free hydroxyl radical which has been demonstrated to influence IL-8 expression (248). Perhaps, the decreased stiffness of the treated discs resulted in less annular wall tension allowing cellular repair mechanisms to engage. However, conclusive evidence establishing a causal relationship between plasma discectomy and the alteration of these cytokines has not been established (234). Elevated TNF levels have been harvested from nuclear material in herniated lumbar intervertebral discs causing radicular pain (218). In O'Neill's animal model, TNF was not elevated and thus not affected by plasma discectomy which may reflect a minimal role of TNF in the animal annular stab model of disc degeneration rather than herniation (234).

Dekompressor Probe™

Animal and human investigations of reduction in intradiscal pressure have been pursued to validate Dekompressor's clinical success (123,189). In a live sheep model, intradiscal pressure was observed to decrease from 44 psi to 0 to 13 psi after 60 seconds of device operation (189). A 1.2-mm piezoelectric pressure transducer was placed through a 17-gauge introducer needle contralateral to the annular region penetrated by the Dekompressor Probe. The quickest rate of reduction occurred within the first 15 seconds of device application and a 36% reduction in intradiscal pressure occurred after 60 seconds of device operation. Intradiscal pressure was reduced by a total of 70% by gently advancing the probe minutely across the nucleus after the initial 60-second time period (189). A control disc was not included that would have allowed the evaluation of change in intradiscal pressure because of annular penetration with the introduction of the two 17-gauge cannulas across the annular fibers without activation of the helical auger tip. However, upon the introduction of movement across the nucleus, a larger reduction in intradiscal pressure was achieved suggesting that more nuclear material was thus removed leading to greater reduction in pressure.

Cadaveric experimentation involving the eviscerated torso of a female body demonstrated similar findings. Pressure monitoring was performed using a new monitoring system in which annular fenestration is not required (189). A piezoelectric pressure transducer was used to measure intrinsic disc pressure and reduction during the decompression (189). A pressure reduction from 15 psi to 7 psi was observed in the lumbar disc after activating the device for two minutes. A reduction from 17 psi to -0.2 psi was observed after 10 seconds of treatment in the thoracic disc. A half to 1 cc of nuclear material was removed from each disc. A total of six discs were investigated, three from both the lumbar and thoracic spines. However, data was only reported from one level in each region without the mention of mean and range data (189).

Alo et al. claimed a reduction in disc herniation size subsequent to the Dekompressor intervention (123). However, inspection of the six images published in his article challenges the authors' contention. Each postprocedure image is an image perspective that is not the same cut as the preprocedure image. For example, inspection of an axial view of a central focal protrusion, the postprocedure axial view is a cut cephalad to the disc space which precludes any definitive comment regarding morphologic change involving that disc after the decompressive procedure. Despite an apparent lack of reduction in disc herniation size, an alteration in annular stiffness, reduction in disc height, and internal disc decompression may explain the biomechanical effect of Dekompressor on contained disc herniations.

Biochemical influences of Dekompressor have not been methodologically studied. In Alo's 50 consecutive patients, the authors report that cellular qualitative and quantitative assessments were performed on the sampled nuclear tissue (123). However, no description of these findings was contained in the paper. Campbell and Slipman documented elevated concentrations of TNF-α obtained during treatment via Dekompressor of disc herniations causing lumbar radiculopathy (218). An experimental investigation involving an animal model has not yet been presented to verify any influence of percutaneous disc decompression with Dekompressor on the expression of inflammatory cytokines in disc herniation.

CLINICAL APPLICATION OF NONENDOSCOPIC PERCUTANEOUS DISC DECOMPRESSION

In the hierarchy of research methodology, randomized, controlled trials are universally accepted as providing evidence of the highest grade. In contrast, observational studies have less validity and are predisposed to overestimating treatment effects (249). The Agency for Health Care and Policy Research (AHCPR) has utilized a rating schema composed of five levels of evidence to evaluate the strength of published articles in determining management guidelines. The five levels are as follows: Level I (conclusive): research-based evidence with multiple relevant and high-quality scientific studies; Level II (strong): research-based evidence from at least one properly designed randomized, controlled trial of appropriate size (≥ 60 patients in each arm), and high-quality or multiple adequate scientific studies; Level III (moderate): evidence from well-designed trials without randomization, single group prepost cohort, time series, or matched case-controlled studies; Level IV (limited): evidence from well-designed nonexperimental studies from more than one center or research group; and Level V (intermediate): opinions of respected authorities, based on clinical evidence, descriptive studies, or reports of expert committees.

Level I evidence exists proving both short- and long-term efficacy of chemonucleolysis in treating lumbosacral radiculopathy owing to a contained disc herniation (81–84). Levels II and III evidences support chemonucleolysis as similarly effective to open surgical discectomy (85,168). Level III evidence has been collected demonstrating that chemonucleolysis is safe with a lower incidence of major complications compared with open surgery (190,191,196). Despite compelling evidence, chemonucleolysis has been abandoned as a percutaneous disc decompression treatment modality because injection of the proteolytic enzyme is less controlled and target-specific and has led to severe and persistent lumbar pain. Major complications such as anaphylaxis can be minimized with pretreatment and testing, and misplacement of the probe and injection of chymopapain can be improved with advancement in operator skill and experience. An interesting and perhaps promising intervention is the combination of chemonucleolysis and mechanical decompression. Endoscopic decompression after pretreatment with low-dose chymopapain has yielded impressive results in large trials (250,251). However, data has not been presented regarding any reduction in the incidence of axial pain. Conceptually, this combined intervention is appealing as it allows a more controlled desiccation and cicatrial process, by injection of a lower chymopapain dose, followed by a quick attrition of these effects by removal of a portion of the proteolyzed nucleus and the proteolytic enzyme. Whether these same results can be achieved by nonendoscopic decompressive subsequent to chemonucleolysis needs further examination.

By virtue of limited, uncontrolled clinical trials, mechanical decompression by Dekompressor and Coblation technologies are suggested to be effective by evidences from Levels III and IV (117–124). Mechanical decompression with Dekompressor may be better supported currently by clinical work that has investigated its utility in well-defined patient population suffering from lumbosacral radiculopathy due to defined disc herniation confirmed unresponsive to selective spinal injections. However, conclusive evidence is lacking precluding a definitive conclusion regarding Dekompressor's efficacy compared with placebo or open surgery. The utility of Coblation decompression in the cervical spine may be better supported than in the lumbar region (121,122) as trials have been pursued investigating the efficacy of Coblation in treating defined cervical radiculopathy. In contrast, less well-defined studies have been engineered in the lumbar spine (117,118). Further investigation via controlled trials are warranted to better define the role of these technologies in percutaneously decompressing disc hernia because their safety has been well documented (120–123,198).

Percutaneous laser disc decompression and automated percutaneous discectomy have been more widely studied owing to their maturity but lack conclusive evidence as no controlled trials have been published or presented. Although large prospective, observational studies have demonstrated successful results (94), APLD was less successful at treating radiculopathy than chemonucleolysis in a well-designed study (99). In a smaller study, open surgery achieved better results than APLD (100). Hence, evidences from Levels II and III exist against APLD compared with chemonucleolysis or open surgical discectomy. Furthermore, observational studies utilizing valid outcome tools have found disparate results (176,177). Altogether, Level III evidence supports APLD but stronger evidence suggests that APLD is less effective than chemonucleolysis. Cervical automated percuatneous decompression data is sparse (97) which precludes a definitive statement regarding the efficacy of this technology in the cervical spine.

Prospective, observational investigations of PLDD have demonstrated variable success rates. Most studies have utilized loosely defined criteria of successful outcome (103–108), and studies using structured outcome tools have a short follow-up interval (106). Therefore, evidences from Levels III and IV have been generated to support PLDD. Cervical laser disc decompression has been employed to treat both cervical radicular and axial symptomatology (109), with loosely defined outcome measures (110,111). Hence, again only Levels III and IV evidences exist supporting cervical laser decompression.

A confounding variable in a cohort of these studies (99) has been treatment of disc reherniation at a previously surgerized level. In this scenario, the intervertebral disc is more degenerated than a comparable herniation in a virgin spine. Hence, a more fortuitous mechanical debridement may be necessary to achieve clinical success. Automated percutaneous lumbar discectomy has been most thoroughly investigated in this patient population with a success rate approaching 80% (97). Decompressive efforts with Coblation^{TM}, laser, and chymopapain may not be able to effect a more degenerate herniated intervertebral disc. The nuclear substrate in this scenario is more fibrocartilaginous and may be more resilient to thermal, enzymatic, and nonthermal treatment. Manual decompression with the Dekompressor warrants further investigation based on this concept. Currently, APLD appears best suited to alleviate persistent radicular symptoms owing to a reherniation after previous open surgical discectomy.

Treatment of discogenic axial pain may be better achieved by the modality that alters cytokine production. Disruption of predisposition to further desiccation and greater annular stress might seem counterintuitive in treating discogenic pain. Nucleoplasty with Coblation technology is the only modality that has in vivo experimental evidence documenting a presumeably healthy change in degenerative discs. However, this is evidence obtained from an animal model requiring extrapolation to humans. Slipman et al. observed a significant difference at six months in patients treated for axial lumbar pain owing to a central focal protrusion (252). However, this difference waned at 12 months after treatment (Slipman, personal communication, 2004). Yet, an improvement sustained at six months may allow certain patients to engage in core stabilization to decrease injurious shear forces and torsional strain across the injured intervertebral segment.

Nonendoscopic percutaneous disc decompression (NEPDD) with chymopapain is effective in treating lumbosacral radiculopathy (80–83). Its safety has been contested but new concepts may provide a mechanism by which these rare complications are further reduced. Nonendoscopic percutaneous disc decompression with other modalities has achieved successful outcomes in 52% to 85% of inspected cases. Despite methodological flaws inherent in some of these audits, NEPDD represents a viable, minimally invasive intervention primarily indicated for treatment of radicular signs and symptoms. Evolution of decompressive technologies reflects entrepreneurial efforts. Persistence and maturation of a technique is a testament to the evidence proving its efficacy and safety.

CONCLUSION

The treatment of radicular signs and symptoms by percutaneous disc decompression has a loosely defined role in the discogenic radiculopathy therapeutic algorithm. The standard treatment for persistent symptoms despite conservative care has been open surgical decompression. However, surgical intervention is not without complications. The complication rate associated with nonendoscopic percutaneous decompressive techniques is much less than that associated with its surgical counterpart. Historically, however, percutaneous techniques have come to be viewed as less effective than the traditional open approach. Yet, if one or two out of three patients can be effectively treated percutaneously and avoid open surgery, certain known complications of open surgery can be avoided. No prospective evidence has been produced demonstrating an accelerated risk of recurrent disc herniation after percutaneous decompression. Furthermore, failed percutaneous treatment does not jeopardize postsurgical outcomes, nor does it stimulate epidural or perineural fibrotic changes.

The typical chronology of four to six weeks of physical therapy, nonsteroidal anti-inflammatory medications, and therapeutic selective nerve root blocks may be beneficial for some individuals but others may not tolerate a protracted treatment course. Perhaps a minimally invasive percutaneous procedure combined with the nerve root block may best benefit the patient by a more rapid recovery and overall diminished cost. Further comparison investigations comparing physical therapy, selective nerve root block, anti-inflammatory medications to these interventions with percutaneous disc decompression are warranted. Numerous studies have evaluated the mechanical decompressive characteristics of certain percutaneous techniques. Although NEPDD can successfully reduce intradiscal pressure, its success may primarily be explained by biochemical alterations within the disc. Further studies need to be engineered to analyze alteration in cytokine expression subsequent to disc decompression, and to correlate these expressions with change in the signs and symptoms of nerve root dysfunction.

REFERENCES

1. Lipetz JS. Pathophysiology of inflammatory, degenerative, and compressive radiculopathies. Phys Med Rehabil Clin N Am 2002; 13:439–449.
2. Carey TS, Garrett J, Jackman A, et al. The outcomes and costs of care for acute low back pain among patients seen by primary care practitioners, chiropractors, and orthopedic surgeons. The North Carolina back pain project. N Engl J Med 1995; 333:913–917.
3. Schwarzer AC, Aprill CN, Derby R, et al. The prevalence and clinical features of internal disc disruption in patients with chronic low back pain. Spine 1995; 20:1878–1883.
4. Kuslich SD, Ulstrom CL, Michael CL. The tissue origin of low back pain and sciatica: a report of pain response to tissue stimulation during operations on the lumbar spine using local anesthesia. Ortho Clin N Am 1991; 22(2):181–187.

5. Stanley D, McLoren MI, Evinton HA, et al. A prospective study of nerve root infiltration in the diagnosis of sciatica. A comparison with radiculopathy, computed tomography and operative findings. Spine 1990; 15:540–543.

6. Mixter WJ, Barr JS. Rupture of the intervertebral disc with involvement of the spinal canal. NEJM 1934; 211(5):210–215.

7. Bogduk N. Low back pain. In: Bogduk N, ed. Clinical Anatomy of the Lumbar Spine and Sacrum. 3rd ed. London: Elsevier Science Limited, 2003:187–213.

8. Kimura J. Radiculopathies and plexopathies. In: Kimura J, ed. Electrodiagnosis in Diseases of Nerve and Muscle: Principles and Practice. New York: Oxford, 2001.

9. Wright A, Mayer T, Gatchel RJ. Outcomes of disabling cervical spine disorders in compensation injuries: a prospective comparison to tertiary rehabilitation response for chronic lumbar spinal disorders. Spine 1999; 24(2):178–183.

10. Adson AW. Diagnosis and treatment of lesions of tumors of the spinal cord. Northwest Med 1925; 24:309–317.

11. Stookey B. Compression of the spinal cord due to ventral extradural cervical chondromas: diagnosis and surgical treatment. Arch Neurol Psychiatry 1928; 20:276–291.

12. Hanflig SS. Pain in the shoulder girdle, arm, and precordium due to cervical arthritis. JAMA 1936; 106:523–527.

13. Semmes RE, Murphey MF. The syndrome of unilateral rupture of the sixth cervical intervertebral disc with compression of the seventh cervical nerve root. A report of four cases with symptoms simulating coronary disease. JAMA 1943; 121:1209–1214.

14. Spurling RG, Scoville WB. Lateral rupture of the cervical intervertebral discs. A common cause of shoulder and arm pain. Surg Gynecol Obstet 1944; 78:350–358.

15. Michelsen JJ, Mixter WJ. Pain and disability of shoulder and arm due to herniaiton of the nucleus pulposus of cervical intervertebral discs. N Engl J Med 1944; 8:279–287.

16. Frykholm R. Deformities of dural pouches and strictures of dural sheaths in the cervical region producing nerve-root compression. A contribution to the etiology and operative treatment of brachial neuralgia. J Neurosurg 1947; 4:403–413.

17. Eaton LM. Neurologic causes of pain in the upper extremities with particular reference to syndromes of protruded intervertebral disk in the cervical region and mechanical compression of the brachial plexus. Surg Clin North Am 1946; 26:810–833.

18. Brain WR, Knight GC, Bull JWD. Discussion on rupture of the intervertebral disc in the cervical region. In: Proceedings of the Royal Society of Medicine, Section of Neurology 1948; 41:509–516.

19. Hunt WE, Miller CA. Management of cervical radiculopathy. Clin Neurosurg 1986; 33(29):485–502.

20. Yu YL, Woo E, Huang CY. Cervical spondylitic myelopathy and radiculopathy. Acta Neurol Scand 1987; 75:367–373.

21. Hitselberger WE, Witten RM. Abnormal myelograms in asymptomatic patients. J Neurosurg 1968; 28:204–206.

22. Saal JA, Saal JS. The nonoperative treatment of herniated nucleus pulposus with radiculopathy: an outcome study. Spine 1989; 14:431–437.

23. Wiesel SW, Tsourmas N, Feffer HL, et al. A study of computer-assisted tomography: I the incidence of postitive CAT scans in an asymptomatic group of patients. Spine 1984; 9(6):549–551.

24. Boden SD, Davis DO, Dina TS, et al. Abnormal magnetic-resonance scans of the lumbar spine in asymptomatic subjects: a prospective investigation. J Bone Joint Surg 1990; 72-A(3):403–408.

25. Maigne JY, Rime B, Delinge B. Computed tomographic follow-up study of forty-eight cases of nonoperatively treated lumbar intervertebral disc herniation. Spine 1992; 17:1071–1074.

26. Delauche-Cavallier MC, Budet C, Laredo JD, et al. Lumbar disc herniation: computed tomography scan changes after conservative treatment of nerve root compression. Spine 1992; 17:927–933.

27. Mixter WJ, Ayer JB. Herniation or rupture of the intervertebral disc into the spinal canal. N Engl J Med 1935; 213:385–395.

28. Saal JS, Franson RC, Dobrow R, Saal JA, White AH, Goldwaite N. High levels of inflammatory phospholipase A2 activity in lumbar disc herniations. Spine 1990; 15(7):674–678.

29. Lindahl O, Rexed B. Histologic changes in spinal nerve roots of operated cases of sciatica. Acta Orthop Scand 1951; 20:215–225.

30. Jensen MC, Brant-Zawadzki MN, Obuchowski N, et al. Magnetic resonance imaging of the lumbar spine in people without back pain. N Engl J Med 1994; 331(2):69–73.

31. Thelander U, Fagerlund M, Friberg S, et al. Straight leg raising test versus radiologic size, shape, position of lumbar disc hernias. Spine 1992; 17:395–399.

32. Bobechko WP, Hirsch C. Auto-immune response to nucleus pulposus in the rabbit. J Bone Joint Surg 1965; 47-B(3):574–580.

33. McCarron RF, Wimpee MW, Hudkins PG, et al. The inflammatory effects of nucleus pulposus: a possible element in the pathogenesis of low back pain. Spine 1987; 12:760–764.

34. Saal JS, Franson R, Myers R, Saal JA. Human disc PLA2 induces neural injury: a histolomorphometric study. Presented at the International Society for the Study of the Lumbar Spine, Annual Meeting, May 20–24, 1992.

35. Chen C, Cavanaugh JM, Ozaktay C, et al. Effects of phospholipase A2 on lumbar nerve root structure and function. Spine 1997; 22:1057–1064.
36. Kang JD, Georgescu HI, Larkin L, et al. Herniated cervical intervertebral discs spontaneously produce matrix metalloproteinases, nitric oxide, interleukin-6, and PGE2. Spine 1995; 20:2373–2378.
37. Kang JD, Georgescu HI, McIntyre-Larkin L, et al. Herniated lumbar intervertebral discs spontaneously produce matrix metalloproteinases, nitric oxide, interleukin-6, and prostaglandin E2. Spine 1996; 21(3):271–277.
38. Kang JD, Stefanovic-Racic M, McIntyre L, et al. Toward a biochemical understanding of human intervertebral disc degeneration and herniation: contributions of nitric oxide, interleukins, prostaglandins, and matrix metalloproteinases. Spine 1997; 22:1065–1073.
39. Weiler C, Nerlich AG, Bachmeier BE, et al. Expression and distribution of tumor necrosis factor alpha in human intertervebral discs: a study in surgical specimen and autopsy controls. Spine 2004; 30(1):44–54.
40. Byrod G, Olmarker K, Konno S, Larsson K, Takahashi K, Rydevik B. A rapid transport route between the epidural space and the intraneural capillaries of the nerve roots. Spine 1995; 20:138–143.
41. Rydevik B, Brown MD, Lundborg G. Pathoanatomy and pathophysiology of nerve root compression. Spine 1984; 9:7–15.
42. Murphy RW. Nerve roots and spinal nerves in degenerative disk disease. Clin Orthop Rel Res 1977; 129:46–60.
43. Goddard MD, Reid JD. Movements induced by straight leg raising in the lumbosacral roots, nerves and plexus, and in the intrapelvic section of the sciatic nerve. J Neurol Neurosurg Psychiatry 1965; 28:12.
44. Howe JF, Loeser JD, Calvin WH. Mechanosensitivity of dorsal root ganglia and chronically injured axons: a physiological basis for the radicular pain of nerve root compression. Pain 1977; 3:25–41.
45. Bradley KE. Stress-strain phenomena in human spinal nerve roots. Brain 1961; 84:120.
46. Bora FW, Pleasure DE, Didizian NA. A study of nerve regeneration and neuroma formation after nerve suture by various techniques. J Hand Surg 1976; 1:138–143.
47. O'Donnell J, O'Donnell AL. Prostaglandin E2 content in herniated lumbar disc disease. Spine 1996; 21(14):1653–1655.
48. Radharkrishnan K, Litchy WJ, O'Fallon WM, et al. Epidemiology of cervical radiculopathy. A population-based study from Rochester, Minnesota, 1976–1990. Brain 1994; 117(Pt 2):325–335.
49. Slipman CW, Chow DW. Therapeutic spinal corticosteroid injections for the management of radiculopathies. Phys Med Rehabil Clin N Am 2002; 13:697–711.
50. Saal JA, Saal JS, Herzog RJ. The natural history of lumbar intervertebral disc extrusions treated nonoperatively. Spine 1990; 15:683–686.
51. Weber H. Lumbar disc herniation. A controlled, prospective study with ten years of observation. Spine 1983; 8:131–140.
52. Bush K, Cowan N, Katz DE. The natural history of sciatica with associated disc pathology: a prospective study with clinical and independent radiologic follow-up. Spine 1992; 17:1205–1212.
53. Saal J, Saal J, Yurth E. Nonoperative management of herniated cervical intervertebral disc with radiculopathy. Spine 1996; 21(16):1877–1883.
54. Heckmann JC, Lang CJ, Zobelein I, et al. Herniated cervical intervertebral discs with radiculopathy: an outcome study of conservatively or surgically treated patients. J Spinal Disord 1999; 12:396–401.
55. Bush K, Hillier S. Outcome of cervical radiculopathy treated with periradicular/epidural corticosteroid injections: a prospective study with independent clinical review. Eur Spine J 1996; 5:319–325.
56. Ito T, Takano Y, Yuasa N. Types of lumbar herniated disc and clinical course. Spine 2001; 26:548–551.
57. Teresi L, Lufkin RB, Reicher MA, et al. Asymptomatic degenerative disk disease and spondylosis of the cervical spine: MR imgaing. Radiology 1987; 164:83–88.
58. Boden SD, McCowin PR, Davis DO, et al. Abnormal magnetic-resonance scans of the cervical spine in asymptomatic subjects. A prospective investigation. J Bone Joint Surg [Am] 1990; 72-A(8):1178–1184.
59. Matsumoto M, Fujimura Y, et al. MRI of cervical intervertebral discs in asymptomatic subjects. J Bone Joint Surg [Br] 1998; 80-B(1):19–24.
60. Jensen MC, Brant-Zawadzki MN, Obuchowski N, et al. Magnetic resonance imaging of the lumbar spine in people without back pain. N Engl J Med 1994; 331(2):69–73.
61. Johnson EW, Fletcher FR. Lumbosacral radiculopathy: review of 100 consecutive cases. Arch Phys Med Rehabil 1981; 62(7):321–323.
62. Lutz GE, Vad VB, Wisneski RJ. Fluoroscopic transforaminal lumbar epidural steroids: an outcome study. Arch Phys Med Rehabil 1998; 79:1362–1366.
63. Weiner BK, Fraser RD. Foraminal injections for lateral lumbar disc herniation. J Bone Joint Surg 1997; 79-B:804–807.
64. Berger O, Dousset V, Delmer O, et al. Evaluation of CT-guided periganglionic foraminal steroid injections for treatment of radicular pain in patients with foraminal stenosis. J de Radiologie 1999; 80:917–925.

65. Vallee JN, Feydy A, Carlier RY, et al. Chronic cervical radiculopathy: lateral approach periradicular corticosteroid injection. Radiology 2001; 218:886–892.
66. Cyteval C, Thomas E, Decoux E, et al. Cervical radiculopathy: open study on percutaneous periradicular foraminal steroid infiltration performed under CT control in 30 patients. Am J Neuroradiol 2004; 25:441–445.
67. Slipman CW, Lipetz JS, Jackson HB, et al. Therapeutic selective nerve root block in the nonsurgical treatment of atraumatic cervical spondylitic radicular pain: a retrospective analysis with independent clinical review. Arch Phys Med Rehabil 2000; 81:741–746.
68. Vad VB, Bhat AL, Lutz GE, et al. Transforaminal epidural steroid injections in lumbosacral radiculopathy: a prospective randomized study. Spine 2002; 27(1):11–15.
69. Ebeling U, Reichenberg W, Reulen HJ. Results of microsurgical lumbar discectomy: review of 485 patients. Acta Neurochir 1986; 81:45–52.
70. Wilson DH, Kenning J. Microsurgical lumbar discectomy: preliminary report of 83 consecutive cases. Neurosurgery 1979; 4:137–140.
71. Ramirez LF, Thisted R. Complications and demographic characteristics of patients undergoing lumbar discectomy in community hospitals. Neurosurgery 1989; 25:226–231.
72. Stolke D, Soltman WP, Seifert V. Intraoperative and postoperative complications associated with lumbar spine surgery. Spine 1989; 14:56–58.
73. Pappas CTE, Harrington T, Sonntag VKH. Outcome analysis in 654 surgically treated lumbar disc herniations. Neurosurgery 1992; 30:862–866.
74. Morgan-Hough CVJ, Jones PW, Eisenstein SM. Primary and revision lumbar discectomy. A 16-year review from one centre. J Bone Joint Surg [Br] 2003; 85-B:871–874.
75. Herron L. Recurrent lumbar disc herniation: results of repeat laminectomy and discectomy. J Spinal Disord 1994; 7:161–166.
76. Keskimaki L, Seitsalo S, Osterman H, et al. Reoperations after lumbar disc surgery. Spine 2000; 25:1500–1508.
77. Carragee EJ, Kim DH. A prospective analysis of magnetic resonance imaging findings in patients with sciatica and lumbar disc herniation. Correlation of outcomes with disc fragment and canal morphology. Spine 1997; 22:1650–1660.
78. Carragee EJ, Han MY, Suen PW, et al. Clinical outcomes after lumbar discectomy for sciatica: the effects of fragment type and anular competence. J Bone Joint Surg [Am] 2003; 85:102–108.
79. Nygaard OP, Kloster R, Solberg T. Duration of leg pain as a predictor of outcome after surgery for lumbar disc herniation: a prospective cohort study with 1 year follow-up. J Neurosurg 2000; 92(2 suppl):131–134.
80. Javid MJ, Nordby EJ, Ford LT, et al. Safety and efficacy of chymopapain (chymodiactin) in herniated nucleus pulposus with sciatica. Results of a randomized, double-blind study. JAMA 1983; 249(18):2489–2494.
81. Dabezies K, Langford K, Morris J, et al. Safety and efficacy of chymopapain (discase) in the treatment of sciatica due to a herniated nucleus pulopsus. Results of a randomized, double-blind study. Spine 1988; 13(5):561–565.
82. Fraser RD. Chymopapain for the treatment of intervertebral disc herniation. The final report of a double blind study. Spine 1984; 9(8):815–817.
83. Gogan WJ, Fraser RD. Chymopapain. A 10 year, double blind study. Spine 1992; 17(4):388–394.
84. Simmons JW, Nordby EJ, Hadjipavlou AG. Chemonucleolysis: the state of the art. Eur Spine J 2001; 10:192–202.
85. Muralikuttan K, Hamilton A, Kernohan W, et al. A prospective randomized trial of chemonucleolysis and conventional disc surgery in single level lumbar disc herniation. Spine 1992; 17:381–387.
86. Tregonning GD, Transfeldt EE, McCulloch JA, et al. Chymopapain versus conventional surgery for lumbar disc herniation. 10 year results of treatment. J Bone Joint Surg [Br] 1991; 73:481–486.
87. Ramirez LF, Javid MJ. Cost effectiveness of chemonucleolysis versus laminectomy in the treatment of herniated nucleus pulposus. Spine 1985; 10(4):363–367.
88. Kim YS, Chin DK, Cho YE, et al. Predictors of successful outcome for lumbar chemonucleolysis: analysis of 3000 cases during the past 14 years. Neurosurgery 2002; 51(2):123–128.
89. McDermott DJ, Agre K, Brin M, et al. Chymodiactin in patients with herniated lumbar intervertebral discs. An open-label, multi-center study. Spine 1985; 10:242–249.
90. Onik G, Helms CA, Ginsburg L, et al. Percutaneous lumbar diskectomy using a new aspiration probe. AJR 1985; 144:1137–1140.
91. Hijikata S, Yamagishi M, Nakayama T, et al. Percutaneous discectomy: a new treatment method for lumbar disc herniation. J Toden Hosp 1975; 5:5–13.
92. Kambin P, Gellman H. Percutaneous lateral discectomy of the lumbar spine. Clin Orthop 1983; 174:127–132.
93. Maroon JC. Current concepts in minimally invasive discectomy. Neurosurgery 2002; 51(2):137–145.
94. Onik G, Mooney V, Maroon JC, et al. Automated percutaneous discectomy: a prospective multi-institutional study. Neurosurgery 1990; 26(2):228–233.

95. Davis GW, Onik G, Helms C. Automated percutaneous discectomy. Spine 1991; 16(3):359–363.
96. Fiume D, Parziale G, Rinaldi A, et al. Automated percutaneous discectomy in herniated lumbar discs treatment: experience after the first 200 cases. J Neurosurg Sci 1994; 38(4):235–237.
97. Bonaldi G. Automated percutaneous lumbar discectomy: technique, indications and clinical follow-up in over 1000 patients. Neuroradiology 2003; 45:735–743.
98. Ramberg N, Sahlstrand T. Early course and long-term follow-up after automated percutaneous lumbar discectomy. J Spinal Disord 2001; 14(6):511–516.
99. Revel M, Payan C, Vallee C, et al. Automated percutaneous lumbar discectomy versus chemonucleolysis in the treatment of sciatica. A randomized multicenter trial. Spine 1993; 18(1):1–7.
100. Chatterjee S, Foy P, Findlay GF. Report of a controlled clinical trial comparing automated percutaneous lumbar discectomy and microdiscectomy in the treatment of contained lumbar disc herniation. Spine 1995; 20(6):734–738.
101. Shapiro S. Long-term follow up of 57 patients undergoing automated percutaneous discectomy. J Neurosurg 1995; 83:31–33.
102. Quigley MR, Shih T, Elrifai A, et al. Percutaneous laser discectomy with the Ho:YAG laser. Laser Surg Med 1992; 12:621–624.
103. Choy DSJ, Ascher PW, Saddekni S, et al. Percutaneous laser disc decompression. A new therapeutic modality. Spine 1992; 17(8):949–956.
104. Choy DSJ. Percutaneous disc decompression (pldd): 352 cases with an 81/2 year follow up. J Clin Laser Med Surg 1995; 13(1):17–21.
105. Choy DSJ. Percutaneous laser disc decompression (pldd): twelve years' experience with 752 procedures in 518 patients. J Clin Laser Med Surg 1998; 16(6):325–331.
106. McMillan MR, Patterson PA, Parker W. Percutaneous laser disc decompression for the treatment of discogenic lumbar pain and sciatica: a preliminary report with 3-month follow-up in a general pain clinic population. Photomed Laser Surg 2004; 22(5):434–438.
107. Casper DG, Mullins LL, Hartman VL. Laser-assisted disc decompression: a clinical trial of the Holmium:YAG laser with side-firing fiber. J Clin Laser Med Surg 1995; 13(1):27–31.
108. Nerubay J, Caspi I, Levinkopf M. Percutaneous carbon dioxide laser nucleolysis with 2- to 5-year followup. Clin Orthop Rel Res 1997; 337:45–48.
109. Knight MTN, Goswami A, Patko JT. Cervical percutaneous laser disc decompression: preliminary results of an ongoing prospective outcome study. J Clin Laser Med Surg 2001; 19(1):3–8.
110. Choy DSJ, Fejos AS. Cervical disc herniations and percutaneous laser disc decompression: a case report. Photomed Laser Surg 2004; 22(5):423–425.
111. Siebert W. Percutaneous laser discectomy of cervical discs: preliminary clinical results. J Clin Laser Med Surg 1995; 13(3):205–207.
112. Harada J, Dohi M, Fukunda K, et al. CT-guided percutaneous laser disc decompression (PLDD) for cervical disk hernia. Radiation Med 2001; 19(5):263–266.
113. Choy DSJ. Percutaneous laser disc decompression: an update. Photomed Laser Surg 2004; 22(5): 393–406.
114. Hellinger J. Technical aspects of the percutaneous cervical and lumbar laser-disc-decompression and nucleotomy. Neurolog Res 1999; 21:99–102.
115. Quigley MR, Maroon JC, Shih T, et al. Laser discectomy. Comparison of systems. Spine 1994; 19(3):319–322.
116. Hellinger J, Linke R, Heller H. A biophysical explanation for Nd:YAG percutaneous laser disc decompression success. J Clin Laser Med Surg 2001; 19(5):235–238.
117. Sharps LS, Isaac Z. Percutaneous disc decompression using nucleoplasty. Pain Physician 2002; 5(2):121–126.
118. Singh V, Piryani C, Liao K. Evaluation of percutaneous disc decompression using Coblation in chronic back pain with or without leg pain. Pain Physician 2003; 6:273–280.
119. Alexandre A, Coro L, Azuelos A, et al. Percutaneous nucleoplasty for discoradicular conflict. Acta Neurochir 2005(suppl); 92:83–86.
120. Slipman CW, DePalma MJ, Bhargava A, et al. Outcomes and side effects following percutaneous cervical disc decompression using Coblation technology: a pilot study. International Society Interventional Spine 12th Annual Meeting, Maui HI, 2004:161.
121. Slipman CW, Tasca P, Frey ME, et al. One-year outcomes following percutaneous cervical disc decompression using Coblation technology: a pilot study. Proceedings of the NASS 20th Annual Meeting, Spine J 2005; 5:2S.
122. Nardi PV, Cabezas D, Cesaroni A. Percutaneous cervical nucleoplasty using Coblation technology. Clinical results in fifty consecutive cases. Acta Neurochir Suppl 2005; 92:73–78.
123. Alo KM, Wright RE, Sutcliffe J, et al. Percutaneous lumbar discectomy: clinical response in an initial cohort of fifty consecutive patients with chronic radicular pain. Pain Prac 2004; 4(1):19–29.
124. Amoretti N, Huchot F, Flory P, et al. Percutaneous nucleotomy: preliminary communication on a decompression probe (Dekompressor) in percutaneous discectomy. Ten case reports. J Clin Imag 2005; 29:98–101.

125. Gower WE, Pedrini V. Age related variation in protein polysaccharides from human nucleus pulposus, annulus fibrosus, and costal cartilage. J Bone Joint Surg 1969; 51A:1154–1162.
126. Inoue H, Takeda T. Three-dimensional observation of collagen framework of lumbar intervertebral discs. Acta Orthop Scandinav 1975; 46:949–956.
127. Naylor A. Intervertebral disc prolapse and degeneration. The biochemical and biophysical approach. Spine 1976; 1:108–114.
128. Urban J, Maroudas A. The chemistry of the intervertebral disc in relation to its physiological function. Clin Rheum Dis 1980; 6:51–76.
129. Roberts S, Menage J, Duance V, et al. Collagen types around the cells of the intervertebral disc and cartilage end plate: an immunolocalization study. Spine 1991; 16:1030–1038.
130. Buckwalter JA, Cooper RR, Maynard JA. Elastic fibers in human intervertebral discs. J Bone Joint Surg 1976; 58A:73–76.
131. Taylor JR. The development and adult structure of lumbar intervertebral discs. J Man Med 1990; 5:43–47.
132. Hickey DS, Hukins DW. Relation between the structure of the annulus fibrosus and the function and failure of the intervertebral disc. Spine 1980; 5:100–116.
133. Jackson MI, Barks JS. Structural changes in the intervertebral disc. Ann Rheum Dis 1973; 32:10–15.
134. Marchand F, Ahmed AM. Investigation of the laminate structure of lumbar disc annulus fibrosus. Spine 1990; 15:402–410.
135. Best BA, Guilak F, Setton LA, et al. Compressive mechanical properties of the human annulus fibrosus and their relationship to biochemical composition. Spine 1994; 19:212–221.
136. Markolf KL, Morris JM. The structural components of the intervertebral disc. J Bone Joint Surg 1974; 56A:675–687.
137. Shah JS, Hampson WG, Jayson MI. The distribution of surface strain in the cadaveric lumbar spine. J Bone Joint Surg 1978; 60B:246–251.
138. Hansson TH, Keller TS, Spengler DM. Mechanical behaviour of the human lumbar spine. II. Fatigue strength during dynamic compressive loading. J Orthop Res 1987; 5:479–487.
139. Brinkmann P, Frobin W, Hierholzer E, et al. Deformation of the vertebral end plate under axial loading of the spine. Spine 1983; 8:851–856.
140. Adams MA, McNally DS, Wagstaff J, et al. Abnormal stress concentrations in lumbar intervertebral discs following damage to the vertebral bodies: a cause of disc failure? Eur Spine J 1993; 1:214–221.
141. Brinkmann P, Grootenboear H. Changes of disc height, radial disc bulge, and intradiscal pressure from discectomy: an in vitro investigation on human lumbar discs. Spine 1991; 16:641–646.
142. Adams MA, Freeman BJC, Morrison HP, et al. Mechanical initiation of intervertebral disc degeneration. Spine 2000; 25:1625–1636.
143. Seroussi RE, Krag MH, Muller DL, et al. Internal deformations of intact and denucleated human lumbar discs subjected to compression, flexion, and extension loads. J Orthop Res 1989; 7:122–131.
144. Handa T, Ishihara H, Ohshima H, et al. Effects of hydrostatic pressure on matrix synthesis and matrix metalloproteinase production in the human lumbar intervertebral disc. Spine 1997; 22:1085–1091.
145. Maroudas A, Stockwell RA, Nachemson A, et al. Factors involved in the nutrition of the human lumbar intervertebral disc: cellularity and diffusion of glucose in vitro. J Anat 1975; 120:113–130.
146. Olmarker E, Blomquist J, Stromberg J, et al. Inflammatogenic properties of nucleus pulposus. Spine 1995; 20:665–669.
147. Gronblad M, Virri J, Ronkko S, et al. A controlled biochemical and immunohistochemical study of human synovial-type (group II) phospholipase A2 and inflammatory cells in macroscopically normal, degenerated, and herniated human intervertebral disc tissues. Spine 1996; 21:2531–2538.
148. Nachemson A, Lewin T, Maroudas A, et al. In vitro diffusion of dye through the endplates and annulus fibrosus of human lumbar intervertebral discs. Acta Orthop Scand 1970; 41:589–607.
149. Hamanishi C, Kawabata T, Yosii T, et al. Schmorl's nodes on MRI: their incidence and clinical relevance. Spine 1994; 19:450–453.
150. Battie MC, Haynor DR, Fisher LD, et al. Similarities in degenerative findings on magnetic resonance images of the lumbar spine of identical twins. J Bone Joint Surg [Am] 1995; 77:1662.
151. Battie MC, Videman T, Gibbons LE, et al. Determinants of lumbar disc degeneration: a study relating lifetime exposures and MRI findings in identical twins. Spine 1995; 20:2601–2612.
152. Ohshima H, Urban JP, Bergel DH. Effect of static load on matrix synthesis rates in the intervertebral disc measured in vitro by a new perfusion technique. J Orthop Res 1995; 13:22–29.
153. Adams MA, Dolan P. Which comes first: disc degeneration or mechanical failure? Proc Spine Society Australia, Cairns, November 1996.
154. Adams MA, McNally DS, Dolan P. Stress distributions inside intervertebral discs. The effects of age and degeneration. J Bone Joint Surg [Br] 1996; 78-B:965–972.
155. Choy DSJ. Familial incidence of intervertebral disc herniation: a hypothesis suggesting that laminectomy and discectomy may be counterproductive. J Clin Laser Med Surg 2000; 18:29–32.
156. Varlotta GP, Brown MD, Kelsey JL, et al. Familial predisposition for herniation of a lumbar disc in patients who are less than twenty-one years old. J Bone Joint Surg [Am] 1991; 73-A:124–128.

157. Kurihara A, Kataoka O. Lumbar disc herniation in children and adolescents. A review of 70 operated cases and their minimum 5-year follow up studies. Spine 1980; 5:443–451.
158. DeOrio JK, Bianco AJ. Lumbar disc excision in children and adolescents. J Bone Joint Surg 1982; 64:991–996.
159. Epstein JA, Epstein NE, Joseph M, et al. Lumbar intervertebral disk herniation in teenage children: recognition and management of associated anomalies. Spine 1984; 9:427–432.
160. McGill S. Normal and injury mechanics of the lumbar spine. In: McGill S, ed. Low Back Disorders. Evidence-Based Prevention and Rehabilitation. 1st ed. United States of America: Sheridan Books, 2002:87–136.
161. Pearcy MJ. Inferred strains in the intervertebral discs during physiological movements. J Man Med 1990; 5:68–71.
162. Farfan HF, Cossette JW, Robertson GH, et al. The effects of torsion on the lumbar intervertebral joints: the role of torsion in the production of disc degeneration. J Bone Joint Surg [Am] 1970; 52-A: 468–497.
163. Shiraz-Adl A. Strain in fibers of a lumbar disc. Analysis of the role of lifting in producing disc prolapse. Spine 1989; 14:96–103.
164. Tsantrizos A, Ito K, Aebi M, et al. Internal strains in healthy and degenerated lumbar intervertebral discs. Spine 2005; 30(19):2129–2137.
165. Jansen EF, Balls AK. Chymopapain: a new crystalline proteinase from papaya lates (letter). J Biol Chem 1941; 137:459–460.
166. Stern IJ, Smith L. Dissolution by chymopapain in vitro of tissue from normal or prolapsed intervertebral disc. Clin Orthop 1967; 50:269.
167. Smith L. Enzyme dissolution of the nucleus pulposis in humans. JAMA 1964; 187:137–140.
168. Nordby EJ, Javid MJ. Continuing experience with chemonucleolysis. Mt Sinai J Med 2000; 67(4): 311–313.
169. Bromley JW, Varma AO, Santoro AJ, et al. Double blind evaluation of collagenase injections for herniated lumbar discs. Spine 1984; 9:486–488.
170. Wittenberg RH, Oppel S, Rubenthaler FA, et al. Five year results from chemonucleolysis with chymopapain or collagenase. A prospective randomized study. Spine 2001; 26(17):1835–1841.
171. Schwetschenau PR, Ramirez A, Johnston J, et al. Double blind evaluation of intradiscal chymopapain for herniated lumbar discs. Early results. J Neurosurg 1976; 45:622–627.
172. Gomez-Castresana FB, Vazquez HC, Baltes HJL. Cervical chemonucleolysis. Orthopedics 1995; 18(3):237–242.
173. Gomez-Castresana FB. Chemonucleolysis for the herniated cervical disc. International Intradiscal Therapy Society, 18th Annual Meeting Final Program, 2005; 27.
174. Haines SJ, Watridge CB. The current status of percutaneous discectomy. Neurosurgery 1994; 4:129–139.
175. Maroon JC, Onik G. Percutaneous automated discectomy: a new method for lumbar disc removal. J Neurosurg 1987; 66:143–146.
176. Teng GJ, Jeffery RF, Guo JH, et al. Automated percutaneous lumbar discectomy: a prospective multi-institutional study. J Vasc Interv Radiol 1997; 8(3):457–463.
177. Grevitt MP, McLaren A, Shackleford I, et al. Automated percutaneous lumbar discectomy. An outcome study. J Bone Joint Surg [Br] 1995; 77-B(4):626–629.
178. Bonaldi G, Ospedali R, Largo B. Percutaneous discectomy for treatment of cervical herniated nucleus pulposis. American Society of Spinal Radiology, Miami, FL, 2004.
179. Choy DJ, Feilding W, Hughes J, et al. Percutenous laser nucleolysis of lumbar discs. Letter. N Eng J Med 1987; 317(12):771–772.
180. Mayer HM, Muller G, Schwetlick G. Lasers in percutaneous disc surgery. beneficial technology or gimmick? Acta Orthop Scand 1993; suppl 251:38–44.
181. Hall DJ, Littlefield PD, Birkmier-Peters DP, et al. Radiofrequency ablation versus electrocautery in tonsillectomy. Otolaryngol Head Neck Surg 2004; 130:300–305.
182. Dreyfuss P, Baker R, Leclaire R, et al. Radiofrequency facet joint denervation in the treatment of low back pain: a placebo-controlled clinical trial to assess efficacy. Spine 2002; 27(5):556–566.
183. Corrado D, Buja G, Basso C, et al. Clinical diagnosis and management strategies in arrhythmogenic right ventricular cardiomyopathy. J Electrocardiol 2000; 33(suppl):49–55.
184. Voloshin I, DeHaven KE, Steadman JR. Second-look arthroscopic observations after radiofrequency treatment of partial thickness articular cartilage defects in human knees: report of four cases. J Knee Surg 2005; 18(2):116–122.
185. Eggers PE, Thapliyal HV, Mathews LS. Coblation: a newly described method for soft tissue surgery. Res Outcomes Arthrosco Surg 1997; 2:1–4.
186. Stadler K, Woloszko J, Brown IG. Repetitive plasma discharges in saline solutions. Appl Phys Lett 2001; 79:4503–4505.
187. Woloszko J, Stalder K, Brown IG. Plasma characteristics of repetitively pulsed electrical discharges in saline solutions used for surgical procedures. IFEE Transac Plasma Sci 2002; 30(3):1376–1383.

188. Singh V. Percutaneous disc decompression using nucleoplasty. In: Annual Meeting of the Florida Pain Society, Miami, FL, June 2001.
189. Initial experience with the dekompressor 1.5 mm percutaneous lumbar discectomy probe. White paper, 6/2002.
190. Bouillet R. Treatment of sciatica. A comparative survey of complications of surgical treatment and nucleolysis with chymopapain. Clin Orthop 1990; 251:144–152.
191. Nordby EJ, Wright PH, Schofield SR. Safety of chemonucleolysis. Adverse effects reported in the United States, 1982–1991 [Review]. Clin Orthop 1993; 13:122–134.
192. Slivers HR. Microsurgical versus standard lumbar discectomy. Neurosurgery 1988; 22:837–841.
193. Davis RJ, North RB, Campbell JN, et al. Multiple cerebral hemorrhages following chymopapain chemonucleolysis. Case report. J Neurosurg 1984; 61:169–171.
194. Leivseth G, Salvesen R, Hemminghytt S, et al. Do human lumbar discs reconstitute after chemonucleolysis?: a 7-year follow up study. Spine 1999; 24(4):342–347.
195. Mall JC, Kaiser JC. Post-chymopapain (chemonucleolysis)—clinical and computed tomography correlation: preliminary results. Skeletal Radiol 1984; 12:270–275.
196. Brown MD. Update on chemonucleolysis. Spine 1996; 21(24S):62S–68S.
197. Onik G, Maroon JC, Jackson R. Cauda equina syndrome secondary to an improperly placed nucleotome probe. Neurosurgery 1992; 30:412–415.
198. Bhargava A, Slipman CW, Frey ME, et al. Early term side effects and complications after lumbar disk decompression using Coblation technology. Arch Phys Med Rehabil 2004; 85(9):E5.
199. Nau WH, Diederich CJ. Evaluation of temperature distributions in cadaveric lumbar spine during nucleoplasty. Phys Med Biol 2004; 49:1583–1594.
200. Lee MS, Cooper G, Lutz GE, et al. Histologic characterization of Coblation nucleoplasty performed on sheep intervertebral discs. Pain Physician 2003; 6:439–442.
201. Chen YC, Lee SH, Saenz Y, et al. Histologic findings of disc, end plate and neural elements after Coblation of nucleus pulosus: an experimental nucleoplasty study. Spine J 2003; 3:466–470.
202. Bradford DS, Oegema TR, Cooper KM, et al. Chymopapain, chemonucleolysis and nucleus pulposus regernation. A biochemical and biomechanical study. Spine 1984; 9:135–147.
203. Watts C. Mechanism of action of chymopapain in ruptured lumbar disc disease. Clin Neurosurg 1983; 30:642–653.
204. Kiester DP, Williams JM, Andersson GB, et al. The dose-related effect of intradiscal chymopapain on rabbit intervertebral discs. Spine 1994; 19:747–751.
205. Sawin PD, Traynelis VC, Rich G, et al. Chymopapain-induced reduction of proinflammatory phospholipase A2 activity and amelioration of neuropathy behavioral changes in an in vivo model of acute sciatica. J Neurosurg 1997; 86:998–1006.
206. Kato F, Mimatsu K, Kawakami N, et al. Serial changes observed by magnetic resonance imaging in the intervertebral disc after chemonucleolysis. A consideration of the mechanism of chemonucleolysis. Spine 1992; 17:934–939.
207. Szypryt EP, Gibson MJ, Mulholland RC, et al. The long-term effect of chemonucleolysis on the intervertebral disc as assessed by magnetic resonance imaging. Spine 1987; 12:707–711.
208. Castro WH, Halm H, Jerosch J, et al. Long-term changes in the magnetic resonance image after chemonucleolysis. Eur Spine J 1994; 3:222–224.
209. Gibson MJ, Buckley J, Mulholland RC, et al. The changes in the intervertebral disc after chemonucleolysis demonstrated by magnetic resonance imaging. J Bone Joint Surg [Br] 1986; 68:719–723.
210. Boumphrey FRS, Bell GR, Modic M, et al. Computed tomography scanning after chymopapain injection for herniated nucleus pulposus. A prospective study. Clin Orthop 1987; 219:120–123.
211. Gentry LR, Turski PA, Strother CM, et al. Chymopapain chemonucleolysis: CT changes after treatment. AJR 1985; 145:361–369.
212. Fraser RD, Sandhu A, Gogan WJ. Magnetic resonance imaging findings 10 years after treatment for lumbar disc herniation. Spine 1995; 20:710–714.
213. McCulloch JA, Macnab I. Sciatica and Chymopapain. Baltimore: Williams and Wilkins, 1983.
214. Krempen JF, Minnig DI, Smith BS. Experimental studies on the effect of chymopapain on nerve root compression caused by intervertebral disk material. Clin Orthop 1975; 106:336–349.
215. Suguro T, Oegema TR, Bradford DS. The effects of chymopapain on prolapsed human intervertebral disc. A clinical and correlative histochemical study. Clin Orthop Rel Res 1986; 213:223–231.
216. Riew KD, Yin Y, Gilula L, et al. The effect of nerve-root injections on the need for operative treatment of lumbar radicular pain. J Bone Joint Surg 2000; 82A:1589–1593.
217. MacMillan J, Schaffer JL, Kambin P. Routes and incidence of communication of lumbar discs with surrounding neural structures. Spine 1991; 16:161–171.
218. Campbell AG, Slipman CW, Mencken S, et al. Tumor necrosis factor-alpha levels in herniated intervertebral discs. Arch Phys Med Rehabil 2005; 86(9):E20.
219. Takahashi H, Surguro T, Okazima Y, et al. Inflammatory cytokines in the herniated discs of the lumbar spine. Spine 1996; 21(2):218–224.
220. Spencer DL, Miller JAA, Bertolini JE. The effect of intervertebral disc space narrowing on the contact force between the nerve root and a simulated disc protrusion. Spine 1984; 9:422–426.

221. Sahlstrand T, Lomtoft M. A prospective study of preoperative and postoperative sequential magnetic resonance imaging and early clinical outcome in automated percutaneous lumbar discectomy. J Spinal Disord 1999; 12(5):368–374.
222. Delamarter RB, Howard MW, Goldstein T, et al. Percutaneous lumbar discectomy. Preoperative and postoperative magnetic resonance imaging. J Bone Joint Surg 1995; 77-A(4):578–584.
223. Castro WHM, Brinckmann P. Changes of lumbar intervertebral disc under the influence of the nonautomized percutaneous discecotmy. A biomechanical study. Acta Orhop Scand 1993; 64(suppl 253):1.
224. Castro WHM, Rondhuis HJ. The influence of automated percutaneous lumbar discectomy (APLD) on the biomechanics of the lumbar intervertebral disc. An experimental study. Acta Orthop Belgica 1992; 58(4):400–405.
225. Shea M, Takeuchi TY, Wittenberg RH, et al. A comparison of the effects of automated percutaneous diskectomy and conventional diskectomy on intradiscal pressure, disk geometry, and stiffness. J Spinal Disord 1994; 7(4):317–325.
226. Lee SH, Derby R, Chen Y, et al. In vitro measurement of pressure in intervertebral discs and annulus fibrosus with and without annular tears during discography. Spine J 2004; 4:614–618.
227. Monteiro A, Lefevre R, Peiters G, et al. Lateral decompression of a pathological disc in the treatment of lumbar pain and sciatica. Clin Orthop 1989; 238:56–63.
228. Gunzburg R, Fraser RD, Moore R, et al. An experimental study comparing percutaneous discectomy with chemonucleolysis. Spine 1993; 18(2):218–226.
229. Pfeiffer M, Schafer T, Griss P, et al. Automated percutaneous lumbar discectomy with and without chymopapain pretreatment versus non-automated, discoscopy-monitored percutaneous lumbar discectomy. Arch Orthop Trauma 1990; 109:211–216.
230. Brinkmann P, Grootenboer H. Change of disc height, radial disc bulge, and intradiscal pressure from discectomy: an in vitro investigation on human lumbar discs. Spine 1991; 16:641–646.
231. Reuber M, Schultz A, Denis F, et al. Bulging of lumbar intervertebral discs. J Biomech Eng 1982; 104:187–192.
232. Falconer MA, McGeorge M, Begg AC. Observations on the cause and mechanism of symptom production in sciatica and low back pain. J Neurol, Neurosurg, Psychiatry 1948; 11:13–26.
233. Kobayashi S, Baba H, Uchida K, et al. Effect of mechanical compression on the lumbar nerve root: localization and changes of intraradicular inflammatory cytokines, nitric oxide, and cyclooxygenase. Spine 2005; 30(15):1699–1705.
234. O'Neill CW, Liu JJ, Leibenberg E, et al. Percutaneous plasma decompression alters cytokine expression in injured porcine intervertebral discs. Spine J 2004; 4:88–98.
235. Yonezywa T, Onumura T, Kosaka R, et al. The system and procedures of percutaneous intradiscal laser nucleotomy. Spine 1990; 15:1175–1187.
236. Turgut M, Aeikgoz B, Kihne K, et al. Effect of Nd:YAG laser on experimental disc degeneration Part I. Biochemical and radiographical analysis. Acta Neurochi 1996; 138:1348–1354.
237. Kutschera HP, Lack W, Buchelt M, et al. Comparative study of surface displacement in discs following chemonucleolysis and laser nucleotomy. Lasers Surg Med 1998; 22:275–280.
238. Kutschera HP, Buchelt M, Lack W, et al. Circumferential measurement of annulus deviation after laser nucleotomy. Lasers Surg Med 1997; 20:77–83.
239. Hellinger J, Linke R, Heller H. A biophysical explanation for Nd:YAG percutaneous laser disc decompression success. J Clin Laser Med Surg 2001; 19(5):235–238.
240. Hellinger J, Wuttge R, Hellinger S. Pre- and postoperative MR-myelography of nonendoscopic multisegmentale percutaneous Nd:YAG laser disc decompression and nucleotomy (PLDN). Eur Spine J 1999; 8:37–38.
241. Chen YC, Lee SH, Chen D. Intradiscal pressure study of percutaneous disc decompression with nucleoplasty in human cadavers. Spine 2003; 28(7):661–665.
242. Ma XC, Gottschall PE, Chen LT, et al. Role and mechanisms of interleukin-1 in the modulation of neurotoxicity. Neuroimmunomodulation 2002; 10(4):199–207.
243. Ozaktay AC, Cavanaugh JM, Asik I, et al. Dorsal root sensitivity to interleukin-1 beta, interleukin-6 and tumor necrosis factor in rats. Eur Spine J 2002; 11(5):467–475.
244. Bruno V, Copani A, Besong G, et al. Neuroprotective activity of chemokines against N-methyl-D-aspartate or beta-amyloid-induced toxicity in culture. Eur J Pharmacol 2000; 399(2–3):117–121.
245. Ahn SH, Cho YW, Ahn MW, et al. mRNA expression of cytokines and chemokines in herniated lumbar intervertebral discs. Spine 2002; 27(9):911–917.
246. Poole S, Cunha FQ, Ferreira SH. Hyperalgesia from subcutaneous cytokines. In: Watkins LR, Maier SF, eds. Cytokines and Pain. Basel: Birkhauser Verlag, 1998:59–88.
247. Hoffmann E, Dittrich-Breiholz O, Holtmann H, et al. Multiple control of interleukin-8 gene expression. J Leukoc Biol 2002; 72(5):847–855.
248. Villarete LH, Remick DG. Nitric oxide regulation of inteluekin-8 gene expression. Shock 1997; 7(1):29–35.
249. Concato J, Shah N, Horwitz RI. Randomized, controlled trials, observational studies, and the hierarchy of research designs. N Engl J Med 2000; 342:1887–1892.

250. Schuber M, Hoogland T. The endoscopic transforaminal nucleotomy in combination of a low-dose chemonucleolysis: results of a prospective study with 2-year follow up. International Intradiscal Therapy Society, 18th Annual Meeting Final Program 2005; 46.
251. Hoogland T. Literature review and alpha klinik experiences of combined chemonucleolysis with endoscopic discectomy in the cervical and lumbar spine. International Intradiscal Therapy Society, 18th Annual Meeting Final Program 2005; 28.
252. Slipman CW, Sharps L, Isaac Z, et al. Preliminary outcomes of percutaneous nucleoplasty. A comparison of patients with and without an associated central focal protrusion. Eur Spine J 2002; 11(4):416–417.

4 | Endoscopic Decompression for Lumbar Spondylolysis: Clinical and Biomechanical Observations

Koichi Sairyo
Department of Orthopedics, University of Tokushima, Tokushima, Japan

Vijay K. Goel and Ashok Biyani
Department of Bioengineering and Orthopedic Surgery, University of Toledo, Toledo, Ohio, U.S.A.

Nabil Ebraheim
Spine Research Center, University of Toledo and Medical University of Ohio, Toledo, Ohio, U.S.A.

Toshinori Sakai
Department of Orthopedics, University of Tokushima, Tokushima, Japan

Daisuke Togawa
Department of Anatomic Pathology and Orthopaedic Surgery and The Spine Institute
The Cleveland Clinic Foundation, Cleveland, Ohio, U.S.A.

INTRODUCTION

Lumbar spondylolysis is considered to be a stress fracture of the pars interarticularis (1–3), which occurs in approximately 6% of the entire population (4,5). This disorder is usually clinically benign (4); however, in certain cases, surgical treatment is required to reduce the symptoms. For surgical treatment of lumbar spondylolysis, various techniques reported in the literature can be grouped into three categories: direct repair of the lysis, lumbar intersegmental fusion, and decompression. Direct repair of spondylolysis has been widely used to treat young patients in which severe disc degeneration and instability are not apparently combined (1,6,7). When severe disc degeneration causing low back pain and/or instability are observed, lumbar intersegmental fusion has been performed (8,9). Gill et al. (10) were the first to describe nonfusion decompressive surgery in patients with radiculopathy as a result of lumbar spondylolysis. The short-term clinical results were reported to be good. However, some authors have reported that the Gill's laminectomy result in further vertebral slippage postoperatively (11–14); therefore, some surgeons have recommended decompression with simultaneous spinal fusion. If there is a minimally invasive decompression surgery that does not alter the lumbar biomechanics after surgery further additional spinal fusion may not be necessary. Based on this concept, we developed minimally invasive decompression of nerve root affected by lumbar spondylolysis using a spinal endoscope. The spinal endoscope for the posterior decompression surgery was first established by Foley and Smith (15) as a technique for discectomy, and currently, this technique has been widely applied to other spinal disorders (16–21).

Thus, in this Chapter, we have introduced our technique and have reported the clinical outcomes. Also, the biomechanical rationale for its effectiveness is described.

SURGICAL INDICATION

Lumbar spondylolysis is comprised of two pathological entities that lead to symptoms, such as low back pain and leg pain: (*i*) pseudoarthrosis of a fractured pars defect produces radiculopathy by compressing the nerve root; and (*ii*) discogenic problems causing instability and low back pain. The surgical strategy should be tailored to these pathological entities. To treat radiculopathy, decompression is required, whereas spinal fusion is necessary to treat discogenic pain and spinal instability. When both these entities are simultaneously present, both decompression and fusion are needed. Furthermore, the age of the patient must be considered because subluxation in young patients with spondylolysis is likely to progress (22–25).

Since Gill et al. (10) first described decompression surgery without fusion in 1955, the technique had been widely used. Osterman et al. (14) reported long-term follow-up data (mean 12 years) obtained in patients in whom the Gill operation was performed, and concluded that the main indication for this procedure was painful spondylolisthesis with nerve root-related symptoms in patients above 40 years of age. Furthermore, the authors emphasized that the operation was basically contraindicated in adolescents. Davis and Bailey (12) reviewed data in 39 patients who underwent the Gill operation and found that spinal fusion is needed in pediatric patients to prevent likely vertebral slippage.

Based on these clinical results, the surgery-related indications for our endoscopic technique were also: (*i*) radiculopathy without low back pain; (*ii*) absence of spinal instability on dynamic radiographs; and (*iii*) more than 40 years of age.

SURGICAL PROCEDURE

This technique is an application of the microendoscopic discectomy (MED) method established by Foley and Smith. Figures 1 and 2 provide a detailed schema of this procedure. A longitudinal skin incision of 16 mm in length was made 1 cm lateral to the affected side from the midline (Fig. 1A), after the spondylolytic level was confirmed under an image intensifier. A guide pin was then placed onto the caudal edge of the cranial adjacent lamina of the spondylolytic level. A tubular retractor was placed to ensure preservation of the surgical space (Fig. 1B, *black circle*). Endoscopically, laminotomy and removal of the ligamentum flavum were conducted (Fig. 2). The affected nerve root was identified after this step (Fig. 2A). Usually, the nerve root is compressed by the proximal stump at the ragged edge of the spondylolytic lesion, and by the fibrocartilaginous mass (10–12,26,27). Thus, to decompress the affected nerve root, these masses are removed (Fig. 2B). In most cases, the osseous ragged edge was seen to compress tightly the nerve root and it was very difficult to remove this bony spur using a rongeur alone. Usually, the osseous edge was thinned using a high-speed drill or a specially made chisel first so that the edge could be safely removed endoscopically. The osseous mass was then safely and completely removed using a Kerrison rongeur or a curved curette.

CLINICAL OUTCOME

Eleven patients who fulfilled these criteria underwent endoscopic decompressive surgery between January 2001 and July 2003. Their mean age was 61.7 (range 42–70 years). Ten patients had bilateral pars defects at L5. No subluxation was present in six patients; whereas Meyerding grade I slippage was demonstrated in four. In the remaining one patient, we observed a two-level bilateral pars defects at L4 and L5 but no subluxation. No patient suffered low back pain, but leg pain was present.

In all patients, a radiculogram of the affected nerve root was conducted before surgery to confirm the impingement of the nerve root by the osseous ragged edge (Fig. 3). The proximal

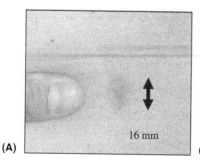
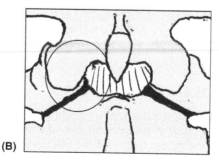

16 mm

(A)　　　　**(B)**

FIGURE 1 Schema of the endoscopic surgery, Part I. (**A**) Skin incision, (**B**) placement of a tubular retractor.

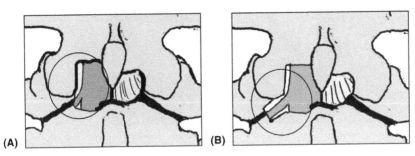

FIGURE 2 Schema of the endoscopic surgery, Part II. (**A**) Identification of compressed nerve root, (**B**) removal of the ragged edge and fibrocartilaginous mass.

stump of the osseous ragged edge of the spondylolytic lesion, which compressed the nerve root, was evaluated by computed tomographic (CT) scan before surgery. Postoperatively, the laminotomy area was assessed using plain anteroposterior radiographs, and resection was confirmed on CT scans. At the final follow-up examination, criteria established originally by Gill were used to evaluate clinical outcome.

Decompression surgery was successfully performed endoscopically for 15 pars defects in 11 patients. We were never required to convert the endoscopic procedure to a conventional open procedure. No complication, such as dural laceration and postsurgical epidural hematoma, was observed intra- or postoperatively. Operative time ranged from 1.5 to 4 hours, and the mean time per level was 2.3 hours. Leg pain disappeared or decreased in all patients, and they returned to their daily activities within three weeks. The follow-up period ranged from 3 to 30 months (mean 10.8 months). Based on Gill criteria, excellent, good and fair clinical outcomes were demonstrated respectively in four, six, and one patients at the final follow-up examination. No patients were in poor outcome. Radiologically, no further slippage appeared after the surgery.

CASE PRESENTATIONS

Figure 3 shows plain radiographs and selective radiculogram from a 60-year-old male patient. Plain radiographs indicated L5 spondylolysis without spondylolisthesis. Right L5 selective

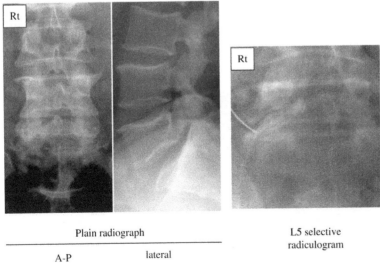

Plain radiograph

A-P   lateral

L5 selective radiculogram

FIGURE 3 Plain radiographs and selective radiculogram from 60-year-old male patient. Plain radiographs indicate L5 spondylolysis. Right L5 radiculogram indicates the nerve root impingement at the proximal edge of the spondylolysis. *Abbreviation*: A-P, anterior-posterior.

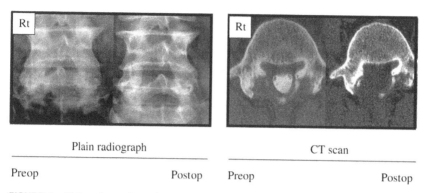

Plain radiograph	CT scan
Preop	Postop	Preop	Postop

FIGURE 4 Plain radiographs and computed tomography (CT) scans pre- and postoperatively. The laminotomized area is observed on the plain radiograph, and on CT scan ragged edge is removed after the surgery.

radiculogram indicated the nerve root impingement at the proximal edge of the spondylolysis. After injection of 1% xylocaine, the pain completely disappeared. Figure 4 shows plain radiographs and CT scans pre and postoperatively. The laminotomized area was observed on the plain radiograph, and on CT scan ragged edge was removed after the surgery. Figure 5 shows CT scans from a 70-year-old male patient, pre- and postoperatively. At the left side, the proximal stump of the osseous ragged edge of the spondylolytic lesion was removed after the surgery.

BIOMECHANICAL EVALUATION

The biomechanical behavior of spines can be studied by

1. quantification of three-dimensional (3D) load-displacement behavior using fresh cadaveric spines (22,28–30), and/or
2. finite element (FE) analyses (29,31–39).

To understand the biomechanical effects of the decompression surgery, we used the second method, FE analysis. Figure 6 demonstrates 3D lumbar FE intact lumbar spine model. The stress concentrations within the spine structures can be calculated using this model. Numerous clinical and biomechanical issues in a variety of spinal disorders have been investigated with this technique (29,31–39).

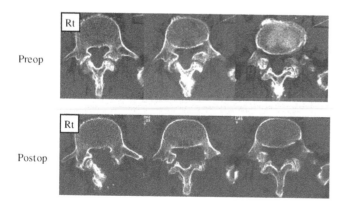

Preop

Postop

FIGURE 5 Computed tomography (CT) scans from 70-year-old male patient, pre- and postoperatively. At the left side, the proximal stump of the osseous ragged edge of the spondylolytic lesion was removed after the surgery.

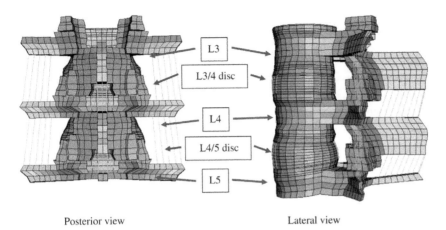

Posterior view   Lateral view

FIGURE 6   Intact nonlinear experimentally validated lumbar three-dimensional finite element model.

Finite Element Model

For the biomechanical study, an experimentally validated 3D nonlinear FE model of the intact ligamentous L3-5 segment was used. This model has been previously used to investigate a number of clinically relevant issues, including biomechanics of spondylolysis (34–39). The intact model was modified to simulate bilateral spondylolysis at L4. Cracks of 1.0 mm were created at both of the pars interarticularis to simulate bilateral spondylolysis (Fig. 7A).

Figure 7B demonstrates the FE model simulating our endoscopic decompression procedure on the left side. According to the procedure, the surgical method involves fenestration at the left L3/4 level, that is, L3 and L4 laminotomy, partial medial facetectomy at L3/4, and curettage of the pars defect. Figure 7C depicts the FE model of Gill's procedure. The loose lamina of L4 is removed. Simultaneously, all surrounding ligaments such as flavum, interspinous, and supraspinous are also removed.

Analysis

Von Mises stress distributions in various structures around L4/5 disc and changes in the intradiscal pressure (IDP) were analyzed in flexion, extension, lateral bending, and axial rotation in response to 400 N of axial compression and 10.6 Nm moment. The IDP and stresses were compared between the models simulating spondylolysis and two surgical procedures.

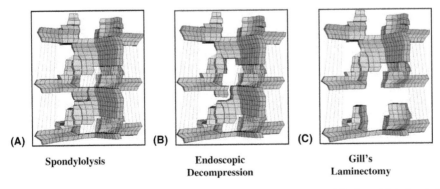

(A)   **(B)**   **(C)**

Spondylolysis   Endoscopic   Gill's
                      Decompression   Laminectomy

FIGURE 7   Lumbar finite element models at L3 to L5 segment. **(A)** Spondylolysis at L4, **(B)** endoscopic decompression, **(C)** Gill's laminectomy.

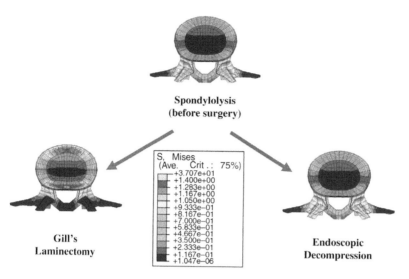

FIGURE 8 The stress distribution of the annulus fibrosus at L4/5.

Stress Distribution

The stresses at the various regions around L4/5 disc were calculated; that is, anterior L4 endplate, posterior L4 endplate, anterior annulus fibrosus, nucleus pulposus, posterior annulus fibrosus, anterior L5 endplate, and posterior L5 endplate. At all evaluated areas, the Von Mises stresses in the Gill's model were the highest among three models during flexion motion. The values in spondylolysis and endoscopic model were similar.

The stresses at the endplates and the intradiscal pressure during flexion motion showed differences among the models. Figure 8 depicts the stress distribution of the annulus fibrosus at L4/5. The anterior area showed an increase in stresses rather than the posterior. The highest stress value for each model was 0.65, 0.65, and 1.25 MPa for spondylolysis, endoscopic decompression, and Gill's laminectomy model, respectively. The stresses at the adjoining endplates showed about twofold increase in the Gill's procedure compared with the other two models (Fig. 9); whereas these stresses for the endoscopic and spondylolysis models were similar. In

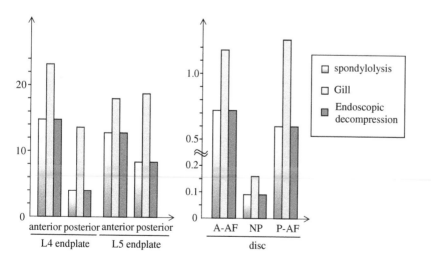

FIGURE 9 Maximum Von Mises stresses at various structures in three models during flexion motion. The stresses at endplate and disc in the Gill's procedure model showed about a twofold increase compared with the other two models. *Abbreviations*: A-AF, anterior annulus fibrosus; NP, nucleus pulposus; P-AF, posterior annulus fibrosus.

the other motions, that is, extension, lateral bending, or axial rotation, the results were similar among the models.

The analyses revealed approximately a twofold increase in the stresses at the anterior spinal column, such as endplates of L4 and L5, the annulus fibrosus, and intradiscal pressure across L4/5 during the flexion motion after Gill's laminectomy. This twofold increase may facilitate disc degeneration, causing forward slippage over time following surgery using Gill's procedure. On the other hand, the endoscopic procedure did not lead to any increase in stresses in various spinal elements and in intradiscal pressure. During the endoscopic surgery, supra- and interspinous ligaments are kept intact. Also, this procedure can be done with minimal invasiveness to the paravertebral muscles. Thus, endoscopic decompression of the spondylolysis is a minimally invasive method to relieve radicular pain without further destabilizing the spine.

CONCLUSION

We introduced our minimally invasive technique to decompress lumbar nerve root affected by spondylolysis. The biomechanical study using FE model supports the concept that endoscopic decompression of the spondylolysis is a minimally invasive method to relieve radicular pain without further destabilizing the spine.

REFERENCES

1. Sairyo K, Katoh S, Sakamaki T, et al. Three successive stress fractures at the same vertebral level in an adolescent baseball player. Am J Sports Med 2003; 31:606–610.
2. Wiltse LL. Spondylolisthesis in children. Clin Orthop 1961; 21:156–163.
3. Wiltse LL, Wildell Jr EH, Jackson DW. Fatigue fracture. The basic lesion in isthmic spondylolisthesis. J Bone Joint Surg [Am] 1975; 57:17–22.
4. Beutler WJ, Fredrickson BE, Murtland A, et al. The natural history of spondylolysis and spondylolisthesis: 45-year follow-up evaluation. Spine 2003; 28:1027–1035.
5. Fredrickson BE, Baker D, McHolick WJ, et al. The natural history of spondylolysis and spondylolisthesis. J Bone Joint Surg 1984; 66A:699–707.
6. Buck JE. Direct repair of the defect in spondylolisthesis. Preliminary report. J Bone Joint Surg 1970; 52B:432–437.
7. Nicol RO, Scott JH. Lytic spondylolysis. Repair by wiring. Spine 1986; 11:1027–1030.
8. DeWald RL, Faut MM, Taddonio RF, et al. Severe lumbosacral spondylolisthesis in adolescents and children. Reduction and staged circumferential fusion. J Bone Joint Surg 1981; 63A:619–626.
9. Seitsalo S. Operative and conservative treatment of moderate spondylolisthesis in young patients. J Bone Joint Surg 1990; 72B:908–913.
10. Gill GG, Manning JG, White HL. Surgical treatment of spondylolisthesis without spine fusion. J Bone Joint Surg 1955; 37A:493–520.
11. Amuso SJ, Neff RS, Coulson DB, et al. The surgical treatment of spondylolisthesis by posterior element resection. A long-term follow-up study. J Bone Joint Surg 1970; 52A:529–536.
12. Davis IS, Bailey RW. Spondylolisthesis. Indications for lumbar nerve root decompression and operative technique. Clin Orthop 1976; 117:129–134.
13. Marmor L, Bechtol CO. Spondylolisthesis. Complete slip following the Gill's procedure. A case report. J Bone Joint Surg 1961; 43A:1068–1069.
14. Osterman K, Lindholm TS, Laurent LE. Late results of removal of the loose posterior element (Gill's operation) in the treatment of lytic lumbar spondylolisthesis. Clin Orthop 1976; 117:121–128.
15. Foley KT, Smith MM. Microendoscopic discectomy. Tech Neurosurg 1997; 3:301–307.
16. Adamson TE. Microendoscopic posterior cervical laminoforaminotomy for unilateral radiculopathy: results of a new technique in 100 cases. J Neurosurg Spine 2001; 95:51–57.
17. Ahn Y, Lee SH, Park WM, et al. Posterolateral percutaneous endoscopic lumbar foraminotomy for L5-S1 foraminal or lateral exit zone stenosis. Technical note. J Neurosurg Spine 2003; 99:320–323.
18. Khoo LT, Fessler RG. Microendoscopic decompressive laminotomy for the treatment of lumbar stenosis. Neurosurgery 2002; 51:146–154.
19. Sairyo K, Katoh S, Sakamaki T, et al. A new endoscopic technique to decompress lumbar nerve roots affected by spondylolysis. Technical note. J Neurosurg 2003; 98(3 suppl): 290–293.
20. Saringer WF, Reddy B, Nobauer-Huhmann I, et al. Endoscopic anterior cervical foraminotomy for unilateral radiculopathy: anatomical morphometric analysis and preliminary clinical experience. J Neurosurg Spine 2003; 98:171–180.

21. Yuguchi T, Nishio M, Akiyama C, et al. Posterior microendoscopic surgical approach for the degenerative cervical spine. Neurol Res 2003; 25:17–21.
22. Sairyo K, Goel VK, Grobler LJ, et al. Pathomechanism of isthmic lumbar spondylolisthesis. A biomechanical study in immature calf spines. Spine 1998; 23:1442–1446.
23. Sairyo K, Katoh S, Ikata T, et al. Development of spondylolytic olisthesis in adolescents. Spine J 2001; 1:171–175.
24. Sairyo K, Katoh S, Sakamaki T, et al. Slippage occurs following epiphyseal separation in immature spine and its occurrence is unrelated to disc degeneration. Spine 2004; 29(5):524–527.
25. Sakamaki T, Sairyo K, Katoh S, et al. The pathogenesis of slippage and deformity in the pediatric lumbar spine: a radiographic and histologic study using a new rat in vivo model. Spine 2003; 28(7):645–650.
26. Edelson JG, Nathan H. Nerve root compression in spondylolysis and spondylolisthesis. J Bone Joint Surg 1986; 68B:596–599.
27. King AB, Baker DR, McHolick WJ. Another approach of the treatment of spondylolisthesis and spondyloschisis. Clin Orthop 1957; 10:257–268.
28. Kajiura K, Katoh S, Sairyo K, et al. Slippage mechanism of pediatric spondylolysis: biomechanical study using immature calf spines. Spine 2001; 26:2208–2212.
29. Konz RJ, Goel VK, Grobler LJ, et al. The pathomechanics of spondylolytic spondylolisthesis in immature primate lumbar spines—in vitro and finite element studies. Spine 2001; 26:E38–E49.
30. Kuroki H, Goel VK, Holekamp SA, et al. Contributions of flexion-extension cyclic loads to the lumbar spinal segment stability following different discectomy procedures. Spine 2004; 29:E39–E46.
31. Goel VK, Monroe BT, Gilbertson LG, et al. Interlaminar shear stresses and laminae separation in a disc: finite element analysis of the L3-4 motion segment subjected to axial compressive loads. Spine 1995; 20:689–698.
32. Goel V, Grauer J, Patel T, et al. Effects of charite artificial disc on the implanted and adjacent spinal segments mechanics using a hybrid testing protocol. Spine 2005; 30(24):2755–2764.
33. Kong WZ, Goel VK. Ability of the finite element models to predict response of the human spine to sinusoidal vertical vibration. Spine 2003; 28:1961–1967.
34. Sairyo K, Katoh S, Sasa T, et al. Athletes with unilateral spondylolysis are at risk of stress fracture at the contralateral pedicle and pars interarticularis: a clinical and biomechanical study. Am J Sports Med 2005; 33(4):583–590.
35. Sairyo K, Goel VK, Masuda A, et al. Biomechanical rationale of endoscopic decompression for lumbar spondylolysis as an effective minimally invasive procedure—a study based on the finite element analysis. Minimally Invasive Neurosurg 2005; 48:119–122.
36. Sairyo K, Katoh S, Komatsubara S, et al. Spondylolysis fracture angle in children and adolescents on CT indicates the facture producing force vector—a biomechanical rationale. Internet J Spine Surg 2005; 1(2), On-line.
37. Sairyo K, Goel VK, Masuda A, et al. Three dimensional finite element analysis of the pediatric lumbar spine: Part I: Pathomechanism of apophyseal bony ring fracture. Eur Spine J 2006; 15:923–929.
38. Sairyo K, Katoh S, Takata Y, et al. MRI signal changes of the pedicle as an indicator for early diagnosis of spondylolysis in children and adolescents. A clinical and biomechanical study. Spine 2006; 31: 206–211.
39. Sairyo K, Goel VK, Vadapalli S, et al. Biomechanical comparison of lumbar spine with or without spina bifida occulta. A finite element analysis. Spinal Cord 2005; Nov 23, On-line.

5 | Improving the Outcome of Discectomy with Specific Attention to the Annulus Fibrosus

Kenneth Yonemura
Department of Neurosurgery, University of Utah, Salt Lake City, Utah, U.S.A.

John Sherman
Orthopedic Consultants PA, Edina, Minnesota, U.S.A.

Walter Peppelman, Jr.
Pennsylvania Spine Institute, Harrisburg, Pennsylvania, U.S.A.

Steven Griffith
Anulex Technologies Inc., Minnetonka, Minnesota, U.S.A.

Reginald Davis
Greater Baltimore Neurosurgical Associates PA, Baltimore, Maryland, U.S.A.

Joseph C. Cauthen III
Neurosurgical and Spine Associates PA, Gainesville, Florida, U.S.A.

INTRODUCTION

The performance of a microdiscectomy procedure for the treatment of a lumbar disc herniation is a well-accepted surgical procedure with a proven track record. In spite of the perceived success rate for this procedure, there remains room to improve clinical outcomes, and ultimately reduce the risk of recurrent disc herniations, thereby reducing the rate of second operative procedures. Clinical research has shown excellent/good results—in some series to be less than 75%, and large population-based studies suggest that reoperation rates after discectomy can range from 9% to 20% within five years. Techniques for the careful repair of the annulus fibrosus after discectomy have included microsurgical suturing, sealants, and more recently, barrier implants. A minimally invasive technique for the repair of soft tissues, such as the annulus fibrosus, utilizing a barrier mesh implant of polyethylene terephthalate (PET) placed in proximity to the inner annular wall and nucleus pulposus has recently been developed. Biomechanics, animal experimentation (with histology), and early clinical experiences have shown this novel approach to be technically feasible. Successful annular repair, reconstruction, and reinforcement potentially can positively affect the ultimate surgical result by enabling a less aggressive discectomy, thus preserving spinal biomechanics; preventing future nucleus pulposus expulsion; or protecting the neural elements from inflammatory mediators that might be implicated in epidural fibrosis or pain.

LUMBAR SPINE DISC HERNIATIONS
Nomenclature, Classification, and Morphology

Herniation of the lumbar intervertebral disc is a common problem of the soft tissue of the spine, and can produce persistent neurologic symptoms that can be relieved by appropriate surgery in carefully selected patients (Fig. 1). Historically, the precise pathology of herniated discs has not always been appreciated. Walter Dandy (1) and Mixter and Barr (2) in the early 1900s are credited with distinguishing herniated intervertebral disc material from tumor tissue. Subsequent refinements in the diagnosis of this pathology and the surgical techniques have been ongoing ever since, particularly in the era of modern imaging techniques.

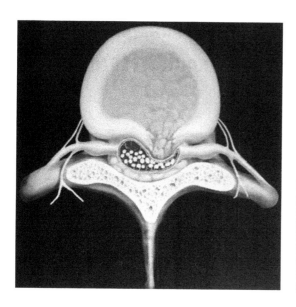

FIGURE 1 Discectomy is a common spine procedure to remove herniated disc material that occurs through fissures and defects in the annulus fibrosus. Mechanisms of symptom production include compression of the neural elements; sensitization of pain-producing nerve endings in the annulus and surrounding tissues; and the release of local chemical mediators of pain, inflammation, and autoimmune responses.

Differences in the surgical outcome of discectomy can be a function of the radiological characteristics of herniation. Morphology of disc herniations, based on medical imaging characteristics with redundant terminology and nomenclature, often creates confusion in the classification schema. It is therefore necessary to have common terminology to facilitate comparative analyses.

A Combined Task Force of the North American Spine Society (NASS), the American Society of Spine Radiology, and the American Society of Neuroradiology has recommended a classification schema that is based on clinical practice (3). This observational and diagnostic schema addresses contour, integrity, organization, and spatial relationships of the lumbar disc. A good understanding of this universally accepted classification scheme is important when considering the repair of the annulus, following a discectomy procedure.

Herniation is defined as a localized displacement of disc material beyond the limits of the intervertebral disc space, as defined by the vertebral body endplates and the outer edges of the vertebral ring apophyses. Disc material that is displaced can include nucleus pulposus, cartilage, fragmented apophyseal bone, annular tissue, or any combination thereof. This localized displacement can be "focal," as defined by significantly less than 25% of the disc circumference, or "broad-based," meaning between 25% and 50% of the circumference (Fig. 2). The presence of disc tissue circumferentially (i.e., 50–100%) beyond the edges of the ring apophyses can be referred to as "bulging," and should not be considered a form of herniation.

Herniated discs can also be described as either protrusions or extrusions (Fig. 3). Protrusion is defined as displaced tissue beyond the disc space that is measurably less than the distance between the outer margin of the disc space. Disc herniations that are classed as protrusions can also be described as contained, if the displaced tissue is covered by the outermost layer of the annulus. Extrusion, in contrast, is defined as tissue that is displaced in at least one plane (either sagittal or axial), and that the disc material is larger than the margins of the site of origin in the same imaging plane. A characteristic mushroom-shaped appearance is indicative of an extruded disc. An extrusion can also be identified on medical imaging as nuclear material that has penetrated the outer annulus fibers, and lies under the posterior longitudinal ligament (PLL). Extrusion can be further subclassified as a sequestration, if the herniated disc material has separated from the parent disc and penetrated through the PLL. This is often referred to as a free fragment when it migrates away from the site of extrusion.

Disc herniations can also be classified according to the location circumferentially around the disc. Herniations are often referred to as: (*i*) central; (*ii*) paracentral or within the lateral recesses; (*iii*) intraforaminal or subarticular; and (*iv*) extraforaminal or far lateral. Generally, most herniations occur at L4-L5 or L5-S1; however, the specific level has not been shown to

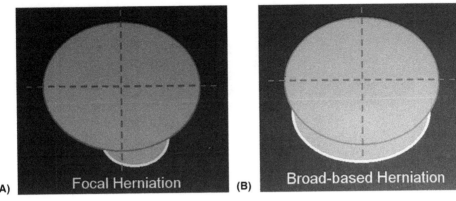

(A) Focal Herniation **(B)** Broad-based Herniation

FIGURE 2 Disc herniations can be classified according to their appearance on an axial image. **(A)** A "focal herniation" involved less than 25% of the disc circumference. **(B)** A "broad-based" herniation involved between 25% and 50% of the disc circumference A "bulging disc" can be described as an extension of disc tissue circumferentially beyond the disc edges (not depicted). *Source*: Adapted from Recommendations of the Combined Task Forces of the North American Spine Society, American Society of Spine Radiology, and American Society of Neuroradiology.

have any predictive value relative to clinical outcome. On the contrary, the circumferential location of the herniation does correlate with outcome with poorer results noted for central disc herniations (4). Carragee et al. (5) also showed other morphometric parameters that were strong predictors of postoperative outcomes. Larger anteroposterior dimension of the disc, a large ratio of disc herniation to spinal canal area, and narrower width of the herniation, were all strong predictors of a good outcome.

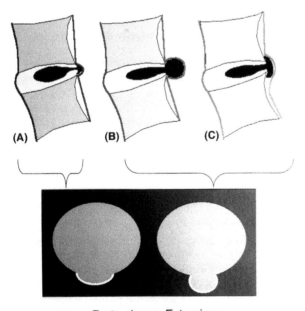

Protrusion vs Extrusion

FIGURE 3 Disc herniations can be classified as protrusions or extrusions on sagittal or axial images. In the sagittal view, disc protrusion **(A)** is described as tissue beyond the boundaries of the disc that is measurably less than the dimension between the disc margins. Extrusions **(B** and **C)** are defined as displaced tissue that is greater than the distance of the edges of the disc space; extrusions can be subclassified as sequestrations (not shown), if the tissue has detached from the parent disc. *Source*: Adapted from Recommendations of the Combined Task Forces of the North American Spine Society, American Society of Spine Radiology, and American Society of Neuroradiology.

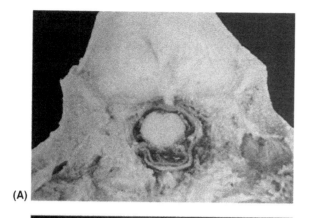

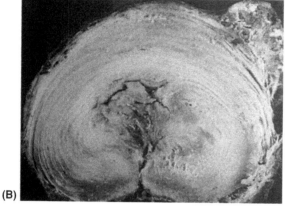

FIGURE 4 Axial views of thoracic (**A**) and lumbar (**B**) discs from cadavers showing midline annular fissures through the posterior annulus fibrosus. *Source*: From HN Herkowitz (ed.) The Lumbar Spine. Courtesy of Lippincott Williams & Williams.

(A)

(B)

The pathway for protruded and extruded herniated tissue is typically through a fissure in the annulus fibrosus (6–8). Annular fissures can be either radial or circumferential in their orientation (9). Radial fissures extend from the nucleus pulposus toward the outer annulus (Fig. 4). Circumferential fissures arise from a delamination of the concentric lamellar layer structure of the annulus fibrosus. These annulus disruption patterns have distinct differences in tissue integrity characteristics, and several authors have suggested differences in postoperative prognosis (4,10–12). It has been reported that contained disc herniations (often a result of circumferential fissures or radial fissures that have not completed reached the outer annulus) or more diffuse, broad-based disc herniation demonstrate poorer prognosis in contrast to more well-defined, focal herniations.

Pathophysiology and Pain Generation Theories

Radicular symptoms from herniated discs can arise from at least two distinct, but related, local mechanisms (13), a chemically mediated inflammatory process and/or pressure hypersensitization. Reference to prolapsed discs, slipped discs, and the like to describe the pathoanatomy of herniated nucleus pulposus (HNP) often creates the illusion that the primary pain stimulus is pressure on the nerve root by the displaced tissue (14). However, it has increasingly become clear that this mechanical pressure is only a secondary contributor to the patient's symptoms, and most likely, the sensitization of neural elements, such as the dorsal root ganglion, is the major contributor. As will be described later in this chapter, if mechanical pressure on the nerves was the only relevant mechanism to produce radicular pain, then theoretically, more of the 20% to 40% of asymptomatic disc herniations seen on medical imaging studies would be symptomatic; but, such is not necessarily the case (15–17). In a study of over 400 symptomatic (i.e., pain, weakness, and dysesthesias) patients, Beattie et al. (18) concluded that the presence of disc extrusion with or without severe nerve compression evidenced on magnetic resonance imaging (MRI) is strongly associated with distal leg pain. Nevertheless, in their study, nerve compression was present in only 37% of the study participants and 18% had severe nerve compression. Mild to moderate nerve compression, disc degeneration or bulging, and spinal stenosis were not significantly associated with specific pain patterns. This further reflects the conundrum facing the surgeon in identifying a neural compression mechanism as the source of pain, and the need to exclude other processes, such as peripheral nerve entrapment syndromes that may mimic a true radiculopathy.

Chemical mediators of pain, inflammation, and autoimmune components have been identified from the nucleus pulposus of the disc (19–21). It has been shown in animal studies that local epidural application of autologous nucleus pulposus can induce morphologic and functional changes in spinal nerve roots (22–24). Additionally, it has been demonstrated that the normally elastic fiber layer surrounding the dorsal root ganglion can undergo disintegration (25,26), thus setting the stage for increased permeability and the possible route for various substances that have been implicated in pain generation (27–29). Cytokines and substances that have been implicated as causative or related agents in the pathophysiology of symptomatic herniated discs include phospholipase A_2 (20,30), tumor necrosis factor-alpha (TNF-α) (25), nitric oxide (19,20,30–32), interleukins-1, -6, and -10 (19,32,33), thromboxane B_2 (34), leukotriene B_4 (34), and prostaglandin E_2 (32,35).

Matrix metalloproteinases (MMPs) have also been identified in herniated disc material, and have been implicated in disc degeneration. Doita et al. (36) demonstrated a relationship between the infiltration of macrophages from herniated disc tissue and the production of MMPs. Ironically, the production of MMPs by activated macrophages attempting to resorb the herniated material may, in fact, be a contributory factor in the patient's pain.

Intervertebral discs contain nerve fibers at the surface of the annulus fibrosus (37–40). It has generally been presumed that these nerve fibers in the disc might contribute to low back pain (39,41–43), but their relevance in radicular symptoms has not been substantiated. Although firing of these nerve endings may play a role, other pathoanatomic theories have been suggested.

IMAGING CHARACTERISTICS PRE- AND POSTDISCECTOMY

There are several imaging techniques available for the evaluation and diagnosis of sciatica. Plain radiographs are easily obtained, and may show narrowing of the disc space, osteophytic changes, or calcifications, but the relationship of the soft tissue components of the spine, the annulus fibrosus, and the nucleus pulposus, with the neural structures cannot be visualized. Computed tomography (CT) can delineate the outer confines of the disc, and therefore, can be helpful with regard to the deformation of the thecal sac by herniations or other processes causing stenosis. However, this requires radiation exposure and often needs a lumbar puncture for injection of a myelographic contrast agent. Discography, with or without CT imaging, can also add additional anatomic information, but this technique is used primarily to determine the site of axial back pain when there is little or no signs of radiculopathy. Magnetic resonance imaging enables detailed distinction between tissues, such as the annulus and the nucleus, making it the current standard of choice for evaluation of symptoms suspected to be due to a disc herniation (Fig. 5). However, even MRI should be viewed cautiously and introspectively, because there are many subtle and potential confounding findings that can affect sensitivity and specificity.

Imaging of Discs in Asymptomatic, Nonoperative Individuals

Research studies using CT or MRI examinations of asymptomatic individuals suggest a high incidence of presumably benign disc abnormalities (15–17,44–46). Weishaupt et al. (46) obtained MR images of 60 volunteers between the ages of 20 and 50. Disc bulging or disc protrusion was seen in approximately two-thirds of the individuals, and 15% of the disc spaces; disc extrusions were far less common (18% of subjects and less than 4% of disc levels). Jensen et al. (16) also examined 98 asymptomatic people with MRI. They noted that approximately one-third of the people had a protrusion, and annular defects were observed in 14%.

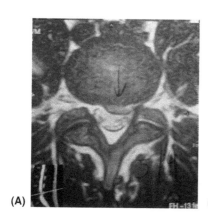
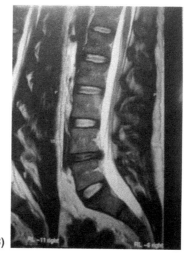

(A)   **(B)**

FIGURE 5   Magnetic resonance images showing typical disc herniation at L4-L5. (**A**) The left image is an axial section of a focal, paracentral herniation compressing the thecal sac. (**B**) The image on the right shows a sagittal view of the herniation.

Boden et al. (15) also reported on the presence of asymptomatic disc herniation evidenced on MRI, noting 20% of people under 60 and more than a third of people over 60 with such a finding. These, and other studies, suggest that radiographic findings, consistent with a significant disc herniation, are common, and the imaging findings need to be critically correlated to the patient's symptoms before surgical intervention is considered.

It might be hypothesized that the observation of radiologic disc abnormalities might be predictive of future symptomatic episodes of either low back pain or sciatica. However, a study by Boos et al. (47) examined 41 asymptomatic patients with MRI during a period of five years. In this study, there was no correlation in the severity of the imaging findings with any functional outcomes, such as symptom initiation or duration and time off work or number of consultations with medical providers. Therefore, an asymptomatic disc herniation is not only relatively common, but when it is seen, it does not necessarily progress over time into a pathologic, symptom-producing condition.

Preoperative Imaging of Symptomatic Individuals

Once the patient's symptoms can be correlated with a radiologic finding, understanding of the natural history of disc herniations is useful, both radiologically and clinically. Studies have shown that in certain patients, spontaneous regression of the herniation can occur with correlative waning of their radicular symptoms (48,49). It has also been suggested that sequestered disc tissue shows a higher propensity for resorption than protruded or extruded discs (50). If the patient can get temporary symptom relief, then conservative nonoperative treatment for at least two months is prudent before considering invasive surgery (51–54).

Postoperative Imaging after Successful (i.e., Asymptomatic) Discectomy

After a successful discectomy procedure that results in a patient satisfied with resolution or diminution of their symptoms, it is unlikely that additional medical imaging is warranted. The exception is a standard office X-ray to assess any potential disc height loss as a result of the nuclectomy. It is, therefore, a rather rare situation where imaging can be justified to examine the radiographic or technical results of discectomy. This information can be obtained in a research setting, and several authors have reported on the postdiscectomy anatomy of the spine and the disc. In the late eighties and early nineties, CT was the modality chosen for many of these investigations (55–57), with MRI becoming the standard in the mid-1990s (58–64).

Montaldi et al. (55) used unenhanced CT and plain radiography to examine 25 patients with good outcome after operation for lumbar disc herniation. These patients had imaging studies before surgery, five to seven days after, and six to seven weeks later. In 44% of the cases, the posterior border showed an image that suggested the persistence of disc herniation. In 84% of the cases, there were major changes in the spinal canal with complete occlusion of the extradural space on the operated side by a heterogeneous material, the attenuation value of which ranged between those of cerebrospinal fluid (CSF) and disc. The outline of the dural sac and of the nerve root was lost, and this aspect did not significantly change between the first and the sixth postoperative week. Heilbronner et al. (57) extended the follow-up period of this original study (55) to three years in 19 of the 25 original patients. Clinical examination, lateral plain X-rays, and CT scans without contrast enhancement of the operated disc were repeated. The results indicated a decrease or even a disappearance of the hyperdense extradural material, thought to represent fibrosis. An image, suggestive of persistent disc herniation, was still present in five of eight patients with this finding on early postoperative CT scans. Persistent intradiscal gas was seen in nearly half of the patients. They concluded that there was no correlation between CT appearance and residual complaints of the patients.

Cervelline et al. (56) also performed CT on asymptomatic postdiscectomy patients. They scanned 20 asymptomatic operated patients and 20 patients with recurrent sciatic nerve pain after disc surgery, who did not have bony stenosis, recurrent disc herniation, or other causes of failed back surgery syndrome. They found no important differences in the degree or type of fibrosis demonstrated by CT between symptomatic and asymptomatic patients, and there was no relationship to recurrent symptoms.

These authors concluded that these early major radiological modifications found in asymptomatic postoperative patients suggest that a positive CT in patients with suspected failed back surgery syndrome may have limited value; myelography, therefore, is preferred as the primary neuroradiological investigation.

Several authors (59–61,65,66) have used MRI, with or without enhancement, to examine anatomic changes that occur as a result of discectomy. Kotilainen et al. (67) showed that postoperative edema at the level of surgery and annular disruption may be important factors leading to increased soft tissue mass. In his study, this mass effect caused compression of the anterior dural sac mimicking preoperative disc herniation. At six months, the mass effect had disappeared in all patients, and the MRI findings in the operated space were read as a prolapsed disc in 15% and a protrusion in 39% of patients. Postoperative scarring was also observed. It is clear that the intervertebral disc may show MRI evidence of a persistent herniation during the early postoperative phase following a successful microdiscectomy procedure.

Van de Kelft et al. (66) and Van Goethem (61) reported a prospective study to establish the normal spectrum of early gadolinium-enhanced MRI findings in patients who had excellent symptom resolution after discectomy. Thirty-four patients had MR examinations six weeks and six months after surgery. Not unexpectedly, all patients showed soft-tissue enhancement along the surgical track. Intrathecal nerve root enhancement was observed in six patients at six weeks. There was only minimal (45%) or no (55%) mass effect on the dural sac associated with epidural scar formation six months after surgery. Nine patients (20%) had residual mass effect on the neural elements with an enhancement pattern, suggestive of a disc fragment.

Floris et al. (59,60) concurred with these findings in their MRI study of patients who underwent successful lumbar microdiscectomy. Early postoperative (within three days) MRI findings consisted of pseudohernia in 80%, annular rent in 80%, and other nonspecific findings. At two months, MRI demonstrated the persistence of pseudohernia in 50% of cases and annular rent in 15%. Because of this normal sequence of changes, MR studies in the early postoperative period are difficult to interpret even when enhanced with gadolinium.

It might be speculated that the healing processes that occur after surgery may alter these radiologic findings. Nakano et al. (68) evaluated the relation between morphologic changes of postoperative intervertebral discs and the clinical outcome after posterior lumbar discectomy. The size of the "bulging disc" was analyzed in randomly selected patients. They concluded that there were three patterns of reduction in the size of the bulge: early reduction (56% of cases), gradual reduction (26% of cases), and late reduction (19% of cases). Late reduction, they suggested, could obviously cause late recovery of subjective symptoms and neurologic disturbance.

Annertz et al. (64) examined patients with successful discectomies in a serial fashion with MRI, preoperatively, at five days, six weeks, and four months after surgery. Pronounced intraspinal changes were seen during follow-up with deformation of the dural sac, apparent in 95% of patients at five days and 60% after four months. Similarly, nerve root involvement was seen in 85% at six weeks and in 75% at four months.

To summarize, it should not be unexpected to see a persistent herniated disc, pseudohernia, dural sac compression, or nerve root involvement on MRI in the early postoperative period. Within one week of surgery, 45% to 95% may, indeed, show persistent disc herniation. After one or two months, the percentage of postsurgery cases that still demonstrate what might be called a herniation drops to 50% to 75%. But even one year after successful discectomy, there may be 25% of cases that radiographically demonstrate an otherwise asymptomatic nerve root displacement or disc herniation (62). Dina (65) concluded that imaging of the lumbar spine after disc herniation surgery is generally an unrewarding challenge. As a constellation of findings is inevitable, determining their significance is often impossible. The challenge is greatest during the first few months following surgery when the rules of scar enhancement, deformity, and mass effect do not apply to help differentiate abnormal from normal findings.

Postoperative Imaging of Discs in Symptomatic Discectomy Patients

In a certain percentage of discectomy patients, residual symptoms of leg pain or back pain require additional imaging. In light of the limitations of medical imaging described earlier (69), it is often difficult to accurately diagnose the anatomic cause of residual postdiscectomy symptoms. Complications that may induce persistent sciatica after discectomy can include not only recurrent/residual disc herniation, but also epidural scar formation, discitis, arachnoiditis, degenerative narrowing of the lateral recess, spinal instability, stress fracture of the remaining neural arch, or pseudomeningocele (70).

Computed tomography with intravenous contrast injection has been shown to be effective in showing the cause of pain recurrence after discectomy. Kotwica et al. (71) suggested that CT was 100% accurate as confirmed at reoperation. Other studies (72,73) have suggested that CT is effective in demonstrating a recurrent disc herniation in 40% to 50% of cases. Gadolinium-enhanced MRI remains the current technique of choice for investigating recurrent symptoms following discectomy (74). Postoperative MRI findings must be interpreted with great care, as the same features described in failed back surgery syndrome (FSBB) are also found at least to some extent in asymptomatic postoperative patients. Imaging findings alone do not constitute an indication for surgical reintervention, or for that matter, for any other therapy.

INFLUENCE OF SURGICAL DISCECTOMY TECHNIQUES AND APPROACH ON OUTCOME

Open lumbar discectomy is, by far, one of the most frequent surgical interventions performed by a spine surgery specialist. Many variations in operative technique and approaches have been proposed over the years, ranging from operating with loupes, to the use of the microscope, to the use of endoscopic visualization, or to percutaneous techniques. Each approach has its own unique challenges, and some have a more profound impact on patient outcome than others.

The historical origin of the surgical technique for lumbar discectomy can be traced to Mixter and Barr (2) when they published their preliminary results for partial discectomy and nerve decompression. They described a laminectomy approach and dural incision for access to the disc space, followed by dissection, curettage, and removal of ruptured fragments. Since then, several variations of the technique have evolved with the most obvious difference being that the dura is no longer intentionally incised. But, the volume of material removed during the surgical procedure has been debated over time. An extensive nuclectomy with near complete removal of the nucleus pulposus, in addition to the herniated tissue, results in many patients with unsuccessful clinical results secondary to persistent low back pain. Progressive degenerative changes are presumably the underlying mechanism of this less-than-optimal result. The advent of percutaneous approaches to the disc (75) caused many surgeons to advocate less extensive extirpation of disc material (76) in an attempt to preserve the inherent function of the disc, at the same time as removing only the offending herniated fragment.

Other modification to the surgical technique emerged when Yasargil reported his results of a discectomy series utilizing the operating microscope and microsurgical techniques (77). Microscopic visualization enables the adoption of an interlaminar approach with limited or no bony resection, except in the presence of osteophytes or where the lamina of involved levels are overlapping. In 1978, Williams (78) reported results from his microsurgical series involving a more defined set of modifications, termed microlumbar discectomy. His minimalist approach included: (*i*) preservation of all laminar and facet bone to prevent osteophyte formation and nerve root entrapment; (*ii*) use of blunt perforation and dilation of the annulus fibrosus rather than scalpel incision, presumably to prevent recurrent herniation; and (*iii*) limited removal of only nuclear elements that could be mobilized easily, to prevent subsequent back pain and sciatica, believed to result from compression of the evacuated disc space secondary to weight bearing activities. These three modifications have, over the years, been debated by others, who contend that adequate bone removal and annular incision are required for proper identification of compressive fragments, and subsequent subtotal (rather than minimal) removal of disc material is necessary to ultimately prevent recurrence (79,80).

Many surgeons now use a portal system in which serial dilators are used to create a percutaneous pathway through the paraspinal muscles to the interlaminar space. Through this portal system, arthroscopic or endoscopic visualization allows disc decompression and fragment removal. The goal of these portal techniques is to reduce approach-related morbidity, and ultimately the discectomy should be equivalent to a standard open procedure.

Regardless of the approach to the disc and the offending herniation, the procedure does not typically include any special attention to the annular defect or the annulotomy. The surgical maneuver involves gaining access to the disc herniation via a laminotomy, and removing the offending disc tissue to ensure adequate nerve decompression, but leaving an annular defect that can often be quite wide. Many authors have suggested that ignoring the pathway through the annulus fibrosus may be a contributing factor in lumbar disc reherniation (6,81–83). Pappas (6) speculated that recurrent herniations less than six months after discectomy occur through the original defect. Matsui et al. (74) also reported a case of lateral disc reherniation within two months after percutaneous discectomy through the annulotomy site. Williams (81) also recognized the possibility of reducing reherniation by suggesting blunt dissection of the annulus rather than incision. This technique is intended for removal of only the symptomatic disc fragment. In an analysis of existing microdiscectomy studies, Apostolides showed that recurrence disc herniation rates were invariably higher for those surgeons who completed only partial removal of disc fragments in contrast to more copious disc excision (84), thus speculating that dilation and spreading of annular fibers by blunt perforation gives only limited access for identification and removal of all disc fragments. Repair, reconstruction, or reinforcement of the annulus fibrosus are clearly areas requiring innovative solutions.

OUTCOMES OF DISCECTOMY

The beneficial result of lumbar discectomy surgery can be described by the patients' clinical outcomes, such as pain relief, or by surgical outcomes, such as the need for future operations. The presence of pain extending to the foot, leg pain on straight leg raise testing, and reflex asymmetry, when present are generally predictive of a good surgical outcome. On the contrary, the presence of a work-related injury or primary back pain can be negative factors in outcome prediction. Radicular pain remains the best predictor of a good outcome, whereas the lack of preoperative radicular pain is a predictor of poor results (85).

The reported clinical success of lumbar discectomy procedures in the literature varies significantly. Publications from single-center studies report success rates greater than 90%. However, more recently, as several controlled, multi-center studies have been performed, the long-term success rate appears to be below 90%, and the true rate may be between 70% and 80% (86).

Clinical Outcomes

Clinical outcomes, such as return to work and pain relief, are important measures for evaluating the success of a lumbar disc intervention, particularly from the perspective of the patient seeking evaluation and treatment. Patients with successful outcomes typically experience immediate pain relief, following a discectomy procedure, and are able to return to work in two to eight weeks. The most commonly reported outcome measure of the patient's pain is with a 10-point visual analog scale (VAS). Typical preoperative VAS scores range from 5 to 7, and immediate postoperative pain scores typically range from 1 to 2, suggesting successful relief of pain (86–89). Less certain, however, is how long this pain relief remains. Long-term studies have shown variable outcomes four to ten years after a discectomy. The Maine Lumbar Spine Study of 507 sciatic patients with disc herniations found that at five years, only 63% of surgical patients were satisfied with their current physical status and 30% still had symptoms of pain (90). Loupasis et al. (91) reported on the outcome of discectomy with 12 years of follow-up data. Results were satisfactory in only 64% of patients, and 28% still complained of significant back or leg pain; yet 94% of the patients were satisfied or very satisfied with their result. Similarly, an outcome study by Woertgen found that approximately 40% of patients experience unfavorable outcomes following surgery (92). Two large reviews have suggested that careful patient selection is critical to consistent success rates for discectomy between 65% and 90% (93,94).

Surgical Outcomes

Both the patient and the surgeon are keenly concerned about the surgical or technical outcome after a discectomy, particularly, the need to ultimately undergo a subsequent operation or other treatment. Radiographic results alone, such as subsequent chronic disc collapse or the extent of dural sac compression or neural impingement, are sometimes interesting to debate, but in most instances, medical imaging after a discectomy is relevant and necessary only if the postoperative patient continues to report persistent or worsening symptoms.

Reoperation can be defined as specifically as the need to remove additional fragment material at the same level as the previous herniation, or as broadly as an arthrodesis at another level. The most commonly published data after lumbar discectomy are technical outcomes defined by the need for additional surgical intervention. Reoperation rates range from as low as 5% to as high as 25%, depending on the design of the study and the length of follow-up. Large, population-based studies show that reoperation rates, irrespective of the reason and the secondary procedure performed, range from 15% to 25% at five to ten years postprocedure (90,95–97). Reasons for reoperation include recurrent reherniation at the same level (42%), recurrence and new herniation (20%), new herniations (23%), epidural fibrosis (5%), and instability (12%) (98).

Postdiscectomy outcome can be affected by proper patient selection, ensuring appropriate pathology and careful surgical technique for annulus incision or disc removal. Many attempts have been made to further improve symptom relief, surgical outcomes, and ultimately patient satisfaction.

REPAIR, RECONSTRUCTION, AND REINFORCEMENT OF THE ANNULUS
Type of Annular Incision and the Role of Annular Integrity

When considering a surgical technique or implant to repair the annulus fibrosus, the influence of the preoperative characteristics of the tissue defect or the integrity of the annulus and the resultant surgical annulotomy is important. A surgical incision through the annulus can alter the biomechanics of the involved disc. Additionally, aggressive nucleus removal can affect postdiscectomy biomechanics, leading to unanticipated effects. It therefore, seems intuitive that the smaller the annular defect that exists, either pathologically or after surgical removal

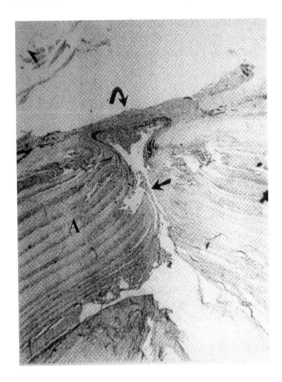

FIGURE 6 Histologic section (10×) of a goat disc four weeks after trocar incision of the annulus. Extravasation of nucleus pulposus (*straight arrow*), and fibrous capping of the exterior tissue surface (*curved arrow*) are seen, but no primary healing was demonstrated. *Source*: From Ref. 100.

of the herniated material, and less-aggressive nucleus removal could result in more positive postsurgery outcomes.

Several authors have used animal models to investigate the influence of different annulotomy incisions (99,100) and repair techniques (101). These studies demonstrated that the technique used to cut through the annulus can indeed affect the timing and strength of any subsequent annular healing and ultimately disc competence. In the goat study by Ethier et al. (100), they demonstrated histologic evidence of "fibrous capping" of the annular fissure created by a trocar (Fig. 6), but they concluded that no primary healing of the fibers occurred after this experimentally produced fissure. A box-type or window annulotomy was shown to result in a significantly weaker healing response than a slit or cruciate incision (99,100). It was therefore speculated that the use of a trocar technique could improve outcomes as a result of stretching rather than lacerating the annulus tissue. It was therefore generally suggested that careful attention to the surgical incision technique could play a role in lessening the risk of recurrent nuclear extrusion through the annulus. In an additional study, Ahlgren et al. (101) examined the healing properties of the intervertebral disc after direct suture repair of different annular defects simulating those that might be made at the time of surgical discectomy. In the case of a box incision, a muscle facial overlay graft was also used. This animal study was unable to identify any influence of direct repair of any typical annulus incision; none of the techniques used were able to change the rate or the strength of the annular healing response. They concluded that preserving as much annular tissue as reasonably possible should be the goal during discectomy in order to prevent recurrence, but they were unable to recommend any specific form of direct surgical repair.

In validation of these animal studies, Carragee et al. (102) evaluated clinical outcomes as a function of intraoperative annular deficiency and the characteristics of the disc herniation fragments. Patients with disc fragments and small annular defects had the best overall outcomes and the lowest rate of reherniation or reoperation. In contrast, patients with no identifiable fragment and a contained disc herniation showed a 10% reherniation rate with a 5% reoperation rate. Furthermore, not surprisingly, those patients with extruded disc fragments and large posterior annular defects had the worst outcome with greater than 20% requiring reoperation.

In addition to careful patient selection and awareness of intraoperative techniques (particularly approach and annulotomy methods), careful repair of the annular fissure may be important. Few investigators have considered techniques for the careful repair, reinforcement, or reconstruction of the annulus fibrosus. These attempts have included suturing concepts, energy deposition, bulking agents or adhesives, and more recently, barrier implants.

Suture Techniques

It may seem intuitive that if a tissue defect is present in the annulus fibrosus either because of a pathological event (i.e., a herniation) or a surgical intervention, then reapproximation of the tissue using sutures might be warranted, but this is currently not the standard of care. Yasargil (103) appears to be one of the first to describe placing a 7-0 suture in the annulus after removal of nucleus pulposus. He claimed that this suturing "may help prevent adhesions," but no mechanism was suggested. Of the 105 patients in Yasargil's microsurgical series, he reported no reherniations, no impairment of neurological symptoms, and no postoperative radiculopathy.

Lehmann et al. (104) also suggested refining the technique to improve discectomy outcome by including a single 4-0 silk suture to close the flaps of the posterior longitudinal ligament, peridural membrane, and outer annulus fibers. His study of 152 patients showed that a greater percentage of those patients that were sutured had less postsurgery pain than those that were not sutured, although statistical significance was not achieved. They did not report the effect of this technique modification on recurrent herniation or reoperation rates.

More recently, Cauthen (105,106) has studied annulus fibrosus suturing in a more extensive manner, with a focus on reducing reoperations. His series of 254 patients suggested a 21% recurrent disc herniation at two years when sutured annulus repair was not performed. Careful microsurgical suturing of the annulus reduced the recurrence rate to less than 10% when one suture was used and to approximately 5% when more than one suture was used.

Few surgeons have adopted this careful and tedious technique of suturing the annulus in spite of the suggestions by these researchers that doing so improves discectomy outcomes. In addition to subtle technique nuances, such as how the annulotomy is created or manually repaired with sutures, other methods of treating and effecting the annulus have been suggested. These have included the deposition of energy to alter tissue characteristics, addition of biocompatible sealing materials, or barrier implants.

Energy Deposition and Tissue Alteration

Recently proposed therapeutic options for altering outcomes in patients with radicular low back pain include intradiscal electrothermal therapy (IDET). This therapy was reported to be successful in 60% to 80% of patients (107) via modulation of collagen tissues, resulting in denaturation, contraction, or shrinkage of the annulus, presumably sealing the defect, and possibly denervating sensitive nociceptors in the layers of the posterior annulus fibrosus. Kleinstueck et al. (108) showed in a cadaveric study that temperatures developed during IDET are insufficient to alter collagen architecture or stiffen the motion segment. Additional studies in sheep by Freeman et al. (109) showed that IDETs thermal necrosis mechanism was not sufficient to cause coagulation of the nociceptors or collagen contraction. They concluded that IDET did not denervate the posterior annulus lesion, and any reported clinical benefit from IDET was most likely related to factors other than denervation and intradiscal repair.

In spite of the lack of understanding of the mechanism of IDET and its impact on clinical outcome, it has been suggested as a method for the repair of the annulus. Cohen et al. (110) reported on a small series of nucleoplasty patients in which 56% had additional IDET added to their procedure. They concluded that the percutaneous removal of nuclear material was not effective in the long term, either with or without the addition of IDET, unless patient criteria was limited to small, contained disc herniations with documented annular integrity by CT discography. In this study, IDET did not appear effective in sealing the annulus or altering outcomes.

Sealant and Bulking Biomaterials

Various biocompatible tissue adhesives and glues have been used in many other soft tissue areas of the body, such as fascial hernia repair, dural repair, or cardiovascular procedures (111–113). The ability to reparatively glue the annulus fibrosus has not been attempted because of the potential untoward adhesive effect that might occur with nearby neural elements or the dural sac. Rather, suggested "sealing" biomaterials have generally been inject-able, cross-linked polymers that cure in situ (114). Conceptually, these bulking hydrogels and polymeric agents are intended to result in a sealant that substantially conforms to the complex and irregular shape of the annulus fibrosus defect, and secondarily may bond strongly to the tissue surrounding the defect. No reported clinical experience with this type of approach to specifically repair the annulus has been made. Rather, these biocompatible materials appear to be more relevant as a complete nucleus pulposus replacement (115–118).

Implantable Devices and Barriers

Implantable barrier-type devices have recently been proposed as an adjunctive therapy after discectomy. Full commercial availability of these concepts has not yet been reached. The ability to ultimately provide a primary barrier to disc re-extrusion seems intuitive, but the ability to provide an efficient method of placing implants on the outside of the annulus or below the surgical surface of the annulus is not without its challenges. Two device concepts in development include a mechanical nitinol-frame barrier (Barricaid™; Intrinsic Therapeutics, Woburn, Massachusetts, U.S.A.) and a polyethylene-terephthalate (PET) mesh (Inclose™ Surgical Mesh System; Anulex Technologies Inc, Minnetonka, Minnesota, U.S.A.).

In vitro biomechanical studies using the Barricaid device have shown its ability to provide stable reinforcement to a large portion of the posterior annulus (119,120). This device substantially covers the better part of the medialateral distance of the posterior annulus, and expands cephalad-caudad after insertion through a 5 × 10-mm annulus defect. Using complex applied loads and measurement of intradiscal pressures in vitro, Yeh et al. (119) reported a twofold increase in the failure pressure when nucleus pulposus extruded. Clinical use of this barrier concept has also been reported (121). When patients who underwent a stan-dard discectomy were compared with those who additionally received the Barricaid annular closure device, maintenance of disc height that was otherwise noted to be lost was achieved. Longer follow-up will be required to conclude that this disc height maintenance can correlate to improved clinical outcomes or the reduction of recurrent herniations.

The Inclose Surgical Mesh System (Fig. 7) is composed of a biocompatible, expandable, braided mesh cylinder of PET. The cylindrical implant is mounted on a delivery tool that allows the device to extend circumferentially out into a barrier by latching the cylinder ends

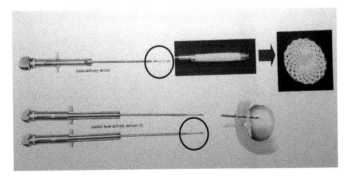

FIGURE 7   The Inclose™ Surgical Mesh System includes a mesh delivery tool with the mesh implanted preattached at the distal end (*upper panel*); upon deployment of the implant, a central latch holds the implant in its final barrier configuration. The system also includes anchor band delivery devices to allow placement of suture anchors/tethers that consist of a distal T-anchor and a proximal pledget. *Source*: Courtesy of Anulex Technologies, Minnetonka, Minnesota, U.S.A.

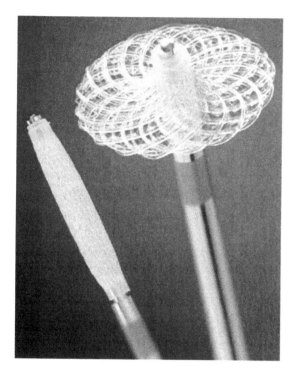

FIGURE 8 A close-up view of the Inclose™ Surgical Mesh implant. In its undeployed configuration (*left*), the implant is a 3-mm cylinder of braided polyethylene terephthalate (PET). When deployed and latched (*right*), the implant expands to cover a 16-mm circumference. *Source*: Courtesy of Anulex Technologies, Minnetonka, Minnesota, U.S.A.

together (Fig. 8). The flexible nature of the braided mesh pattern and the characteristics of the PET allow it to conform to the available anatomic constraints. The mesh implant can be inserted through any tissue aperture, such as an annular defect, and after deployment into position, it can be secured to remaining tissues by suture tethers (Fig. 9).

An in vitro biomechanics study (122) demonstrated that segmental spinal biomechanics were unaffected as a result of placement of Inclose (Fig. 10). This study additionally demonstrated that the implant remains where it was placed beneath the surface of the annulus, even after complex cyclic loading. Theoretically, a biomechanically stable spinal motion segment might reduce the possibility of herniation at an adjacent disc location by avoiding redistribution of stresses. Furthermore, effective repair of annular defects by a device that does not alter disc or motion segment biomechanics may indirectly preclude the excessive removal of nucleus material that is often the case as the surgeon attempts to mitigate recurrent disc herniations.

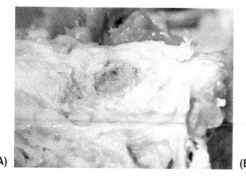

(A)

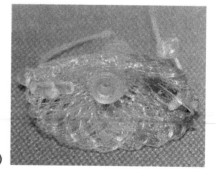

(B)

FIGURE 9 In cadaveric experiments, (**A**) the Inclose™ Surgical Mesh can be seen from the back after placement in tissue and (**B**) after careful removal. Tissue has been removed to facilitate visualization. Distal T-anchors and proximal, circular pledgets can be seen going through the implant, holding it in proximity to the tissue. The characteristic of the braided pattern allows the implant to take the shape of the confines of the available tissue space. *Source*: Courtesy of Anulex Technologies, Minnetonka, Minnesota, U.S.A.

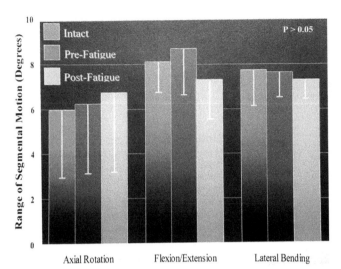

FIGURE 10 In vitro biomechanical experiments conducted in cadaveric spines, demonstrated no effect of the Inclose™ Surgical Mesh (Anulex Technologies, Minnetonka, Minnesota, U.S.A.) on segmental flexibility. The intact condition represents normal, nonimplanted spines (L3-Sacrum), "prefatigue" is after insertion of the Inclose Mesh at L4-L5, and "postfatigue" is after 30,000 bending cycles. The implant remained in place and there was no difference in the biomechanics measured. *Source*: From Ref. 122.

Animal studies of intradiscal implants of any type, and specifically annular repair concepts of implantable barriers, are often hindered by requirements to downsize the device to accommodate relative small tissue areas (Fig. 11). The small cow has been suggested as a model for lumbar intervertebral disc replacement (123), but practically, no reasonable animal model exists that represents typical disc space characteristics that could correlate to clinical use in humans or mimics in situ biomechanics. Furthermore, no large animal model, specifically for disc herniations, has been reported (either naturally-occurring or experimentally produced).

In spite of these limitations, animal experiments were attempted to examine the surgical techniques for Inclose implantation and the histological response to the PET mesh. Studies in the disc space of the Nubian crossbred goat were performed by Peppelman et al. (124). They demonstrated in this goat model that: (*i*) the mesh barrier could be safely placed in proximity to the annulus via a lateral approach (Fig. 12); (*ii*) when properly positioned and affixed, the device remained in position (as assessed by radiographs) over the course of 12 weeks; and (*iii*) the implant histologically incorporated into the annulus tissue without deleterious effects on the surrounding tissues (Fig. 13).

Reports of the earliest clinical use of the Inclose system after discectomy have been promising (125). Following discectomy of L4-L5 or L5-S1 through an endoscopic portal system, the Inclose device was used in less than 10 patients. Minimal disruption of the

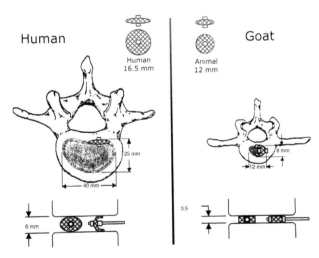

FIGURE 11 Developing technology to repair, reinforce, or reconstruct the annulus is limited by the availability of an appropriate animal model. Farm animals such as goats and sheep have less than half of the disc space height available compared to typical human spines, thus requiring appropriate downsizing of implants. In spite of best efforts to select a model with very large discs and downsized implants, it is often difficult to simulate realistic human clinical usage.

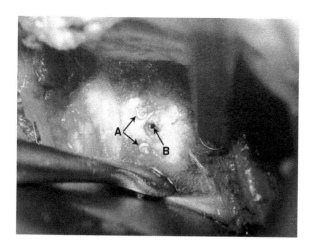

FIGURE 12 An intraoperative view of the Inclose™ Surgical Mesh (Anulex Technologies, Minnetonka, Minnesota, U.S.A.) after implantation in annulus fibrosus of a goat disc model. The implant was placed via a lateral approach. The circular pledgets (**A**) can be seen on the outer soft tissue surface and the latch of the Mesh implant (**B**) can be seen below the tissue surface.

annulus was needed to insert the implant, with access greater than 3 mm, but less than 8 mm. Although none of the patients in this series required re-exploration of the spine at the time of this report, the length of follow-up on this limited series was inadequate to examine the implant's long-term effect on recurrence or reoperation rate. The best technical result was achieved in those patients with focal, protruded, and/or extruded herniations rather than broad-based or bulging discs.

SUMMARY

Discectomy is a common procedure and postsurgery outcomes are generally perceived to be positive in the right patient at the right time, operated on by a qualified and experienced surgeon. Historical efforts to improve outcomes have focused on subtle surgical techniques or modifications, such as the approach (i.e., open discectomy versus the use of an operating portal), and careful attention to such intraoperative technical characteristics as the annular

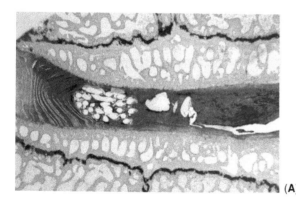

(**A**)

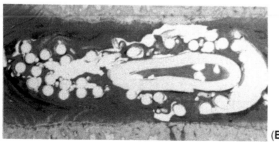

(**B**)

FIGURE 13 Histologic result of the Inclose™ Surgical Mesh (Anulex Technologies, Minnetonka, Minnesota, U.S.A.) after eight weeks in a goat disc model. (**A**) Undecalcified section with Sanderson bone stain shows the soft tissue of the disc (*black*) and the trabecular bone (*gray*). The Inclose™ Surgical Mesh is seen in proximity to the annulus fibers. (**B**) Higher magnification shows the implant's mesh structure surrounded by fibrous tissue and extracellular matrix in close approximation. No inflammatory response or deleterious tissue response is noted.

incision method (i.e., box annulotomy vs. blunt dissection) or the amount of nucleus material removed.

Limited clinical success has been demonstrated by some surgeons that have suggested suture reapproximation of the annulus tissues. However, the fastidious methods required for this additional surgical benefit has reduced the overall adaptability of these techniques. Additionally, some in vitro experiments have questioned the viability of these suturing techniques. Altering the collagen structures of the annulus fibrosus with such energy deposition techniques as intradiscal electrothermal therapy has also shown limited success as a means of repairing or treating annulus defects. Although adhesives or other bulking biomaterials, such as hydrogels have been contemplated, for inherent technical reasons these appear to be less of a focus than the barrier-type implantable devices. Recent developments in the ease of insertion of barrier implants, such as the Inclose Surgical Mesh, has caused spine surgeons to contemplate improving discectomy outcomes by better patient satisfaction and symptom resolution or avoiding reoperations by preventing recurrent disc herniations.

REFERENCES

1. Dandy W. Loose cartilage from intervertebral disc simulating tumor of the spinal cord. Arch Surg 1929; 19:660–672.
2. Mixter W, Barr J. Ruptures of the intervertebral disc with involvement of the spinal canal. NEJM 1934; 211:210–214.
3. Fardon D, Herzog R, Mink J, Simmons J, Kahanovitz N, Haldeman S. Nomenclature of lumbar disc disorders. In: Garfin S, Vaccaro A, eds. Orthopaedic Knowledge Update—Spine. Rosemount, IL: American Academy of Orthopaedic Surgeons, 1997:A3–A14.
4. Knop-Jergas BM, Zucherman JF, Hsu KY, DeLong B. Anatomic position of a herniated nucleus pulposus predicts the outcome of lumbar discectomy. J Spinal Disord 1996; 9(3):246–250.
5. Carragee EJ, Kim DH. A prospective analysis of magnetic resonance imaging findings in patients with sciatica and lumbar disc herniation: correlation of outcomes with disc fragments and canal morphology. Spine 1997; 22(14):1650–1660.
6. Pappas CTE, Harrington T, Sontag VKH. Outcome analysis in 654 surgically treated lumbar disc herniations. Neurosurgery 1992; 30(6):862–866.
7. Matsui H. Lateral disc herniation following percutaneous lumbar discectomy. Int Orthop 1997; 21:169–171.
8. Kayam S, Konno S, Olmarker K, et al. Incision of the annulus fibrosus induces nerve root morphologic, vascular, and functional changes—an experimental study. Spine 1996; 21:2539–2543.
9. Ito S, Yamada Y, Tsubio S, Yamada Y, Muro T. An observation of ruptured annulus fibrosus in lumbar discs. J Spinal Disord 1991; 4(4):462–464.
10. Spangler E. The lumbar disc herniation—a computer-aided analysis of 2,504 operations. Acta Orthop Scand Suppl 1972; 142:1–95.
11. Hasenbring M, Marienfeld G, Kuhlendahl D, et al. Risk factors of chronicity in lumbar disc patients. A prospective investigation of biologic, physiologic, and social predictors of therapy outcome. Spine 1994; 19:2759–2765.
12. Thelander U, Fagerlund M, Friberg S, et al. Straight leg raising test versus radiologic size, shape, and position of lumbar disc hernias. Spine 1992; 17:395–399.
13. Olmarker K, Myers RR. Pathogenesis of sciatic pain: role of herniated nucleus pulposus and deformation of spinal nerve root and dorsal root ganglion. Pain 1998; 78(2):99–105.
14. Hou SX, Tang JG, Chen HS, Chen J. Chronic inflammation and compression of the dorsal root contribute to sciatica induced by the intervertebral disc herniation in rats. Pain 2003; 105(1–2):255–264.
15. Boden SD, Davis DO, Dina TS, et al. Abnormal magnetic-resonance scans of the lumbar spine in asymptomatic subjects: a prospective investigation. J Bone Joint Surg Am 1990; 72:403–408.
16. Jensen MC, Brant-Zawadzki MN, Obuchowski N, et al. Magnetic resonance imaging of the lumbar spine in people without back pain. N Engl J Med 1994; 331:69–73.
17. Boos N, Reider R, Schade V, et al. Volvo Award in clinical sciences. The diagnostic accuracy of magnetic resonance imaging, work perception, and psychosocial factors in identifying symptomatic disc herniations. Spine 1995; 20:2613–2625.
18. Beattie PF, Meyers SP, Stratford P, Millard RW, Hollenberg GM. Associations between patient report of symptoms and anatomic impairment visible on lumbar magnetic resonance imaging. Spine 2000; 25(7):819–828.
19. Kang JD, Stefanovic-Racic M, McIntyre L, Georgescu HI, Evans CH. Toward a biochemical understanding of human intervertebral disc degeneration and herniation. Spine 1997; 22(10):1065–1073.

20. Kawakami M, Tamaki T, Hayashi N, Hashizume H, Nishi H. Possible mechanism of painful radicu-lopathy in lumbar disc herniation. Clin Orthop Relat Res 1998; 351:241–251.
21. Specchia N, Pagnotta A, Toesca A, et al. Cytokines and growth factors in the protruded interverteb-ral disc of the lumbar spine. Eur Spine J 2002; 11:1145–1151.
22. Olmarker K, Rydevik B, Nordborg C. Autologous nucleus pulposus induces neurophysiologic and histologic changes in porcine cauda equina nerve roots. Spine 1993; 18:1425–1432.
23. Olmarker K, Brod G, Cornefjold M, Nordborg C, Rydevic B. Effects of methyl-prednisolone on nucleus pulposus-induced nerve root injury. Spine 1994; 19:1803–1808.
24. Kawakami M, Tamaki T, Weinstein JN, et al. Pathomechanism of pain-related behavior produced by allografts of intervertebral disc in the rat. Spine 1996; 21:2101–2107.
25. Olmarker K. Neovascularization and neoinnervation of subcutaneously placed nucleus pulposus and the inhibitory effects of certain drugs. Spine 2005; 30(13):1501–1504.
26. Murata Y, Rydevik B, Takahashi K, Larsson K, Olmarker K. Incision of the intervertebral disc induces disintegration and increases permeability of the dorsal root ganglion capsule. Spine 2005; 30(15):1712–1716.
27. Yabuki S, Kikuchi S, Olmarker K, et al. Acute effects of nucleus pulposus on blood flow and endo-neurial fluid pressure in rat dorsal root ganglia. Spine 1998; 23:2517–2523.
28. Otani K, Arai I, Mao GP, et al. Nucleus pulposus-induced nerve root injury: relationship between blood flow and motor nerve conduction velocity. Neurosurgery 1999; 45:614–619.
29. Olmarker K, Storkson R, Berge O. Pathogenesis of sciatic pain—a study of spontaneous behavior in rats exposed to experimental disc herniation. Spine 2002; 27:1312–1317.
30. Kawakami M, Tamaki T, Hashizume H, Weinstein JN, Meller ST. The role of phospholipase A2 and nitric oxide in pain-related behavior produced by an allograft of intervertebral disc material to the sciatic nerve of the rat. Spine 1998; 22(10):241–251.
31. Hashizume H, Kawakami M, Nishi H, Tamaki T. Histochemical demonstration of nitric oxide in herniated lumbar discs—a clinical and animal model study. Spine 1997; 22(10):1080–1084.
32. Kang JD, Georgescu HI, McIntyre-Larkin L, Stefanovic-Racic M, Donaldson WF, Evans CH. Herniated lumbar intervertebral discs spontaneously produce matrix metalloproteinases, nitric oxide, interleukin-6, and prostaglandin E_2. Spine 1996; 21(3):271–277.
33. Kawakami M, Matsumoto T, Kuribayashi K, Tamaki T. mRNA expression of interleukins, phospho-lipase A2, and nitric oxide synthase in the nerve root and dorsal root ganglion induced by autolo-gous nucleus pulposus in the rat. J Orthop Res 1999; 17:941–949.
34. Nygaard OP, Mellgren SI, Osterud B. The inflammatory properties of contained and noncontained lumbar disc herniations. Spine 1997; 22:2484–2488.
35. O'Donnell JL, O'Donnell AL. Prostaglandin E2 content in herniated lumbar disc disease. Spine 1996; 21:1653–1656.
36. Doita M, Kanatani T, Ozaki T, et al. Influence of macrophage infiltration of herniated disc tissue on the production of matrix metalloproteinases leading to disc resorption. Spine 2001; 26:1522–1527.
37. McCarthy PW, Carruthers B, Martin D, et al. Immunohistochemical demonstration of sensory nerve fibers and endings in lumbar intervertebral discs of the rat. Spine 1991; 16:653–655.
38. Coppes MH, Marani E, Thomeer RT, et al. Innervation of "painful" lumbar discs. Spine 1999; 22:2342–2349.
39. Palmgren T, Gronblad M, Virri J, et al. An immunohistochemical study of nerve structures in the annulus fibrosus of human normal lumbar intervertebral discs. Spine 1999; 24:2075–2079.
40. Ohtori S, Takahashi Y, Takahashi K, et al. Sensory innervation of the dorsal portion of the lumbar intervertebral disc in rats. Spine 1999; 24:2295–2299.
41. Freemont AJ, Peacock TE, Goupille P, et al. Nerve ingrowth into diseased intervertebral disc in chronic back pain. Lancet 1997; 350:178–181.
42. Freemont AJ, Watkins A, LeMaitre C, et al. Nerve growth factor expression and innervation of the painful intervertebral disc. J Pathol 2002; 197:286–292.
43. Freeman BJ, Walters RM, Moore RJ, Fraser RD. Does intradiscal electrothermal therapy denervate and repair experimentally induced posterolateral annular tears in an animal model? Spine 2003; 28(33):2602–2608.
44. Weisel SW, Twourmas N, Feffer HL, et al. A study of computer-assisted tomography. I. The inci-dence of positive CAT scans in an asymptomatic group of patients. Spine 1984; 9:549–551.
45. Greenberg JO, Schnell RG. Magnetic resonance imaging of the lumbar spine in asymptomatic adults. J Neuroimag 1991; 1:2–7.
46. Weishaupt D, Zanaetti M, Hodler J, Boos N. MR imaging of the lumbar spine prevalence of interver-tebral disk extrusion and sequestration, nerve root compression, end plate abnormalities, and osteo-arthritis of the facet joints in asymptomatic volunteers. Radiology 1998; 209(3):661–666.
47. Boos N, Semmer N, Elfering A, et al. Natural history of individuals with asymptomatic disc abnorm-alities in magnetic resonance imaging: predictors of low back pain-related medical consultation and work incapacity. Spine 2002; 21:1484–1492.
48. Komori H, Shinomiya K, Nakai O, et al. The natural history of herniated nucleus pulposus with radiculopathy. Spine 1996; 21:225–229.

49. Bozzao A, Gallucci M, Masciocchi C, et al. Lumbar disc herniation: MR imaging assessment of natural history in patients treated without surgery. Radiology 1992; 185:135–141.
50. Ahn SH, Ahn MW, Byun WM. Effect of the transligamentous extension of lumbar disc herniations on their regression and the clinical outcome of sciatica. Spine 2000; 25:475–480.
51. Dullerud R, Nakstad PH. CT changes after conservative treatment for lumbar disk herniation. Acta Radiol 1994; 17:927–933.
52. Ellenburg MR, Ross ML, Honet JC, et al. Prospective evaluation of the course of disc herniations in patients with proved radiculopathy. Arch Phys Med Rehabil 1993; 74:3–8.
53. Saal J, Saal J. Nonoperative treatment of herniated lumbar intervertebral disc with radiculopathy: an outcome study. Spine 1989; 14:431–437.
54. Saal J, Saal J, Herzog RJ. The natural history of lumbar intervertebral disc extrusions treated nonoperatively. Spine 1990; 15:683–686.
55. Montaldi S, Fankhauser H, Schnyder P, de Tribolet N. Computed tomography of the postoperative intervertebral disc and lumbar spinal canal: investigation of twenty-five patients after successful operation for lumbar disc herniation. Neurosurgery 1988; 22(6):1014–1022.
56. Cervelline P, Curri D, Volpin L, Bernardi L, Pinna V, Benedetti A. Computed tomography of epidural fibrosis after discectomy: a comparison between symptomatic and asymptomatic patients. Neurosurgery 1988; 23(6):710–713.
57. Heilbronner R, Fankhauser H, Schnyder P, de Tribolet N. Computed tomography of the postoperative intervertebral disc and lumbar spinal canal: serial long-term investigation in 19 patients after successful operation for lumbar disc herniation. Neurosurgery 1991; 29(1):1–7.
58. Kotilainen E, Alanen A, Erkintalo M, Valtonen S, Kormano M. Magnetic resonance image changes and clinical outcome after microdiscectomy or nucleotomy for ruptured disc. Surg Neurol 1992; 41(6):432–440.
59. Floris R, Spallone A, Aref TY, et al. Early postoperative MRI findings following surgery for herniated lumbar disc. Acta Neurochir 1997; 139(3):169–175.
60. Floris R, Spallone A, Aref TY, et al. Early postoperative MRI findings following surgery for herniated lumbar disc part II: a gadolinium-enhanced study. Acta Neurochir 1997; 139(12):1101–1107.
61. Van Goethem JW, Van de Kelft E, Biltjes IG, et al. MRI after successful lumbar discectomy. Neuroradiology 1996; 38(Suppl 1):S90–S96.
62. Nygaard OP, Jacobsen EA, Solberg T, Kloster R, Dullerud R. Postoperative nerve root displacement and scar tissue. A prospective cohort study with contrast-enhanced MR imaging one year after microdiscectomy. Acta Radiol 1999; 40(6):598–602.
63. Awwad EE, Smith KR Jr. MRI of marked dural sac compression by Surgical® in the immediately postoperative period after uncomplicated lumbar laminectomy. J Compt Assist Tomogr 1999; 23(6):969–975.
64. Annertz M, Jonsson B, Stromqvist B, Holtas S. Serial MRI in the early postoperative period after lumbar discectomy. Neuroradiology 1995; 37(3):177–182.
65. Dina TS, Boden SD, Davis DO. Lumbar spine after surgery for herniated disk: imaging findings in the early postoperative period. Am J Roentgenol 1995; 163(30):665–671.
66. van de Kelft JZ, VanGoethem JWM, de la Port C, Verlooy JSA. Early postoperative gadolinium-DTPA-enhanced MR imaging after successful lumbar discectomy. Br J Neurosurg 1996; 10(1):41–49.
67. Kotlainen E, Alanen A, Erkintalo M, Helenius H, Valtonen S. Postoperative hematomas alter successful lumbar microdiscectomy or percutaneous nucleotomy: a magnetic resonance imaging study. Surg Neurol 1994; 41(2):98–105.
68. Nakano M, Matsui H, Ishihara H, Kawaguchi Y, Gejo R, Hirano N. Serial changes of herniated intervertebral discs after postoperative lumbar discectomy: the relation between magnetic resonance imaging of the postoperative intervertebral discs and clinical outcome. J Spinal Disord 2001; 14(4):293–300.
69. VanGoethem JWM, Parizel PM, Jinkins JR. Review Article: MRI of the postoperative lumbar spine. Neuroradiology 2002; 44(9):723–739.
70. Laredo JD, Wybier M. Imaging of the lumbar spine after discectomy. Ann Radiol 1995; 38(4):161–168.
71. Kotwica Z, Chmielowski M, Andrzejak S, Hupalo M. Computed tomography CT is effective in the diagnosis of pain recurrence after surgical removal of herniated lumbar disc. Rev Rheum Med Ser Neurol Psychiatr 1989; 27(3):223–224.
72. Burval S, Nekula J, Vaverka M, Veleeskove J. Computed tomography in the diagnosis of recurrent herniated disks following prior lumbar intervertebral disk operations. Rofo 1992; 156(5):433–436.
73. Burval S, Nekula J, Vaverka M, Veleeskove J, Klaus E. Value of computed tomography in the differential diagnosis of postoperative lumbar disc herniation recurrence and fibrotic changes. Acta Univ Palacki Olomuc Fac Med 1993; 135:37–41.
74. Babar S, Saifuddin A. MRI of the post-discectomy lumbar spine. Clin Radiol 2002; 57(11):969–981.
75. Suezawa Y, Jacob HAC. Percutaneous nucleotomy: an alternative to spinal surgery. Arch Orthop Trauma Surg 1986; 105:287–295.

76. Mochida J, Nishimura K, Nomura T, Toh E, Chiba M. The importance of preserving disc structure in surgical approaches to lumbar disc herniation. Spine 1996; 21(13):1556–1564.
77. Yasargil MG. Microsurgical operation of herniated lumbar disc. Proceedings of the 27th Annual Meeting of the Deutsche Gesellschaft fur Neurochirurgie, Berlin, Germany, September 12–15, 1976.
78. Williams R. Microlumbar discectomy: a conservative surgical approach to the virgin herniated lumbar disc. Spine 1978; 3:175–182.
79. Hudgins WR. The role of microdiscectomy. Orthop Clin North Am 1983; 14:589–603.
80. Wilson D, Harbaugh R. Microsurgical and standard removal of the protruded lumbar disc: a comparative study. Neurosurgery 1981; 8:422–427.
81. Williams R. Microdiskectomy: myth, mania, or milestone? An 18-year surgical adventure. Mt Sinai J Med 1991; 58(2):139–145.
82. Suk K-S, Lee H-M, Moon S-H, Kim N-H. Recurrent lumbar disc herniation: results of operative management. Spine 2001; 26(6):672, 676.
83. Matsui H. Lateral disc herniation following percutaneous lumbar discectomy. Int Orthop 1997; 21:169–171.
84. Apostolides P. Lumbar discectomy microdiscectomy: the "gold standard." Clin Neurosurg 1996; 43:228–238.
85. Abramovitz JN, Neff SR. Lumbar disc surgery: results of the prospective lumbar discectomy study of the joint section on disorders of the spine and peripheral nerves of the American Association of Neurological Surgeons and the Congress of Neurological Surgeons. Neurosurgery 1991; 29(2):301–307.
86. Asch HL, Lewis PJ, Moreland DB, Egnatchik JG, Yu YJ, Clabeaux DE, Hyland AH. Prospective multiple outcomes study of outpatient lumbar microdiscectomy: should 75 to 80% success rates be the norm? J Neurosurg 2002; 96(1 Suppl):34–44.
87. Tureyen K. One-level one-sided lumbar disc surgery with and without microscopic assistance: 1-year outcome in 114 consecutive patients. J Neurosurg 2003; 99(3 Suppl):247–250.
88. Kahanovitz N, Viola K, MuCulloch J. Limited surgical discectomy and microdiscectomy. Spine 1989; 14(1):79–81.
89. Buttermann GR. Treatment of lumbar disc herniation: epidural steroid injection compared with discectomy. J Bone Joint Surg Am 2004; 86-A(4):670–679.
90. Atlas SJ, Keller RB, Chang Y, Deyo RA, Singer DE. Surgical and nonsurgical management of sciatica secondary to a lumbar disc herniation: five-year outcomes from the Maine lumbar spine study. Spine 2001; 26(10):1179–1187.
91. Loupasis GA, Stamos K, Katonis PG, et al. Seven- to 20-year outcome of lumbar discectomy. Spine 1999; 24:2313–2317.
92. Woertgen C, Rothoerl RD, Breme K, Altmeppen J, Holzschuh M, Brawanski A. Variability of outcome after lumbar disc surgery. Spine 1999; 24(8):807–811.
93. Hoffman RM, Wheeler KJ, Deyo RA. Surgery for herniated lumbar discs: a literature synthesis. J Gen Int Med 1993; 8:487–496.
94. Stevens CD, Dubois RW, Larequi-Lauber T, et al. Efficacy of lumbar discectomy and percutaneous treatments for lumbar disc herniation. Soz-Prvedtivmed 1997; 42:367–379.
95. Malter AD, McNeney B, Loeser JD, Deyo RA. 5-year reoperation rates after different types of lumbar surgery. Spine 1998; 23:814–820.
96. Atlas SJ, Keller RB, Wu YA, Deyo RA, Singer DE. Long-term outcomes of surgical and nonsurgical management of sciatica to a lumbar herniation: 10 year results from the Maine lumbar spine study. Spine 2005; 30:927–935.
97. Osterman H, Sund R, Seitsalo S, Keskimaki I. Risk of multiple reoperations after lumbar discectomy: a population based study. Spine 2003; 28:621–627.
98. Fritsch EW, Heisel J, Rupp S. The failed back surgery syndrome. Reasons, intraoperative findings, and long-term results: a report of 182 operative treatments. Spine 1996; 21:626–633.
99. Ahlgren BD, Vasavada V, Brower RS, Lydon C, Herkowitz HN, Panjabi MM. Anular incision technique on the strength and multidirectional flexibility of the healing intervertebral disc. Spine 1994; 19(8):948–954.
100. Ethier DB, Cain JE, Yaszemki MJ, et al. The influence of anulotomy selection on disc competence. Spine 1994; 19(18):2071–2076.
101. Ahlgren BD, Lui W, Herkowitz HN, Panjabi MM, Guiboux JP. Effect of anular repair on the healing strength of the intervertebral disc—a sheep model. Spine 2000; 25(17):2165–2170.
102. Carragee EJ, Han MY, Suen PW, Kim D. Clinical outcome after lumbar discectomy for sciatica: the effects of fragment type and anular competence. J Bone Joint Surg Am 2003; 85-A(1):102–108.
103. Yasargil MG. Microsurgical operation of herniated lumbar disc. Adv Neurosurg 1977; 4:81.
104. Lehmann TR, Titus MK. Refinements in technique for open lumbar discectomy. Proceedings of the International Society for the Study of the Lumbar Spine (ISSLS), June 1997.

105. Cauthen J. Microsurgical annular reconstruction (annuloplasty) following lumbar microdiscectomy: preliminary report of a new technique. Proceedings of the AANS/CNS Joint Section on Spine and Peripheral Nerves. Orlando, Florida, 1999.

106. Cauthen J. Chapter 11—Microsurgical anular reconstruction (anuloplasty) following lumbar micro-discectomy. In: Guyer RD, Zigler JE, eds. Spinal Arthroplasty: A New Era in Spine Care. St. Louis MO: Quality Medical Publishing, 2005:157–177.

107. Wetzel FT, McNally TA. Treatment of chronic discogenic low back pain with intradiscal electrother-mal therapy. J Am Acad Orthop Surg 2003; 11(1):6–11.

108. Kleinstueck FS, Diedrich CJ, Nau WH, et al. Acute biomechanical and histological effects of intradis-cal electrothermal therapy on human lumbar discs. Spine 2001; 26(20):198–207.

109. Freeman BJ, Walters RM, Moore RJ, Fraser RD. Does intradiscal electrothermal therapy denervate and repair experimentally induced posterolateral annular tears in an animal model? Spine 2003; 28(23):2602–2608.

110. Cohen SP, Williams S, Kurihara C, Griffith S, Larkin TM. Nucleoplasty with or without intradiscal electrothermal therapy (IDET) as a treatment for lumbar herniated disc. J Spinal Disord Tech 2005; 18:S119–S224.

111. Miyano G, Yamataka A, Kato Y, et al. Laparoscopic injection of dermabond tissue adhesive for the repair of inguinal hernia: short- and long-term follow-up. J Pediatr Surg 2004; 39(12):1867–1870.

112. Kato Y, Yamataka A, Miyano G, et al. Tissue adhesives for repairing inguinal hernia: a preliminary study. J Laparoendosc Adv Surg Tech A. 2005; 15(4):424–428.

113. Basu S, Marini CP, Bauman FG, et al. Comparative study of biological glues: cryoprecipitate glue, two-component fibrin sealant, and "French" glue. Ann Thorac Surg 1995; 60(5):1255–1262.

114. Haldimann D. System for repairing intervertebral discs. US Patent 6,428,576 B1, August 6, 2002.

115. Bao QB, Yuan HA. New technologies in spine: nucleus replacement. Spine 2002; 27:1245–1247.

116. Bao QB, Yuan HA. Prosthetic disc replacement: the future? Clin Orthop Rel Res 2002; 394:139–145.

117. Carl A, Ledet E, Yuan H, Sharan A. New developments in nucleus pulposus replacement technology. Spine J 2004; 4:S325–S329.

118. Sieber AN, Kostuik JP. Concepts in nuclear replacement. Spine J 2004; 4:S322–S324.

119. Yeh O, Chow S, Small M, Einhorn J, Lambrecht G. Novel approach to closing anular defects: a bio-mechanical study. Proceedings of the Fifth Global Symposium on Motion Preservation Technology. Spine Arthroplasty Society (SAS), New York NY, 2005.

120. Einhorn J, Yeh O, Kamaric E, Chow S, Small M, Lambrecht G. Stability of a mechanical barrier used to seal annular defects. Proceedings of the Fifth Global Symposium on Motion Preservation Technol-ogy. Spine Arthroplasty Society (SAS), New York NY, 2005.

121. Kamaric E, Yeh O, Velagic A, et al. Restoration of disc competency by increasing disc height using an annular closure device. Proceedings of the Fifth Global Symposium on Motion Preservation Tech-nology. Spine Arthroplasty Society (SAS), New York NY, 2005.

122. Cunningham BC, Hu N, Beatson H, McAfee P. Acute in vitro stability of an anular repair device after multi-directional cyclic fatigue evaluated in human specimens. Proceedings of the Fifth Global Sym-posium on Motion Preservation Technology. Spine Arthroplasty Society (SAS), New York NY, 2005.

123. Mendenhall M. The small cow as an animal model for lumbar intervertebral disc replacement. Pro-ceedings of the North American Spine Society 20th Annual Meeting. Spine J 2005; 5(4S):S121–S122.

124. Peppelman WC, Davis R, Sherman J, Yonemura K, Griffith SL, Cauthen J. Feasibility results of a novel anular repair device in a goat model. Proceedings of World Spine III. Rio de Janeiro, Brazil, 2005.

125. Bajaras G, Perez-Olivia A. A pilot study evaluating a novel device for anular repair following spinal discectomy. Proceedings of the Fifth Global Symposium on Motion Preservation Technology. Spine Arthroplasty Society (SAS), New York NY, 2005.

6 The Lumbar Alligator Spinal System™— A Simple and Less Invasive Device for Posterior Lumbar Fixation

Takeshi Fuji and Noboru Hosono
Department of Orthopaedic Surgery, Osaka Koseinenkin Hospital, Osaka, Japan

Yasuji Kato
Department of Orthopaedic Surgery, Toyonaka Municipal Hospital, Toyonaka, Japan

INTRODUCTION

Spinal fusion is an important procedure for various kinds of instability in the lumbar spine, such as spondylolisthesis, degenerative disc disease, fracture/dislocation, infection, or trauma. The rate of union, however, was not necessarily high in the fusion operation without the aid of instrumentation (1–3).

Pedicle screw system has been used widely as a posterior augmentation for the arthrodesis of the lumbar spine. The rate of union has become extremely higher with the use of pedicle screw system. However, it has some disadvantages–misinsertion of the screw (4), inadvertent destruction of suprajacent facet joints, and extreme damage of the paraspinal muscles.

The prototype of spinous process plate was devised as a simple implant to stabilize the spinal segment half a century ago (5,6). Most types of the spinous process plate consisted of one or two plates and some screws connecting them. These spinous process plates clamp the spinous processes and therefore the stabilization force was derived solely by the friction between plates and the spinous processes. To increase the pinch force, we developed a new spinous process plate with large spikes, which bite tightly into the spinous processes, and named it the Lumbar Alligator Spinal System™ (Showa Ika Kohgyo Co. Ltd, Hongo, Meito-ku, Nagoya, Aichi, Japan) (7). The aim of this Chapter is to introduce our new spinous process plate, and demonstrate the usefulness of this instrumentation.

LUMBAR ALLIGATOR SPINAL SYSTEM™ AND OPERATIVE TECHNIQUE

Lumbar Alligator Spinal System (LA) has been developed from the Alligator Plate™ (Mizuho Ikakogyo Co. Ltd, Hongo, Bunkyo-ku, Toko, Japan) for cervical spine (8). The LA is a kind of clamping plate for the spinous processes, and stabilizes the lumbar spinal segments from posterior. This system is composed of two plates positioned on both sides of the spinous process, and two or three transverse systems that connect these plates. The cut surface of the plate is in contact with the base of the spinous processes. The inside of the plate has two rows of triangular spikes that bite into the cortex and clamp the spinous process. Square-shaped prominences of the outsides help the transverse system to be held in position (Fig. 1). An L-shaped plate has a small hole at the end of its projection, and an I-shaped plate is introduced into this hole. In this manner, two plates are connected at the cephalic end. Additional transverse systems are applied between the two plates (Fig. 2).

The plate has only one length, and can be cut to the appropriate size. A pair of plates and two or three transverse systems are all the implants needed. After exposing the laminae and spinous processes in a conventional manner, check the length spanning the spinous processes to be fused by aligning the L-shaped plate. Cut the L-shaped plates to the appropriate

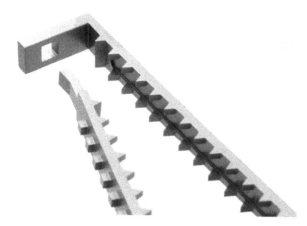

FIGURE 1 The Lumbar Alligator Spinal System™ (Mizuho Ikakogyo Co. Ltd, Hongo, Bunkyo-ku, Toko, Japan) is composed of two plates: L-shaped plate and I-shaped plate. The inside of the plate has two rows of triangular spikes. The outside of the plate has square-shaped prominences to hold the transverse system in position.

size. Cut the I-shaped plate to the same length. The L-shaped plate is installed at the base of the spinous processes. Interspinous ligaments can be partially lacerated to pass the projection of the L-shaped plate and transverse systems. But they should be preserved as much as possible to prevent the adjacent troubles thereafter. The I-shaped plate is installed on the opposite side of the spinous processes, the tip of which is inserted to the hole of the L-shaped plate. The V-shape of the two plates is first closed manually, followed by further compression force by special pliers until the inner spikes of the plate bite into the spinous processes (Fig. 3).

The transverse system is composed of two kinds of hooks (initial and second) and a transverse pin that connects them. A transverse pin is first fixed on an initial hook. This complex is placed on the outside of the plate between spinous processes so that the transverse pin penetrates the interspinous ligament. From the opposite side, the second hook is inserted, which accepts the transverse pin and tightly fix it with a nut (Fig. 4). Compression pliers can approximate two hooks before tightening a nut (Fig. 5). Cut off any portion of the transverse pin protruding from the hook.

Surgical instruments used for surgery consist of a plate holder, hook holder, compression pliers, pin holder, nut driver, and transverse compressor. When viewed from posterior, the

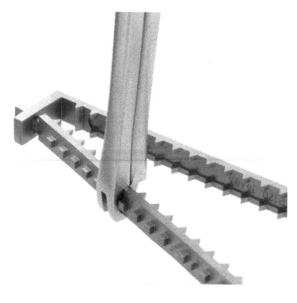

FIGURE 2 An L-shaped plate has a small hole at the end of its projection, and an I-shaped plate is introduced into this hole. In this manner, two plates are connected at the cephalic end.

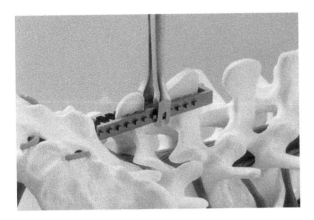

FIGURE 3 The V-shape of the two plates is first closed manually followed by further compression force by special pliers until the inner spikes of the plate bite into the spinous processes.

plates and transverse systems seem to form a ladder, demonstrating that the spinous process is clamped securely. Because of its small size and location, just beside the spinous processes, the LA might damage back muscles less aggressively than pedicle screw systems, which are installed far from the midline under muscles (Figs. 6 and 7).

The LA can be used for various pathologies of the lumbar spine with instability. Surgical procedures using the LA as an augmentation include anterior interbody fusion, posterior interbody fusion, and anterior fusion using strut graft. The LA is a less invasive instrumentation than pedicle screw system.

CLINICAL STUDY: PATIENTS AND METHODS

Between January 2000 and August 2004, lumbar spinal fusion using the LA was performed in 107 patients: single-level posterior lumbar interbody fusion (PLIF) in 75 patients, double-level PLIF in 18, and anterior spinal fusion in combination with posterior augmentation by the LA in 14. A pair of titanium cages packed with iliac bone was implanted between the vertebral bodies after complete curettage of disc material in all patients.

The union rate and surgical complications were assessed. The presence of bony bridge between vertebral bodies on lateral and/or anteroposterior radiographs was interpreted as solid union.

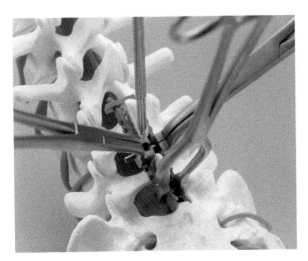

FIGURE 4 The transverse system is composed of two kinds of hooks (initial and second) and a transverse pin that connects them. The transverse system is installed through the interspinous ligament placed on both sides of the spinous processes.

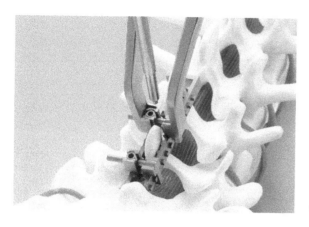

FIGURE 5 Compression pliers can approximate two hooks before tightening a nut.

CLINICAL RESULTS

In patients who underwent PLIF, solid union was achieved in 73.3% at one year after operation—89.4% in single-level PLIF. The union rate increased to 88.7% two years postoperatively—97.9% in single-level PLIF (Figs. 8–12). The union rate was 100% one year after anterior fusion except for seven patients, who underwent surgery owing to osteoporotic vertebral collapse, where union rate was only 71.4%. In four out of seven patients with osteoporotic vertebral collapse, kyphotic deformity occurred. Three of them eventually attained solid fusion, but the last patient required additional surgery owing to nonunion two years after the index surgery. Fracture of the spinous process occurred in three patients in PLIF operation owing to large amount of excision of the laminae.

BIOMECHANICAL STUDY: MATERIALS AND METHODS

Five functional spinal units (FSUs) were used out of three calf lumbar spines to supply biomechanical data for the LA (Figs. 13 and 14). Tests were performed in the order of pure

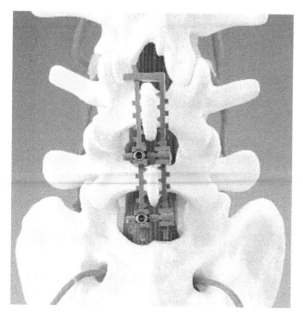

FIGURE 6 When viewed from posterior, the plates and transverse systems seem to form a ladder.

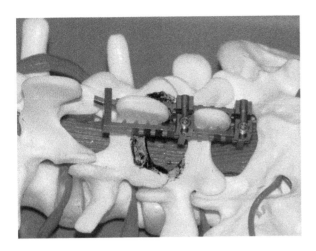

FIGURE 7 The spinous process is clamped securely by the Lumbar Alligator™.

compression, flexion-compression, extension-compression, both lateral bending and both axial rotation, with material testing machine under the load-control method (Fig. 15). The load–displacement curve and the load–angle curve were recorded. All spinal units were tested at intact (INT) first, then after the insertion of a pair of Bagby and Kuslich (BAK) cages, and finally after augmentation by the LA (B + LA). Tests were performed five times in each condition, and we used the data of second, third, fourth, and fifth tests. The data were normalized by the mean stiffness of the intact spines.

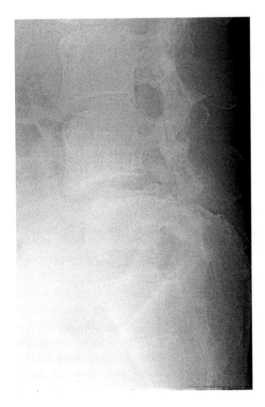

FIGURE 8 A 65-year-old male suffered from intermittent claudication because of degenerative spondy-lolisthesis. Lateral radiograph shows the spondylolisthesis of L4.

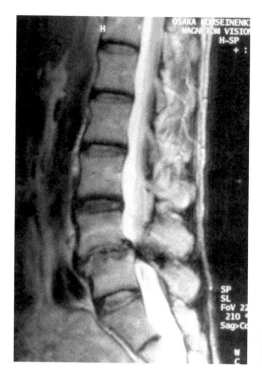

FIGURE 9 T2-weighted magnetic resonance imaging sagittal view revealed the stenosis of the spinal canal of L4/5.

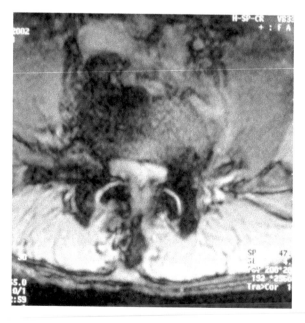

FIGURE 10 T2-weighted image of axial magnetic resonance imaging of L4/5 level. Severe spinal canal stenosis and joint fluid of the facet joints were visible.

BIOMECHANICAL STUDY: RESULTS

The results are shown in Table 1. Compression stiffness was 1.19 at "BAK" and 1.12 at "B + LA." The flexion stiffness is 0.70 at "BAK" and 0.79 at "B + LA." Extension stiffness is 0.97 at "BAK" and 2.26 at "B + LA." Lateral bending stiffness is 2.40 at "BAK" and 2.53 at "B + LA." The rotation stiffness is 1.02 at "BAK" and 1.09 at "B + LA." Therefore, LA gives the stability in extension stiffness.

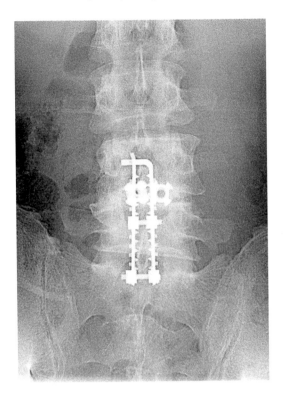

FIGURE 11 Anteroposterior radiograph of the lumbar spine three years after the operation. Bony bridge was seen outside the cages.

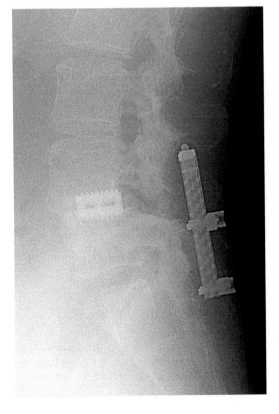

FIGURE 12 Lateral radiograph shows the bony fusion between two vertebrae at the front of the cages.

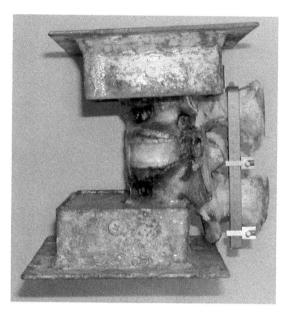

FIGURE 13 A functional spinal unit of calf lumbar spine.

DISCUSSION

Various methods of posterior lumbar fixation have been proposed so far. Each method has its advantages and disadvantages. Pedicle screw fixation is the most rigid fixation system, but it has some disadvantages, such as misinsertion of the screw, damage to the paraspinal muscles, and inadvertent destruction of the suprajacent facet joints. Hook and rod system has been used for a long time, but its technique is slightly complicated. In spinal fusion longer than two levels, pedicle screw system or hook and rod system

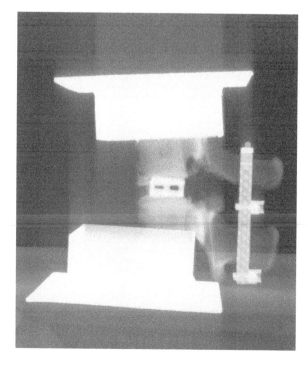

FIGURE 14 Lateral radiograph of the functional spinal unit after the insertion of a pair of Bagby and Kuslich (BAK) cages, followed by augmentation with Lumbar Alligator™.

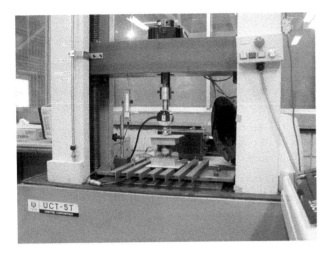

FIGURE 15   A material-testing machine.

is necessary to attain secure fusion. However, in single-level fusion or cases with less segmental instability, recommended is an easy, simple, and less invasive fixation method like the LA of ours.

Lumbar Alligator™ is a kind of spinous process plate, a prototype of which was developed in 1950s. In most types of commercially available spinous process plates, two plates are connected by small screws and nuts, which is often difficult to introduce to the plate in the bottom of the operation field. In contrast, LA has quite unique original implants for combining two plates. An L-shaped plate has small hole, and an I-shaped plate is introduced into this hole. In this manner, two plates are connected and additional transverse systems are applied between two plates.

The indications of LA are PLIF using threaded interbody cages and single-level anterior fusion. The LA is useful especially for infectious cases, because the LA, placed exclusively on the posterior elements of the spine is not likely to disseminate organisms that form infection lesions in the vertebral bodies.

CONCLUSIONS

The LA spinal system is a newly designed instrument for posterior spinal fixation of the lumbar spine. For relatively less spinal instability, LA is a promising alternative to stabilize the segment with its simple application technique and less invasiveness to back muscles.

TABLE 1   Biomechanical Study of the Lumbar Alligator™

Test	INT	BAK	B + LA
Compression stiffness	1	1.19	1.12
Flexion stiffness	1	0.70	0.79
Extension stiffness	1	0.97	2.26
Lateral bending stiffness	1	2.40	2.53
Rotation stiffness	1	1.02	1.09

Abbreviations: B + LA, after augmentation by LA; BAK (Bagby and Kuslich), after the insertion of a pair of BAK cages following curettage of disc material; INT, intact.

REFERENCES

1. Cleveland M, Bosworth DM, Thompson FR. Pseudarthrosis in the lumbosacral spine. J Bone Joint Surg 1948; 30-A:302–312.
2. Thompson WAL, Ralston EL. Pseudarthrosis following spine fusion. J Bone Joint Surg 1949; 31-A: 400–405.
3. Fuji T, Oda T, Kato Y, Fujita S, Tanaka M. Posterior lumbar interbody fusion using titanium cylindrical threaded cages: is optimal interbody fusion possible without other instrumentation? J Orthop Sci 2003; 8:142–147.
4. Esses SI, Sachs BL, Dreyzin V. Complications associated with the technique of pedicle screw fixation. A selected survey of ABS members. Spine 1993; 18(15):2231–2239.
5. Wilson PD, Straub LR. Lumbosacral fusion with metallic plate fixation. Instr Course Lect 1952; 9:52–57.
6. Bostman O, Myllynen P, Riska EB. Posterior spinal fusion using internal fixation with the Daab plate. Acta Orthop Scand 1984; 55:310–314.
7. Fuji T, Ishikawa M, Shigi T, Kanazawa A, Owada T. Posterior lumbar interbody fusion using lumbar alligator spinal system—preliminary report. Cent Japan J Orthop Surg Trauma (Jpn) 2002; 45:97–98.
8. Fuji T, Tanaka M, Hirota S, Masuhara K, Mitsuoka T, Hamada H. Posterior spinal fusion of the cervical spine using the alligator plate: operative technique and clinical results. Eur Spine J 1993; 2:169–174.

7 | Functional Spinal Stability: The Role of the Back Muscles

Lieven A. Danneels and Guy G. Vanderstraeten
Department of Rehabilitation Sciences and Physiotherapy, Ghent University, Ghent, Belgium

Hugo J. De Cuyper
Hospital Jan Palfijn—Campus Gallifort, Antwerp, Belgium

INTRODUCTION

Low back pain (LBP) has become epidemic throughout the western society (1–4). Disorders of the low back and spine make up the largest fraction of musculoskeletal disorders and are among the leading causes of disability in people of working age (5). Estimates of lifetime incidence of LBP range from 60% to 80% (6,7) and, although most LBP episodes (90%) subside within two to three months, recurrence is common (8). As a consequence, chronic low back pain (CLBP) has become a major problem, which affects the availability of health care resources in all industrialized nations (9,10).

Although in recent years great advances have been made in our basic knowledge of the structure and function of the vertebral column, and a considerable body of further evidence has been gathered to acquire a better understanding of the pathogenesis of LBP, in most cases a definitive diagnosis is difficult to achieve (11). As a result, 85% of the CLBP population are classified as having "nonspecific LBP" (7,12).

The huge socioeconomic impact and the complexity of the LBP disorder have led to the development of a variety of differing treatment approaches (7,13–16). Inspired by different viewpoints and findings, therapists have searched for the most efficient treatment. In recent years, it has become clear that physical activity is beneficial to patients with back pain (17–21). There is no evidence that prolonged rest or avoidance of exercise/activity brings about a reduction in chronic back pain (16). A number of studies suggest that prolonged inactivity may even accentuate the problem and increase the severity of the pain (22). We are now much more aware of the beneficial effects of exercise programs for the management of LBP (13,16,22–28). Rehabilitation programs that emphasize exercise and active patient participation appear not only to restore function, but in many cases also alleviate pain (29–34). However, despite the increasing consensus in the literature supporting the need for active exercise therapy in the treatment of CLBP (35), scientific evidence for this approach is lacking. It is still unclear whether one specific exercise is more effective than another (22).

In the past, the management of patients with CLBP by using exercise therapy has been founded largely on empirical knowledge and clinical observations, rather than on research findings regarding the function and dysfunction of the muscular system (36). Last decade however, clinical studies confirmed the presence of muscle dysfunctions in LBP and the effectiveness of therapeutic exercises that are focusing on the control and the coordination of the muscle system in order to obtain functional spinal stability.

In this Chapter, an attempt is made to obtain a better insight into the concept of functional spinal stability, the normal functioning of back muscles, and the characteristics of muscle dysfunction in LBP. Furthermore, different rehabilitation strategies are discussed.

FUNCTIONAL SPINAL STABILITY

Biomechanically, the human spine is a remarkable structure that must meet two seemingly contradictory requirements: the achievement of sufficient stability and the provision of adequate mobility. In protecting the delicate spinal cord and nerve roots, providing adequate support/stability/load-bearing capacity and allowing motion in multiple planes, the spine performs seemingly conflicting functions. Functional stability, both static and dynamic, is required to satisfy these demands. The osteoligamentous spine alone cannot perform all these functions, and, as such, the muscles and their ability to achieve stability and balance assume prime importance (37–41).

The biomechanical research of Panjabi and others introduced a new framework for a more comprehensive interpretation and understanding of spinal intersegmental stabilization and its relationship to back pain (42,43). Rather than limiting the definition of instability to an osteoligamentous insufficiency resulting in abnormally large intersegmental displacements, they described three systems that contribute to spinal intersegmental stabilization: a passive subsystem, an active subsystem, and a control subsystem. The passive subsystem comprises of the osseous and articular structures, the spinal ligaments, and their restriction of segmental movement. The active subsystem refers to the muscles themselves, which stabilize the spinal segment mechanically. The muscles must have adequate endurance and strength to perform this function satisfactorily. The control subsystem refers to the control of the muscles that provide this spinal support (42,43). Neuromuscular control provides a concerted action between the afferent input (proprioception) and the efferent output of the nervous system (coordination), and allows the muscles to contract with the required strength and at the appropriate time (refer to the subsection on "Neuromuscular Control—Muscle Functional Characteristics").

In this Chapter, the concept of intersegmental stabilization is extended to a more global model of functional spinal stability determined by four elements: the passive structures, muscle functional characteristics, neuromuscular control, and postural control (44). The fourth element, postural control, is the capacity to keep the projection of the body's center of gravity within the base of support. In contrast to the concept of spinal intersegmental stabilization (42,43), postural control has in our opinion an important function within the framework of a more general concept of functional spinal stability, as described in the subsection on "Postural Control." Analogous to the models described in the literature (42), Figure 1 provides a simple depiction of functional spinal stability. These four elements constantly interact to offer adequate stability to the spine during changes of posture and static and dynamic loading (44).

This description of the concept of functional spinal stability is followed by a discussion of the different components that determine its quality (subsections on "Passive Structures," "Muscle Functional Characteristics and Neuromuscular Control," and "Postural Control").

Passive Structures

Passive structures of the spine, that is, the vertebral bodies, zygapophyseal joints, capsules, spinal ligaments, and discs, provide a certain amount of mechanical stability. However, they do not confer any significant stability on the spine in the vicinity of the neutral position. It is only toward the ends of the range of motion that these structures develop reactive forces that resist spinal motion.

Dysfunction of the passive structures may be caused by mechanical injury, such as overstretching of the ligaments, development of tears and fissures in the annulus, development of

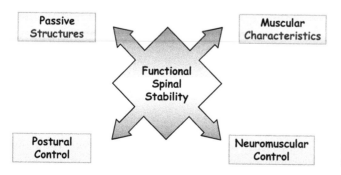

FIGURE 1 Model of functional spinal stability. *Source*: From Ref. 44.

microfractures in the endplates, and extrusion of disc material into the vertebral bodies. Injury may result from overloading of a normal structure or normal loading of a weakened structure. A passive structure can be weakened by degeneration or disease. In general, all these factors decrease the load-bearing and stabilizing capacity of the passive structures. This may require compensatory changes in the active structures (42).

It has also been hypothesized that insufficient neuromuscular control, resulting in a momentary loss of spinal stability, can lead to unexpected displacements, causing either initial trauma or reinjury of previously damaged tissues (45). Although important, the contribution of the passive structures to functional spinal stability will not be further investigated within the context of the present Chapter. This text intended, instead, to focus on the role of the back muscles.

Neuromuscular Control—Muscle Functional Characteristics

Without the influence of muscles, the osteoligamentous spine is unstable at very low compressive loads (37). As such, it is generally accepted that a combination of muscle forces are employed to stabilize the spine dynamically during the various demands that accompany the performance of activities of daily living. There is growing evidence to indicate that the neuromuscular system employs complex and varied strategies of trunk muscle cocontraction in order to provide stiffness and dynamic stability to the spine while simultaneously initiating movement (42).

Proprioception and coordination can be considered as the basic elements for neuromuscular control (46). The two most relevant muscle functional characteristics are endurance and strength (47,48).

Proprioception
Proprioception is a feedback mechanism supplied by specialized nerve terminals and mechanoreceptors in articular capsules, ligaments, skin, and muscles, which give afferent information necessary for the control of posture and movement (46,49).

Coordination
Coordination is defined as the process that results in the generation of patterns of co-contraction of many motor units from multiple muscles with the appropriate force, combination, and sequence of activation and the simultaneous inhibition of other muscles in order to carry out the desired activity (50).

Endurance
Endurance is mechanically defined as either the point of isometric fatigue, where the contraction can no longer be maintained at a certain level, or as the point of dynamic fatigue, where repetitive work can no longer be sustained at a certain force level (51,52).

Strength
The strength of a muscle reflects its ability to generate force. However, assessments of maximal strength can be made with the muscles operating isometrically, concentrically, or eccentrically, and the latter two actions may be performed at a wide range of velocities. All these factors influence the mechanical output and, as such, an infinite number of values may be obtained for the maximal strength of an isolated muscle or for a human movement, depending on the type of action, the velocity of the action, and the length of the muscle(s) (53).

Postural Control

In addition to the aforementioned characteristics (passive structures, neuromuscular control, and muscle functional capacity), the functional stability of the spine during static and dynamic postures in load-bearing and nonload-bearing situations is also determined by postural control. Balance or postural control concerns the ability to maintain equilibrium or to maintain the center of gravity over the base of support. Maintaining posture and balance requires sensory, biomechanical, and motor-processing strategies as well as the anticipation of events and past experiences. The main sensory inputs in the postural control system are

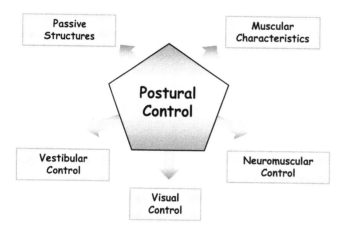

FIGURE 2 The five elements determining the quality of postural control. *Source:* From Ref. 44.

the visual, vestibular, and the neuromuscular (proprioception) control mechanisms (54–58). The interdependence of the sensory systems makes it possible to prepare, maintain, and regain body position in response to unexpected events. In most circumstances, their interactive nature also makes adequate compensation possible, in the case of loss of any one particular modality (56).

Obviously, the passive structures and good muscle functional capacity are also required for the control and maintenance of postural balance (Fig. 2). Abnormalities of the passive structures can result in disturbed joint stiffness and increased segmental mobility. Segmental instability and/or associated pain can impair postural control. With regard to muscle functional characteristics, it has been shown that good muscle condition is essential, as the adaptive response to perturbations or unexpected events may be less effective when the trunk muscles are fatigued (59).

If postural control is impaired, functional spinal stability may be compromised. During activities of daily life, insufficient postural control frequently places the spine in unstable positions and makes the different structures more vulnerable to stress and repetitive strain. Hence, decreased postural stability may increase the risk of injurious loading of the spine (59). Low back pain among industrial workers often occurs because of losses of balance in connection with slips and trips while handling loads (60,61). When balance is impaired or temporarily lost, the recovery strategy must include the maintenance of lumbar spine stability to avoid injuries to that region (33).

MUSCLE FUNCTION

Contributing to functional lumbopelvic stability, a body of knowledge exists about the importance of the paravertebral and abdominal muscles (39,62,63), and increasing evidence is gathered about the muscles of the pelvic floor and the diaphragm being an integral part of the muscular mechanism (64,65). However, in this Chapter major attention has been given to the back muscles.

The following subsections deal first with the functional subdivision of the trunk muscles. Then, the most important back muscles will be described. Finally, different components of muscle function will be dealt with, in relation to the development of a strategy for muscle rehabilitation.

Muscular Subdivision

The provision of functional spinal stability involves a complex interaction between many muscles of the trunk and limb girdles. While some muscles perform and control the primary action, other muscles must work in synergy to balance any asymmetrical forces, control unwanted movements, and offer support to articular structures (7).

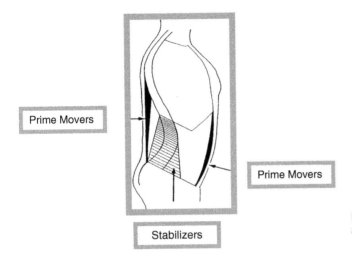

Prime Movers

Prime Movers

Stabilizers

FIGURE 3 A simple depiction of the local and global muscle system. *Source*: From Ref. 44.

Leonardo da Vinci was the first to suggest that some muscles surrounding the spine were primarily concerned with stability (66). In describing muscles of the neck, he suggested that the more central muscles stabilize the spinal segment while the more lateral muscles control the neck orientation (66). In subsequent years, it was realized that the way in which muscles support and stabilize the spine was far more intricate than this simple model would suggest. Nevertheless, it is pertinent to address the issue of local (stabilizers) and global (prime movers) muscles for a better understanding of muscle function in relation to functional spinal stability (Fig. 3).

Bergmark (62) proposed the concept of different trunk muscles playing different roles in the provision of dynamic stability to the lumbar spine and introduced the concept of two muscular systems: the global and the local systems. The global muscle system consists of large, torque-producing muscles that act on the trunk and spine without being directly attached to it. In addition to allowing movement of the spine, the global muscles provide general trunk stabilization, but they do not have a direct influence on the spinal segments. The local muscular system consists of muscles that directly attach to the lumbar vertebrae and are responsible for providing segmental stability and directly controlling the lumbar segments (62,67).

The addition of muscle action imparts stability to the passive structures (39). In this manner, it appears that the local and global muscles of the trunk combine to exert compressive loading of the spine, thereby enhancing its stiffness and functional stability. However, it is the muscles of the local system that have the greatest potential to prevent segmental buckling and control the motion segment (63).

The Lumbar Paravertebral Muscles: The Multifidus and Erector Spinae
The Lumbar Multifidus
The lumbar multifidus is the most medial of the lumbar muscles, and has the unique arrangement of predominantly vertebra-to-vertebra attachments within the lumbar spine and between the lumbar and sacral vertebrae (68). The muscle has five separate bands, each consisting of a series of fascicles that stem from the spinous processes and laminae of the lumbar vertebrae (69) (Fig. 4).

The attachment of the lumbar multifidus to the spinous process provides a strong lever arm for spinal extension. During forward bending motions, this muscle contributes in controlling the rate and magnitude of flexion and anterior shear. Because of its deep location, short-fiber span, and oblique orientation, the multifidus is thought to stabilize against flexion and rotation forces on the lumbar spine (70). Several studies have illuminated its relationship with the vertebral segment. The phenomenon of dysfunction of this muscle and its effect on recurrence of LBP is discussed next.

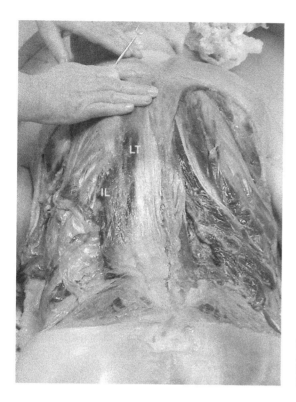

FIGURE 4 A posteral caudalcranial view of the back muscles. On the left side the thoracic parts of the longissimus thoracis (LT) and the iliocostalis lumborum (IL).

Within the pelvis, the multifidus muscle also attaches to the laminae of the posterior thoracodorsal fascia at a raphe that separates it from the gluteus maximus muscle. Fibers from the multifidus pass beneath the posterior sacroiliac ligaments to merge with the sacrotuberous ligament. The interconnections of the multifidus muscle facilitate its contribution to stability of the low back and pelvis (71).

The unique segmental arrangement of the multifidus fascicles in the lumbar region indicates that it has the capacity for fine control of the movements of the individual lumbar vertebrae. This is reflected in its segmental innervation. Each fascicle of the lumbar multifidus and the zygapophyseal joint of that level are innervated by the medial branch of the dorsal ramus. Each nerve innervates only those fascicles that arise from the spinous process or lamina of the vertebrae with the same segmental number as the nerve, illustrating the direct relationship between a particular segment and its multifidus muscle. This suggests that the segmental multifidus can adjust or control a particular segment to match the applied load (70).

The Erector Spinae

The lumbar erector spinae lies lateral to the multifidus and forms the prominent dorsolateral contour of the back muscles in the lumbar region. It consists of two muscles: the longissimus thoracis and the iliocostalis lumborum. Furthermore, each of these muscles has two components: a lumbar part, consisting of fascicles arising from the lumbar vertrebrae, and a thoracic part, consisting of fascicles arising from thoracic vertebrae or ribs (68,72). These four parts may be referred to, respectively, as longissimus thoracis pars lumborum, iliocostalis lumborum pars lumborum, longissimus thoracis pars thoracis, and iliocostalis lumborum pars thoracis.

Even though the thoracic erector spinae have no essential attachments to the lumbar spine, they have an optimal lever arm for lumbar extension. By pulling the thorax posteriorly, they create an extension moment at the lumbar spine. They function eccentrically to control descent of the trunk during forward bending and isometrically to control the position of the lower thorax with respect to the pelvis during functional movements (73). The lumbar erector spinae have a poor lever arm for spine extension but are aligned to provide a dynamic counterforce to the anterior shear force imparted to the lumbar spine from gravitational force.

Owing to their morphology, the thoracic parts of the erector spinae can be considered global muscles. On the other hand, the lumbar parts are well suited for the role of a segmental stabilizer. In consequence, they can be assumed as local muscles.

Strategy for Muscle Rehabilitation

In this section, the different components of muscle function (proprioception—coordination—endurance—strength) will be discussed, in relation to the development of a strategy for muscle rehabilitation.

Rehabilitation of the trunk muscle system is one of the most important aspects of treatment undertaken by physical therapists to help LBP patients regain function and to prevent the recurrence of further back pain episodes. A vital function of the muscle system is to support and control the back in static and dynamic postures during both load-bearing and nonload-bearing activities. A systematic progression is imperative in the rehabilitation of the neuromuscular control system and the muscle functional characteristics (63,64). Proprioception and coordination can be considered as the foundations for efficient neuromuscular control (46). The superstructure consists of the two most relevant muscle functional characteristics: endurance and strength (44,47,48) (Fig. 7).

Proprioception and Coordination

Proprioception and coordination exercises are essential components of the rehabilitation program and form the foundation for both the static and dynamic motor programs necessary to generate and maintain functional spinal stability. Recent evidence exists of the effectiveness of therapeutic strategies that aim at coordinating the local and global muscles (efferent pathways of coordination) in order to compensate for the changing demands (via afferent pathways of proprioception) associated with activities of daily life, and to ensure that dynamic stability of the spine is preserved (37,45). This process can also be described as stabilization training (46). Analogous to the model described previously, Figure 8 illustrates that stabilization training covers proprioception as well as coordination, and establishes the basis for traditional endurance and strength in training.

At the start of stabilization training, static exercises develop coordinated muscle patterns that stabilize the spine in a neutral position. The neutral position is defined as the most comfortable, least painful position of the spine, and preferably reflects a lumbar lordosis within the mid-range position. Theoretically, the stabilization concept works by minimizing repetitive end-range loading and torsional stress of the spine. This can help in preventing LBP and allowing healing, and can potentially alter the spinal degenerative process. Once the achievement of

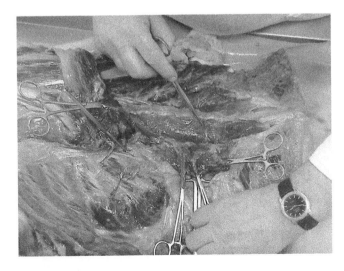

FIGURE 5 A posterolateral view of the multifidus with repeating series (five separate bands) of fascicles which stem from the top and the lateral side of the spinous processes of the lumbar vertebrae and exhibit a constant pattern of attachments caudally.

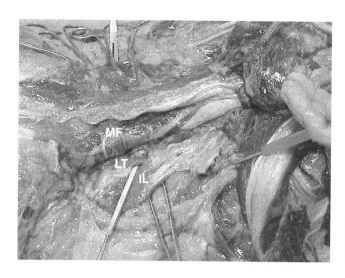

FIGURE 6 A posterolateral view of the multifidus (MF) and the lumbar parts of the longissimus thoracis (LT) and the iliocostalis lumborum (IL).

stability has been learned and practiced through static stabilization exercises, the program progresses to incorporate dynamic movements of the trunk with appropriate activation of the supporting muscles (7).

Endurance and Strength

For strength and endurance training, the intensity can objectively be quantified by controlling exercise intensity (percentage of repetition maximum), volume (sets of repetitions), and frequency. The resistance is based on the maximum number of repetitions performed before fatigue prevented completion of an additional repetition. This is referred to as the repetition maximum (1-RM), and generally reflects the intensity of the exercise (74). To train for basic strength, subjects generally train at 70% of the 1-RM (74). This allows 15 to 18 repetitions until muscular fatigue (75,76). In each training session, subjects are required to perform three sets of each exercise.

To train endurance in a dynamic way, no special exercise recommendations are needed, because the dosage can be modified for exercises prescribed for strength training. A higher number of repetitions are performed (25–30) with lower resistance (at 50–60 of the 1-RM).

Reconditioning requires a careful examination so that the rehabilitation program is focused on the specific muscles in need of training endurance and/or strength. The program has to be initiated at the appropriate level of difficulty.

The dilemma with most strengthening exercises is that the exercise is often performed at a higher level than the muscles can safely execute the movement. When one synergist of a muscle group is relatively weak during performance of a movement, the other synergists often produce the necessary force required to perform the desired movement, thereby reinforcing the muscle imbalance and increasing the risk of injury of the lumbopelvic region.

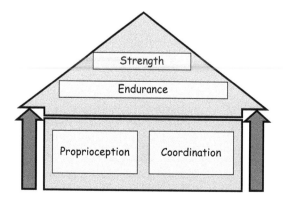

FIGURE 7 Strategy in muscle rehabilitation *Source*: From Ref. 44.

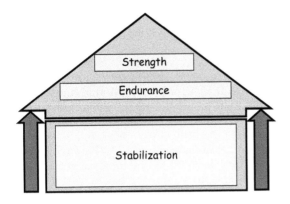

FIGURE 8 Stabilization training establishes the basis for traditional endurance and strength training. *Source*: From Ref. 44.

Subdividing the muscle rehabilitation strategy into different categories of exercise may to some extent seem artificial and rigid. However, in the evaluation of muscle function (section on "Evaluation of Functional Spinal Stability") and in the identification of muscle dysfunction this model provides a certain structure and can shed light on this complex matter.

In the rehabilitation of muscle dysfunction (section on "Rehabilitation of Functional Spinal Stability"), the model serves as a guideline and allows the physical therapist to develop a structured approach. Nonetheless, it must also be emphasized that each muscle dysfunction requires individual assessment and rehabilitation.

MUSCLE DYSFUNCTION IN LOW BACK PAIN

Trunk muscle dysfunction is being increasingly implicated as a contributory factor in the development or recurrence of subacute and chronic mechanical back complaints (77). Factors such as the degree of trunk muscle strength (19,74,78–82) and endurance (83–87), as well as coordination (36,88–90) and proprioceptive awareness (91,92), have been shown to be influenced by the presence of LBP.

Strength, endurance, coordination, and proprioception are mentioned in the same chronological sequence in which they have received attention in the literature. Interestingly, however, this order is the reverse of that proposed in the previous muscle rehabilitation strategy. A number of studies have shown that CLBP patients have significantly lower trunk strength when compared with healthy controls (74,80–82,93–95), while other authors reported that trunk strength is not significantly affected in CLBP patients (85–87,96–98). Even so, controversy exists about the contribution of trunk muscle weakness to the development of LBP. According to some authors, weak trunk muscle strength is one of the strongest risk factors for LBP (19,78), whereas others suggest that trunk muscle weakness does not increase the risk of developing LBP (99,100). An important finding within this context is that differences seem to exist between back and abdominal muscles. Different studies have demonstrated that extensor strength is reduced more than flexor strength in patients with CLBP (81,93–95,101). From a five-year prospective study, it was concluded that an imbalance of trunk muscle strength, that is, extensor strength lower than flexor strength, and not the absolute strength of each muscle group, was a risk factor for the development of first-time LBP (102).

Decreased back muscle endurance has not only been identified as a predictor of first-time occurrence of LBP, but has also been demonstrated in persons with CLBP compared with those with healthy backs (52,97,98). Although most studies provide data on gross muscle function, more specific information is required concerning the pattern and degree to which individual muscles contribute to the dysfunction. In the previous decade, researchers have found that the muscular response to back pain may not be uniform among all muscles of the back; it is mainly the action of the deep muscle system that is disturbed and inhibited in the presence of LBP (8,103–107).

Several investigators have studied the response of the multifidus in LBP and found that the fatigue rate of the multifidus muscle was greater in patients with chronic back pain compared with control subjects without back pain, while no such difference was evident for the thoracic part of the iliocostalis lumborum (77). Others noted that the multifidus becomes inhibited and reduces in size in LBP (8,79,103,106,107).

Within this context, our research group demonstrated an atrophy of the multifdus and not of the lumbar erector spinae and hip flexor muscles in normal active CLBP patients. As disuse and immobilization related to back pain leads to atrophy of flexors and extensors (106), the question arises as to whether reflex inhibition, pain, and/or inflammation arising in the lumbar spine could hamper activation of the multifidus and thus have caused the observed selective atrophy of this muscle. Using real-time ultrasound imaging, Hides et al. (103) detected unilateral wasting of the multifidus in acute and subacute LBP patients. The fact that reduced cross-sectional area was unilateral and isolated to one level suggested that the mechanism of wasting was not generalized disuse atrophy or spinal reflex inhibition. Inhibition as a result of perceived pain, via a long loop reflex, which targeted the vertebral level of pathology to protect the damaged tissues, was the likely mechanism of wasting in the acute stage. In a following study, Hides et al. (8) showed that multifidus recovery did not occur spontaneously on remission of painful symptoms.

Therefore, based on the available literature, we suggested that after the pain onset and possible pain inhibition of the multifidus, in the subacute and chronic stage, a combination of reflex inhibition and changes in coordination of the trunk muscles work together (106). The reflex inhibition hampers alpha motor neuron activity in the anterior horn of the spinal cord and inhibits accurate activity of the multifidus. Moreover, already in the early stage, different recruitment patterns install, other muscles become active and try to substitute for the stabilizing muscles, particularly the multifidus (36). This mechanism becomes chronic and results in selective atrophy of the multifidus. Diminished ability to recruit the multifidus, as found in another study of a chronic LBP population, supports these results (79). Another explanation could be that the atrophy of the multifidus is not secondary to LBP, but that there is an etiological relationship. Further prospective studies are required to resolve this question (106).

Dysfunction of the local and global muscles in LBP may be related not only to neural inhibition patterns but also other mechanisms such as the adoption of guarded movements and disuse. Guarded movements appear to be particularly important, and could be closely linked to psychological processes. These movements bear little relationship to current pain, but are strongly related to fear avoidance. Fear of pain or reinjury, and the patients' own perception of their ability—or lack of ability—to perform movements and activities despite pain may all lead to guarded movements. Exacerbations of back pain are common and may further reinforce this conditioning. These patterns may develop as a physiologic response to injury or primary dysfunction, but seem to persist because of psychophysiological rather than physiologic processes. They may be executed subconsciously and independently of existing back pain, and may result in neurophysiological and physical changes, such as disturbed proprioception, coordination and postural control, reduced range of movement, loss of strength, and fatigue (5).

Guarded movements and the lack of normal muscle use lead in turn to physical deconditioning. The "disuse syndrome" that develops is the direct consequence of reduced activity and illness behavior. Disuse has a profound effect on the physical condition of the back, which can aggravate and maintain the muscle dysfunction, and lead to more severe disability (4).

EVALUATION OF FUNCTIONAL SPINAL STABILITY

Physical therapists address the often complex muscle dysfunction in patients suffering from LBP. Currently, muscle dysfunction is more and more assumed to be involved in acute LBP (8) and chronic LBP (36,77,79,85,89,95,106). Every muscle dysfunction requires a systematic yet specific approach. Systematic because we should aim at a progressive exercise program, specific because each patient has to be individually assessed and rehabilitated.

In clinical practice, there is an increasing need for objective assessment. At our department, a test battery of exercises is used to diagnose and treat a possible dysfunction of the different components contributing to functional spinal stability (108).

Proprioception

Proprioception is evaluated by performing a position–reposition task, that is, reposition accuracy, for the pelvis and lumbar spine. This is a method to evaluate the position sense. Three-dimensional data of the pelvis and the lumbar region are collected using an ultrasonic movement analysis system (Zebris CMS 50®, Isny, Germany). Three ultrasound microphones determining a local coordinate system are used to track the ultrasonic markers on the back and pelvis with an absolute accuracy better than 0.6 mm. Spatial marker positions are derived by triangulation and used for the standardization of net angular displacements of the pelvis and the lumbar spine in the sagittal, transverse, and frontal planes.

The criterion position is determined by the tester. Starting from a relaxed posture, the test subjects are placed in a physiological lordosis (sitting: about half way between full extension and a flat position of the spine—standing: determined by a horizontal alignment between the anterior-superior iliac spine and the posterior-superior iliac spine). For measuring the repositioning accuracy, the subjects are asked to maintain the criterion position while the position of the markers is determined. Afterwards, they have to tilt their pelvis three times forward and backward, after which they have to try to reproduce the criterion position.

Coordination, Stabilization, Endurance, and Strength

The objective measurement of back muscle dysfunction has become an important aspect in the evaluation of low back disability. Although increasing evidence shows that a functional subdivision exists between the local and the global muscles, the mechanism of dysfunction has rarely been approached for the two muscle groups separately. In order to objectively identify the mechanism of back muscle dysfunction, this functional test battery evaluates the electromyogram (EMG) activity of a representative of the two muscle systems. The test subjects are asked to perform a set of exercises, subdivided into four categories: coordination, stabilization, endurance, and strength exercises. The myoelectric signals of a local back muscle, the multifidus, and a global back muscle, the iliocostalis lumborum pars thoracis, are analyzed.

In our opinion, EMG measurements of muscle function are an excellent tool for identifying and subsequently guiding treatment strategies designed to remedy back muscle dysfunction. The subdivision into different categories of exercises gives us a better understanding of muscle dysfunction, if any, and illustrates in which category(ies) the patient fails.

In the first category, the coordination abilities to activate the back muscles in order to obtain a physiological (appropriate neutral) lumbar lordosis, are evaluated in sitting and standing positions (63,64). Starting from a relaxed posture, the test subjects are asked to assume a physiological lordosis, sustain this posture and relax. As a specific part of the coordination exercises, a flexion–relaxation test is performed to evaluate the capacity of the back muscles to relax during flexion.

In the second category, the stabilization exercises are aimed at evaluating the holding capacity of the back muscles. In contrast to the former category, the subjects are first asked to assume a physiological lordosis before starting the exercise. In a first set of stabilization exercises, the back muscle activity in the neutral position of the lumbar spine is tested in a variety of body positions in conjunction with leg- and arm-loading activities. In a second set of stabilization exercises, the physiological lordosis has to be assumed and maintained during slow controlled movements of the trunk (63).

Endurance of the trunk extensors is measured using the Sorensen Test. The Sorensen Test measures the trunk extensors' capability of sustaining an antigravity position over time. During this test, subjects lie prone with the pelvis at the edge of a table. Our patients are instructed to maintain their body in the horizontal position for as long as they could tolerate that position (109). Endurance is monitored by time and power spectral analysis of the EMG signals.

The strength exercises consist of a maximal voluntary isometric contraction (MVIC) of the back muscles. For the maximal effort each subject lay prone, with the hands on the forehead and the feet strapped to the examination table. The subjects are asked to produce the maximal isometric extension effort while resistance is given to the scapular region by the examiner or, if necessary with use of a belt.

Postural Control

A Balance Master® dual force plate (Neurocom International Inc., Packomas, OR, U.S.A.) is used for data collection of postural control. Data are sampled at the rate of 100 Hz. An accompanying software program (110) calculates the position of the center of pressure relative to the platform coordinates. From the center of pressure data, the software then calculated an estimate of the center of gravity (COG) based on the subject's height.

The center of pressure is equal and opposite to the average of all downward acting forces on the force plate. The center of pressure represents the neuromuscular response at the ankles to imbalances in the body's COG (54,111).

The subjects are asked to stand on one leg, with the other leg in hip and knee flexion. The following conditions are applied: eyes open left leg stance, eyes closed left leg stance, eyes open right leg stance, and eyes closed right leg stance. The COG way velocity (deg/sec), the ratio of the distance travelled by the COG to the time of the trial are calculated for each trial of 10 seconds.

Reliability

We evaluated the reliability of measuring the EMG activity of the back muscles during coordination, stabilization, and strength exercises (108). The results demonstrated that when back muscle function is evaluated during coordination, stabilization, and strength exercises, the amplitude EMG parameter has acceptable reproducibility over time when assessed by the same operator. They also indicated that the reliability was better for the multifidus than for the iliocostalis lumborum pars thoracis, and also for exercises at higher loads (strength exercises).

The reliability of using the power spectral analysis for evaluating fatigue for back muscles has been investigated and found to be acceptable (86,112–114) and previous studies have demonstrated the validity and reliability of the Balance Master dual force plate and the protocol used in the test battery (115).

Relevance

The development of a test battery to identify dysfunctions in back pain patients can be important for clinical, economic, and scientific reasons. First, within its limitations, the battery gives a better understanding of dysfunction, if any, and illustrates in which category(ies) the patient fails. The quality of each separate exercise can also be determined. Starting from the test findings, the clinician can set up an individualized exercise routine.

Second, CLBP places an increasing economical burden on the health budget (9). As a result, objective tests become necessary to measure in what way LBP patients need and will benefit from physical therapy.

Finally, many researchers emphasize the need for the identification of different subgroups within "the nonspecific LBP" population (116–118). The successful management of CLBP and the homogeneity of the results among randomized controlled trials (116,117) greatly depend on the accurate identification of subgroups within this population (118). The combination of an accurate physical examination with a functional test battery allows subdividing "the nonspecific LBP" population into subgroups. Based on the findings of the physical examination and the quality of performance during the different functional tests, an objective evaluation of the different elements contributing to functional spinal stability is possible.

REHABILITATION OF FUNCTIONAL SPINAL STABILITY

A recent focus in the physiotherapeutic management of patients with CLBP has been the specific training of muscles surrounding the lumbar spine, the primary role of which is considered to be the provision of dynamic stability and segmental control to the spine (64). Recent studies have shown that the lumbar multifidus is one of the most important muscles for lumbar segmental stability (39,41,42,73). Precisely, this muscle was found to be atrophied in (sub)acute (103) and chronic (106) back pain patients.

The use of static stabilization training has been advocated by Jull and Richardson (67) as an ideal means of improving the recruitment of the multifidus. On the other hand, many others support the role of high-loaded dynamic exercises in the successful management of back pain (26). Although courses of vigorous physical training have been undertaken in CLBP and produced obvious improvements (26,119,120), little information is available on the effects of different contraction modalities of the paravertebral muscles. Nevertheless, the type of muscle work seems to be important. Eccentric muscle contractions seem to be essential to obtain an optimal hypertrophy in response to resistance training (121,122), and a combined dynamic–static training mode has been recommended in order to recruit as many motor units as possible. The efficacy of exercises in the conservative management of CLBP is well documented, but many questions remain regarding their prescription and method of application.

Stabilization Vs. Traditional Resistance Training

Strength and endurance training has long formed the basis for therapeutic exercise, while coordination and stabilization training has only gained importance over the last decade. In this Chapter, a strategy of back muscle rehabilitation was presented in which the traditional strength and endurance exercises are combined with the rather new concept of stabilization training (refer to the subsection on "Strategy for Muscle Rehabilitation").

It has been argued in the literature that the local muscle system is most affected in the CLBP patient, and that it is the functional impairment of this system that is linked to the high recurrence rate seen in CLBP. As such, it is recommended that the local muscle system be trained first, using the appropriate physiotherapeutic regimen, until adequate stabilization is achieved. Retraining of proprioception and coordination then provides a foundation for the safe performance of more general exercise programs directed at general endurance and strength (44,63,67).

At our department, an experiment was conducted to determine whether strength training is beneficial in addition to stabilization training, that is, whether strength training has further effect over and above that of stabilization training. Moreover, information relating to the effect of different contraction modalities of the back muscles is lacking. It remains unclear whether any specific type of contraction is superior to another in back muscle rehabilitation. In this experiment, the effects of two commonly used strength-training regimes (dynamic and dynamic–static) were compared.

Chronic low back pain patients were randomized to 10-week stabilization training (group I), 10-week stabilization training combined with dynamic resistance training (group II), or 10-week stabilization training combined with dynamic–static resistance training (group III). Prior to, and after 10 weeks of training, the size of the total paraspinal muscle mass and the isolated multifidus were measured from standard computed tomography (CT) images at three different spinal levels. In addition, pain relief, and short- and long-term functional outcomes were evaluated.

The results indicated that significant hypertrophy of the paravertebral muscles was observed in groups II and III compared with group I. The hypertrophy of the multifidus was found to be significantly greater in group III than in groups I and II. All groups showed a significant reduction in pain and functional disability levels, with no significant difference among the three groups. During the 12-month follow-up, the self-reported disability statistically increased in the stabilization group, whereas long-term gains were achieved with both strengthening programs.

In conclusion, the findings of this study indicate that strengthening exercises are essential to achieve a volume-growing effect of the paravertebral muscles in CLBP patients, without a difference between the dynamic and dynamic–static modes. On the other hand, the static-holding component seems to be critical to induce hypertrophy of the multifidus. Besides these morphological changes of the back muscles, all groups showed a statistically significant reduction in pain and functional disability levels, whereas the long-term gains in self-reported disability favored intensive strengthening training without a significant difference between the dynamic and the dynamic–static modes.

The differences between the effects of dynamic and dynamic–static strengthening training on hypertrophy incite us to further investigate the mechanical and metabolic characteristics of the described strengthening modes, and their different impacts on the different back muscles. Moreover, in our experiment no other effects of parameters, such as proprioception, coordination, and strength were measured. Future experiments in which the different training modalities will be evaluated by means of the functional test battery, could give relevant information. Furthermore, the optimum frequency, intensity, and duration of these exercises need to be determined.

Although many recent literature reports stress the importance of the incorporation of stabilization training, the benefits of stabilization training as a foundation for strength training should be pointed out. Therefore, on this moment a randomized clinical trial is conducted comparing the efficacy of combined stabilization–strength training with that of isolated strength training. Once more, it has to be mentioned that greater differences in outcome between the different rehabilitation programs are expected if in future interventions the CLBP patients would be categorized into different subgroups.

Giving a better insight into the concept of functional spinal stability and normal back muscle function, characterizing possible dysfunctions of the elements contributing to functional spinal stability, and providing evaluation and rehabilitation strategies, this Chapter aims at making a valuable contribution to the quality of the daily work of everyone concerned with the LBP patient.

SUMMARY

Biomechanically, the human spine is a remarkable structure that must meet two seemingly contradictory requirements: the achievement of sufficient stability and the provision of adequate mobility. In protecting the delicate spinal cord and nerve roots, providing adequate support/stability/load-bearing capacity, and allowing motion in multiple planes, the spine performs seemingly conflicting functions. Functional stability, both static and dynamic, is required to satisfy these demands.

Without the influence of muscles, the osteoligamentous spine is unstable at very low compressive loads. As such, it is generally accepted that a combination of muscle forces are employed to stabilize the spine dynamically during the various demands that accompany the performance of activities of daily living. There is growing evidence to indicate that the neuromuscular system employs complex and varied strategies of trunk muscle co-contraction in order to provide stiffness and dynamic stability to the spine while simultaneously initiating movement.

Based on the literature, own research, and clinical experience this Chapter has dealt on the importance of the back muscles in relation to low back pain. Giving a better insight into normal back muscle function, characterizing back muscle dysfunction, and providing evaluation and rehabilitation strategies, this Chapter aims at making a valuable contribution to the quality of the daily work of therapists.

ACKNOWLEDGMENTS

The authors wish to express their sincere appreciation to Dr. Ann Cools for her contribution to many conceptual ideas presented in this chapter, Dr. Peter O'Sullivan for sharing constructive ideas, Dr. Anne Mannion for the most interesting discussions and for her efforts in proofreading some parts of this work, and Mrs. Iris Wojtowicz for the linguistic corrections.

REFERENCES

1. Andersson G. The epidemiology if spinal disorders. In: Frymoyer JW, ed. The Adult Spine: Principles and Practice. New York: Ravel Press, 1991:107–146.
2. Leboeuf I, Kyvik K. At what age does low back pain become a common problem? A studie of 424 individuals aged 12–41 years. Spine 1998; 23:228–234.

3. Volinn E. The epidemiology of low back pain in the rest of the world. A review of surveys in low- and middle-income countries. Spine 1997; 22:1747–1754.
4. Waddell G. A new clinical model for the treatment of low-back pain. Spine 1987; 12:632–644.
5. Waddell G. The back pain revolution. London: Churchill Livingstone, 1998.
6. Long D, BenDebba M, Torgenson W. Persistent back pain and sciatica in the United States: patient characteristics. J Spinal Disord 1996; 9:40–58.
7. Twomey L, Taylor J. Spine update. Exercise and spinal manipulation in the treatment of low back pain. Spine 1995; 20:615–619.
8. Hides J, Richardson C, Jull G. Multifidus recovery is not automatic following resolution of acute first episode of low back pain. Spine 1996; 21:2763–2769.
9. Indahl A, Velund L, Reikeras O. Good prognosis for low back pain when left untampered. Spine 1995; 20:473–477.
10. Spzalski M, Nordin M, Skovron ML, Melot C, Cukier D. Health care utilization for low back pain in Belgium. Spine 1995; 20:431–442.
11. Waddell G. Modern management of spinal disorders. J Manipulative Physiol Ther 1995; 18:590–596.
12. Dillingham T. Evaluation and management of low back pain: an overview. State Art Rev 1995; 9:559–574.
13. Koes B, Bouter L, Beckerman H, van der Heijden G, Knipschild P. Physiotherapy exercises and back pain: a blinded review. Br Med J 1991; 302:1572–1576.
14. Mc Kinnon M, Vickers M, Ruddock V, Townsend J, Meade T. Community studies of the health service implications of low back pain. Spine 1997; 22:2116–2166.
15. Scheer S, Watanabe T, Radack K. Randomized controlled trials in industrial low back pain. Part 3. Subacute/chronic pain interventions. Arch Phys Med Rehabil 1997; 78:414–423.
16. Twomey L, Taylor J, eds. Physical Therapy of the Low Back. 2nd ed. New York: Churchill Living- stone, 1994.
17. Abenheim L, Rossignol M, Valat J-P, et al. The role of activity in the therapeutic management of back pain. Report of the International Paris Task Force on back pain. Spine 2000; 25:1–33.
18. Battié M. Aerobic fitness and its measurement. Spine 1991; 16:677–678.
19. Biering-Sorensen F, Thomsen C, Hilden J. Risk indicators for low back trouble. Scand J Rehabil Med 1989; 21:151–157.
20. Frost H, Klaber Moffett J, Moser J, Fairbank J. Randomised controlled trial for evaluation of fitness programme for patients with chronic low back pain. Br Med J 1995; 310:151–154.
21. Mannion A, Müntener M, Taimela S, Dvorak J. 1999 Volvo award winner in clinical studies. A ran- domized clinical trial of three active therapies for chronic low back pain. Spine 1999; 24:2435–2448.
22. Van Tulder M, Koes B, Bouter L. Conservative treatment of acute and chronic nonspecific low back pain. A systematic review of randomized controlled trials of the most common interventions. Spine 1997; 22:2128–2156.
23. Edwards B, Zusman M, Hardcastle P, Twomey L, O'Sullivan P, McLean N. A physical approach to the rehabilitation of patients disabled by chronic low back pain. Med J Austr 1992; 156:167–172.
24. Elnaggar I, Nordin M, Sheikhzzadeh A, Parnianpour M, Kahanovitz N. Effects of spinal flexion and extension exercises on low-back pain and spinal mobility in chronic mechanical low back pain patients. Spine 1991; 16:967–972.
25. Lindström I, Ohlund C, Eek C, Wallin L, Peterson L. Mobility, strength and fitness after a graded activity program of patients with subacute low back pain. A randomized prospective clinical study with a behavioral therapy approach. Spine 1992; 17:641–652.
26. Manniche C, Hesselhoe G, Bentzen L, Christensen I, Lundberg E. Clinical trial of intensive muscle training for chronic low back pain. Lancet 1988; 2:1473–1476.
27. Mitchell R, Carmen G. Results of a multicenter trial using an intensive active exercise program for the treatment of acute soft tissue and back injuries. Spine 1990; 15:514–521.
28. Stankovic R, Johnell O. Conservative treatment of acute low back pain: a prospective randomized trial—McKenzie method of treatment versus patient education in mini back school. Spine 1990; 15: 120–123.
29. Hazard R, Fenwick J, Kalisch S, et al. Functional restoration with behavioral support. A one-year prospective study of patients with chronic low-back pain. Spine 1989; 14:157–161.
30. Hildebrandt J, Pfingsten M, Saur P, Jansen J. Prediction of success from a multidisciplinary treat- ment programme for chronic low back pain. Spine 1997; 22:990–1001.
31. Mayer T, Gatchel R, Kishino N, et al. Objective assessement of spine function following industrial injury. A prospective study with comparison group and one-year follow-up. Spine 1985; 10:482–493.
32. O'Sullivan P, Phyty G, Twomey L, Allison G. Evaluation of specific stabilizing exercise in the treat- ment of chronic low back pain with radiologic diagnosis of spondylolysis or spondylolisthesis. Spine 1997; 22:2959–2967.
33. Oland G, Tveiten G. A trial of modern rehabilitation for chronic low-back pain and disability. Vocational outcome and effect of pain modulation. Spine 1991; 16:457–459.

34. Smith S, Mayer T, Gatchell R, Becker T. Quantification of lumbar function. Part 1: isometric and multispeed isokinetic trunk strength measures in sagittal and axial planes in normal subjects. Spine 1985; 10:757–764.
35. Carpenter DM, Nelson BW. Low back strengthening for the prevention and treatment of low back pain. Med Sci Sports Exerc 1999; 31:18–24.
36. O'Sullivan P, Twomey L, Allison G. Dysfunction of the neuro-muscular system in the presence of low back pain—implications for physical therapy management. J Man Manip Ther 1997; 5:20–26.
37. Gardner-Morse M, Stokes I, Laible J. Role of muscles in lumbar spine stability in maximum extension efforts. J Orthop Res 1995; 13:802–808.
38. Gardner-Morse M, Stokes I. The effects of abdominal muscle coactivation on lumbar spine stability. Spine 1998; 23:86–92.
39. Goel V, Kong W, Han J, Weinstein J, Gilbertson L. A combined finite element and optimization investigation of lumbar spine mechanics with and without muscles. Spine 1993; 18:1531–1541.
40. Kaigle A, Holm S, Hansson T. Experimental instability in the lumbar spine. Spine 1995; 20:421–430.
41. Wilke H, Wolf S, Claes L, Arand M, Wiesend A. Stability increase of the lumbar spine with different muscle groups. A biomechanical in vitro study. Spine 1995; 20:192–198.
42. Panjabi M. The stabilising system of the spine: Part I, function, dysfunction, adaptation and enhancement. Part II, neutral zone and instability hypothesis. J Spinal Disord 1992; 5:383–397.
43. Quint U, Wilke H-J, Shirazi-Adl A, Parnianpour M, Löer F, Claes LE. Importance of the intersegmental trunk muscles for the stability of the lumbar spine. A biomechanical study in vitro. Spine 1998; 23:1937–1945.
44. Danneels L. Evaluation and rehabilitation of functional spinal stability. Doctoral dissertation, Ghent University, 2001.
45. Cholewicki J, McGill SM. Mechanical stability of the in vivo lumbar spine: implications for injury and chronic low back pain. Clin Biomech 1996; 11:1–15.
46. Lephart S, Fu F. Proprioception and neuromuscular control in joint stability. Hum Kinet, USA, 2000.
47. Cools A, Witvrouw E, Cambier D, Vanderstraeten G. Conservatieve behandeling bij schouderinstabiliteit: belang van functionele neuromusculaire training. Vlaams Tijdsschrift voor Sportgeneeskunde en Wetenschappen 1999; 81:16–30.
48. Danneels L, De Cuyper H, Vanderstraeten G, Cambier D, Witvrouw E. Spierreëducatie bij lage rugklachten. Vlaams Tijdsschrift voor Sportgeneeskunde en Wetenschappen 1999; 81:32–37.
49. Dietz V. Human neuronal control of automatic functional movements: interaction between central programs and afferent input. Physiol Rev 1992; 72:33–69.
50. Kottke F. Therapeutic exercise to develop neuromuscular coordination. In: Kottke F. Lehman, ed. Krusen's Handbook of Physical Medicine and Rehabilitation. Philadelphia: WB Saunders Company, 1990:452–479.
51. Alaranta H, Hurri H, Heliovaara M, Soukka A, Harju R. Non-dynamometric trunk performance tests: reliability and normative data. Scand J Rehabil Med 1994; 26:211–215.
52. Moffroid M. Endurance of trunk muscles in persons with chronic low back pain: assessment, performance, training. J Rehab Res Dev 1997; 34:440–447.
53. Knuttgen H, Komi P. Basic definitions for exercise. In: Komi P, ed. Strength and Power in Sport. Oxford: Blackwell Scientific Publications, 1992:3–6.
54. Alaranta H, Moffroid M, Elmqvist LG, Held J, Pope M, Renstorm P. Postural control of adults with musculoskeletal impairment. Crit Rev Phys Rehab Med 1994; 6:337–370.
55. Alexander K, Kinney LaPier T. Differences in static balance and weight distribution between normal subjects and subjects with chronic unilateral low back pain. JOSPT 1998; 28:378–383.
56. Luoto S, Aalto H, Taimela S, Hurri H, Pyykkö I, Alaranta H. One-footed and externally disturbed two-footed postural control in patients with low back pain and healthy control subjects. Spine 1998; 23:2081–2090.
57. Luoto S, Taimela S, Hurri H, Aalto H, Pyykkö I, Alaranta H. Psychomotor speed and postural in chronic low back pain patients: a controlled follow-up study. Spine 1996; 21:2621–2627.
58. Mientjes M, Frank J. Balance in chronic low back pain patients compared to healthy people under various conditions in upright standing. Clin Biomech 1999; 14:710–716.
59. Sparto P, Parnianpour M, Reinsel T, Simon S. The effect of fatigue on multijoint kinematics, coordination, and postural stability during a repetitive lifting test. JOSPT 1997; 25:3–12.
60. Omino K, Hayashi Y. Preparation of dynamic posture and occurrence of low back pain. Ergonomics 1992; 35:693–707.
61. Troup J, Martin J, Lloyd D. Back pain in industry. A prospective survey. Spine 1981; 6:61–69.
62. Bergmark. Stability of the lumbar spine. A study in mechanical engineering. Acta Orthop Scand 1989; 60:20–24.
63. O'Sullivan P, Twomey L, Allison G. Dynamic stabilization of the lumbar spine. Crit Rev Phys Rehab Med 1997; 9:315–330.
64. Richardson C, Jull G, Hodges P, Hides P. Therapeutic exercise for spinal segmental stabilisation in low back pain. Scientific Basis and Clinical Approach. London: Churchill Livingstone, 1999.

65. Vleeming A, Lee D. In: Proceedings of the Seventh Scientific Conference of the International Federation of Orthopaedic Manipulative Therapists, Perth, Austnepie, 2000:465–491.
66. Crisco J, Panjabi M. The intersegmental and multisegmental muscles of the spine: a biomechanical model comparing lateral stabilising potential. Spine 1991; 7:793–799.
67. Richardson C, Jull G. Muscle control—pain control. What exercises would you prescribe? Manual Ther 1995; 1:2–10.
68. Macintosh J, Valencia F, Bogduk N, Munro R. The morphology of the human lumbar multifidus. Clin Biomech 1986; 1:196–204.
69. Danneels L. Clinical anatomy of the multifidus. In: Vleeming, Stoeckaert, eds. Movement, Stability and Low Back Pain. Elsevier, 2005, in press.
70. Aspden R. Review of the functional anatomy of spinal ligaments and the lumbar erector spinal muscles. Clin Anat 1992; 5:372–387.
71. Vleeming A, Mooney V, Dorman T, Snijders C, Stoeckart R, eds. Movement, Stability and Low Back Pain. The Essential Role of the Pelvis. Edinburgh: Churchill Livingstone, 1997.
72. Bogduk N. Clinical Anatomy of the Lumbar Spine and Sacrum. Edinburgh: Churchill Livingstone, 1997.
73. Danneels L, Vanderstraeten G, Cambier, et al. A functional subdivision of hip, abdominal, and back muscles during asymmetric lifting. Spine 2001; 26:E114–E121.
74. Pollock M, Leggett S, Graves J, et al. Effect of resistance training on lumbar extension strength. Am J Sports Med 1989; 17:624–629.
75. Danneels LA, Vanderstraeten GG, Cambier DC, et al. The effects of three different training modalities in the cross-sectional area of the lumbar multifidus. Brit J Sports Med 2001; 35:186–191.
76. Danneels LA, Vanderstraeten GG, Cambier DC, Witvrouw EE, Bourgois J, De Cuyper HJ. The effects of three different training modalities in the cross-sectional area of the paravertebral muscles and hip flexors. Scand J Sci Sports Med 2001; 11:335–341.
77. Biedermann H. A method for assessing the equivalence of repeated measures of muscle fatigue rates estimated from EMG power spectrum analysis. J Electr Kinet 1991; 1:288–292.
78. Chaffin D, Herrin G, Keyserling W. Preemployment strength testing—an updated position. J Occup Med 1978; 6:403–408.
79. Danneels L, Coorevits P, Cools A, et al. Differences in multifidus and iliocostalis lumborum activity between healthy subjects and patients with subacute and chronic low back pain. Eur Spine J 2002; 11:13–19.
80. Hasue M, Masatoshi F, Kikuch S. A new method of quantitative measurement of abdominal and back muscle strength. Spine 1980; 5:143–148.
81. Mayer T, Smith S, Keeley J, Mooney V. Quantification of lumbar function. Part 2: sagittal plane trunk strength in chronic low-back patients. Spine 1985; 10:765–772.
82. Nordgren B, Scheile R, Linroth K. Evaluation and prediction of back pain during military field service. Scand J Rehabil 1980; 12:1–7.
83. Cooper R, Stokes M, Sweet C, Taylor R, Jayson M. Increased central drive during fatiguing contractions of the paraspinal muscles in patients with chronic low back pain. Spine 1993; 18:610–616.
84. DeLuca C. Use of the surface EMG signal performance evaluation of back muscles. Muscle Nerve 1993; 16:210–216.
85. Nicholaison T, Jorgenson K. Trunk strength, back muscle endurance and low back trouble. Scand J Rehab Med 1985; 17:121–127.
86. Roy S, De Luca C, Casavant D. Lumbar muscle fatigue and chronic lower back pain. Spine 1989; 14:992–1001.
87. Roy S, Luca C, Snyder-Mackler L, Emley M, Crenshaw R, Lyons J. Fatigue, recovery, and low back pain in varsity rowers. Med Sci Sports Exerc 1990; 22:463–469.
88. Hodges P, Richardson C. Delayed postural contraction of the transversus abdominis in low back pain associated with movement of the lower limb. J Spinal Disord 1998; 11:46–56.
89. Hodges P, Richardson C. Inefficient muscular stabilization of the lumbar spine associated with low back pain: a motor control evaluation of transversus abdominis. Spine 1996; 21:2640–2650.
90. Luoto S, Hurri H, Alaranta H. Reaction time in patients with chronic low-back pain. Eur J Phys Med Rehabil 1995; 5:47–50.
91. Brumagne S, Cordo P, Lysens R, Verscheuren S, Swinnen S. The role of paraspinal spindles in lumbosacral position sense in individuals with and without low back pain. Spine 2000; 25:989–994.
92. Gill K, Callaghan M. The measurement of lumbar proprioception in individuals with and without low back pain. Spine 1998; 23:371–377.
93. Addison R, Schultz A. Trunk strengths in patients seeking hospitalisation for chronic low back pain. Spine 1980; 5:539–544.
94. Beimborn D, Morrissey M. A review to the literature related to trunk muscle performance. Spine 1998; 13:655–660.
95. McNeill T, Warwick D, Anderson G, Schultz A. Trunk strengths in attempted flexion, extension and lateral bending in healthy subjects and patients with low-back disorders. Spine 1980; 5:529–538.

96. Grabiner M, Koh, T, Ghazawi AE. Decoupling of bilateral paraspinal excitation in subjects with low back pain. Spine 1992; 17:1219–1223.
97. Holmstrom E, Moritz U, Andersson M. Trunk muscle strength and back muscle endurance in construction workers with and without back pain disorders. Scand J Rehabil Med 1992; 24:3–10.
98. Suzuki N, Endo S. A quantitative study of trunk muscle strength and fatigability in the low-back-pain syndrome. Spine 1983; 8:69–74.
99. Mostardi R, Noe D, Kovacik M, Porterfield J. Isokinetic lifting strength and occupational injury: a prospective study. Spine 1992; 17:189–193.
100. Newton M, Thow M, Somerville D, Henderson I, Waddell G. Trunk strength testing with iso-machines. Part 2: experimental evaluation of Cybex II Back Testing System in normal subjects and patients with chronic low back pain. Spine 1993; 18:812–824.
101. Takemasa R, Yamamoto H, Tani T. Trunk muscle strength in and effect of trunk muscle exercises for patients with chronic low back pain: the differences in patients with and without organic lumbar lesions. Spine 1995; 20:2322–2330.
102. Lee J-H, Hoshino Y, Nakamura K, Kariya Y, Saita K, Ito K. Trunk muscle weakness as a risk factor for low back pain. A 5-year prospective study. Spine 1999; 24:54–57.
103. Hides J, Stokes M, Saide M, Jull G, Cooper D. Evidence of lumbar multifidus muscle wasting ipsilateral to symptoms in patients with acute/subacute low back pain. Spine 1994; 19:165–172.
104. Hodges P, Richardson C. Inefficient muscular stabilization of the lumbar spine associated with low back pain: a motor control evaluation of transversus abdominis. Spine 1996; 21:2640–2650.
105. Hodges P, Richardson C. Delayed postural contraction of the transversus abdominis in low back pain associated with movement of the lower limb. J Spinal Disord 1998; 11:46–56.
106. Danneels LA, Vanderstraeten GG, Cambier DC, Witvrouw EE, De Cuyper HJ. CT imaging of trunk muscles in chronic low back pain patients and healthy control subjects. Eur Spine J 2000; 9:266–272.
107. Barker KL, Shamley DR, Jackson D. Changes in cross-sectional area of multifidus and psoas in patients with unilateral back pain. The relation to pain and disability. Spine 2004; 29:E515–E519.
108. Danneels LA, Cagnie B, Cools A, et al. Intra-operator and inter-operator reliability of surface electromyography in clinical evaluation of back muscles. Manual Ther 2001; 6:145–153.
109. Moffroid MT, Reid S, Henry SM, et al. Some endurance measures in persons with chronic low back pain. J Orthop Sports Phys Ther 1994; 20:81–87.
110. Neurocom® International, Inc. Balance Master Operator's Manual, Version 6.1. Clackamas, OR: Neuromcom® International, Inc., 1998.
111. Brouwer B, Culham E, Liston R, Grant T. Normal variability of postural measures: implications for the reliability of relative balance performance outcomes. Scand J Rehabil Med 1998; 30:131–137.
112. Thompson D, Biedermann H. EMG power spectrum analysis of the paraspinal muscles: long-term reliability. Spine 1993; 18:2310–2313.
113. Mannion A, Dolan P. Electromyographic median frequency changes during isometric contraction of the back extensors to fatigue. Spine 1994; 19:1223–1229.
114. Ng JK-F, Richardson C. Reliability of EMG power spectral analysis of back muscle endurance in healthy subjects. Arch Phys Med Rehabil 1996; 77:259–264.
115. Liston R, Brouwer B. Reliability and validity of measures obtained from stroke patients using the Balance Master. Arch Phys Med Rehabil 1996; 77:425–430.
116. Bogduk N. The anatomical basis for spinal pain syndromes. J Manip Physiol Ther 1995; 18:603–605.
117. Coste J, Paolaggi J, Spira A. Classification of non-specific low back pain II. Clinical diversity of organic forms. Spine 1992; 17:1038–1042.
118. O'Sullivan P. Lumbar segmental instability: clinical presentation and specific stabilizing exercise management. Manual Ther 2000; 5:2–12.
119. Mooney V, Kron M, Rummerfield P, et al. The effect of workplace-based strengthening on low back injury rates: a case study in the strip mining industry. J Occup Rehabil 1995; 5:157–168.
120. Risch S, Norvell N, Pollock M. Lumbar strengthening in chronic low back pain patients: physiologic and psychological benefits. Spine 1993; 18:232–238.
121. Hather B, Tesch P, Buchanan P, et al. Influence of eccentric actions on skeletal muscle adaptations to resistance training. Acta Physiol Scand 1991; 143:177–185.
122. Walker P, Brunotte F, Rouhier-Marcer I, et al. Nuclear magnetic resonance evidence of different muscular adaptations after resistance training. Arch Phys Med Rehabil 1998; 79:1391–1398.

8 Influence of Injury or Fusion of a Single Motion Segment on Other Motion Segments in the Spine

Yuichi Kasai and Atsumasa Uchida
Department of Orthopaedic Surgery, Mie University Graduate School of Medicine, Tsu, Mie, Japan

Takaya Kato, Tadashi Inaba, and Masataka Tokuda
Department of Mechanical Engineering, Mie University, Tsu, Mie, Japan

INTRODUCTION

Since the 1980s, spinal fusion using a pedicle screw system has widely been implemented all over the world, yet many cases with postoperative adjacent segment degeneration have been reported (1–3). An accelerated degenerative change caused by increased motion or load on the motion segments adjacent to the fixed vertebrae is considered to lead to such adjacent segment degeneration (4,5). Changes in adjacent motion segments, such as degeneration of the intervertebral disc and facet joint and segmental instability, occur at the early stage, and failures including spinal canal stenosis, spondylosis, spondylolisthesis, and fracture of the vertebral body are observed at the progressive stage (6).

Among the changes in the motion segments adjacent to the fixed vertebrae, the differentiation between adjacent segment degeneration and adjacent segment disease is required (7). Adjacent segment degeneration refers to a change demonstrated only by image analyses using X-ray examination and magnetic resonance imaging without any clinical symptoms; adjacent segment disease refers to a change with postoperative symptoms newly developed by adjacent segment degeneration. Ghiselli et al. (8) reported that of 215 patients who underwent lumbar spinal fusion, 59 (27.4%) had adjacent segment disease and that additional surgery was performed in 16.5% of the patients five years after surgery and 36.1% 10 years after surgery. Etebar et al. (9) described that 18 (14.4%) of 125 patients who received lumbar spinal fusion had adjacent segment disease that developed mainly on the cranial side of the fixed vertebrae at a mean postoperative time of 26.8 months. They also reported that 4 of the 18 patients with adjacent segment disease developed degeneration of the intervertebral disc, bone fracture, scoliosis, and spondylolisthesis in not only the motion segments adjacent to the fixed vertebrae but also in the motion segments apart from the adjacent motion segments. As shown in this report, fixation of a single motion segment may cause adjacent segment degeneration and adjacent segment disease not only in the adjacent motion segments but also in the motion segments apart from the adjacent motion segments.

In general, biomechanical tests for the spine are carried out to target a single motion segment as a single functional spinal unit but rarely to target multiple motion segments. Therefore, in this study, we conducted a simple compression test on seven consecutive motion segments to investigate the influence of injury or fusion of a single motion segment on other motion segments by examining the effect of spinal deformation generated by compressive pressure on an impaired or fixed motion segment and adjacent motion segments as well as motion segments apart from adjacent motion segments.

METHODS

Thoracolumbar vertebrae harvested from 10 fresh cadaveric wild boars were used in this study. The thoracolumbar vertebrae were first stored and frozen at $-80°C$, and then gradually thawed at room temperature before study. The vertebrae T10 to L5 were carved out and the soft tissue

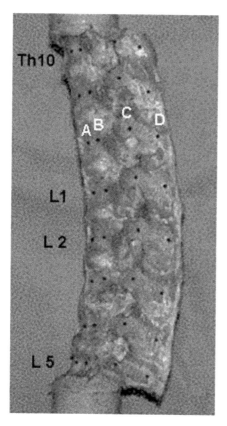

FIGURE 1 Thoracolumbar vertebrae of a cadaveric wild boar.

and muscles surrounding the vertebrae were removed with conservation of the constitutional elements of the functional spinal unit. Because the thoracolumbar vertebrae harvested from wild boars naturally have a kyphotic form, in this study we designated T10/11 as the first motion segment, T11/12 as the second, T12/L1 as the third, L1/2 as the fourth, L2/3 as the fifth, L3/4 as the sixth, and L4/5 as the seventh motion segments to create a series of motion segments to be tested (Fig. 1). Four sites (site A, the anterior vertebral body; site B, the posterior vertebral body; site C, the facet joint; and site D, the tip of the spinous process) were marked with a permanent marker, resulting in markings on eight vertebrae and 32 sites overall.

The three animal models used in this study were as follows: (*i*) normal model, (*ii*) impaired model with total resection of the supraspinous and interspinous ligaments and bilateral facet joints in the fourth motion segment (L1/2), and (*iii*) fusion model of an impaired model that received spinal instrumentation using a pedicle screw system. Texas Scottish Rite Hospital (TSRH®) instrumentation (Medtronic®, Memphis, Tennessee, U.S.A.) were used as the pedicle screw system; this system had a rod that was 4 cm long and 6.3 mm in diameter and a screw that was 30 mm long and 6.5 mm in diameter. During fusion, two screws were inserted into each vertebral body and two rods were attached, followed by the application of compression to the impaired vertebrae (L1/2).

The vertebral subjects to be tested were mounted at both ends with a dental resin (C.G. Dental Product Co. Ltd., Tokyo, Japan) and placed firmly on the Autograph® AG-G precision universal tester (Shimadzu Co., Kyoto, Japan) (Fig. 2). The maximum compressive load was 1000 Newton and loading and unloading were repeated three times at a speed of 0.4 mm/ min, the lowest possible speed, to minimize the relaxation effect derived from viscoelasticity. In the third repetition of 1000 N loading and unloading, digital photos were taken laterally to include all 32 markers on the subjects, with a stationary digital camera.

The digital photos were downloaded into the Microsoft Office Visio® business and technical diagramming program to measure the distance (*d*) between markers on the cranial and

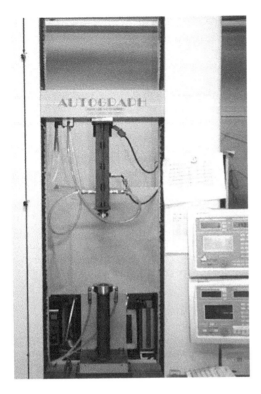

FIGURE 2 Autograph® AG-G.

caudal sides of the adjacent vertebrae (Fig. 3). The displacement magnitude of the distance between markers on the vertebrae was calculated using the following formula: Δd (mm) $= d2 - d1$, where Δd was the displacement magnitude of the distance between markers, $d1$ was the distance between the markers in the unloading condition, and $d2$ was the distance between the markers under 1000 N loading condition. Two researchers uncommitted to this study measured these parameters and the mean values were accepted as Δd. Negative Δd values indicated that motion segments were compressed and positive Δd values indicated that motion segments were extended. For instance, when the displacement magnitude (L1/2D Δd) of the distance between two of the D sites on L1 and L2 was calculated

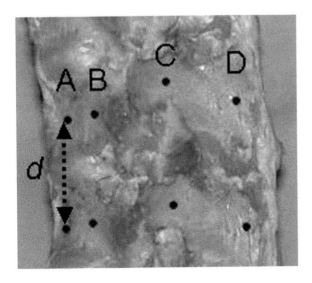

FIGURE 3 The distance (d) of each marker on the cranial or caudal sides of the vertebrae adjacent to each other.

under the condition that $d1$ was 17.28 mm and $d2$ was 12.66 mm, the calculation was as follows: L1/2D $\Delta d = 12.66 - 17.28 = -4.62$ mm, indicating that the motion segment between L1 and L2 was compressed by 1000 N loading to become shorter by 4.62 mm. In this manner, the displacement magnitude of the distance between each pair of specified sites A, B, C, and D on all eight vertebrae was calculated and the spinal deformation generated by a simple compression of 1000 N was evaluated in the seven motion segments. The Student's t-test was used for statistical analyses; P values <0.05 were considered to indicate statistical significance.

RESULTS

The thoracolumbar vertebrae from 10 fresh cadaveric wild boars have a tendency to be compressed in a kyphotic position by a simple compression of 1000 N. The results of a simple compression test for the fourth motion segment (L1/2), the third and fifth motion segments (T12/L1 and L2/3), the second and sixth motion segments (T11/12 and L3/4), and the first and seventh motion segments (T10/11 and L4/5), are shown next. If the difference between the Δd values measured by the two researchers was 0.5 mm or more, it was considered to be "inconsistent;" if the difference was less than 0.5 mm, it was considered to be "consistent." As a result, the Δd values measured by the two researchers were completely consistent (100%).

The Fourth Motion Segment (L1/2)

In the fourth motion segment, L1/2, each of the three models showed negative A Δd and positive D Δd and this motion segment was displaced toward the kyphotic position by 1000 N loading (Fig. 4). When the L1/2D Δd values were compared between the models, the values increased by approximately 2 mm on average in the impaired model compared with the normal model, and the displacement magnitude toward the kyphotic position increased significantly in the impaired model ($P < 0.05$). The L1/2D Δd values decreased approximately by 2 mm on average in the fusion model compared with the normal model and the displacement magnitude toward the kyphotic position decreased significantly in the fusion model ($P < 0.05$). The L1/2D Δd value was significantly greater in the impaired model than in the fusion model ($P < 0.01$).

The Third and Fifth Motion Segments (T12/L1 and L2/3)

In T12/L1 and L2/3, the motion segments adjacent to the impaired or fused vertebrae, each model showed negative A Δd and positive D Δd and all models of T12/L1 and L2/3 were displaced toward the kyphotic position by 1000 N loading (Figs 5, 6). When the T12/L1 D Δd values and L2/3D Δd values were compared between the models, the values increased by approximately 2 mm on average in the impaired model compared with the normal model and the displacement magnitude toward the kyphotic position increased significantly in the impaired model ($P < 0.05$). The D Δd values increased approximately by 3 mm on average

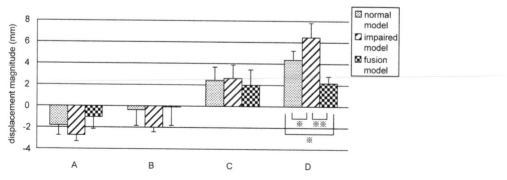

FIGURE 4 Results of the fourth motion segment (L1/2); *$P < 0.05$, **$P < 0.01$. Error bars represent standard deviation. Data of negative A Δd and positive D Δd mean displacement toward kyphotic position.

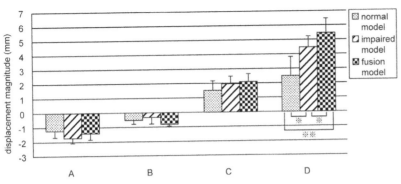

FIGURE 5 Results of the third motion segment (Th12/L1); *P < 0.05, **P < 0.01. Data of negative A Δd and positive D Δd mean displacement toward kyphotic position.

in the fusion model compared with the normal model and the displacement magnitude toward the kyphotic position increased significantly in the fusion model (*P* < 0.01). The D Δd values were significantly greater in the fusion model than in the impaired model (*P* < 0.05).

The Second and Sixth Motion Segments (T11/12 and L3/4)

In T11/12 and L3/4, the motion segments apart from the adjacent motion segments toward the cranial and caudal sides, each model showed negative A Δd and a greater negative D Δd compared with the A Δd, and the motion segments of T11/12 and L3/4 were compressed and slightly displaced toward the lordotic position by 1000 N loading (Figs 7, 8). When the T11/12D Δd values and L3/4D Δd values were compared between the models, the values decreased approximately by 3 mm on average in the impaired model compared with the normal model and the displacement magnitude toward the kyphotic position decreased significantly in the impaired model (*P* < 0.01). The D Δd values decreased by approximately 1 mm in the fusion model compared with the normal model and the displacement magnitude toward the kyphotic position decreased significantly in the fusion model (*P* < 0.05).

The First and Seventh Motion Segments (T10/11 and L4/5)

In T10/11 and L4/5, the motion segments farthest apart from the adjacent motion segments, each model showed negative A Δd and greater negative D Δd compared with the A Δd, and the motion segments of T10/11 and L4/5 were compressed and slightly displaced toward the lordotic position by 1000 N loading (Figs 9, 10). When the T10/11D Δd values and L4/5D Δd values were compared between the models, there was no significant difference.

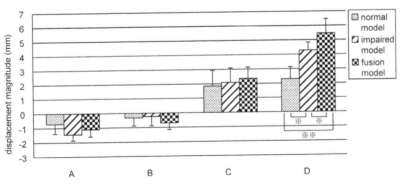

FIGURE 6 Results of the fifth motion segment (L2/3); *P < 0.05, **P < 0.01. Data of negative A Δd and positive D Δd mean displacement toward kyphotic position.

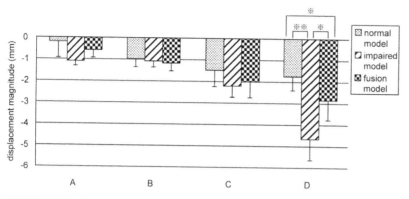

FIGURE 7   Results of the second motion segment (Th11/12); *$P < 0.05$, **$P < 0.01$. Data of negative A Δd and a greater negative D Δd mean displacement toward lordotic position.

DISCUSSION

Lumbar fusion is known to generate adjacent segmental degeneration and adjacent segmental disease in the motion segments adjacent to the fused vertebrae (7,10). Rahm et al. (11) reported that adjacent segmental degeneration occurred in 17 (35%) of 49 patients who received spinal fusion and instrumentation, and Aota et al. (12) described that symptomatic adjacent segment instability appeared in 16 (25%) of 65 patients who underwent spinal fusion. Such failure of the motion segments adjacent to the fused vertebrae has also been observed in the cervical vertebrae. Kulkari et al. (13) reported that 33 (75%) of 44 patients who received anterior cervical discectomy and fusion (ACDF) had degeneration two years after surgery, and Ishihara et al. (14) described that 19 (17%) of 112 patients who underwent ACDF developed symptomatic degeneration, with disease-free survival rates of 89% five years after surgery and 84% 10 years after surgery.

The cause of these changes, which occurred in the motion segments of the lumbar and cervical vertebrae adjacent to the fixed vertebrae, is considered not to be aging but to be an accelerated spinal degeneration induced by the altered movement of the facet joint or the internal pressure of the intervertebral disc, disorders which were because of solid spinal fusion (7,8). It is believed that because the motion segments fixed locally in a kyphotic position can lead to a slightly excessive lordotic position of the motion segment adjacent to the cranial side of a fixed vertebra, contracture of the facet joint and failure of the posterior ligamentous complex may easily occur (15,16).

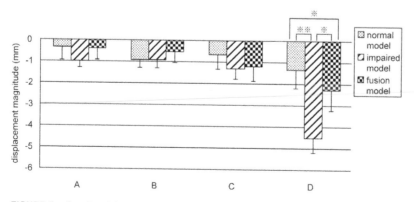

FIGURE 8   Results of the sixth motion segment (L3/4); *$P < 0.05$, **$P < 0.01$. Data of negative A Δd and a greater negative D Δd mean displacement toward lordotic position.

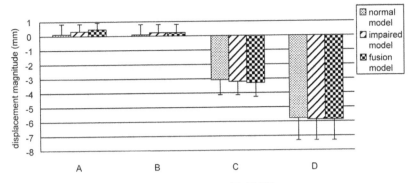

FIGURE 9   Results of the first motion segment (Th10/11).

Numerous factors reported to render the adjacent motion segments degenerative (9,17,18) may be classified into two groups: factors not directly affecting the adjacent motion segments and factors contained in the adjacent motion segments themselves before surgery. Factors not directly affecting the adjacent motion segments include advanced age, female sex, menopause, osteoporosis, patients receiving interbody fusion, patients with a long follow-up period after surgery, patients undergoing multiple operations, and patients undergoing multiple intervertebral fusion. Factors involving the adjacent motion segments themselves include preoperative instability of motion segments, a high degeneration of the intervertebral disc, spinal canal stenosis, degeneration of the facet joint, and localized kyphosis and/or scoliosis.

The results obtained in this study showed that in T12/L1 and L2/3, the motion segments adjacent to the fused vertebrae, the impaired and fusion models showed negative A Δd and positive D Δd; these data indicate that elevation of the internal pressure of the intervertebral disc in the adjacent motion segments and failure of the posterior ligamentous complex may readily occur in the impaired and fusion models. In T11/T12 and L3/4, the motion segments apart from the adjacent motion segments, the impaired and fusion models showed significantly negative D Δd compared with the normal model, indicating that there is an influence of injury or fusion on the motion segments apart from the adjacent motion segments.

Our results showed that owing to injury of a single motion segment, the displacement magnitude toward the kyphotic position increases in an impaired motion segment and its adjacent motion segments and decreases in the motion segments apart from the adjacent motion segments; furthermore, because of fixation of an impaired motion segment with a pedicle screw system, the displacement magnitude toward the kyphotic position slightly decreases in the fixed motion segments, largely increases in the adjacent motion segments, and decreases in the motion segments apart from the adjacent motion segments. These results reveal that a displacement occurring in a single motion segment generates another displacement of other

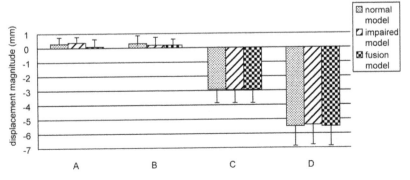

FIGURE 10   Results of the seventh motion segment (L4/5).

motion segments that can adjust the aberrant position of the single motion segment to normal. Untch et al. (19) performed an in vitro study using cadaveric human lumbar vertebrae and showed that the range of motion of L3/L4 increased by approximately 15% in an L4/S1 fusion model compared with an L4/L5 fusion model. These results indicate that an increase in the range of motion may result from the adjustment effect mentioned here. Taken together, such increase in the range of motion burdens the adjacent motion segments with a high load and adjacent segmental degeneration may progress.

In this study, the results from the tests using the first and seventh motion segments were considered to be affected by the experimental condition that these motion segments were located at the ends of the entire vertebral column used and were mounted and held firmly at both ends. Thus, creating a longer series of motion segments using 10 vertebrae (from T9 to L6) and mounting T9 and L6 with resin to fix them on an experimental board may reduce such unfavorable influence. The thoracolumbar vertebrae of the wild boar used in this study naturally have a kyphotic form; thus, for further studies, we will use human thoracolumbar vertebrae and carry out similar biomechanical studies using multiple motion segments.

CONCLUSIONS

Our results showed that deformity or displacement caused by injury or fusion of a single motion segment generates another displacement of other motion segments, which can adjust the aberrant position of the single motion segment to normal, and that injury or fusion of a single motion segment has an influence on not only the adjacent motion segment but also on the motion segments apart from the adjacent motion segments.

REFERENCES

1. Brunet JA, Wiley JJ. Acquired spondylosis after spinal fusion. J Bone Joint Surg (Br) 1984; 66(5):720–724.
2. Lehmann TR, Spratt KF, Tozzi JE, et al. Long-term follow-up of lower lumbar fusion patients. Spine 1987; 12(2):97–104.
3. Brodsky AE, Hendricks RL, Khalil MA, et al. Segmental ("floating") lumbar spine fusions. Spine 1989; 14(4):447–450.
4. Ha KY, Schendel MJ, Lewis JL, et al. Effect of immobilization and configuration on lumbar adjacent segment biomechanics. J Spinal Disord 1993; 6(2):99–105.
5. Weinhoffer SL, Guyer RD, Herbert M, et al. Intradiscal pressure measurements above an instrumented fusion. A cadaveric study. Spine 1995; 20(5):526–531.
6. Eck JC, Humphreys SC, Hodges SD. Adjacent segment degeneration after lumbar fusion: a review of clinical, biomechanical, and radiologic studies. Am J Orthop 1999; 28(6):336–340.
7. Hilibrand AS, Robbins M. Adjacent segment degeneration and adjacent segment disease: the consequences of spinal fusion? Spine J 2004; 4(6 suppl):190S–194S.
8. Ghiselli G, Wang JC, Bhatia NH, et al. Adjacent segment degeneration in the lumbar spine. J Bone Joint Surg Am 2004; 86-A(7):1497–1503.
9. Etebar S, Cahill DW. Risk factors for adjacent segment failure following lumbar fixation with rigid instrumentation for degenerative instability. J Neurosurg (Spine 2) 1999; 90:163–169.
10. Chen WJ, Lai PL, Tai CL, et al. The effect of sagittal alignment on adjacent joint mobility after lumbar instrumentation—a biomechanical study of lumbar vertebrae in a porcine model. Clin Biomech 2004; 19(8):763–768.
11. Rahm MD, Hall BB. Adjacent segment degeneration after lumbar fusion with instrumentation: a retrospective study. J Spinal Disord 1996; 9(5):392–400.
12. Aota Y, Kumano K, Hirabayashi S. Postfusion instability at the adjacent segments after rigid pedicle screw fixation for degeneration lumbar spinal disorders. J Spinal Disord 1995; 8(6):464–473.
13. Kulkarni V, Rajshekhar V, Raghuram L. Accelerated spondylotic changes adjacent to the fused segment following central corpectomy: magnetic response imaging study evidence. J Neurosurg 2004; 100(1 suppl Spine):2–6.
14. Ishirara H, Kanamori M, Kawaguchi Y, et al. Adjacent segment disease after anterior cervical interbody fusion. Spine J 2004; 4(6):624–628.
15. Umehara S, Zindrick MR, Patwardhan AG, et al. The biomechanical effect of postoperative hypolordosis in instrumented lumbar fusion on instrumented and adjacent spinal segments. Spine 2000; 25(13):1617–1624.

16. Lai PL, Chen LH, Niu CC, et al. Relation between laminectomy and development of adjacent segment instability after lumbar fusion with pedicle fixation. Spine 2004; 29(22):2527–2532.

17. Oda I, Cunningham BW, Buckley RA, et al. Does spinal kyphotic deformity influence the biomechanical characteristics of the adjacent motion segments? An in vivo animal model. Spine 1999; 24(20):2139–2146.

18. Sudo H, Oda I, Abumi K, et al. In vitro biomechanical effects of reconstruction on adjacent motion segment: comparison of aligned/kyphotic posterolateral fusion with aligned posterior lumbar interbody fusion/posterolateral fusion. J Neurosurg 2003; 99(2 suppl):221–228.

19. Untch C, Liu Q, Hart R. Segmental motion adjacent to an instrumented lumbar fusion: the effect of extension of fusion to the sacrum. Spine 2004; 29(21):2376–2381.

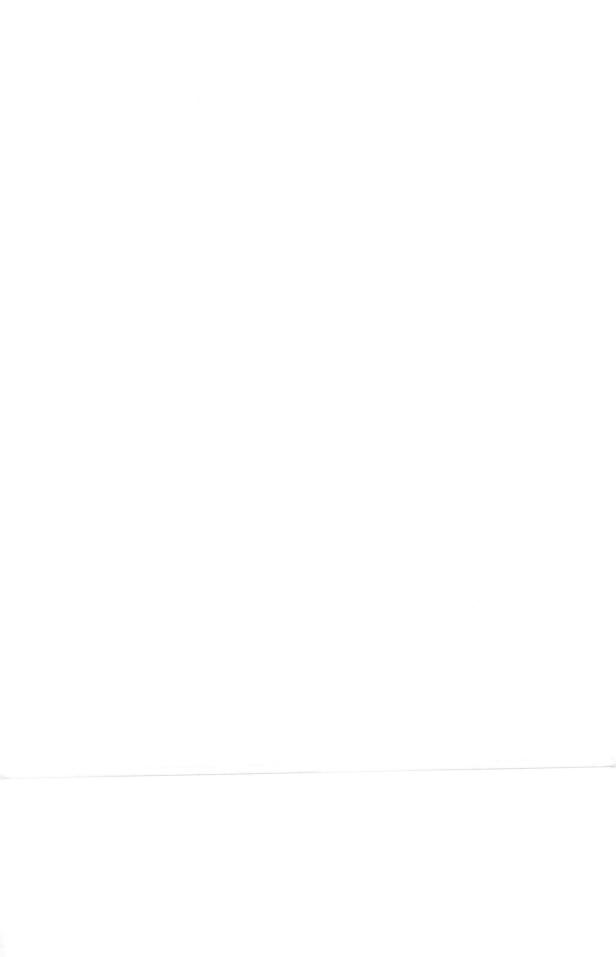

9 Degenerative Disease Adjacent to Spinal Fusion

Patrick W. Hitchon, Timothy Lindley, and Stephanie Beeler
Department of Neurosurgery, University of Iowa, Carver College of Medicine, Iowa City, Iowa, U.S.A.

Brian Walsh
University of Wisconsin, Madison, Wisconsin, U.S.A.

Ghassan Skaf
American University of Beirut, Beirut, Lebanon

INTRODUCTION

Adjacent degenerative disease (ADD) to spinal fusion has long been recognized and suspected (Figs. 1,2). With the advancement of spinal instrumentation, ADD has become an issue with which to contend when recommending spinal fusion to patients who are candidates for spinal fusion. In 1988, Lee (1) reported on 18 patients who had developed ADD at least one year following lumbar fusion. The range prior to the development of ADD was 3 to 38 years with a mean of 15.2 years. Eleven of these patients had developed new symptoms within five years of their fusion. With the exception of one, the rest had developed ADD above the lumbar fusion. Nine patients were treated with extension of the initial spinal fusion to include the adjacent level. Four of these same cases required a third operation for ADD above the second fusion.

In 1994, Whitecloud et al. (2) reported on 14 patients who required decompression and fusion for ADD. Surgery was undertaken at an average of 11.5 years from the first operation with a range of 3 to 29 years. The first five revision surgeries consisted of noninstrumented fusion with four of the five patients developing psudoarthrosis. Three of the five went on to undergo instrumented revisions. Thus, the next nine patients underwent instrumented fusion of the adjacent degenerated level.

Two years later, Schlegel et al. (3) reported 58 patients who presented with pathology adjacent to a previous thoracic or lumbar fusion after a symptom-free period of 13.1 years. The diagnoses of ADD included stenosis, disc herniation, and instability. Thirty-seven of these patients had a two-year follow-up. Fourteen of these underwent decompression and fusion, whereas 23 underwent decompression only. Seven of these required further surgery. In three, decompression was performed followed at a later time by fusion. Two underwent decompression and fusion that required revision. The last two had their hardware removed. Outcomes were described as good to excellent in 70%.

In 1998, Hambly et al. (4) reported on a retrospective study in which 42 patients who had undergone a posterolateral lumbar fusion and were followed for a mean of 22.6 years. Fusion patients were compared with a gender-matched cohort that had not undergone surgery. The comparison revealed an increase in the range of motion at the first and second adjacent levels in the fusion group compared with the control, although the difference was not significant. An increase in the development of osteophytes at the first and second levels above the fusion was noted compared with controls. This increase reached significance at the second level above the fusion. Unfortunately the control group, though nonoperative, were patients under the care of Dr. Wiltse for back pain, ant their exact number is unclear.

Adjacent degenerative disease has also been described in the cervical spine. In 1999, Hillibrand et al. (5) described 374 patients who underwent 409 anterior cervical fusions for degenerative disease. There were 168 one-level fusions, 131 two-level fusions, 37 three-level fusions, 2 four-level fusions, and 71 who underwent corpectomy and fusion.

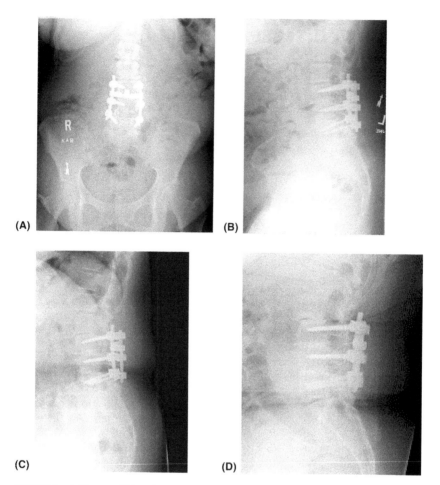

FIGURE 1 A 77-year-old female presents with neurogenic claudication, back and leg pain. The magnetic resonance image (MRI) from August 20, 2003 showed stenosis at L4-5. Plain films demonstrated instability at L3-4 as well as L4-5. On October 17, 2004, she underwent L3, L4, and L5 laminectomy, L3-4 and L4-5 discectomy, interbody fusion, pedicle screw fixation, and posterolateral fusion. (**A**) and (**B**) show anteroposterior or lateral radiographs obtained 5 days postoperative. (**C**) Five months later, she is symptomatic with lumbar pain aggravated by exercise. Gradual degeneration at L2-3 is noted with loss in height and the development of osteophytes (March 1, 2005). (**D**) A year later, her symptoms are worsening. Radiographs demonstrate progressive degeneration at L2-3 (October 24, 2005). She was offered extension of her fusion but declined.

Symptomatic ADD developed at adjacent levels in 55 of the 374 patients for an overall prevalence of 14.2%. New ADD developed at a rate of 2.9% per year, for a prevalence of 12% at five years and 19% at 10 years. Forty-six of the 55 patients had a two-year follow-up, and of these 27 required surgery. Kaplan-Meir survivorship analysis suggests that subsequent to anterior cervical fusion, 14% of patients will develop ADD within five years, and 26% within 10 years.

CLINICAL MATERIALS AND METHODS

To explore the incidence of ADD at our institution, lumbar fusions undertaken between 2000 and 2002 were reviewed. A total of 58 lumbar spine fusions were performed in 20 males and 38 females, with a mean age of 54 years. There were 50 posterior and 8 anterior fusions. During 46.2 months of follow-up, reoperation for adjacent degenerative disease was undertaken in four patients, and reinstrumentation at the same level in two, for an overall reoperation rate of 10% at a mean of 18 months. Examples of the need for extension of spinal fusion are shown in Figures 1 and 2. Both these patients are not included in our patient population described previously as they underwent surgery subsequent to 2002. Three patients (5.2%) required reoperation for infection, seroma, or dural repair. Over the same period, laminectomy was performed in 103 patients, 60 males, and 43 females, with a mean age of 67. Of these, reoperation was required in four (4%) at a mean of 11.4 months with instrumentation being used in all. Though this a small series with a relatively short follow-up, the results suggest that fusion is twice as likely as laminectomy to require subsequent surgery. The majority of reoperations in fused cases were for ADD.

DISCUSSION

The basis of ADD lies in the hypermobility and stress at adjacent levels as a result of spinal instrumentation and eventual fusion. Over the past 20 years, this has been demonstrated in

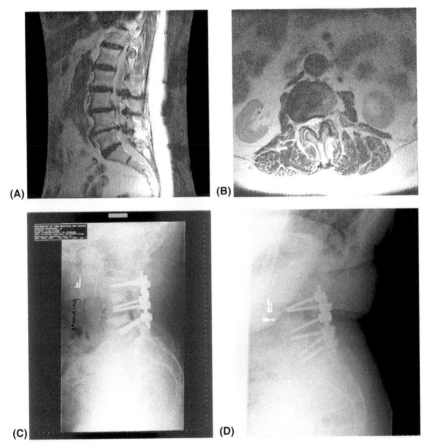

FIGURE 2   (**A**) 82-year-old female with neurogenic claudication, low back pain with radiation into the left leg. Magnetic resonance image (MRI) from August 1, 2003 reveals a grade-one spondylolisthesis of L3 on L4. There is advanced degenerative disease and disc desiccation at L3-4 and L4-5. There is also a herniated disc at L3-4 on the left side. (**B**) The L2-3 level on MRI from August 1, 2003 is of normal caliber without stenosis. (**C**) On August 22, 2003, the patient underwent L3-L4-L5 laminectomies, interbody fusion, pedicle screw fixation, and posterolateral fusion. (**D**) She had been doing well up until a month before her return on June 9, 2005. She then started experiencing pain, aggravated by walking and standing. She had been to the emergency room twice, and was started on hydrocodone. (**E**) Lumbar sagittal MRI on June 9, 2005 shows stenosis at L2-3, which had not been noted on earlier studies. (**F**) Axial MRI on June 9, 2005 shows L2-3 stenosis. (**G**) On June 14, 2005, the patient underwent L2-3 interbody fusion with extension of her fusion to L1. Following a month's stay in skilled care, the patient's symptoms improved. She is off narcotics and still lives on her own. Radiographs from August 4, 2005 are shown. (*E, F, and G on next page.*)

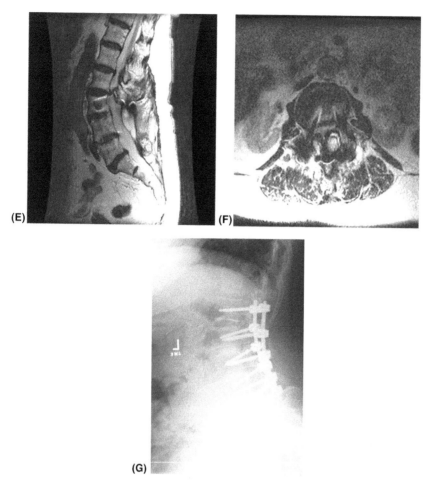

FIGURE 2 *Continued.*

many in vitro studies with both human and calf spines. In 1984, Lee et al. (6) studied 16 human cadaveric spines. Spines from L3 to S2 were subjected to displacement-controlled flexion to 20° while applying a dead weight of 29 lbs anteriorly, and 21 lbs posterior to the specimens. Spines were tested in the intact state and after anterior, posterior, or lateral instrumentation at L5-S1. With this paradigm, an increase in motion in mm, though inconsistent, was noted at both L3-4 and L4-5.

A second study by Yogandan et al. (7) was conducted in seven T11-L5 cadaveric spines subjected to compressive fractures at L1, L2, or L3. The spines were retested under the same compressive load after pedicle screw instrumentation one level proximal and one level distal to the fracture. Anterior and posterior motions of the vertebrae were measured with retroreflective markers in mm. Under loading, a decrease in motion of the disc spaces across the fixated levels was noted. An increase in anterior and posterior motions was seen at levels proximal and distal to fixation. Fixation of the spine thus resulted in an increase in motion at adjacent levels, which the authors believed could contribute to "hypermobility and degeneration."

Intradiscal pressure readings have been taken in cadaveric spines adjacent to instrumentation (8). Six spines with intradiscal pressure transducers placed at L3-4 and L4-5 underwent displacement-controlled flexion of 20° to 40°. Measurements were made in the intact state and after pedicle screw fixation first at L5-S1, and again after L4-S1. In this set-up, with flexion, intradiscal pressure increased more than in the intact state as the number of levels of fixation increased. To the authors, this increase in intradiscal pressure was a reflection of the increase in flexibility above instrumentation. The authors hypothesized that "this force transmission may also account for the many reports of accelerated degeneration in adjacent discs."

In the study by Chow et al. (9), six cadaveric spines from L1 to S3 were tested in the intact state, after L4-5, and L4-S1 anterior interbody fixation. Pressure transducers were inserted into the L1-2, L2-3, L3-4 disc spaces, and into L5-S1 when simulating an L4-5 fusion. The spines were subjected to controlled flexion of 20°, and extension of 10°. An increase in segmental mobility and intradiscal pressure at L1-2, L2-3, L3-4, and L5-S1 was noted in flexion and extension. With the fusion extended to include L5-S1, the increases in flexion and extension motions and intradiscal pressure were greater than had been noted with a single-level simulated fusion. The interpretation of the authors was that "fusion of part of the spine throws extra stress onto neighboring unfused segments, and that the longer and stiffer the fusion mass, the greater the stress."

Motion at levels adjacent to instrumentation was conducted in 18 calf spines from L3 to the sacrum (10). Displacement-controlled axial rotation, flexion and extension, and lateral bending were applied before and after posterior instrumentation at L4-5, L4-L6, and L4-S1. Instrumented constructs produced higher displacement values in all three planes at the rostral adjacent mobile segment. The caudal mobile segment also showed increased rotation with instrumentation. The longer instrumented constructs were associated with greater motion at the adjacent mobile segments. Thus, "application of instrumentation changes the motion pattern of adjacent segments, and these changes become more distinct with the extent and rigidity of the construct."

Similar studies have been performed in the cervical cadaveric spine by Eck et al. (11). Six cadaveric spines were fixed at T1 and underwent controlled flexion at C3 of 20°, and controlled extension of 15°. Intradiscal pressures were recorded at C4-5 and C6-7 in the intact state and after anterior plating at C5-6. Motion increased above and below the instrumented segment in both flexion and extension. Also, intradiscal pressures increased at adjacent levels in flexion and extension. The authors concluded that by "eliminating motion, fusion shifts the load to adjacent levels causing earlier disc degeneration."

SUMMARY

This review of our clinical material and the literature, reveals unequivocally that spinal fusion is associated with an increased need to undergo further surgery and or fusion in the following 5 to 10 years. This rate of reoperation is in the order of 10% to 20%. The biomechanical data attributes ADD to stresses upon adjacent levels brought about by increased motion and intradiscal pressure adjacent to the fusion. It is this need for additional surgery that should temper the enthusiasm of a surgeon to offer, and the patient to accept, spinal fusion as a treatment modality for spinal disease. Spinal instrumentation and fusion remains a valuable tool in the treatment of degenerative disease or instability when associated with severe and intractable pain, or is accompanied with neurological deficit.

REFERENCES

1. Lee CK. Accelerated degeneration of the segment adjacent to lumbar fusion. Spine 1988; 13(3):375–377.
2. Whitecloud TS, Davis JM, Olive PM. Operative treatment of the degenerated segment adjacent to a lumbar fusion. Spine 1994; 19(5):531–536.
3. Schlegel JD, Smith JA, Schleusener RL. Lumbar motion segment pathology adjacent to thoracolumbar, lumbar, and lumbosacral fusions. Spine 1996; 21(8):970–981.
4. Hambly MF, Wiltse LL, Raghavan N, et al. The transition zone above a lumbosacral fusion. Spine 1998; 23(16):1785–1792.
5. Hilibrand AS, Carlson GD, Palumbo MA, et al. Radiculopathy and myelopathy at segments adjacent to the site of previous anterior cervical arthrodesis. J Bone Joint Surg Am 1999; 81-A(4):519–528.
6. Lee CK, Langrana NA. Lumbosacral spinal fusion. Spine 1984; 9(6):574–581.
7. Yoganandan N, Pintar F, Maiman DJ, et al. Kinematics of the lumbar spine following pedicle screw plate fixation. Spine 1993; 18(4):504–512.

8. Weinhoffer SL, Guyer RD, Herber M, et al. Intradiscal pressure measurements above an instrumented fusion. Spine 1995; 20(5):526–531.
9. Chow DH, Luk KD, Evans JH, et al. Effects of short anterior lumbar interbody fusion on biomechanics of neighboring unfused segments. Spine 1996; 21(5):549–555.
10. Shono Y, Kaneda K, Abumi K, et al. Stability of posterior spinal instrumentation and its effects on adjacent motion segments in the lumbosacral spine. Spine 1998; 23(14):1550–1558.
11. Eck JC, Humphreys SC, Lim TH, et al. Biomechanical study on the effect of cervical spine fusion on adjacent-level intradiscal pressure and segmental motion. Spine 2002; 27(22):2431–2434.

10 | Adjacent Segment Degeneration

Adrian P. Jackson
Premier Spine Care, Overland Park, Kansas, U.S.A.

Joseph H. Perra
Twin Cities Spine Center, Minneapolis, Minnesota, U.S.A.

For as long as spinal fusions have been performed, there have been questions regarding the fate of the segments adjacent to the fusion. The term "adjacent segment degeneration" is loosely defined as degenerative changes that occur at the mobile spinal segment immediately above or below a previously fused segment or segments. The first published report of adjacent segment degeneration was in 1956 (1). Since that time, there have been more than 300 articles published pertaining to the definition, diagnosis, outcomes, and treatment of adjacent segment degeneration. There are several reports that have described degeneration adjacent to noninstrumented fusions (2,3,4), but the large majority of the descriptions refer to segments adjacent to an instrumented fusion (5,6,7,8). Recent advances in motion-sparing surgery have spurned even more interest in risk factors for and treatment of adjacent segment degeneration. The industry for disc arthroplasty has described motion preservation as a primary advantage of the artificial disc over fusion for degenerative conditions. Data exists both supporting and refuting this claim, but a question remains. Does fusion truly increase the rate of adjacent segment degeneration, or is it just a passive player present in a patient that is "preprogrammed" to degenerate at those levels regardless?

The first issue addressed should be the definition of adjacent segment degeneration. This can be somewhat problematic as there is a lack of uniformity in the literature. The broad definition includes any abnormality in the mobile segment adjacent to a previous spinal fusion. Disc degeneration (9,10,11), instability (12), facet arthrosis (13), scoliosis (14), and spinal stenosis (15) were the most common pathologies identified at the adjacent segment. In a few select publications, adjacent segment degeneration was not identified in the most adjacent mobile segment, rather in segments separated from the fusion by other segments, with or without degeneration (16,17). This highlights the lack of a uniform definition in the current literature.

Possible risk factors include instrumented fusion, fusion length (6,13,18), sagittal contour (15), degenerative disc disease, spinal stenosis, preexisting degenerative disc disease at the adjacent segment (19,20), age (21,22), facet joint injury (8,22), interbody fusion (21), and postmenopausal females (7). There are several proposed etiologies for adjacent segment degeneration. Mechanical, biological, and iatrogenic causes have all been considered. Instrumented fusions have also been proposed to increase the risk of adjacent segment degeneration compared with uninstrumented fusions, although this remains marginally supported in the literature and reports to the contrary exist.

Postsurgical sagittal malalignment has been shown to change the loading characteristics of a cadaveric model, shifting the shear forces to the adjacent intervertebral disc, and excessive loading of the posterior column, particularly the facet joints (23,24,25). Most surgeons would agree with the biomechanical conclusion that fusion places additional stress on the adjacent mobile segments, and at least in theory, contributes to the degeneration of those levels. In 1984, Lee and Langrana examined the mechanical effects of a midline, anterior interbody, and posterior intertransverse lumbosacral fusion in a cadaveric model on the adjacent motion segment (26). Compression–flexion loads were exerted on the L3-S1 cadaveric spine before and after the simulated fusion. Flexion to 20°, followed by extension to neutral was performed. They noted a shift in the center of rotation in the fused models increasing the stresses on both the adjacent intervertebral disc and facet joints. Furthermore, in a cadaveric model, Cunningham found a significant increase in intradiscal pressures adjacent to pedicular instrumented lumbar spines (23). Up to 45% increased pressures were demonstrated with the simulated instrumented posterior spinal fusions. Numerous other in vitro studies have shown similar conclusions in both human cadaveric models and in animal models. More importantly, Dekutoski, in an in vivo dog model demonstrated increased facet motion at the proximal adjacent segment with lumbar fusion (12). In an in vivo mouse model, static compressive loading of the disc causing increased intradiscal pressure led to the development of disc degeneration (27). As may be expected based on the cadaveric and animal studies, radiographic analyses of posterior fusion patients likewise showed an increase in mobility at the segments adjacent to the fusion, particularly the cephalad-adjacent segment. In a prospective clinical study, Axelsson radiographically demonstrated increased mobility in the cephalad-adjacent segment after an uninstrumented posterior intertransverse spinal fusion (28). The fusion of more than two segments has been thought to lead to adjacent segment degeneration more often than single-level fusions. The extended lever arm of a long fusion has been biomechanically shown to increase the stress at the adjacent motion segment (13). Based on a mechanical theory of wear with increased repetitive motion, one may assume an increased rate of adjacent segment degeneration. This assumption remains to be demonstrated conclusively in the literature. The majority of the literature on adjacent segment degeneration is Class III data. There is a lack of reliable Class I data demonstrating a link between the mechanical alterations of lumbar spinal fusion and the development of adjacent segment degeneration.

Degenerative disc disease or spinal stenosis as an etiology for the index fusion procedure has been shown to predispose to future adjacent segment surgery, which supports the theory that a disc that has pre-existing degenerative changes will continue to deteriorate under additional stress (20). Penta evaluated 108 patients who underwent anterior lumbar interbody fusion with both magnetic resonance imaging (MRI) and plain radiographs at a minimum of 10 years postfusion (29). The plain radiography was used to determine fusion status, and the MRI to assess the adjacent disc integrity. The incidence of adjacent segment disc pathology was found to be independent of the presence of a solid anterior interbody fusion, fusion to the sacrum, or the length of the fusion. Similar conclusions have been reached by Lehmann and Frymoyer in independent studies (30,31). Lehmann reported an incidence of cephalad-adjacent segment spinal stenosis of 30% at 21-year follow-up. At 10-year follow-up, Frymoyer reported 5% radiographic adjacent segment disc disease following spinal fusion. Interestingly, in 1992, Van Horn retrospectively evaluated an age and gender matched pair of patients at 16-year follow-up after anterior spinal fusion (32). They demonstrated radiographic degenerative changes in the adjacent discs at rates comparable with the general population. Seitsalo evaluated 227 patients with surgically and conservatively managed spondylolisthesis with no significant difference in adjacent segment disease (33). Hambly reached a similar conclusion in 42 patients with a posterolateral spinal fusion (34). Most spinal fusions are performed for severe degenerative disease that is unlikely isolated to only the treated segment(s). Many authors have reached the conclusion that adjacent segment disease is nothing more than a continuation of normal degenerative changes, independent of the biomechanical changes associated with spinal fusion. The truth probably lies somewhere in between.

Age-related changes have often been implicated in the development of adjacent segment degeneration. Aota found that the incidence of adjacent segment degeneration was much higher in patients over 55 years of age at the time of the index fusion (8). A recent meta-analysis explored the published risk factors contributing to adjacent segment disease following a lumbar fusion. Age was the only consistent, uncontradicted risk factor for radiographic adjacent segment degeneration. Proponents of adjacent segment degeneration's independence to fusion attribute this finding to a likely continuum of the degenerative disease process. Instrumented arthrodesis, length of fusion, sagittal alignment, degenerative disc disease, spinal stenosis, pre-existing degenerative disc disease, facet joint injury, interbody fusion, and the postmenopausal osteoporotic female were all relative risks, but contradictory reports exist for all but age. One of the long established, proposed risk factors is the presence of an instrumented arthrodesis. However, Wiltse found a decreased incidence of adjacent segment degeneration in patients who underwent instrumented arthodesis compared with uninstrumented spinal fusion (22). Small differences in patient groups, including age and length of follow-up have been proposed as possibilities for these results and those of other contradictory studies. However, this raises the possibility that instrumented arthrodesis or length of arthrodesis may be independent variables in their contribution to adjacent segment degeneration.

Iatrogenic facet joint injury has also been implicated as a factor in facet joint degeneration. Placement of pedicle screws at the cephalad junctional segment can injure either the facet capsule or the inferior articular process of the superior adjacent segment, leading to facet arthrosis. As established by biomechanical studies, fusion alters the normal axis of flexion and extension of the lumbar spine. This leads to increased stress transferred to the posterior column, most notably the facet joints (13). Increased load at an iatrogenically injured facet joint may contribute to accelerated degeneration of that level. This is theorized to be a contributing factor to the increased rate of adjacent segment degeneration seen at the cephalad segment as compared with the caudad segment with pedicular instrumented spinal fusion (8). With this in mind, surgeons should be vigilant in the preservation of the cephalad-adjacent facet joint and capsule during pedicle screw placement.

Another difficulty in quantifying the clinical significance of adjacent segment degeneration is uniformity in the outcomes measures. Most published reports of adjacent segment disease assess radiographic pathology. There are few reports that correlate radiographic disease with clinical impact, which is ultimately the measure of importance. Interbody fusion combined with posterolateral arthrodesis demonstrated an increased risk for adjacent segment degeneration in several reports. This was, in theory, the result of increased rigidity. These studies were all based on radiographic changes and not clinical outcome. In 2004, Okuda attempted to limit clinical variables by reviewing patients who underwent posterior lumbar interbody fusion (PLIF) without posterolateral fusion at L4/5 for degenerative spondylolisthesis (35). At a minimum of two-year follow-up, 29% of the 87 patients showed radiographic signs of increased/continued degeneration at L3/4. Sixty-seven percent of the original group showed no radiographic progression of L3/4 degeneration. None of the patients demonstrated progression of degeneration below the L4/5 fusion. In the final analysis, there was no correlation of radiographic findings to clinical outcome. There is a consistent conclusion of radiographic degeneration after a lumbar arthrodesis, in retrospective reviews. Radiographic evidence of adjacent segment degeneration has never been clearly correlated to clinical outcome. There is an assumption that radiographic evidence of adjacent segment degeneration precedes symptomatic adjacent segment degeneration. It is fairly well accepted in the literature that sagittal instability is present when there is radiographic translation of 3–4 mm or angular changes of 10° to 15° with flexion/extension (36). Even when radiographic instability is present, there is no consistent correlation to a poor clinical outcome. The question remains—when does adjacent segment degeneration matter? There is little debate that adjacent segment degeneration happens. It is unclear in the current literature, however, when and why it happens?

One interesting issue not addressed in the current literature is whether nonfusion lumbar spinal surgery predisposes to adjacent segment degeneration. Currently, unpublished data suggests that at 10-year follow-up, the rates of adjacent segment fusion for adjacent segment degeneration are similar with both fusion and nonfusion index procedures, 20% and 17%, respectively (37,38). In addition, the only risk factors that were predictive of adjacent segment fusion were preoperative disc desiccation at the adjacent segment and a positive smoking history at the time of the index procedure. The fact is, no surgeon currently knows how to accurately predict which patient is likely to develop symptomatic adjacent segment degeneration or how to avoid its development. The increased interest in alternative procedures to fusion has been largely driven by the hope that this will limit or eliminate adjacent segment degeneration by preserving motion. This fact remains to be shown conclusively.

REFERENCES

1. Anderson CE. Spondyloschisis following spine fusion. J Bone Joint Surg Am 1956; 38:1142–1146.
2. Axelsson P, Johnsson R, Stromqvist B, et al. Posterolateral lumbar fusion. Outcome of 71 consecutive operations after 4 (2–7) years. Acta Orthop Scand 1994; 65:309–314.
3. Brodsky AE. Post-laminectomy and post-fusion stenosis of the lumbar spine. Clin Orthop 1976; 115:130–139.

4. Lorenz M, Zindrick M, Schwaegler P, et al. A comparison of single-level fusions with and without hardware. Spine 1991; 16:S455–458.
5. Lee CK. Accelerated degeneration of the segment adjacent to a lumbar fusion. Spine 1988; 13:375–377.
6. Schlegel JD, Smith JA, Schleusener RL. Lumbar motion segment pathology adjacent to thoracolumbar, lumbar, and lumbosacral fusions. Spine 1996; 21:970–981.
7. Etebar S, Cahill DW. Risk factors for adjacent-segment failure following lumbar fixation with rigid instrumentation for degenerative instability. J Neurosurg 1999; 90:163–169.
8. Aota Y, Kumano K, Hirabayashi S.'Postfusion instability at the adjacent segments after rigid pedicle screw fixation for degenerative lumbar spinal disorders. J Spinal Disord 1995; 8:464–473.
9. Miyakoshi N, Abe E, Shimada Y, et al. Outcome of one-level posterior lumbar interbody fusion for spondylolisthesis and postoperative intervertebral disc degeneration adjacent to the fusion. Spine 2000; 25:1837–1842.
10. Kim YE, Goel VK, Weinstein JN, et al. Effect of disc degeneration at one level on the adjacent level in axial mode. Spine 1991; 16:331–335.
11. Phillips FM, Reuben J, Wetzel FT. Intervertebral disc degeneration adjacent to a lumbar fusion. An experimental rabbit model. J Bone Joint Surg Br 2002; 84:289–294.
12. Dekutoski MB, Schendel MJ, Ogilvie JW, et al. Comparison of in vivo and in vitro adjacent segment motion after lumbar fusion. Spine 1994; 19:1745–1751.
13. Nagata H, Schendel MJ, Transfeldt EE, et al. The effects of immobilization of long segments of the spine on the adjacent and distal facet force and lumbosacral motion. Spine 1993; 18:2471–2479.
14. Kumar MN, Baklanov A, Chopin D. Correlation between sagittal plane changes and adjacent segment degeneration following lumbar spine fusion. Eur Spine J 2001; 10:314–319.
15. Phillips FM, Carlson GD, Bohlman HH, et al. Results of surgery for spinal stenosis adjacent to "previous lumbar fusion. J Spinal Disord 2000; 13:432–437.
16. Hsu K, Zucherman J, White A, et al. Deterioration of motion segments adjacent to lumbar spine fusions. Ortho Transact 1988; 12:605–606.
17. Umehara S, Zindrick MR, Patwardhan AG, et al. The biomechanical effect of postoperative hypolordosis in instrumented lumbar fusion on instrumented and adjacent spinal segments. Spine 2000; 25:1617–1624.
18. Chow DH, Luk KD, Evans JH, et al. Effects of short anterior lumbar interbody fusion on biomechanics of neighboring unfused segments. Spine 1996; 21:549–555.
19. Hsu K, Zucherman J, White A.'The long-term effect of lumbar spine fusion: deterioration of adjacent motion segments. In: Yonenobu K, Ono K, Takemitsu Y, eds. Lumbar Fusion and Stabilization. Tokyo: Springer, 1993:54–64.
20. Nakai S, Yoshizawa H, Kobayashi S.'Long-term follow-up study of posterior lumbar interbody fusion. J Spinal Disord 1999; 12:293–299.
21. Rahm MD, Hall BB. Adjacent-segment degeneration after lumbar fusion with instrumentation: a retrospective study. J Spinal Disord 1996; 9:392–400.
22. Wiltse LL, Radecki SE, Biel HM, et al. Comparative study of the incidence and severity of degenerative change in the transition zones after instrumented versus noninstrumented fusions of the lumbar spine. J Spinal Disord 1999; 12:27–33.
23. Cunningham BW, Kotani Y, McNulty PS, et al. The effect of spinal destabilization and instrumentation on lumbar intradiscal pressure: an in vitro biomechanical analysis. Spine 1997; 22:2655–2663.
24. Chen CS, Cheng CK, Liu CL, et al. Stress analysis of the disc adjacent to interbody fusion in lumbar spine. Med Eng Phys 2001; 23:483–491.
25. Weinhoffer SL, Guyer RD, Herbert M, et al. Intradiscal pressure measurements above an instrumented fusion. A cadaveric study. Spine 1995; 20:526–531.
26. Lee CK, Langrana NA. Lumbosacral spinal fusion. A biomechanical study. Spine 1984; 9:574–581.
27. Lotz JC, Colliou OK, Chin JR, et al. Compression-induced degeneration of the intervertebral disc: an in vivo mouse model and finite-element study. Spine 1998; 23:2493–2506.
28. Axelsson P, Johnsson R, Stromqvist B.'The spondylolytic vertebra and its adjacent segment. Mobility measured before and after posterolateral fusion. Spine 1997; 22:414–417.
29. Penta M, Sandhu A, Fraser RD. Magnetic resonance imaging assessment of disc degeneration 10 years after anterior lumbar interbody fusion. Spine 1995; 20:743–747.
30. Lehmann TR, Spratt KF, Tozzi JE, et al. Long-term follow-up of lower lumbar fusion patients. Spine 1987; 12:97–104.
31. Frymoyer JW, Hanley E, Howe J, et al. Disc excision and spine fusion in the management of lumbar disc disease. A minimum ten-year follow-up. Spine 1978; 3:1–6.
32. Van Horn JR, Bohnen LM. The development of discopathy in lumbar discs adjacent to a lumbar anterior interbody spondylodesis. A retrospective matched-pair study with a postoperative follow-up of 16 years. Acta Orthop Belg 1992; 58:280–286.
33. Seitsalo S, Schlenzka D, Poussa M, et al. Disc degeneration in young patients with isthmic spondylolisthesis treated operatively or conservatively: a long-term follow-up. Eur Spine J 1997; 6:393–397.

34. Hambly MF, Wiltse LL, Raghavan N, et al. The transition zone above a lumbosacral fusion. Spine 1998; 23:1785–1792.
35. Okuda S, Iwasaki M, Miyauchi A, et al. Risk factors for adjacent segment degeneration after PLIF. Spine 2004; 29:1535–1540.
36. Wiltse LL and Winter RB. Terminology and measurement of spondylolisthesis. J Bone Joint Surg Am 1983; 65:768–772.
37. MacDougall JB, Perra JH, Pinto MR, et al. Incidence of adjacent segment degeneration at ten years after lumbar spine fusion: an epidemiologic study. Presented at NASS, 2002.
38. Jackson AP, Perra JH. Operative adjacent segment disease. Currently unpublished.

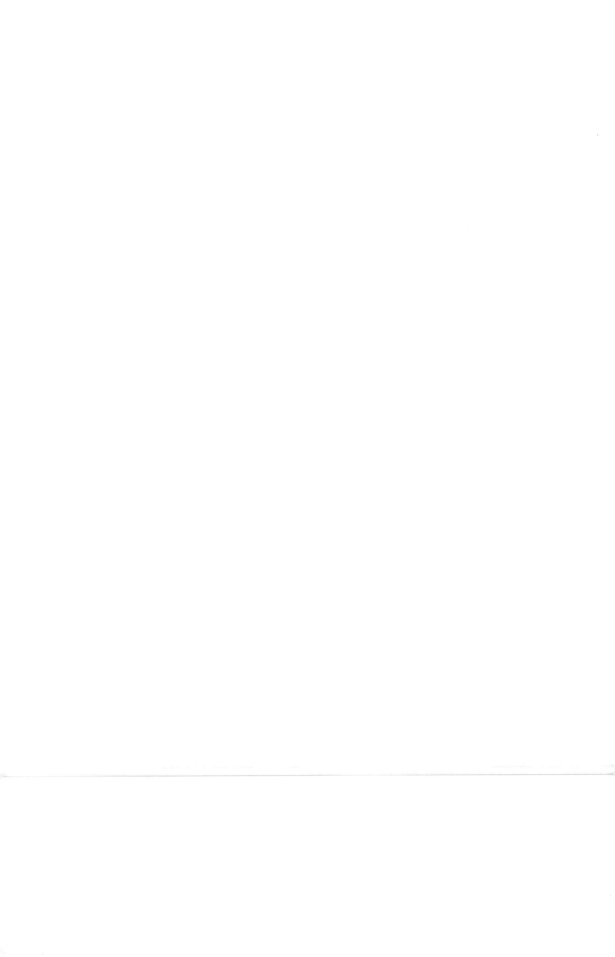

11 | Quantifying the Surgical Risk Factors for Adjacent Level Degeneration in the Lumbar Spine: A Meta-Analysis of the Published Literature

Christopher M. Bono
Department of Orthopaedic Surgery, Harvard Medical School, Brigham and Women's Hospital, Boston, Massachusetts, U.S.A.

Michael Alapatt
Boston University School of Medicine, Boston, Massachusetts, U.S.A.

Chelsey Simmons
Harvard University, Cambridge, Massachusetts, U.S.A.

Hassan Serhan
DePuy Spine, Raynham, Massachusetts, U.S.A.

INTRODUCTION

The movement toward motion-preserving technology, such as disc replacement and posterior dynamic stabilization, as an alternative to lumbar fusion has been driven by the recognition of the potential deleterious effects of adjacent segment degeneration (ASD) (1–5). Despite the continually expanding market of motion preservation devices, a clear understanding of the predisposing factors and the clinical significance of ASD in the lumbar spine is still lacking. It was the authors' purpose in this Chapter to review the published literature from the past 25 years to gain a better understanding of the incidence and risk factors for ASD. Although previous studies have compiled lists of risk factors, it was this study's goal to perform a meta-analysis of the data from the available literature to determine the incidences of ASD for various subgroups of patients. In particular, the authors were interested in the influence of controllable surgical factors, such as fusion method and the use of pedicle screws.

MATERIALS AND METHODS

A PubMed/Medline search of all articles published up to and including December, 2004, was performed using various combinations of the keywords *lumbar, fusion, arthrodesis, adjacent segment degeneration, adjacent segment disease, adjacent level degeneration,* and *adjacent level disease*. The abstracts of all "hits" were analzyed for eligibility by two reviewers (Bono and Simmons). The a priori inclusion criteria for article eligibility were that: (*i*) the study must be a clinical series of human patients who underwent lumbar fusion for any clinical indication; (*ii*) the incidence/rate of ASD must be documented; (*iii*) the data must be reported in a manner that enables calculation of the number of patients with and without evidence of ASD at final radiographic follow-up. The fully published manuscripts of potentially eligible articles were then reviewed in detail by three reviewers (Alapatt, Simmons, and Bono).

Various data from the articles were extracted and recorded in a Microsoft Access database. These included:

- fusion method,
- clinical indications for fusion,
- use of pedicle screws,

- total number of patients with radiographic follow-up,
- number of patients with and without ASD (either calculated from the data or directly reported within the article),
- predisposing factors for ASD (as per the original authors),
- radiographic criteria for ASD,
- number of patients with clinical symptoms from ASD,
- number of patients who underwent a reoperation for ASD, and
- presence/absence of clinical correlation with ASD.

After compiling these data, various subgroups were extracted using filters. Analysis was then made to compare the incidence of ASD between these subgroups. The subgroups were organized by fusion method [anterior lumbar interbody fusion (ALIF) and posterolateral fusion (PLF)], whether or not pedicle screws were used. In addition, comparison was made of the incidence of ASD in patients who were radiographically followed for more than or less than five years (60 months).

By pooling the data using simple summation techniques, the incidence of ASD was calculated for the entire study group and for each of the subgroups. Using a chi-squared test, the incidence of ASD was statistically compared between the subgroups. A *P*-value less than 0.05 was considered statistically significant. When available, the percentages of patients with clinical symptoms and those who were reoperated were also calculated; however, statistical analysis was not attempted because of the inconsistency of these reported values. To determine if a relationship existed between the duration of radiographic follow-up and the incidence of ASD, a linear regression analysis was performed.

RESULTS

After review of all abstracts, 36 articles were reviewed in detail. Thirty-one of these articles satisfied the inclusion criteria (6–36). Information from these 33 articles was used in the present study, which included data from 2228 patients. The year of publication of the articles varied from 1979 to 2004. Seventeen articles reported results of PLF, eight with posterior lumbar interbody fusion (PLIF), five with ALIF, one with ALIF or PLIF [Bagby and Kuslich (BAK) cages], and one with circumferential fusion. One article did not report the method of fusion. Sixteen studies documented the use of pedicle screws, whereas 10 reported no use of screws. The remainder of the articles did not specify if screws were used, or they reported data for instrumented and noninstrumented cases together, which did not permit subgroup calculation.

The radiographic criteria for ASD varied among the studies. Surprisingly, two studies reported the incidence of ASD without clearly stating what criteria were used. The most common criterion was disc height loss, which was used in 14 of the studies. The next most common one was new onset spondylolisthesis at the adjacent segment, which was used in eight of the studies. Other criteria included mobility or instability (five studies), spurs or sclerosis (three studies), stenosis (two studies), herniated disc (two studies), and abnormal sagittal alignment (one study). A common, but unclear criterion, was the so-called presence of disc degeneration (five studies), without any further descriptors.

The disorders treated were mostly degenerative in nature, although spondylolisthesis (either degenerative or isthmic) was the most common one. In two studies, primary fusion was performed for the treatment of a herniated disc. In one study, fusion was performed for a burst fracture. Only six manuscripts directly analyzed the correlation between ASD and clinical symptoms. Of these, only one found a relationship between symptoms and the presence of ASD, with a reported correlation of 20% (7).

The rates of ASD varied widely (0–100%) among the studies. On the whole, the incidence of ASD was 25.6% among the 2228 study patients. Only nine studies documented the incidence of clinically significant ASD, which varied from 0% to 19%. For the group as a whole, clinical symptoms from ASD were uncommon, averaging only 2.0%. Interestingly, the rate of reoperations from ASD was higher, averaging 4.9%. This was partly because two additional studies reported this information, increasing the number of patients included in this analysis. If the

TABLE 1 General Comparison of Adjacent Segment Degeneration with Different Fusion Methods (Instrumented and Noninstrumented Cases)

Fusion method	Rate of ASD (%)
PLIF	47
ALIF	29
PLF	24
Statistical Comparisons (chi-squared test)	*P-value*
ALIF vs. PLIF	0.15
PLIF vs. PLF	0.0041
PLF vs. ALIF	0.083

Abbreviations: ASD, adjacent segment degeneration; ALIF, anterior lumbar interbody fusion; PLF, posterolateral fusion; PLIF, posterior lumbar interbody fusion.

seven studies that reported both the incidence of clinical symptoms and the number of reoperations were analyzed, the former was 2.6% and the latter 2.3%.

Only six of the reviewed studies identified a risk factor for ASD based on their original analysis. For a variety of reasons, these data could not be pooled for meta-analysis. These risk factors included smoking, older age, preoperative hypermobility of the adjacent segment, sagittal misalignment, postmenopausal status, female sex, and decompressive surgery performed for spinal stenosis (in comparison with discogenic low back pain).

Comparative analysis of the pooled data from various subgroups yielded a number of interesting findings. The incidence of ASD was lowest for PLF (24%) and highest for PLIF (47%). Anterior lumbar interbody fusion had a 29% rate of ASD. Statistical comparison between these groups demonstrated no difference between ALIF and PLIF ($P = 0.15$), and only a trend toward significance between ALIF and PLF ($P = 0.083$). However, a highly significant difference was detected between PLIF and PLF ($P = 0.0041$) (Table 1).

The influence of pedicle screws on ASD also appeared to be significant. For all types of fusion, the use of pedicle screws demonstrated a 28% incidence; uninstrumented fusions had a 20% incidence. This difference was marginally statistically significant ($P = 0.053$) (Table 2). To eliminate the confounder of posterior surgical exposure, a comparison was made of instrumented versus uninstrumented fusions only in those patients who underwent a PLF or PLIF. In this group, the use of screws displayed a trend toward higher rates of ASD (30%) compared with noninstrumented cases (24%) ($P = 0.10$) (Table 3).

Linear regression analysis demonstrated a poor relationship between the duration of follow-up and the incidence of ASD demonstrated ($r = 0.22$). However, subgroup analysis using five years as a dividing point between so-called long and short follow-up demonstrated a statistically significant difference, with the former having an incidence of 35%, and the latter an incidence of 18%. This difference was highly statistically significant ($P = 0.0029$) (Table 4).

DISCUSSION

In his landmark article, Lee (37) retrospectively described the development of degenerative changes at a nonfused level adjacent to various types of lumbar fusion in 18 patients. Changes included severe disc degeneration, facet joint arthritis, and newly acquired spondylolysis. With this work, spinal practitioners became increasingly aware of this phenomenon,

TABLE 2 General Comparison of Adjacent Segment Degeneration Between Instrumented Vs. Noninstrumented Fusions

Fusion method	Rate of ASD (%)
Instrumented	28
Noninstrumented	20
Statistical comparisons (chi-squared test)	*P-value*
Instrumented vs. noninstrumented	0.053

Abbreviation: ASD, adjacent segment degeneration.

TABLE 3 Subgroup Comparison of Adjacent Segment Degeneration Between Instrumented Vs. Noninstrumented Posterior Fusions (Posterior Lumbar Interbody Fusion and Posterolateral Fusion Only)

Fusion method	Rate of ASD (%)
Instrumented PLIF or PLF	30
Noninstrumented PLIF or PLF	24
Statistical comparisons (chi-squared test)	*P-value*
Instrumented vs. noninstrumented PLIF or PLF	0.10

Abbreviations: ASD, adjacent segment degeneration; PLF, posterolateral fusion; PLIF, posterior lumbar interbody fusion.

commonly known as ASD. As Lee's study examined only those 18 cases, the overall incidence of ASD was not reported. Since its publication in 1988, many subsequent studies have documented widely varied incidences of ASD following numerous types of lumbar fusion (7,10,11,13,18,19,38).

Despite this seeming plethora of information, the role of suspected predisposing factors for ASD remains unclear. Individual studies have suggested certain factors as being more or less important (6–11,14). In an excellent review of the literature, Park et al. (39) compiled a list of potential risk factors for ASD as purported by the authors of the articles they analyzed. These included posterior lumbar interbody fusion, unfused facet joint injury from pedicle screw insertion, increasing fusion length, sagittal alignment, pre-existing disc degeneration, lumbar stenosis, age, osteoporosis, female gender, and postmenopausal state (39). Of particular interest are those factors that may be surgically controllable, such as the choice of fusion method, fusion length, alignment, and use of pedicle screws.

Without detracting from the importance of Park et al. (39) work, the present authors were interested to see if any trends in the rates of ASD could be recognized if the body of literature was considered as a whole. Using meta-analytical techniques, the data from the studies reviewed in Park et al. (39) article in addition to nine others that fulfilled inclusion criteria were pooled using summation methods. Inherent in this method of data analysis, only those identified risk factors that were common to the various studies could be statistically evaluated. These included the use of pedicle screws and the type or method of fusion (PLIF, ALIF, or PLF). Despite the numerous other potential risk factors recognized in the current literature search in addition to previous reviews (39,40), they were not consistently reported in all of the studies. As the majority of studies clearly documented what type of fusion was performed, and whether it was instrumented or noninstrumented, these risk factors were most easily analyzed. Because of the complexity of such an analysis, the influence of the number of levels on the rate of ASD could not be analyzed using meta-analysis. In order for this to have been possible, each study would have had to report data in such a manner that would have enabled the calculation of the number of patients who developed ASD in relation to the number of segments fused (9,22,31).

One of the more interesting findings from the current study was the difference in the rate of ASD between PLIF and PLF. To the authors' knowledge, only one previous study has identified the use of PLIF as a risk factor for ASD. Rahm et al. (22), using a logistic regression analysis, found that those who underwent PLIF were more at risk for ASD than those who underwent PLF ($P = 0.02$). In the current study, comparison of the pooled results of the

TABLE 4 Subgroup Comparison of Adjacent Segment Degeneration Between Fusion Followed for Less Than Five Years and Fusion Followed for Five Years or More

Duration of follow-up	Rate of ASD (%)
< 5 years	18
≥5 years	36
Statistical comparisons (chi-squared test)	*P-value*
< 5 years vs. ≥5 years	0.0021

Abbreviation: ASD, adjacent segment degeneration.

seven studies that reported the results of PLIF, compared with the 17 studies of PLF, demonstrated a highly significant difference (47% and 24%, respectively, P-value = 0.0041).

Among other factors, one of the potential confounding variables in such an analysis could have been a disproportionate use of pedicle screws in the PLIF versus PLF groups. In anticipation of this, an analysis of only those cases of PLIF and PLF that used screws was performed. Although the incidence of ASD with PLIF was unchanged (as they all used instrumentation), it was slightly lower for instrumented PLF (23%). The difference of ASD between instrumented PLIF and PLF remained statistically significant ($P = 0.0056$). Thus, it would appear that PLIF is a risk factor for ASD, independent from the use of pedicle screws.

The increased stiffness of a PLIF compared with a PLF could help explain the difference in ASD rates. According to this logic, ALIF and PLIF should result in comparable rates of ASD. In the current study, ALIF was associated with a 29% incidence. Although substantially lower than the rate of ASD for PLIF, the difference was not statistically significant ($P = 0.157$). The chance for beta (type II) error in this analysis was considerable, as the number of patients who underwent ALIF ($n = 134$) was much lower than for PLIF ($n = 369$). Thus, one might conclude that a trend toward lower rates of ASD was true for ALIF.

One may ask the question, based on these trends, why would ALIF result in a lower rate of ASD than PLIF. Biomechanical studies (41,42) have clearly demonstrated that a solid ALIF and PLIF result in comparable rigidity. Thus, one may speculate that the surgical approach and use of pedicle screws with PLIF may be a clear disadvantage with regard to the incidence of ASD. This may also help explain why the rates of ASD for PLF and ALIF are more comparable; the contribution of pedicle screws (i.e., facet injury) to the development of ASD may be nearly equivalent to the contribution of the stiffness of interbody fusion. Instrumented PLIF, in following, suffers from both of these negative risk factors.

Naturally, this leads to a discussion of the influence of pedicle screws. In addition to the added stiffness that pedicle screw supply to a fusion, it is widely believed that it is the potential facet injury during pedicle screw insertion that may be a more important contributing factor to ASD. The data, at first, appear to support the notion that instrumented fusions lead to a higher rate of ASD. Considering all the fusion methods, the use of pedicle screws was associated with a 28% rate of ASD compared with a 20% rate if screws were not used—a difference that was marginally statistically significant ($P = 0.053$). To eliminate the confounding variable of the surgical approach by considering only those cases of PLF and PLIF, the rate of ASD with instrumented fusion was 30% compared with 24% for noninstrumented fusions. This difference was not statistically significant ($P = 0.10$) (Table 5).

Considering the higher rates of ASD with PLIF, one can take this analysis one step further. A more "pure" comparison was made of only those cases of PLF. Instrumented PLIF had a 23% incidence of ASD, and uninstrumented PLIF had a 24% rate (Table 6). As one would expect, this was not statistically significant ($P = 0.54$). Though limited by the pitfalls of meta-analysis, these findings might help relieve culpability from pedicle screws as being a risk factor for ASD and point more toward fusion method. It also underscores the tendency to draw potentially incorrect conclusions from generalized analyses, oftentimes fueled by surgeon's guilt (for having to burr so close to the suprajacent unfused joint to place a screw!).

TABLE 5 Subgroup Comparison of Adjacent Segment Degeneration with Posterolateral Fusion and Posterior Lumbar Interbody Fusion (Instrumented Cases Only)

Fusion method	Rate of ASD (%)
PLIF	47
PLF	23
Statistical comparisons (chi-squared test)	*P-value*
PLIF vs. PLF	0.0056

Abbreviations: ASD, adjacent segment degeneration; PLF, posterolateral fusion; PLIF, posterior lumbar interbody fusion.

TABLE 6 Subgroup Comparison of Adjacent Segment Degeneration
Between Instrumented Vs. Noninstrumented

Fusion method	Rate of ASD (%)
Instrumented PLF	23
Noninstrumented PLF	24
Statistical comparisons (chi-squared test)	*P-value*
Instrumented vs. noninstrumented PLF	0.54

Abbreviations: ASD, adjacent segment degeneration; PLF, posterolateral fusion; PLIF,
posterior lumbar interbody fusion.

Studies of the rates of ASD have varied follow-up intervals. Although it seems intuitive
that the longer one follows a group of patients the higher the rate of ASD would be, this
relationship has not been examined previously. Using linear regression analysis, the present
study found a poor correlation between time to follow-up, and the incidence of ASD, with
an *r*-value (slope of the curve) of only 0.22. In a distinct, but potentially related phenomenon,
Park et al. (39) found little consistency between studies concerning the interval between fusion
and the development of ASD.

In a separate analysis, the incidence of ASD was compared between two subgroups; those
patients who were followed for less than five years, and those who were followed for five years
or more. Although somewhat arbitrary, the five-year mark has appeared to be a point of distinction for some studies of ASD (10). The current data found that the rate of ASD in the former
group was 18%, whereas that in the latter group was 36%. This difference was highly statistically significant ($P = 0.0021$). Notwithstanding the number of covariates that were not included
in this analysis (including use of screws and fusion method), these data strongly suggest that
the studies of ASD should have follow-up periods of at least five years.

An understanding of the relationship, or lack thereof, between adjacent segment degeneration and clinical symptoms is important (39,40). In a recent publication, Hilibrand and
Robbins (40) distinguished between adjacent segment *degeneration* (a radiographic finding)
and adjacent segment *disease*, which is the constellation of clinical symptoms that are variably
associated with degeneration. Various individual studies have suggested that there it little
association between a poor clinical outcome and the presence of radiographic adjacent
degeneration (14,18,43). Notwithstanding this trend, individual cases of ASD can be clinically
present in a variety of manners, such as spinal stenosis, axial discogenic back pain, and facet
syndrome (37). Various studies have used the need for subsequent surgery as a clinical indicator of adjacent segment disease (10,44), with reported rates as low as 3% (7) and as high as
26% (10) at follow-up greater than five years after surgery.

Accordingly, the present authors felt it important to examine the rates of symptomatic
ASD in the reviewed studies. Unfortunately, not all the papers reported these data. In fact,
only 17 studies provided any information concerning clinical symptoms; 12 studies reported
reoperation rates (which varied from 0% to 26%); eight reported the rate of symptomatic
ASD (which varied from 0% to 19%). Only seven of the reviewed studies reported both the
rate of reoperation and the rate of symptoms from ASD. Pooling the data from these studies,
the rate of radiographic ASD was 32%; the rate of symptomatic ASD was 9%; and the rate of
reoperation was 8%. Confirming previous authors' conclusions, these data do not support a
relationship between ASD and symptoms or the need for further surgery.

Whereas these data and analyses appear to show a number of trends and interesting
findings, the authors highlight a number of factors that might limit the accuracy of the pooled
data. First, the radiographic criteria used were varied and inconsistent. Even if one were to consider the most commonly used criterion (disc height, used in 14 of the studies), this is a radiographic measurement that is prone to interobserver/intraobserver error. In order for better
comparison of future studies of ASD, it would be important that the same or similar methods
of measurement be used, and that these measurements be performed by a uniform system to
ensure optimum reproducibility and reliability. The variability of the ASD criteria used in the
studies reviewed in the current meta-analysis undoubtedly affected the rates of ASD reported.

Another potential confounder that the authors recognize is the diagnostic subgroups treated with fusion. As surgery for lumbar stenosis has been recognized as a potential risk factor for ASD (45), comparing groups of patients with "like" disorders would allow a better analysis of the surgical risk factors for ASD. Although the authors considered performing such a subgroup analysis, the diagnoses treated were mixed and would not have permitted meaningful comparisons.

REFERENCES

1. Sengupta DK, Mulholland RC. Fulcrum assisted soft stabilization system: a new concept in the surgical treatment of degenerative low back pain. Spine 2005; 30:1019–1029.
2. Sengupta DK. Dynamic stabilization devices in the treatment of low back pain. Orthop Clin N Am 2004; 35:43–56.
3. deKleuver M, Oner FC, Jacobs WCH. Total disc replacement for chronic low back pain: background and a systematic review of the literature. Eur Spine J 2003; 12:108–116.
4. Cinotti G, David T, Postacchini F. Results of disc prosthesis after a minimum follow-up period of 2 years. Spine 1996; 21:995–1000.
5. Buttner-Janz K, Schellnack K, Zippel H, et al. Experience and results with the SB Charite lumbar intervertebral endoprosthesis. Z Klin Med 1988; 43:1785–1789.
6. Aota Y, Kumano K, Hirabayashi S. Postfusion instability at the adjacent segments after rigid pedicle screw fixation for degenerative lumbar spinal disorders. J Spinal Disord 1993; 8:464–473.
7. Brantigan JW, Stefee AD, Lewis ML, et al. Lumbar interbody fusion using the Brantigan I/F cage for posterior lumbar interbody fusion and the variable pedicle screw placement system. Spine 2000; 25:1437–1446.
8. Chou W, Hsu C, Chang W, et al. Adjacent segment degeneration after lumbar spinal posterolateral fusion with instrumentation in elderly patients. Acta Orthop Trauma Surg 2002; 122:xx.
9. Etebar S, Cahill DW. Risk factors for adjacent-segment failure following lumbar fixation with rigid instrumentation for degenerative instability. J Neurosurg 1999; 90:163–169.
10. Ghiselli G, Wang JC, Bhatia NN, et al. Adjacement segment degeneration in the lumbar spine. J Bone Joint Surg Am 2004; 86-A:1497–1503.
11. Ghiselli G, Wang JC, Hsu WK, et al. L5-S1 segment survivorship and clinical outcome analysis after L4-L5 isolated fusion. Spine 2003; 28:1275–1280.
12. Hambly MF, Wiltse LL, Raghavan N, et al. The transition zone above a lumbosacral fusion. Spine 1998; 23:1785–1792.
13. Kanayama M, Hashimoto T, Shigenobu K, et al. Adjacent-segment morbidity after Graf ligamento-plasty compared with posterolateral lumbar fusion. J Neurosurg 2001; 95:5–10.
14. Kumar MN, Baklanov A, Chopin D. Correlation between sagittal plane changes and adjacent segment degeneration following lumbar spine fusion. Eur Spine J 2001; 10:314–319.
15. Kumar MN, Jacquot F, Hall H. Long-term follow-up of functional outcomes and radiographic changes at adjacent levels following lumbar spine fusion for degenerative disc disease. Eur Spine J 2001; 10:309–313.
16. Lai P, Chen L, Niu CC, et al. Effect of postoperative lumbar sagittal alignment on the development of adjacent instability. J Spinal Disord Tech 2004; 17:353–357.
17. Lai P, Chen L, Niu CC, et al. Relation between laminectomy and development of adjacent segment instability after lumbar fusion with pedicle fixation. Spine 2004; 29:2527–2532.
18. Miyakoshi N, Abe E, Shimada Y, et al. Outcome of one-level posterior lumbar interbody fusion for spondylolisthesis and postoperative disc degeneration adjacent to the fusion. Spine 2000; 25:1837–1842.
19. Miyakoshi N, Abe E, Shimada Y, et al. Anterior decompression with single segmental spinal inter-body fusion for lumbar burst fracture. Spine 1999; 24:67–73.
20. Okuda S, Iwasaki M, Miyauchi A, et al. Risk factors for adjacent segment degeneration after PLIF. Spine 2004; 14:1535–1540.
21. Penta M, Avninder S, Fraser RD. Magnetic resonance imaging assessment of disc degeneration 10 years after anterior lumbar interbody fusion. Spine 1995; 20:743–747.
22. Rahm MD, Hall BB. Adjacent-segment degeneration after lumbar fusion with instrumentation: a retrospective study. J Spinal Disord 1996; 9:392–400.
23. van Horn JR, Bohnen LM. The development of discopathy in lumbar discs adjacent to a lumbar anterior interbody spondylodesis, a retrospective matched-pair study with a postoperative follow-up of 16 years. Acta Orthop Belg 1992; 58:280–286.
24. Ishihara H, Osada R, Kanamori M, et al. Minimum 10-year follow-up study of anterior lumbar interbody fusion for isthmic spondylolisthesis. J Spinal Disord 2001; 14:91–99.
25. Kuslich SD, Danielson G, Dowdle JD, et al. Four-year follow-up results of lumbar spine arthrodesis using the Bagby and Kuslich lumbar fusion cage. Spine 2000; 25:2656–2662.

26. Booth DC, Bridwell KH, Eisenberg BA, et al. Minimum 5-year results of degenerative spondylolisthesis treated with decompression and instrumented posterior fusion. Spine 1999; 24:1721–1727.

27. Nakai S, Yoshizawa H, Kobayashi S. Long-term follow-up study of posterior lumbar interbody fusion. J Spinal Disord 1999; 12:293–299.

28. Chen WJ, Niu CC, Chen LH, et al. Survivorship analysis of DKS instrumentation in the treatment of spondylolistehsis. Clin Orthop 1997; 339:113–120.

29. Guigui P, Lambert P, Lassale B, et al. [Long-term outcome at adjacent levels of lumbar arthrodesis]. Rev Chir Orthop Reparatrice Appar Mot 1997; 83:685–696.

30. Seitsalo S, Schlenzka D, Poussa M, et al. Disc degeneration in young patients with isthmic spondylolisthesis treated operative or conservatively: a long-term follow-up. Eur Spine J 1997; 6:393–397.

31. Wimmer C, Krismer M, Gluch H, et al. Autogenic versus allogenic bone grafts in anterior lumbar interbody fusion. Clin Orthop 1999; 360:122–126.

32. Pihlajamaki H, Bostman O, Ruuskanen M, et al. Posterolateral lumbosacral fusion with transpedicular fixation. Acta Orthop Scand 1996; 67:63–68.

33. Axelsson P, Johnsson R, Stromqvist B, et al. Posterolateral lumbar fusion. Acta Orthp Scand 1994; 65:309–314.

34. Lehmann TR, Spratt KF, Tozzi JE, et al. Long-term follow-up of lower lumbar fusion patients. Spine 1987; 12:97–104.

35. Frymoyer JW, Hanley EN, Howe J, et al. A comparison of radiographic findings in fusion and nonfusion patients ten or more years following lumbar disc surgery. Spine 1979; 4:435–440.

36. Leong JC, Chun SY, Grange WJ, et al. Long-term results of lumbar intervertebral disc prolapse. Spine 1983; 8:793–799.

37. Lee CK. Accelerated degeneration of the segment adjacent to a lumbar fusion. Spine 1988; 13:375–377.

38. Kuslich SD, Ulstrom CL, Grifith SL, et al. The Bagby and Kuslich method of lumbar interbody fusion. History, techniques, and 2-year follow-up results of a United States prospective, multicenter trial. Spine 1998; 23:1267–1278.

39. Park P, Garton HJ, Gala V, et al. Adjacent segment disease after lumbar or lumbosacral fusion; review of the literature. Spine 2004; 29:1938–1944.

40. Hilibrand AS, Robbins M. Adjacent segment degeneration and adjacent segment disease: the consequences of spinal fusion? Spine J 2004; 4:190S–194S.

41. Bono CM, Khanda A, Vadapalli S, et al. Residual angular motion after simulated solid lumbar fusion: a finite element analysis with implications on interpreting flexion-extension radiographs. Spine J 2005; 5:23S.

42. Bono CM, Bawa M, White K, et al. Lumbar arthrodesis: how much radiographic motion is present after solid fusion? International Society for the Study of Lumbar Surgery. Vancouver, 2003.

43. Throckmorton TW, Hilibrand AS, Mencio GA, et al. The impact of adjacent level disc degeneration on health status outcomes following lumbar fusion. Spine 2003; 28:2596–50.

44. Gillet P. The fate of the adjacent motion segments after lumbar fusion. J Spinal Disord Tech 2005; 16:338–345.

45. Guigi P, Chopin D. Assessment of the use of the Graf ligamentoplasty in the surgical treatment of lumbar spinal stenosis. Apropos of a series of 26 patients. Rev Chir Orthop Reparatrice Appar Mot 1994; 80:681–688.

12 | Transition Zone Failure in Patients Undergoing Instrumented Lumbar Fusions from L1 or L2 to the Sacrum

Michael L. Swank, Adam G. Miller, and Leslie L. Korbee
Cincinnati Orthopaedic Research Institute, Cincinnati, Ohio, U.S.A.

INTRODUCTION

The long-term success of arthrodesis for degenerative conditions in the lumbar spine depends on many factors, including the effects of arthrodesis on the transition zone between the last fused level and the next untreated level. As rigid internal fixation with spinal instrumentation has been performed, there has been interest in the effects the arthrodesis has on accelerating transition zone degeneration (1–3). These changes are summarized as adjacent segment disease (ASD), and include: listhesis, scoliosis, instability, herniated disc, osteophyte formation, arthritis, stenosis, and vertebral compression fracture (4). Hardware, the approach used, and the level of instrumentation have been the reported causes of accelerated degeneration above and below instrumented fusions (4). Other reports have indicated that the degenerative changes may not be greater than those expected with the natural history of the degenerative process, as degenerative disease is not expected to be isolated to one level (4–7). Reports that have suggested an increased risk of adjacent segment degeneration indicate that there are several risk factors for this condition, including age, gender, bone quality, levels of instrumentation, associated degenerative changes at the time of index surgery, history of previous surgeries, and so on (8–12). Owing to the lack of understanding of ASD etiology, incidence rates have been reported between 8% and 100%, using radiographic criteria and between 5.2% and 18.5%, using symptomatic criteria (4). However, few have looked specifically at multilevel arthrodesis as a risk factor for accelerated transition zone degeneration at the cephalad end vertebra and the effects on both radiographic and clinical criteria.

Although etiology is still being hypothesized, stress and movement in noninstrumented levels play a role. Following lumbar fusion, pressure, flexion, and extension increase at the transition zone (13). Theoretically, as more levels are involved, fewer segments are available to dissipate the mechanical stresses at the transition zone, which could accelerate degenerative changes at this level. The following study was conducted to evaluate the incidence and types of transition zone failure relating to ASD following instrumented lumbar fusion surgery (ILFS).

METHODS

From 1994 to 2000, a single surgeon performed 257 ILFS for a variety of spinal conditions, including postlaminectomy syndrome, spondylolisthesis, scoliosis, spinal stenosis, and pseudarthrosis. Of these, 18 patients with degenerative spinal stenosis were instrumented from L5 or S1 to L1 or L2.

Clinical Presentation

These patients represent a complex group of spinal disorders (Table 1). The average age at presentation was 64 ± 11.4 (range 41–84 years). Unilateral radiculopathy or neurogenic claudication was a presenting condition in all the 18 patients. Two of the patients had a partial cauda equina syndrome. The average symptom duration at presentation was 4.7 ± 3.2 years (range

TABLE 1 Preoperative Data

Pt. no.	BMI (kg/m²)	First-degree symptom	Second-degree symptom	SYMD (yr)	X-ray Dx	MRI/myelo. Dx	Comorbidities	Prev. spinal surg.
1	28.4	Radiculopathy	Claudication	2	Spondy	Stenosis	HTN	0
2	26.7	Radiculopathy	Claudication	12	Spondy/scoli	Stenosis	CS	0
3	29.0	Back pain	Claudication	1	DDD	Stenosis	HTN, cardiac, CS	0
4	38.2	Back pain	Claudication	3	Scoliosis	Stenosis	Diabetes, smoker	0
5	24.7	Radiculopathy	Claudication	6	Spondy	Stenosis	HTN, diabetes, cardiac	0
6	31.2	Claudication	Back pain	2	Spondy	Block L3/4	CS	0
7	26.2	Radiculopathy	Back pain	1	Spondy	Block L3/4	HTN	0
8	34.1	Back pain	Claudication	6	Spondy/scoli	Stenosis	CS	1
9	22.6	Radiculopathy	Back pain	6	Spondy	Stenosis	None	1
10	39.8	Radiculopathy	Back pain	10	Spondy	Stenosis	None	1
11	32.7	Radiculopathy	Back pain	2	DDD	Stenosis	HTN, diabetes	1
12	25.0	Claudication	Back pain	6	Spondy	Stenosis	HTN, smoking	1
13	35.2	Radiculopathy	Back pain	4	Scoliosis	Stenosis	HTN, diabetes, cardiac, CS	1
14	29.1	Radiculopathy	Back pain	3	DDD	Stenosis	HTN	2
15	28.1	Cauda equina	Claudication	3	Spondy	Block L4/5	HTN, diabetes, cardiac, CS	2
16	32.5	Claudication	Back pain	5	DDD	Block L2/3	None	2
17	36.0	Radiculopathy	Claudication	10	DDD	Stenosis	HTN, diabetes, cardiac CS	2
18	30.0	Cauda equina	Radiculopathy	3	Scoli/spondy	Block L2/3	HTN, CS	3

Note: Average age was 64 (41–84). Seventy-two percent were women. Patients were referred by primary care physician (3), neurosurgeon (11), and orthopedic surgeon (4).
Abbreviations: BMI, body mass index; DX, diagnosis; MRI, magnetic resonance imaging; SYMD, symptom duration; spondy, spondylolisthesis; scoli, scoliosis; DDD, degenerative disc disease; HTN, hypertension; CS, cervical spondylosis.

1 to 12 years). Sixty-one percent (11 of 18) of the patients had a prior laminectomy and 6% (1 of 18) had prior lumbar fusion.

Radiographic Presentation

All patients had spinal stenosis on magnetic resonance imaging (MRI) or computer tomography (CT) myelogram, and five patients had a myelographic block at L4 or higher preoperatively. Five patients had degenerative disc disease (DDD), 11 had spondylolisthesis, and 5 had degenerative scoliosis.

Index Procedure

The index procedure for these patients was an instrumented lumbosacral fusion in which the most cephalad segment was either L1 or L2, and the most caudad segment was L5 or S1. The author's surgical philosophy at the time of index procedure was to perform a wide decompression of all involved levels and obtain a rigid arthrodesis over the levels that were decompressed. Only the levels that were decompressed or directly involved in the deformity were included in the instrumented arthrodesis in an attempt to avoid fusion of normal spinal motion segments.

   All patients had three or more instrumented levels. The average number of levels decompressed was 4 ± 0.6 (range 3–5 levels). The average number of levels fused with posterolateral fusion was 3.8 ± 0.9 (range 1–5 levels). The average number of interbody fusions was 2.8 ± 1.9 (range 0–5 levels) (Table 2).

Outcome Measures

All data were prospectively collected in a computerized database at the time of each visit, and reviewed retrospectively. Patient assessment includes numerical rating scale for pain, medication usage, satisfaction surveys, daily life questionnaire, radiographic analysis, and incidence of complications. Data was taken during preoperative, six-month, one-year, and two-year

TABLE 2 Operative Procedures

Pt. no.	Cephalad vertebrate	Caudad vertebrate	ALIF levels	PLIF levels	PLF levels	Laminectomy levels	Total levels
1	L2	L5	0	2	3	1	3
2	L2	L5	3	0	3	2	3
3	L1	S1	0	5	5	5	5
4	L1	S1	0	5	3	3	5
5	L2	L5	0	1	3	3	3
6	L2	S1	0	4	4	4	4
7	L2	S1	0	1	4	3	4
8	L2	S1	0	4	4	4	4
9	L2	L5	0	3	3	3	3
10	L2	S1	0	4	4	4	4
11	L2	S1	0	0	4	4	4
12	L2	S1	0	4	4	4	4
13	L1	S1	0	5	5	5	5
14	L1	S1	0	5	5	5	5
15	L2	S1	0	0	4	4	4
16	L2	L5	0	1	1	1	3
17	L2	S1	0	0	4	4	4
18	L2	S1	0	4	4	4	4

Abbreviations: ALIF, anterior lumbar interbody fusion; PLF, posterolateral lumbar fusion; PLIF, posterior lumbar interbody fusion.

visits. Subsequent follow-up visits were also documented for various patients after 24 months. All patients attended an initial preoperative visit and at least one final postoperative visit.

RESULTS
Clinical Outcome
Pain Scores
Thirteen of the 18 patients reported decreased back pain, and 15 reported decreased leg pain (Table 3). The average pain score for back pain was 7.4 ± 2.3 (range 4–10), preoperatively.

TABLE 3 Clinical Results

Pt. no.	Follow-up (mo)	Final satisfaction	Back pain		Leg pain	
			Pre	Post	Pre	Post
1	65	5	10	2	10	4
2	32	1	6	6	8	7
3	34	1	8	8	8	7
4	9	1	7	7	6	7
5	35	5	8	8	9	9
6	6	6	8	3	8	0
7	86	2	6	5	7	5
8	57	1	6	4	5	0
9	41	5	6	3	7	0
10	63	2	4	3	8	5
11	3	1	10	8	10	8
12	24	1	10	7	10	7
13	59	1	8	6	8	9
14	7	4	10	7	10	3
15	52	4	6	5	3	7
16	45	2	10	8	10	8
17	46	1	2	2	10	2
18	56	1	10	0	10	3

Note: Follow-up time measured from date of surgery to final visit. Final satisfaction measured from internal questionnaire on a scale of 0 to 6: 0, extremely unsatisfied; 1, very unsatisfied; 2, unsatisfied; 3, neutral; 4, satisfied; 5, very satisfied; 6, extremely satisfied. "Prepain" scores taken at time of preoperative visit. "Postpain" scores taken at time of last follow-up visit.

Back and Leg Pain

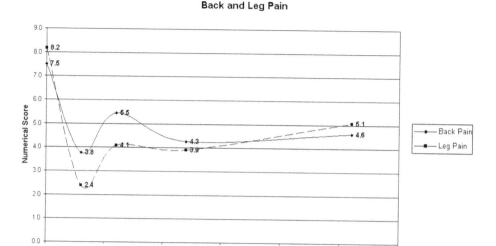

FIGURE 1 Average pain scores from patients reporting at specified times with: 100% preop; 72% six months; 61% 12 months; 61% 24 months; 72% >24 months visit compliance. Average ">24 months" visit at 4.3 years follow-up.

At the final follow-up visit for all patients, the average back pain score significantly decreased to 5.1 ± 2.5 (range 2–8), postoperatively ($P = 0.01$). The average preoperative pain score for leg pain was 8.1 ± 2.0 (range 3–10), and dropped to 5.1 ± 3.1 (range 3–9), postoperatively, at the final visit ($P < 0.01$). These reductions represent a statistically significant drop in pain for most patients. Evaluating pain scores chronologically yields a gradual increase in pain from six months to two years and beyond (Fig. 1). Whereas these increases are statistically insignificant, they represent no improvement in pain beyond six months, postoperatively.

Medication Usage
Fifteen patients were taking daily narcotics and nine were taking nonsteroidal anti-inflammatory drugs (NSAIDs) at the time of their index procedure. At the final follow-up, 12 required daily narcotics and six were taking daily NSAIDs at final follow-up (Fig. 2).

Satisfaction
At final follow-up, patients rated their satisfaction with their condition on a questionnaire ranging from "very satisfied" to "very unsatisfied" (Table 3). Thirty-three percent of patients rated their condition as satisfactory or better. Fifty percent of the patients were reported to be "very unsatisfied" with the state of their condition.

Daily Life
Employment, walking, and device assistance were assessed. Of the two employed patients at the time of surgery, only one returned to a vocation. Ambulatory status improved in only one patient, changing from a lack of ambulation preoperatively to ambulation in a community setting. All other patients maintained their original status. Three patients were able to stop their cane usage and walk without assistance. One patient moved from a wheelchair to walker usage. Three patients regressed to a walker from a cane or no support. All other patients experienced no significant change in device usage.

Radiographic Outcome
No patients had a radiographic pseudarthrosis over the levels instrumented. Both patients who had instrumentation removal for infection developed increasing deformity, one a worsening

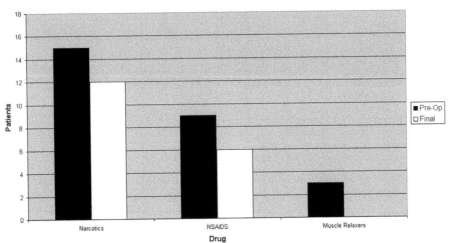

FIGURE 2 Medication usage measured preoperatively and at time of final visit. Average of final follow-up visit was 3.3 (0.5–7) years.

kyphoscoliosis and one an increased scoliosis, but both patients went on to a subsequent arthrodesis. Other patient complications were confirmed diagnostically as needed.

Complications

Fourteen patients experienced 45 complications related to the index surgery. Only three patients did not develop any significant complications. Complications were evaluated in six categories: reoperations, medical complications, infection, instrumentation failure, fracture/avascular necrosis (AVN), and adjacent segment degeneration (Tables 4, 5). Minor complications, such as urinary tract infections and adverse reactions to pain medicine were not evaluated.

TABLE 4 Complications

Pt. no.	Medical complications	Infection	Construct failure	Fracture AVN	DDD at TZ
1	Yes		Yes	Yes	Yes
2					Yes
3	Yes			Yes	Yes
4		Yes	Yes		
5	Yes				
6					
7					Yes
8			Yes		Yes
9				Yes	Yes
10					Yes
11					
12	Yes				Yes
13	Yes	Yes		Yes	Yes
14		Yes			
15	Yes				Yes
16					Yes
17	Yes	Yes		Yes	Yes
18					
Total	7	3	3	5	12

Abbreviations: AVN, avascular necrosis; DDD at TZ, degenerative disc disease at transition zone.

TABLE 5 Reoperations

Pt. no.	Reoperations	Reoperation reason			
		First	Second	Third	Fourth
1	2	Extended fusion	Adjust construct		
3	2	Battery pack removal	Extend fusion		
4	4	Debridement	Debridement	Implant removal	Debridement
13	3	Debridement	Debridement	Implant removal	
14	1	Debridement			
17	5	Battery pack removal	Extend fusion	Debridement	Laminectomy/debridement

Note: Reoperations listed for patients in chronological order.

Reoperations

Six patients (33%) underwent at least one reoperation within the follow-up period related to their lumbar fusion (Table 5). Two additional patients have been recommended for extension of the fusion at their last office visit. Four patients underwent debridement for infection—two with implant removal. Three patients underwent extension of the fusion for kyphotic angulation at or above the most cephalad instrumented level.

Medical Complications

Seven patients experienced significant medical complications requiring either a medical intervention or increased hospital stay. Three patients developed a postoperative cardiac abnormality—two required angioplasty and stent placement and one required a pacemaker. None actually sustained a myocardial infarction. Two patients developed a gastrointestinal bleeding episode requiring endoscopy, despite the fact that all patients received H2 antagonist prophylaxis. Two patients developed a postoperative pneumonia requiring extended antibiotics and increased hospitalization.

Infections

Four patients developed an acute postoperative wound infection (onset less than six weeks, postoperatively) requiring eight additional surgeries. Additionally, two patients underwent eventual implant removal to clear the infection. Two infected patients were able to retain the construct. All patients eventually had an apparent arthrodesis, although the two patients who underwent implant removal had increased spinal deformity.

Construct Failure

Three instrumentation changes occurred. One patient experienced screw fixation loss at upper levels of the fusion, and subsequently underwent the removal of cephalad ends of rods. Two patients developed asymptomatic instrumentation failure at the instrumented levels. One presented as a failure of an S1 screw rod coupling mechanism, whereas another showed screws backed out at the cephalad end. These two defects did not lead to any specific intervention, and a solid arthrodesis was maintained.

Fractures/Avascular Necrosis

A commonality in this series is a high incidence of fracture or AVN of the cephalad-most vertebral body. Five patients developed fracture or AVN at either the cephalad-most vertebral body or the vertebral body disc complex immediately adjacent to it. Four of these underwent surgery, and one was treated nonoperatively. Three patients developed a pedicle fracture, which started at the most cephalad level, usually within the first three months, postoperatively (Figs. 3–5). The clinical sequence was a stress fracture of the cephalad-most pedicles, followed by progressive kyphotic angulation of the transition zone and ultimate collapse of the anterior part of the cephalad, instrumented vertebral body.

Degenerative Disc Disease

Twelve patients showed progressive degenerative changes at the transition zone, with three patients developing a retrolisthesis and spinal stenosis (Figs. 6, 7). Although this is relatively

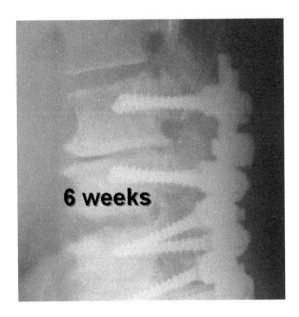

FIGURE 3 Six-week postop film reveals normal clinical alignment.

asymptomatic in most patients, two patients who developed a retrolisthesis with spinal stenosis have been recommended for extension of their fusion into the thoracic spine.

DISCUSSION

Transition zone changes and the incidence of ASD after ILFS are a frequent, yet not completely understood phenomenon. The literature has been unclear as to the exact role of instrumentation length and number of interbody fusions in accelerating the rates of degeneration beyond that of natural history (6,12). This work represents an attempt to demonstrate degenerative changes in ILFS performed for degenerative, multilevel, spinal stenosis that extend into the upper lumbar spine with the cephalad-end vertebra at L1 or L2. In this series, multilevel (three or more) arthrodesis leads to higher complication rates than have been reported for single- and two-level fusions—83.3% of patients experienced some complication.

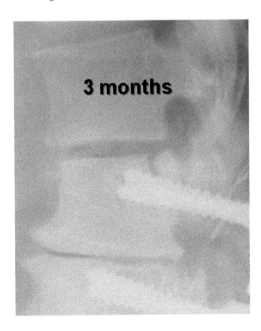

FIGURE 4 Three-month postop film reveals pedicle fracture and screw pullout.

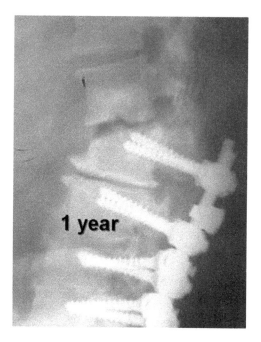

FIGURE 5 One-year postop film reveals healed pedicle fracture and collapse of anterior body with kyphotic angulation.

Sixty-six percent of patients had DDD postoperatively on radiographic evaluation. This rate is higher than most reports and reflects the length and level of the arthrodesis. Guigui reported one of the higher incidence rates of DDD at 49% (14). Instability at the adjacent level was also significant with 27.7% of patients experiencing a fracture or necrosis, leading to kyphotic angulation. These results for instability are consistent with other studies. A study done by Chou presents instability with adjacent segment saggital translation (>4 mm) to be 21.4% in long fusion (three or more level) cases (15). Kumar reports instability following postero-lateral fusion to be 14.2%, although the length of arthrodesis was less (16). The case series presented here suggests that complication rates may be higher for long-instrumented fusions.

The surgeon's philosophy at the time of index surgery was to include only the diseased levels, and perform extensive decompressions and circumferential arthrodesis in an attempt to

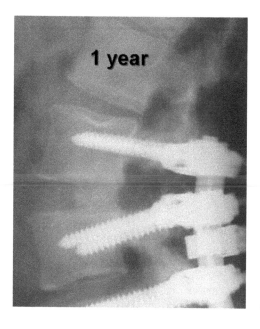

FIGURE 6 One-year postop film reveals correct clinical alignment.

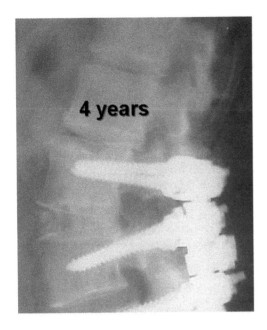

FIGURE 7 Four-year postop film reveals degenerative collapse and retrolisthesis in transition zone.

eliminate both back and leg pain. This series represents a very complex group of older patients with degenerative spinal stenosis. Preoperatively, 5 of the 18 patients had complete myelographic block, 11 had prior laminectomy, and 9 had significant motor defects. Eighty-three percent of patients were taking daily narcotics at the time, prior to surgery, and all had failed a trial of physical therapy and epidural steroid injections. Comorbidities existed in all but two patients, and only two patients had symptoms present less than two years (Table 1).

The clinical outcome mildly improved overall with respect to total medication usage in this series (Fig. 1). Yet those who continued narcotic use had little change in dosage at final follow-up. In regard to pain scores, 5 of the 18 patients did not improve in pain scores for back or leg pain from the initial visit to the final follow-up. Pain scores collected over time amplify the finding of accelerated degeneration (Fig. 1). The initial drop in back and leg pain from a preoperative visit to six-month follow-up is statistically significant ($P < 0.01$). However, the gradual increase in average pain scores during subsequent visits—though not statistically significant—demonstrates a lack of improvement past six months postoperatively, and possibly an increase in pain. Daily life, in terms of employment, ambulation, and assistive device use changed little in this series. Confounding factors during recovery and beyond the index procedure may influence these findings; nevertheless, little improvement in daily life measures was documented.

In addition, the number of major complications and need for significant postoperative intervention are unacceptably high. Disc degeneration is the most common abnormality associated with ASD (4). Our experience was no different. With such a high incidence rate, some suggest that disc degeneration arises from increases in disc pressure (17,18). Furthermore, disc pressure has been said to increase following adjacent fusion (19).

Only three patients did not experience significant complications in the follow-up period. Noteworthy in this series is the high incidence of adjacent segment kyphotic angulation. Five of the 18 patients experienced this problem, which appeared to start with pedicle fatigue failure at the cephalad instrumented level and progressed to collapse of the cephalad-most vertebral body in four. This data appears to support Chow's findings that the mechanical stress from the relatively rigid thoracic spine and lumbosacral fusion was too great to be dissipated over the remaining noninstrumented motion segments—especially in a multilevel fusion (13). In addition, radiographic analysis shows an increase in mobility in noninstrumented segments after posterior fusions (20,21). Whereas the mechanism for the degeneration of the transition zone segment can only be hypothesized, it appears that the length of the fusion, the use of interbody and posterolateral fusion techniques with instrumentation, and the cephalad vertebra at

L1 or L2 leads to unfavorable transition zone mechanics, which appear to accelerate degenerative changes radiographically and symptomatically. In this series, 83.3% of the patients had transition zone changes within a two-year follow-up period. Further surgical treatment for these difficult patients remains unclear and cannot be pursued without conclusive alternatives.

CONCLUSIONS

A single surgeon treated patients with degenerative spinal stenosis. Long instrumented lumbar fusion surgeries with posterolateral and posterior interbody fusion techniques began at L1 or L2 and extended into L5 or S1. Many of these patients developed early onset of transition zone changes, which frequently require additional surgery. Clinical measures improved slightly at best. Furthermore, these accelerated changes resulted in an unacceptably high complication rate in this population with degenerative multilevel spinal stenosis. This correlation suggests that rigid instrumented arthrodesis extending from the upper lumbar spine to the lumbosacral junction cannot be recommended for degenerative spinal conditions.

REFERENCES

1. Aota Y, Kumano K, Hirabayashi. Postfusion instability at the adjacent segments after rigid pedicle screw fixation for degenerative lumbar spinal disorders. J Spinal Disord 1995; 8(6):464–473.
2. Bohnen IM, Schaafsma J, Tonino AJ. Results and complications after posterior lumbar spondylodesis with the "Variable Screw Placement Spinal Fixation System." Acta Orthop Belg 1997; 63(2);67–73.
3. Pihlajamaki H, Myllynen P, Bostman O. Complications of transpedicular lumbosacral fixation for non-traumatic disorders. J Bone Joint Surg Br 1997; 79(2):183–189.
4. Park P, Garton HJ, Gala EC, et al. Adjacent segment disease after lumbar or lumbosacral fusion: review of the literature. Spine 2004; 29(17):1938–1944.
5. Hambly MF, Wiltse LL, Raghavan N, et al. The transition zone above a lumbosacral fusion. Spine 1998; 23(16):1785–1792.
6. Lee CK. Accelerated degeneration of the segment adjacent to a lumbar fusion. Spine 1988; 13(3): 375–377.
7. Wiltse LL, Radecki SE, Biel HM, et al. Comparative study of the incidence and severity of degenerative change in the transition zones after instrumented versus noninstrumented fusions of the lumbar spine. J Spinal Disord 1999; 12(1):27–33.
8. Chen WJ, Lai PL, Niu CC, et al. Surgical treatment of adjacent instability after lumbar spine fusion. Spine 2001; 26(22):E519–524.
9. Eck JC, Humphreys SC, Hodges SD. Adjacent-segment degeneration after lumbar fusion: a review of clinical, biomechanical, and radiologic studies. Am J Orthop 1999; 28(6):336–340.
10. Etebar S, Cahill DW. Risk factors for adjacent-segment failure following lumbar fixation with rigid instrumentation for degenerative instability. J Neurosurg 1999; 90(4 suppl):163–169.
11. Niu CC, Chen WJ, Chen LH, et al. Reduction-fixation spinal systems in spondylolisthesis. Am J Orthop 1996; 25(6):418–424.
12. Rahm MD, Hall BB. Adjacent-segment degeneration after lumbar fusion with instrumentation: a retrospective study. J Spinal Disord 1996; 9(5):392–400.
13. Chow DH, Luke KD, Evans JH, et al. Effects of short anterior lumbar interbody fusion on biomechanics of neighboring unfused segments. Spine 1996; 21(5):549–555.
14. Guigui P, Lambert P, Lassale B, et al. [Long-term outcome at adjacent levels of lumbar arthrodesis.] Rev Chir Orthop Reparatrice Appar Mot 1997; 83:685–696.
15. Chou WY, Hsu CJ, Chang WN, et al. Adjacent segment degeneration after lumbar spinal posterolateral fusion with instrumentation in elderly patients. Arch Orthop Trauma Surg 2002; 122(1):39–43.
16. Kumar MN, Baklanov A, Chopin D. Correlation between sagittal plane changes and adjacent segment degeneration following lumbar spine fusion. Eur Spine J 2001; 10:314–319.
17. Chen CS, Cheng CK, Liu CL, et al. Stress analysis of the disc adjacent to interbody fusion in lumbar spine. Med Eng Phys 2001; 23:483–491.
18. Kim YE, Goel VK, Weinstein JN, et al. Effect of disc degeneration at one level on the adjacent level in axial mode. Spine 1991; 16:331–335.
19. Cunningham BW, Kotani Y, McNulty PS, et al. The effect of spinal destabilization and instrumentation on lumbar intradiscal pressure: an in vitro biomechanical analysis. Spine 1997; 22:2655–2663.
20. Frymoyer JW, Hanley EN Jr, Howe J, et al. A comparison of radiographic findings in fusion and nonfusion patients ten or more years following lumbar disc surgery. Spine 1979; 4:435–440.
21. Stokes IA, Wilder DG, Frymoyer JW, et al. Assessment of patients with low-back pain by biplanar radiographic measurement of intervertebral motion. Spine 1981; 6:233–240.

13 | Adjacent Intervertebral Disc Lesions Following Anterior Cervical Decompression and Fusion: A Minimum 10-Year Follow-up

Shunji Matsunaga
Department of Orthopaedic Surgery, Imakiire General Hospital, Kagoshima, Japan

Yoshimi Nagatomo, Takuya Yamamoto, Kyoji Hayashi, Kazunori Yone, and Setsuro Komiya
Department of Orthopaedic Surgery, Graduate School of Medical and Dental Sciences, Kagoshima University, Kagoshima, Japan

INTRODUCTION

Anterior cervical decompression and fusion was introduced by Robinson and Smith (1) and Cloward (2,3) in the 1950s and became a common procedure because of the excellent clinical results achieved (4–10). However, the influence of anterior cervical decompression and fusion on the unfused segments of the spine has become clear through long-term follow-up studies (11–15). Examination by routine radiography showed the development of degeneration (11,14). Recently, artificial intervertebral disc replacement has developed as a substitute for anterior decompression and fusion (16,17). The authors have investigated the occurrence of herniation of the unfused intervertebral discs on magnetic resonance imaging (MRI) following anterior cervical decompression and fusion to elucidate the influence of this surgery on the unfused segments of the spine.

SUBJECTS AND METHOD

Forty-six patients (31 men, 15 women) subjected to anterior cervical decompression and fusion for herniation of intervertebral discs was examined by MRI pre and postoperatively and post-surgical occurrence of disc herniation were examined with a minimum of 10-year follow-up. Their age at the time of operation ranged from 29 to 71 years (average age 41.3 years old). Anterior decompression and fusion was carried out according to Cloward technique in 28 patients, Robinson technique in four patients, and subtotal vertebrectomy in 14 patients. The range of fusion comprised one segment in 26 patients, two segments in 16 patients, and three segments in four patients. The portions of fusion were C3/4 in 10, C4/5 in 20, C5/6 in 26, C6/7 in 13, and C7/T1 in one patients. Postoperative follow-up was 16.5 years (average ranging from 10–26 years). Disc herniation was defined as the bulging annulus that encroaches on the thecal sac in T1-weighted MRI according to Maruyama's criteria (18). Clinical symptoms were evaluated by the criteria for cervical myelopathy established by the Japanese Orthopaedic Association (JOA score) (19) and the criteria for pain established by White (20). Postoperative results were assessed according to the neuralgic recovery rate of Hirabayashi (21), and were classified according to a four-grade scale into: poor (improvement rate below 25%), fair (26% to 50%), good (51% to 75%), and excellent (more than 76%). Relief of pain was classified using four-grade scale into: poor, fair, good, and excellent according to White's criteria.

STATISTICAL ANALYSIS

Categorical variables were analyzed using χ-square analysis or Fisher's exact test. All values were expressed as means with 95% confidence intervals.

TABLE 1   Characteristics of Patients Showing the Occurrence of Herniation of Intervertebral Discs Postoperatively

Case	Sex	Age (yr)	Fused discs	Procedure	Level of disc herniation	Onset of herniation after surgery (mo)
1	M	31	C4/5	Cloward	C3/4, C6/7[a]	37
2	M	66	C4/5	Cloward	C3/4	51
3	F	29	C5/6	Cloward	C6/7	38
4	F	41	C5/6	Cloward	C6/7	44
5	M	49	C3/4, C4/5	Cloward	C5/6, C6/7	29
6	M	61	C3/4, C4/5, C5/6	Cloward	C6/7	56
7	M	54	C3/4, C4/5	SV	C5/6, C6/7	31
8	F	46	C3/4, C4/5	SV	C5/6	23
9	M	71	C4/5, C5/6	SV	C6/7	42
10	M	50	C4/5, C5/6	SV	C3/4	210
11	F	58	C3/4, C4/5	SV	C5/6	64
12	M	49	C3/4, C4/5	SV	C5/6	68
13	M	52	C5/6, C6/7	SV	C7/T1	69
14	F	39	C5/6, C6/7	SV	C4/5	112
15	M	41	C5/6, C6/7	SV	C4/5	281
16	M	40	C3/4, C4/5, C5/6	SV	C6/7	26

[a]Shows the disc herniation on nonadjacent segment to fusion.
Abbreviations: M, male; F, female; Cloward, Cloward's anterior discectomy and fusion; SV, subtotal vertebrectomy.

RESULTS

Herniation of unfused intervertebral discs was detected in 16 patients (19 discs) out of the 46 patients who underwent MRI examination postoperatively (Fig. 1). The segment affected was C3/4 in three cases, C4/5 in two, C5/6 in five, C6/7 in eight, and C7/T in one. In all but one cases, disc herniation was found on the segments adjacent to anterior decompression and fusion (Table 1). Herniation of unfused intervertebral disc occurred more frequently within five years after surgery (Fig. 2) (22). In case of double- and triple-level fusion, herniation of

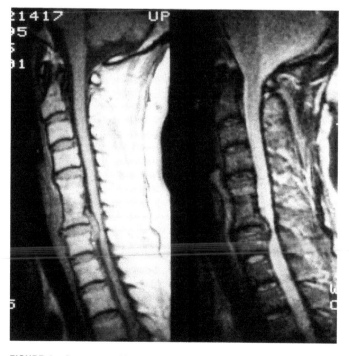

FIGURE 1   Occurence of herniation of unfused intervertebral disc. Massive herniation of C6/7 intervertebral disc was recognized in a 44 year-old woman who had undergone C5/6 anterior decompression and fusion 44 months previously.

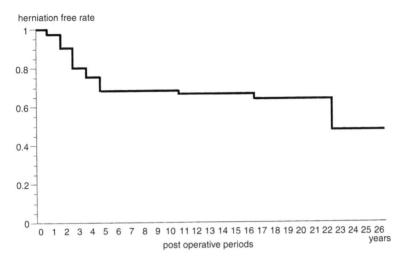

FIGURE 2   Herniation-free rate calculated by Kaplan–Meier method following anterior decompression and fusion.

unfused intervertebral disc occurred more frequently than in the case of single-level fusion (Table 2).

The final recovery rate for myelopathy and pain is shown in Table 3. The rate of relief of pain was superior to that of recovery of myelopathy. The average recovery rate of myelopathy of patients with postoperative disc herniation was 21.9%. This rate was significantly ($P < 0.01$) low when compared with the rate (58.4%) of patients who did not develop disc herniation postoperatively.

DISCUSSION

Anterior cervical decompression and fusion is an established surgical procedure and many researchers have reported good results with this surgery for the treatment of cervical lesions. However, long-term follow-up evaluation of anterior cervical decompression and fusion revealed degenerative changes at levels above and below the fusion. Many claims about the influence of anterior cervical fusion on the unfused segments of the spine have been made. Capen et al. (14) reported that degenerative changes above and below the fusion were detected in 36 of 59 patients treated by anterior surgery after long-term follow-up. Baha et al. (11) noted that cervical flexion/extension resulted in significantly increased movement about the vertebral interspace at the upper adjacent level following anterior cervical fusion. Whether the degenerative changes of the nonfused discs are the body's response to altered mechanical forces on joints next to a fused spinal segment or whether the changes merely represent the natural progression of the degenerative disease process is difficult to ascertain. Gore et al. (23) reviewed the pre- and postoperative lateral cervical roentgenograms of 90 patients who had undergone anterior cervical fusion and compared their findings with age- and sex-matched people without neck problems. They concluded that there was no difference in the incidence of degenerative change between the operated and control group at the levels above and below the fusion. Cherubimo et al. (24) reported that in spite of the worsening of the radiographic findings, from a clinical standpoint there was a significant improvement in

TABLE 2   Relationship Between Occurrence of Herniation and Number of Fusion Discs

Number of fusion discs	Patients	Patients with occurrence of disc herniation (%)	P
One segment	26	4 (15.4)	—
Two segments	16	10 (62.5)	<0.01
Three segments	4	2 (50)	<0.01

TABLE 3 Surgical Results of Myelopathy and Pain

	Patients with adjacent disc herniation [mean (SD)]	Patients without adjacent disc herniation [mean (SD)]
No. of patients	16	30
Recovery rate of myelopathy (%)	21.9 (52.8)	58.4 (34.8)
Grading of recovery of myelopathy		
Excellent	1	9
Good	3	16
Fair	7	4
Poor	5	1
Relief of pain		
Excellent	0	15
Good	4	9
Fair	7	5
Poor	5	1

the symptomatology of 86.5% of the patients. They concluded that degenerative change following anterior cervical fusion was not clinically important. However, patients with postoperative disc herniation of unfused segments showed significantly poor clinical results in the current study. The influence of anterior cervical decompression and fusion on unfused segments cannot be ignored. Recently, artificial intervertebral disc replacement has developed as a substitute for anterior decompression and fusion.

A biomechanical analysis is necessary after anterior cervical decompression and fusion to elucidate its influence on adjacent segments. We had reported that the change of distribution of discs strain following anterior cervical decompression and fusion by individual plane X-ray films of the cervical spine (25). In this study, no statistical increase of shear strain was observed postoperatively in case of single-level fusion. In case of double- and triple-level fusion, however, shear strain was increased at one year postoperatively. Thereafter, the shear strain decreased gradually both in one-level fusion and multi-level fusion. The postoperative herniation occurred more frequently within five years after surgery, and the rate of herniation decreased with time. These changes of shear strain on the intervertebral disc may impact the development of disc herniation following anterior cervical decompression and fusion.

There are many reports about evaluation of disc degeneration by MRI (18,26,27). However, the correlation between histological changes and MRI findings has not yet been established. Maruyama (18) examined 210 cervical discs histologically and by MRI, and established a relationship between types of findings. He emphasized the risk of false-positive posterior protrusion on MRI. We could not determine whether all cases of herniation on MRI in our study represented herniation in the strict sense. However, Maruyama (18) reported that the bulging annulus that encroaches on the thecal sac in T1-weighted MRI corresponded to protrusion-type herniation of the disc in the histological examination in 79.3% of the cases. In our study, nine of 16 patients with disc herniation on MRI showed worsening of clinical symptoms. The development of herniation on postoperative MRI should not be ignored.

REFERENCES

1. Robinson RA, Smith GW. Anterolateral cervical disc removal and interbody fusion for cervical disc syndrome. Bull Johns Hopkins Hosp 1955; 96:223–224.
2. Cloward RB. The anterior approach for removal of ruptured cervical discs. J Neurosurg 1958; 15:602–617.
3. Cloward RB. History of the anterior cervical fusion technique. J Neurosurg 1985; 63:817–818.
4. Connoly Es, Seymour RJ, Adams JE. Clinical evaluation of anterior cervical fusion for degenerative cervical disc disease. J Neurosurg 1965; 23:431–437.
5. Gore DR, Sepic SB. Anterior cervical fusion for degenerated or protruded discs. A review of one hundred forty-six patients. Spine 1984; 9:667–671.
6. Green PW. Anterior cervical fusion. A review of thirty-three patients with cervical disc degeneration. J Bone Joint Surg [Br] 1977; 59:236–240.

7. Herkowitz HN, Kurz LT, Overholt DP. Surgical management of cervical soft disc herniation. A comparison between the anterior and posterior approach. Spine 1990; 10:1026–1030.
8. Lindberg L. Anterior cervical fusion for cervical rhizopathies. A follow-up study. Acta Orthop Scand 1970; 41:312–519.
9. Moussa AH, Nitta M, Symon L. The results of anterior cervical fusion in cervical spondylosis. Review of 125 cases. Acta Neurochir Wien 1983; 68:277–288.
10. Wiersma JA. Anterior cervical fusion: long-term follow-up of 48 patients. J Am Osteopath Assoc 1976; 75:564–568.
11. Baba H, Furusawa N, Imura S, Kawahara N, Tsuchiya H, Tomita K. Late radiographic findings after anterior cervical fusion for spondylotic myeloradiculopathy. Spine 1993; 18:2167–2173.
12. Braunstein EM, Hunter LY, Bailey RW. Long term radiographic changes following anterior cervical fusion. Clin Radiol 1980; 31:201–203.
13. Brunton FJ, Wilkinson JA, Wise KS, Simonis RB. Cine radiography in cervical spondylosis as a means of determining the level for anterior fusion. J Bone Joint Surg [Br] 1982; 64:399–404.
14. Capen DA, Garland DE, Waters RL. Surgical stabilization of the cervical spine. A comparative analysis of anterior and posterior spine fusions. Clin Orthop 1985; 196:229–237.
15. Hunter LY, Braunstein EM, Bailey RW. Radiographic changes following anterior cervical fusion. Spine 1980; 5:399–401.
16. Wigfield CC, Gill SS, Nelson RJ, Metcalf NH, Robertoson JT. The new Frenchay artificial cervical joint results from a pilot study. Spine 2002; 27:2446–2452.
17. Pickett GE, Rouleau JP, Duggal N. Kinematic analysis of the cervical spine following implantation of an artificial cervical disc. Spine 2005; 30:1949–1954.
18. Maruyama Y. Histological, magnetic resonance imaging, and discographic findings on cervical disc degeneration in cadaver spines: a comparative study. J Jpn Orthop Assoc 1995; 69:1102–1112.
19. Yone K, Sakou T, Yanase M, Ijiri K. Preoperative and postoperative magnetic resonance imaging evaluations of the spinal cord in cervical myelopathy. Spine 1992; 17:S388–S392.
20. White AA III, Southwick WO, Deponte RJ, Gainor JW, Hardy R. Relief of pain by anterior cervical fusion for spondylosis. A report of sixty-five patients. J Bone Joint Surg 1973; 55A:525–534.
21. Hirabayashi K, Miyakawa J, Satomi K, Maruyama T, Wakano K. Operative results and postoperative progression of ossification among patients with ossification of cervical posterior longitudinal ligament. Spine 1981; 6:354–364.
22. Kaplan EL, Meier P. Nonparametric estimation from incomplete observation. J Am Stat Assoc 1958; 53:457–481.
23. Gore DR, Gardner GM, Sepic SB, Murray MP. Roentgenographic findings following anterior cervical fusion. Skeletal Radiol 1986; 15:556–559.
24. Cherubimo P, Benazzo F, Borromeo U, Perle S. Degeneration arthritis of the adjacent spinal joints following anterior cervical spinal fusion: clinicoradiologic and statistical correlations. Ital J Orthop Traumatol 1990; 16:533–543.
25. Matsunaga S, Kabayama S, Yamamoto T, Yone K, Sakou T, Nakanisshi K. Strain on interbertebral discs after anterior cervical decompression and fusion. Spine 1999; 24:670–675.
26. Finelli DA, Hurst GC, Karaman BA, Simon JE, Duerk JL, Bellon EM. Use of magnetization transfer for improved contrast on gradient-echo MR images of the cervical spine. Radiology 1994; 193:165–171.
27. Modic MT, Masaryk TJ, Mulopulos GP, Bundschuh C, Han JS, Bohlman H. Cervical radiculopathy: prospective evaluation with surface coil MR imaging, CT with metrizamide, and metrizamide myelography. Radiology 1986; 161:753–759.

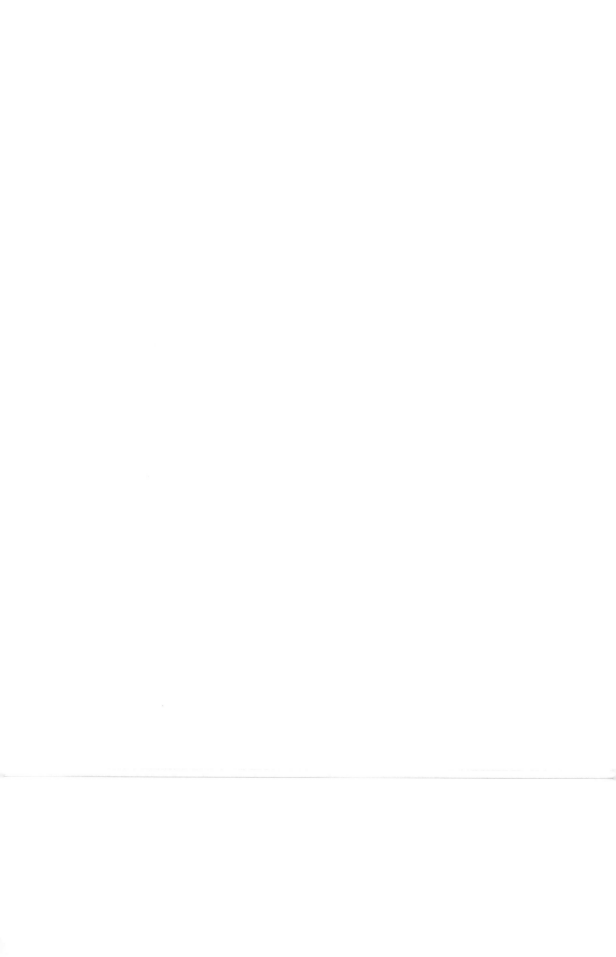

14 | The Role of Biologics in Lumbar Interbody Fusions

Donald W. Kucharzyk
The Orthopaedic, Pediatric and Spine Institute, Crown Point, Indiana, U.S.A.

Low back pain is one of the most commonly cited reasons for patients to schedule an appointment with a physician. It has been cited as the most common cause for lost work and wages in the workforce in the United States (1,2). Despite the frequency of visits to the physician and the economic impact, there is no clear consensus on the appropriate management and treatment of patients with lumbar back pain (3). Surgical and nonsurgical options exist and in most situations, conservative care can avail a patient to an asymptomatic result. But when a patient fails supportive conservative care, surgical intervention in the form of spinal surgery and fusion is indicated (4). With the goal being the elimination of the offending disc and pain generator and stabilization of an unstable spine coupled with the rebalancing and re-establishment of appropriate balance of the spine. This has been accomplished through a variety of means including posterior spinal instrumentation alone, anterior interbody fusion alone, and a combination of both, the 360° fusion (5–7).

The bottom line is a solid, stable arthrodesis of the spinal segments that will be able to sustain loads, maintain disc height and realign, and provide sagittal plane balance. This is the emerging role of interbody fusion in instrumented lumbar fusion surgery (8,9). In patients who have persistent back pain because of a variety of reasons and for which they are appropriate candidates for spinal fusion surgery, commonly the intervertebral disc heights are diminished, loss of lumbar lordosis is apparent, and sagittal plane balance is lost. This is where interbody fusion is most indicated and will allow one to reestablish intervertebral disc height, which translates into adequate decompression of the neural structures and maintenance of neural foraminal patency. It will also allow one to reconstruct segmental lordosis of the individual disc space and maintain overall sagittal plane balance of the operative levels. This in principle should prevent eccentric loading on adjacent segments and prevent degeneration of adjacent segments. Also, interbody fusion and support increases the construct stiffness and provides maintenance of the deformity correction through anterior column support (10–12).

A variety of devices have been developed for interbody and anterior column support. These include autograft, allograft, metallic spacers, biologics, bioabsorbables, and composites. Autograft is the most readily available and can be harvested from the iliac crest in any size, shape, or form for the specific disc space. It can be shaped to establish that degree of lordosis specific for the intervertebral disc and which is necessary to establish the appropriate sagittal plane balance. Unfortunately, it has its share of complications and these include persistent pain, numbness, bleeding, infection, and increased morbidity and mortality.

Allograft is readily available in various forms from freeze-dried to fresh frozen and in various shapes from wedges to femoral rings. The advantages include the availability of significant quantities for multilevel fusions and the ability to contour and shape the allograft. When femoral rings are used, one can contour and shape the graft to match the specific lordosis of the disc space, which is extremely beneficial especially at L5S1. It does provide significant structural support and also provides a bed to insert Demineralized Bone Matrix (DBM), autograft, or bone morphogenetic protein (BMP). Disadvantages include the quality of the graft, preparation of the graft, and the possibility of disease transmission.

Grafts that have been developed incorporate segmental lordosis in addition to providing varying heights and depths in their design. The lordosis is typically 6° and heights range from 7 mm to 13 mm with depths being from 21 mm to 24 mm. These grafts allow placement of local

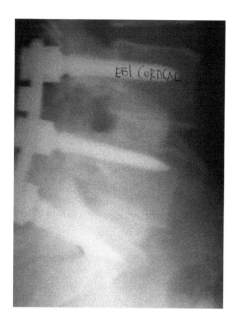

FIGURE 1 Twelve months postop with allograft (EBI, Parsippany, New Jersey, U.S.A.) cortical bone graft with 6° lordosis.

bone, autograft, DBM, or BMP for a complete circumferential interbody fusion. These grafts are available as tangent cortical grafts or EBI cortical (PLIF) posterior lumbar interbody fusion bone (Fig. 1).

In the ever-changing environment of spinal surgery, metallic interbody devices were developed. The first was the Bagby and Kuslich (BAK) device, which was a metallic cylinder that provided stability of the disc space either through anterior or posterior approaches, direct end-plate contact, and a place for bone graft. The disadvantage is that there is no lordosis built into the device. The Ray Cage was next in the evolution and included the same benefits and disadvantages as with the BAK device. To address the need for segmental lordosis, the LT cage was developed, which provided direct end-plate contact with segmental lordosis built into the prosthesis. This took the advantages of the BAK and Ray Cages and added this benefit, which as we know now is important for overall sagittal plane balance.

It allowed for the use of autograft, local bone, and BMP and can function well as a stan-dalone device but it is limited to pure anterior approach and offers no flexibility in being per-formed as a PLIF or transforaminal interbody fusion (TLIF). The EBI, ESL™ (Parsippany, New Jersey, U.S.A.) (endplate sparing lordotic) metallic spacer allows one to insert a spacer that is end-plate sparing, reestablishes segmental lordosis, provides a bed for circumferential bone grafting, and may be inserted via an anterior or posterior approach (Fig. 2).

Biologics in orthopedics has been around for a long time especially in sports medicine, but its role in the spine has only until recently been emerging. Biologics offer the advantage of providing structural support, anterior and lateral column support, and an abundant area for bone grafting. These implants should provide segmental lordosis as well as guard against migration with ease of insertion either via anterior or posterior approach. Biologics that offer this are the PEEK™ (Zimmer Inc., Warsaw, Indiana, U.S.A.) implant and Hourglass, which incorporates all the features as cited here with either 3° or 6° of lordosis as needed for the reconstruction of the sagittal plane balance. PEEK is 3° and Hourglass is in either 3° or 6°. PEEK is a polyetheretherketone polymer that features high tensile strength, high modulus of elas-ticity, is biocompatible, and it features bone-like strength and stiffness.

The implant features segmental lordosis, serrations to prevent migration, as well as ample space for bone graft that will allow for incorporation. Preliminary results in a study of the first 25 patients performed by the author revealed an increase in the anterior disc height by 7 mm, an increase in the posterior disc height of 5 mm, and an increase in the lordotic angle of 6°. Clinical success at 30 months of follow-up was 96% with no implant failure and 100% incorporation of the interbody graft (Fig. 3).

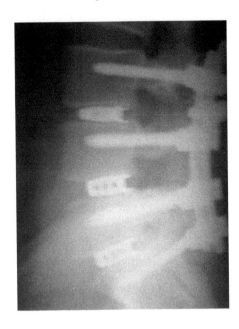

FIGURE 2   Six months postop with EBI, ESL™ (Parsippany, New Jersey, U.S.A.) implant with posterior spinal instrumentation.

Hourglass is a PEEK polymer implant that allows one even greater versatility in determining the degrees of lordosis that the surgeon desires to use. The implant comes in lordotic angles of 3° and 6° with varying heights and lengths. Also, it features an ease of insertion through even a minimally invasive approach by being inserted on its side and then rotating it into position. This allows it to be the perfect choice for either a PLIF or a TLIF approach to the disc space. It also features serrations to prevent migration and provides ample space for grafting (Fig. 4).

Bioabsorbables are an interesting concept for implantation in the intervertebral disc space in spinal fusion cases. If a bioabsorbable would work, it should provide a structural support until the graft has a chance to incorporate, provide adequate strength to support the anterior column and participate in load sharing, and once the absorption process begins feature a low inflammatory rate. Hydrosorb is a bioabsorbable that offers these features (13). It is a PLDLA implant that is 70% poly-L-lactide crystalline with 30% poly-D,L-lactide in a noncrystalline PLA copolymer. This combination provides high strength, slower degradation, slower resorption rates, and a low inflammatory response rate (14,15). Hydrosorb incorporates via bulk hydrolysis with both surface and internal resorption with the end products of this process being CO_2 and H_2O. Numerous studies have evaluated hydrosorb from a TLIF and

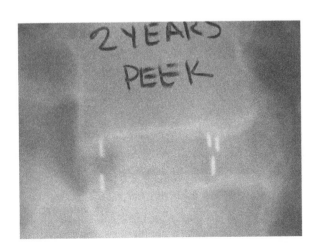

FIGURE 3   Two-years postop polyetheretherketone polymer (PEEK™, Zimmer Inc., Warsaw, Indiana, U.S.A.) interbody implant.

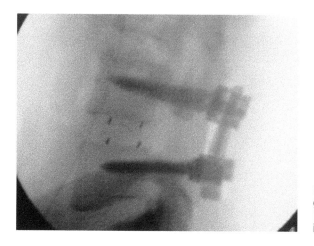

FIGURE 4 Postoperative radiograph of Hour-glass™ interbody implant (Cytori Therapeutics Inc., San Diego, California) with posterior instrumentation.

PLIF device design approach and results have shown favorable results. In TLIF studies, the fusion rates have been reported in follow-up of up to 18 months from 97% to 100% with no long-term implant complications. In PLIF studies, at longest follow-up of 32 months, fusion rates ranged from 96% to 100% with no implant complications in one and a 7% complication rate reported by Couture and Branch.

And when one combines all the studies involving hydrosorb with greater than one year follow-up, fusion rates have been reported at 97% with an implant complication rate of only 1.7% (16). In a study of 20 patients undertaken at our institution, we observed that the anterior disc height was increased by 7.5 mm, the posterior disc height was increased by 5.5 mm, and the segmental lordosis was increased by seven degrees. The results have been promising with reference to the ability to reestablish the sagittal alignment and disc heights but complications have occurred with this implant. Complications seen have arisen from the aggressive hydrolysis of the implant that causes an apparent appearance of a recurrent disc and at time of re-exploration it was a fluid collection and was because of the slower than normal reabsorption of the fluid (17–20). Also, we have seen nonunions of the graft in most recent follow-up at 24 months with poor incorporation of the grafts seen and a nonunion rate of 8% in our current study (Fig. 5).

If one could combine two emerging technologies and provide an excellent scaffold for incorporation, this could meet a need in spine fusion technology. Such a combination exists in the form of BioPlex. This is a combination of a PLDLLA™ polymer (hydrosorb) coupled with coralline hydroxyapatite (ProOsteon 500R). This combination provided improved strength, slower degradation rates, and improved ingrowth throughout the implant (21). This was far superior to that of PLDLA alone and when one analyzed the amount of new

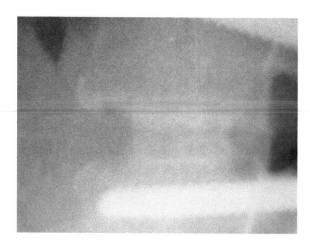

FIGURE 5 Twelve months postop with hydrosorb interbody implant and posterior instrumentation revealing incorporation of graft and bridging bone with no evidence nonunion.

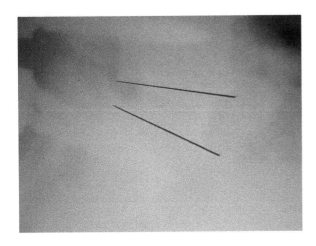

FIGURE 6 Six months postop with BioPlex™ (Interpore Cross International, Irvine, California) interbody graft with posterior spinal instrumentation.

bone formation in BioPlex compared with PLDLA alone, there was significantly greater new bone formation with a stronger implant–bone interface (21). This stabilizes the implant at the site and prevents migration. In addition, BioPlex features no significant inflammatory reactions or bone resorption and had a high degree of biocompatibility at long-term follow-up. Its design features parallel end-plates but recent changes now allow an implant with 6° of lordosis with again varying heights and depths for customization specific for the patient (Fig. 6) (22).

As technology continues, newer implants involving bioabsorbables and biologics will be seen possibly including the BMP technology. But with any implant, it must stand up to the gold standard autograft and to a certain extent allograft. The implant must provide the surgeon with ease of insertion, applicability via either an anterior or posterior approach, minimal trauma to the spinal cord and nerve roots, re-establish segmental lordosis, reconstruct sagittal plane balance, maintain disc height, feature a low incidence of subsidence with no migration, incorporate with ingrowth of new bone, and most importantly maintain the decompression of the neuroforaminae. If these devices can provide this, then they have met the criteria and can enhance a lumbar fusion with the understanding that these devices are not standalone devices and will require supplemental posterior instrumentation.

REFERENCES

1. Deyo RA, Tsui-Wu YJ. Descriptive epidemiology of low back pain and its related medical care in the United States. Spine 1987; 12:264–268.
2. Bentkover JD, Sheshinski RH, Hedley-Whyte J, Warfield CA, Mosteller F. Lower back pain: laminectomies, spinal fusion, demographics, and socioeconomics. Int J Technol Assess Health Care 1992; 8:309–317.
3. Holbrook TL, Glazier K, Kelsey JL, Stauffer RN. The socioeconomic impact of selected musculoskeletal disorders. Am Acad Orthop Surg Chicago 1984.
4. Turner JA, Ersek M, Herron L, et al. Patient outcomes after lumbar spinal fusions. JAMA 1992; 268:907–911.
5. Zdeblick TA. A prospective randomized study of lumbar fusion. Spine 1993; 18:983–991.
6. Hanley EN. The indications for lumbar spinal fusion with and without instrumentation. Spine 1995; 20(suppl 24):S143–S153.
7. Sonntag VK, Marciano FF. Is fusion indicated for lumbar spinal disorders? Spine 1995; 20(suppl 24):S138–S142.
8. Humphreys SC, Hodges SD, Patwardham AG, et al. Comparison of posterior and transforaminal approaches to lumbar interbody fusion. Spine 2001; 26:567–571.
9. Stonecipher T, Wright S. Posterior lumbar interbody fusion with facet screw fixation. Spine 1989; 14:468–471.
10. Booth KC, Bridwell KH, Lenke LG, et al. Complications and predictive factors for the successful treatment of flatback deformity (fixed sagittal imbalance). Spine 1999; 24:1712–1720.
11. Enker P, Steffee AD. Interbody fusion and instrumentation. Clin Orthop 1994; 300:90–101.
12. Gelb DE, Lenke LG, Bridwell KH, et al. An analysis of sagittal spinal alignment in 100 asymptomatic middle and older aged volunteers. Spine 1995; 20:1351–1358.

13. Kulkarni RK, Pani KC, Neuman C, Leonard F. Polylactic acid for surgical implants. Arch Surg 1966; 93:839–843.
14. Leenslag JW, Pennings AJ, Bos RR, Rozema FR, Boering G. Resorbable material of poly-L-lactide plates and Screwsa for internal fracture fixation. Spine 1987; 8:70–77.
15. Vainionpaa S, Kilpikari J, Laiho J, Helevirta P, Rokkanen P, Tormala P. Strength and strength retention in vitro of absorbable self reinforced PGA rods for fracture fixation. Spine 1987; 8:46–48.
16. Borden M, BioPlex Technology Overview, BioMet, EBI, InterporeCross Oct 2004.
17. Bostman OM. Reaction to biodegradable implants. J Bone Joint Surg Br 1993; 75:336–337.
18. Bostman OM. Intense granulomatous inflammatory lesions associated with absorbable internal fixation devices made of polyglycolide in ankle fractures. Clin Orthop 1998; 348:193–199.
19. Bostman OM. Osteoarthritis of the ankle after foreign body reaction to absorbable pins and screws. J Bone Joint Surg Br 1998; 80:333–338.
20. Bostman OM, Pihlajamaki HK. Adverse tissue reactions to bioabsorbable fixation devices. Clin Orthop 2000; 372:216–227.
21. Thomson RC, Yaszemski MJ, Powers JM, Mikos AG. Fabrication of biodegradable polymer scaffolds to engineer trabecular bone. J Biomater Sci Polym Ed 1995; 7:23–38.
22. Toth JM, Wang M, Scifert JL, et al. Evaluation of 70/30 DLPLA for use as a resorbable interbody fusion cage. Orthopaedics 2002; 25:1121–1130.

15 | Current Perspectives on Biologic Strategies for the Therapy of Intervertebral Disc Degeneration

Helen E. Gruber and Edward N. Hanley, Jr.
Carolinas Healthcare System, Charlotte, North Carolina, U.S.A.

INTRODUCTION

Promising new approaches for the biologic treatment of disc degeneration are evolving from a number of current scientific fronts, including: (*i*) an improved understanding of the function of the disc cell in vivo; (*ii*) advances in tissue engineering, (*iii*) advances in gene therapy techniques, and (*iv*) recognition of the potential value of stem cells in cell-based therapies. Biologic approaches to disc therapy are important as current methods of treatment, including fusion, disc spacers and disc replacement, are not physiologic, limit motion, and place excess stress on adjacent spinal segments. Methods which manipulate and modulate disc cell function open exciting and challenging new therapeutic possibilities. In this Chapter, we provide a current perspective on the progress relevant to biologic treatments for disc degeneration, as demonstrated by progress from basic science contributions toward the understanding of disc cell biology, manipulation of disc cells, and new biologic strategies for the therapy of intervertebral disc degeneration (Fig. 1).

DISC CELL FUNCTION
Basic Science Contributions Toward the Understanding of Disc Cell Biology

In spite of the large health care costs associated with low back pain and disc degeneration, much less is currently known about the regulation of the disc extracellular matrix (ECM) and disc cell biology compared with our understanding of the bone and cartilage matrices, or chondrocyte, osteoblast, or osteoclast cell behavior.

It is critically important to understand disc biology because ultimately it is the ECM which fails in disc degeneration; dehydration and matrix fraying culminate in the formation of tears within the annulus during biomechanical loading and torsion. The nucleus and disc material rupture through these tears, impinging on nerves and causing pain. The life-time prevalence of low back pain in the general population is about 80%. It is a primary cause of disability and plays a major role in this country's medical, social, and economic structure. Estimated costs related to low back disorders are in the range of $50–100 billion per year in the United States alone. In spite of these highly relevant health care statistics, the structural integrity of the intervertebral disc ECM, and the complex interaction between disc cells and the ECM they produce and remodel, remain poorly understood.

Recent reviews summarizing important advances in disc cell biology were published in 2003 (1–3). Here, we will highlight relevant new research (2003 to August 2005) which expands our understanding of the biology of the disc.

It is now known that the ECM can modulate cell function via growth factor/bioactive agents bound within in it and thus influence cell proliferation and gene expression. A protein known to regulate the ECM, secreted protein, acidic, and rich in cysteine (SPARC, also called osteonectin and BM-40), is a "matricellular protein" that in itself is not a structural component of the ECM. Instead, this protein mediates cell–ECM interactions and ECM production/assembly. Recent work by Gruber et al. (4) documented that SPARC is present in the human disc, and suggests the significance of future studies to identify its role and function in the disc ECM homeostasis.

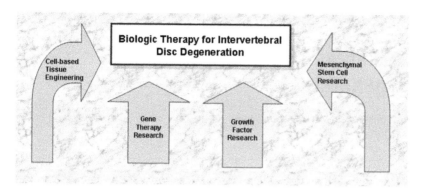

FIGURE 1   Schematic diagram presenting the major components providing essential scientific information for biologic therapy for disc degeneration.

Manipulation of Disc Cells In Vitro
Monolayer and Three-Dimensional Cell Culture
Relevant current research efforts involving development of techniques to culture disc cells in vitro in monolayer and three-dimensional (3D) construct are important not only for in vitro experiments, but also because such studies can lead to carrier material for cell implantation. Such "cell carrier" constructs can not only provide a physical support system for cells, but can also provide specific microenvironments and molecules designed to direct cell proliferation or ECM product or to influence cell signaling pathways. Important cell carrier characteristics include the ability to support disc cell attachment and the ability to provide a microenvironment, which allows expression of desired gene products. Carriers which are to be implanted should also undergo biologic degradation but not produce inflammatory or giant cell host responses, and also should not produce degradation products which lower pH as this could have adverse effects on implanted cells. An interesting current developmental area in tissue engineering involves formulation of "smart materials" to serve as cell scaffolds (5). Rosso et al. (5) explain that these scaffolds may contain oligopeptide cleaving sequences for biologically relevant molecules such as matrix metalloproteinases, integrin-binding site, or growth factors, thus providing the ability to present these materials directly to cells seeded within them.

Cell carrier materials with recent disc applications include the atelocollagen scaffold used by Sato et al. (6) for in vitro studies and implantation into the rabbit disc. A porous calcium polyphosphate substrate has been investigated by Séguin et al. (7) with studies of bovine caudal disc cells, and Yang et al. (8) used a gelatin/chondroitin-6-sulfate copolymer scaffold to culture human disc cells. Alginate culture of rabbit disc cells was used by Anderson et al. (9) to show that fibronectin fragments appear to have a detrimental role on disc cell function. Shen et al. (10) used agarose disc culture to demonstrate that interleukin-1β can induce matrix metalloproteinase-2 and -3 activities in ovine disc cells. A collagen-hyaluronan scaffold was used by Alini et al. (11) to culture bovine disc cells for long-term studies. Gruber et al. (12) showed that media supplementation with insulin, transferring and sodium selenite, insulin-like growth factor-1 (IGF-1) and transforming growth factor-β1 (TGF-β1) could modulate human disc cell ECM production in agarose culture. Extracellular matrix production and human disc cell gene expression were tested by Gruber et al. (13) in a comparison of collagen sponge, collagen gel, alginate, agarose, and fibrin culture microenvironments; the collagen sponge provides superior ECM production and gene expression results.

Zhang et al. (14) chose alginate beads to assess the effects of growth factor osteogenic protein-1 on bovine disc cells (15). Masuda et al. (16) also used alginate beads to show that recombinant osteogenic protein-1 upregulates ECM metabolism in rabbit disc cells. Wiseman et al. (17) demonstrated variation in metabolic function in cells derived from sequential bovine caudal discs and then cultured in alginate beads. Yoon et al. (18) used monolayer cell culture to show that bone morphogenetic protein-2 induces rat disc cells to produce more

ECM and enhance cell proliferation. Monolayer culture was also used by Johnson et al. (19) to demonstrate that aggrecan derived from the human disc is inhibitory for endothelial cell migration.

Whole-Organ Disc Culture

Whole-organ culture of discs is a laboratory technique which is receiving increased attention. With this technique, loss of proteoglycans from the disc can be prevented because the disc is left intact surrounded by adjacent vertebral endplates and soft tissue. Two recent publications have used this specialized culture technique. Ariga et al. (20) have harvested mouse coccygeal discs and applied static compression loads; loaded discs showed the presence of apoptotic cells when compared with unloaded discs. Risbud et al. (21) used a disc organ culture system to assess rat lumbar discs; cells were metabolically active producing type II collagen, aggrecan, and decorin after one week in culture.

Growth Factor Studies

Two excellent reviews on growth factors and the intervertebral disc were published by Masuda et al. in 2004 (22,23); the interested reader is referred to these summaries for detailed information. Table 1 summarizes the major growth factors studied to date with relevance to disc cell biology. Both in vivo and in vitro experimental evidence points to the potential value of recombinant growth factors in treating disc degeneration. As delineated in Masuda et al., osteogenic protein-1, IGF-1, growth differentiation factor-5 (GDF-5), and TGF-β appear to have had the most utilization as applied to in vitro and in vivo models. Application of growth factors following induction of disc degeneration in animal models has also been tested, as illustrated by the study of Walsh et al. in which degeneration was induced in murine caudal discs by static compression, and GDF-5, IGF-1, or basic fibroblast growth factor (bFGF) injected into the disc (24). These researchers found the most prominent positive effects following administration of GDF-5 and TGF-β, a lesser effect with IGF-1, and little effect with bFGF.

   Growth factor research as related to the disc is an exciting current avenue of research; much further work is needed to elucidate the effects of growth factors on disc cells, both in vivo and in vitro.

Animal Models

Phillips et al. have recently observed that it is unfortunate that the majority of current animal models for disc degeneration involve infliction of a physical or chemical injury to the disc; as this may not accurately replicate the degenerative process(es) in the human disc, this caveat should be kept in mind (25). Commonly employed current models utilize a stab injury to

TABLE 1 Selected Growth Factors with Relevance to Disc Cell Biology

Growth factor	Effect on cell proliferation	Effect on proteoglycan production	Comments
TGF-β, TGF-β1	Increases	Increases	Studied in vitro and in vivo
IGF-1	Increases	Increases	Decreases apoptosis in vitro; studied in vitro and in vivo
PDGF	—	—	Decreases apoptosis in vitro
OP-1, BMP-7	—	Increases	Studied in vitro and in vivo
BMP-2	—	Increases	Increases collagen production in vitro
BMP-12	—	Increases	Increases collagen production in vitro
GDF-5	—	—	Increased cell population in vivo
bFGF	Increases	Increases	Studied in vitro and in vivo
EGF	Increases	Increases	Organ culture (in vitro)

Abbreviations: bFGF, basic fibroblast growth factor; BMP, bone morphogenetic protein; EGF, epidermal growth factor; GDF-5, growth differentiation factor-5; IGF-1, insulin-like growth factor-1; OP-1, osteogenic protein-1; PDGF, platelet-derived growth factor; TGF, transforming growth factor.
Source: From Refs. 22, 23.

the disc, or apply mechanical compression. It is worth noting here that the sand rat model (*Psammomys obesus*) is a spontaneous, age-related animal model of disc degeneration which has an extremely reliable pattern of disc degeneration (26,27). The sand rat model been used successfully in autologous disc cell implantation implanting cells either by injection or via cell placement within a collagen carrier (28).

Nonhuman primates are costly research models, but there has been one study by Pfeiffer et al. that tested whether hyaluronic acid could influence the degenerative changes in discs following nucleotomy (29). Favorable outcomes were seen with this implant material as assessed with radiography, magnetic resonance imaging (MRI) and computed tomography (CT). Canine is another large animal model which has been used in disc research, as illustrated by the studies of Ganey et al., which employed autologous chondrocytes reimplanted in the donor animal and assessed after 12 weeks (30). This technique was deemed technically feasible and retarded disc degeneration. Haro et al. also used the canine model to test the effects of recombinant human matrix metalloproteinases on disc resorption (31). Rabbits, another popular animal model, continue to be used by a number of groups active in the gene therapy field.

Another approach utilizing animal models in the study of disc degeneration is to use an animal, usually a mouse, with a known single molecular defect. There are two recent examples of such animal models. Li et al. have utilized disc cells harvested from GDF-5 $(-/-)$ and $(+/+)$ mice, and assessed the cellular in vitro response to recombinant GDF-5 (32). Treatment produced upregulation of aggrecan and type II collagen. Gruber et al. have explored the role of SPARC in disc biology by examining SPARC null and wild-type mice; they found that when SPARC was absent, lumbar discs underwent accelerated degeneration and contained herniations and abnormal matrix collagen fibrils (33). The use of such knock-out (null) animal models adds a new, important tool with which new research possibilities open for the disc.

BIOLOGIC STRATEGIES FOR THE THERAPY OF INTERVERTEBRAL DISC DEGENERATION
Tissue Engineering Involving Cellular Transplantation

As the human disc is avascular by young adulthood (and thus may be "immuno-privileged"), the disc appears well-suited for cell-based application of tissue engineering either by application of cells alone or by cells in combination with a carrier material or scaffold. As the aging and degenerating disc has a declining number of cells, augmentation of the cell population is a desirable goal, as is the direction of gene expression and protein production of desired ECM components. As pointed out by Bertram et al. in their rabbit studies, development and choice of appropriate matrix substitutes is an important issue to ensure transplanted cell survival in the avascular disc (34). Progress on disc tissue engineering involving cell transplantation has advanced because of progress in the fields of gene therapy, the action of growth factors on disc cells, and mesenchymal stem cell research; each of these topics is discussed subsequently. These are other aspects of orthopedic gene therapy and has also been reviewed by Evans et al. (35).

Gene Therapy

Gene therapy efforts directed toward biologic therapy for disc degeneration are based on selection of genes with specific products and attributes, which favor improvement of the disc tissue. Such genes are delivered via disc cells, which have first been altered in vitro and then are implanted into the disc. Selection of the gene of interest may be either designed to enhance matrix synthesis (anabolic), or to prevent matrix degradation (catabolic); thus the reader can readily appreciate how critical it is to expand our basic science knowledge base on disc matrix formation and turnover.

Six recent review articles have focused on the current advances in gene therapy as related to therapeutic approaches for disc degeneration (36–41). These articles summarize both researches with animal and human cells in vitro and animal in vivo studies. Adenoviral vectors have been studied both in vivo and in vitro; as noted by Lattermann et al., concerns do exist about immunogenicity and potential safety in the clinical therapeutic setting as spinal applications near the central nervous system could have potentially toxic or immunologic side effects. Because of these issues, Lattermann et al. have investigated the adeno-associated viral vector methodology (42). These vectors were studied in designs where the vector carried various marker genes, and were used to transduce both human and rabbit disc cells. The in vivo and in vitro findings showed that this technique holds significant promise for future gene therapy research. Other recent gene therapy studies evaluated GDF-5, TGF-β, LMP-1, SOX9, and tissue inhibitor of matrix metalloproteinase-1 (TIMP-1) (22,43–46).

Stem Cell Applications

Although scientific utilization of fetal stem cells remains controversial, mesenchymal stem cells have gained prominence because these uncommitted pluripotent stem cells are present in skeletal muscle, dermis, bone marrow, fat, and synovial membranes of adults. The use of such stem cells represents the newest area of interest in tissue engineering. Mesenchymal stem cells (MSCs) are high clonogenic cells with the capacity of self-renewal and multilineage differentiation (47–49). Such adult stem cells are being investigated for applications in orthopedic tissue engineering, such as the chondrogenic differentiation studies by Awad et al. which utilized adipose-derived MSCs (47).

Mesenchymal Stem Cells for Disc Research

Since the earlier 2003 reviews (1–3), increasing interest has developed regarding the use of MSCs in disc applications (50–52). Sakai et al. have used autologous rabbit MSCs and implanted them into the donor disc in a collagen gel (53); the stem cell implantation was successful and there was evidence of proteoglycan production. Steck et al. used human bone marrow-derived MSCs that were cultured to develop disc-like cells as assessed with gene array profiles (54). Rat MSCs were cultured by Risbud et al. in a study which used hypoxia and TGF-β to differentiate cells to a disc-like phenotype (55). Crevensten et al. also used the rat model in their studies which injected MSCs in a gel into the disc; cells remained viable and proliferated (56). Yamamoto et al. used a coculture experimental technique and found that direct cell–cell contact between rabbit nucleus pulposus cells and bone marrow-derived MSCs increased cell proliferation and proteoglycan synthesis (57). Rabbits were also used by Zhang et al. in a study which showed that bone marrow-derived MSCs that were transplanted into the disc increased proteoglycan production (58).

Considerable optimism exists for the potential contribution of MSCs in biologic therapy of disc degeneration. Progress in other areas of disc cell biology, such as characterization of disc cell phenotypes, cell carrier materials, and growth factors beneficial to disc cell survival, proliferation and ECM production, will benefit future MSC disc research.

CONCLUSIONS AND FUTURE DIRECTIONS

- Enthusiasm continues to be high for biologic approaches to treat disc degeneration.
- Potential biologic therapies include cell-based tissue engineering, gene therapy, and the application of adult MSCs.
- Information obtained from basic science studies of the disc, disc cells, and animal models of disc degeneration plays an important role in obtaining information critical for successful biologic therapies for disc degeneration.

REFERENCES

1. Gruber HE, Hanley EN, Jr. Recent advances in disc cell biology. Spine 2003; 28:186–193.
2. Gruber HE, Hanley EN Jr. Current perspectives on novel biologic therapies for intervertebral disc degeneration. Minerva Ortopedica e Traumatologica 2003; 54:297–303.
3. Gruber HE, Hanley EN Jr. Biologic strategies for the therapy of intervertebral disc degeneration. Expert Opin Biol Ther 2003; 3:1209–1214.

4. Gruber HE, Ingram JA, Leslie K, Hanley EN Jr. Cellular, but not matrix, immunolocalization of SPARC in the human intervertebral disc—decreasing localization with aging and disc degeneration. Spine 2004; 29:2223–2228.
5. Rosso F, Marino G, Giordano A, Barbarisi M, Parmeggiani D, Barbarisi A. Smart materials as scaffolds for tissue engineering. J Cell Physiol 2005; 203:465–470.
6. Sato M, Asazuma T, Ishihara M, Kikuchi T, Kikuchi M, Fujikawa K. An experimental study of regeneration of intervertebral disc with an allograft of cultured annulus fibrosus cells using a tissue enginering method. Spine 2003; 28:548–553.
7. Séguin Cagmdprmwsdkra. Tissue engineered nucleus pulposus tissue formed on a porous calcium polyphosphate substrate. Spine 2004; 29:1299–1307.
8. Yang S-H, Chen P-Q, Chen mYF, Lin F-H. Gelatin/chondroitin-6-sulfate copolymer scaffold for culturing human nucleus pulposus cells in vitro with production of extracellular matrix. J Biomed Mater Res Part B: Appl Biomater 2005; 74B:488–494.
9. Anderson DG, Li X, Balian G. A fibronectin fragment alters the metabolism by rabbit intervertebral disc cells in vitro. Spine 2005; 30:1242–1246.
10. Shen B, Melrose J, Ghosh P, Taylor TKF. Induction of matrix metalloproteinase-2 and -3 activity in ovine nucleus pulposus cells grown in three-dimensional agarose gel culture by interleukin-β: a potential pathway of disc degeneration. Eur Spine J 2003; 12:66–75.
11. Alini M, Li W, Markovic P, Aebi M, Spiro RC, Roughley PJ. The potential and limitations of a cell-seeded collagen/hyaluronan scaffold to engineer an intervertebral disc-like matrix. Spine 2003; 28:446–454.
12. Gruber HE, Norton HJ, Leslie K, Hanley EN, Jr. Clinical and demographic prognostic indicators for human disc cell proliferation in vitro: a pilot study. Spine 2001; 26:2323–2327.
13. Gruber HE, Leslie K, Ingram J, Norton HJ, Hanley EN, Jr. Cell-based tissue engineering for the intervertebral disc: in vitro studies of human disc cell gene expression and matrix production within selected cell carriers. Spine J 2004; 4:44–55.
14. Zhang Y, An HS, Song S, et al. Growth factor osteogenic protein-1. Differing effects on cells from three distinct zones in the bovine intervertebral disc. Am J Phys Med Rehabil 2004; 83:515–521.
15. Ahang Y, An HS, Toofanfard M, Li Z, Andersson GBJ, Thonar EJMA. Low-dose interleukin-1 partially counteracts osteogenic protein-1-induced proteoglycan synthesis by adult bovine intervertebral disc cells. Am J Phys Med Rehabil 2005; 84:322–329.
16. Masuda K, Takegami K, An H, et al. Recombinant osteogenic protein-1 upregulates extracellular matrix metabolism by rabbit annulus fibrosus and nucleus pulposus cells cultured in alginate beads. J Orthop Res 2003; 21:922–930.
17. Wiseman MA, Birch HL, Akmal M, Goodship AE. Segmental variation in the in vitro cell metabolism of nucleus pulposus cells isolated from a series of bovine caudal intervertebral discs. Spine 2005; 30:505–511.
18. Yoon ST, Kim KS, Li J, et al. The effect of bone morphogenetic protein-2 on rat intervertebral disc cells in vitro. Spine 2003; 28:1773–1780.
19. Johnson WEB, Caterson B, Eisenstein SM, Roberts S. Human intervertebral disc aggrecan inhibits endothelial cell adhesion and cell migration in vitro. Spine 2005; 30:1139–1147.
20. Ariga K, Yonenobu K, Nakase T, et al. Mechanical stress-induced apoptosis of endplate chondrocytes in organ-cultured mouse intervertebral discs—an ex vivo study. Spine 2003; 28:1528–1533.
21. Risbud MV, Izzo MW, Adams CS, et al. An organ culture system for the study of the nucleus pulposus: description of the system and evaluation of the cells. Spine 2003; 28:2652–2658.
22. Masuda K, Oegema TR, Jr., An HS. Growth factors and treatment of intervertebral disc degeneration. Spine 2004; 29:2757–2769.
23. Masuda K, An HS. Growth factors and the intervertebral disc. Spine J 2004; 4:S330–S340.
24. Walsh AJL, Bradford DS, Lotz JC. In vivo growth factor treatment of degenerated intervertebral discs. Spine 2004; 29:156–163.
25. Phillips FM, An H, Kang JD, Boden SD, Weinstein J. Biologic treatment for intervertebral disc degeneration—summary statement. Spine 2003; 28:S99.
26. Gruber HE, Johnson T, Norton HJ, Hanley EN, Jr. The sand rat model for disc degeneration: radiologic characterization of age-related changes. Cross-sectional and prospective analyses. Spine 2002; 27:230–234.
27. Gruber HE, Gordon B, Williams C, Norton HJ, Hanley EN, Jr. Bone mineral density of lumbar vertebral end plates in the aging male sand rat spine. Spine 2003; 28:1766–1772.
28. Gruber HE, Johnson TL, Leslie K, et al. Autologous intervertebral disc cell implantation: a model using *Psammomys obesus*, the sand rat. Spine 2002; 27:1626–1633.
29. Pfeiffer M, Boudriot U, Pfeiffer D, Ishaque N, Goetz W, Wilke A. Intradiscal application of hyaluronic acid in the non-human primate lumbar spine: radiologic results. Eur Spine J 2003; 12:76–83.
30. Yamamoto Y, Fujimura M, Nishita T, Nishijima K, Atoji Y, Suzuki Y. Immunohistochemical localization of carbonic anhydrase isozymes in the rat carotid body. J Anat 2003; 202:573–577.

31. Haro H, Komori H, Kato T, et al. Experimental studies on the effects of recombinant human matrix metalloproteinases on herniated disc tissues-how to facilitate the natural resorption process of herniated discs. J Orthop Res 2005; 23:412–419.
32. Li X, Leo BM, Beck G, Balian G, Anderson DG. Collagen and proteoglycan abnormalities in the GDF-5-deficient mice and molecular changes when treating disc cells with recombinant growth factor. Spine 2004; 29:2229–2234.
33. Gruber HE, Sage EH, Norton HJ, Funk S, Ingram J, Hanley EN, Jr. Targeted deletion of the SPARC gene accelerates disc degeneration in the aging mouse. J Histochem Cytochem 2005; 53:1131–1138.
34. Bertram H, Kroeber M, Wang H, et al. Matrix-assisted cell transfer for intervertebral disc cell therapy. Biochem Biophys Res Commun 2005; 331:1185–1192.
35. Evans CH, Ghivizzani SC, Robbins PD. The 2003 Nicolas Andry Award: orthopaedic gene therapy. Clin Orthop 2004; 429:316–329.
36. Yoon ST. The potential of gene therapy for the treatment of disc degeneration. Orthop Clin N Am 2004; 35:95–100.
37. Chadderdon RC, Shimer AL, Gilbertson LG, Kang JD. Advances in gene therapy for intervertebral disc degeneration. Spine J 2004; 4:S341–S347.
38. Shimer AL, Chadderdon RC, Gilbertson LG, Kang JD. Gene therapy approaches for intervertebral disc degeneration. Spine 2004; 29:2770–2778.
39. Wallach CJ, Gilbertson LG, Kang JD. Gene therapy applications for intervertebral disc degeneration. Spine 2003; 28:S93–S98.
40. Sobajima S, Kim JS, Gilbertson LG, Kang JD. Gene therapy for degenerative disc disease. Gene Ther 2004; 11:390–401.
41. Levicoff EA, Gilbertson LG, Kang JD. Gene therapy to prevent or treat disc degeneration: is this the future? SpineLine 2005; VI:10–16.
42. Lattermann C, Oxner WM, Xiao X, et al. The adeno associated viral vector as a strategy for intradiscal gene transfer in immune competent and pre-exposed rabbits. Spine 2005; 30:497–504.
43. Wang H, Kroeber M, Hanke M, et al. Release of active and depot GDF-5 after adenovirus-mediated overexpression stimulates rabbit and human intervertebral disc cells. J Mol Med 2004; 82:126–134.
44. Yoon ST, Park JS, Kim KS, et al. ISSLS prize winner: LMP-1 upregulates intervertebral disc cell production of proteoglycans and BMPs in vitro and in vivo. Spine 2004; 29:2603–2611.
45. Paul R, Haydon RC, Cheng HW, et al. Potential use of Sox9 gene therapy for intervertebral degenerative disc disease. Spine 2003; 28:755–763.
46. Wallach CJ, Watanabe Y, Gilbertson LG, Kang JD. Gene transfer of the catabolic inhibitor tissue inhibitor of metalloproteinase-1 increases measured proteoglycans in cells from degenerated human intervertebral discs. Spine 2003; 28:2331–2337.
47. Conrad C, Huss R. Adult stem cell lines in regenerative medicine and reconstructive surgery. J Surg Res 2005; 124:201–208.
48. Jorgensen C, Gordeladze J, Noel D. Tissue engineering through autologous mesenchymal stem cells. Curr Opin Biotechnol 2004; 15:406–410.
49. Roberts I. Mesenchymal stem cells. Vox Sang 2004; 87:38–41.
50. Mochida J. New strategies for disc repair: novel preclinical trials. J Orthop Sci 2005; 10:112–118.
51. Risbud MV, Shapiro IM, Vaccaro AR, Albert TJ. Stem cell regeneration of the nucleus pulposus. Spine J 2004; 4:S348–S353.
52. Brisby H, Tao H, Ma DDF, Diwan AD. Cell therapy for disc degeneration—potentials and pitfalls. Orthop Clin N Am 2004; 35:85–93.
53. Sakai D, Mochida J, Yamamoto Y, et al. Transplantation of mesenchymal stem cells embedded in Atelocollagen® gel to the intervertebral disc: a potential therapeutic model for disc degeneration. Biomaterials 2003; 24:3531–3541.
54. Steck E, Bertram H, Abel R, Chen BH, Winter A, Richter W. Induction of intervertebral disc-like cells from adult mesenchymal stem cells. Stem Cells 2005; 23:403–411.
55. Risbud MV, Albert TJ, Guttapalli A, et al. Differentiation of mesenchymal stem cells towards a nucleus pulposus-like phenotype in vitro: implications for cell-based transplantation therapy. Spine 2004; 29:2627–2632.
56. Crevensten G, Walsh AJL, Ananthakrishnan D, et al. Intervertebral disc cell therapy for regeneration: mesenchymal stem cell implantation in rat intervertebral discs. Ann Biomed Eng 2004; 32:430–434.
57. Yamamoto Y, Mochida J, Sakai D, et al. Upregulation of the viability of nucleus pulposus cells by bone marrow-derived stromal cells—significance of direct cell-to-cell contact in coculture system. Spine 2004; 29:1508–1514.
58. Zhang YG, Guo XO, Xu P, Kang LL, Li J. Bone mesenchymal stem cells transplanted into rabbit intervertebral discs can increase proteoglycans. Clin Orthop 2005; 430:219–226.

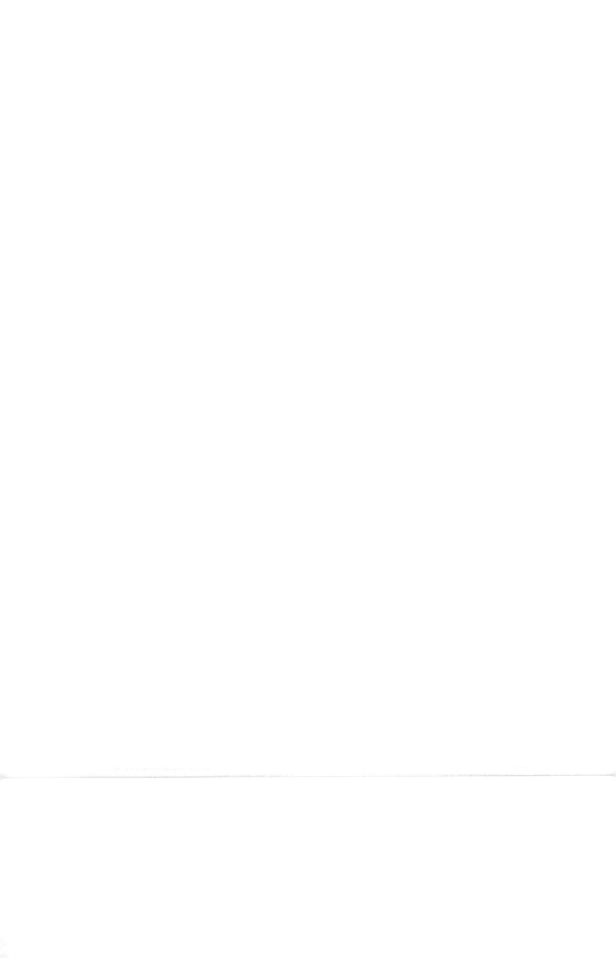

16 | Intervertebral Disc Growth Factors

Mats Grönblad
Division of Physical Medicine and Rehabilitation, University Central Hospital, Helsinki, Finland

Jukka Tolonen
Department of Internal Medicine, University Central Hospital, Helsinki, Finland

INTRODUCTION

Growth factors are important regulators of the intervertebral disc extracellular matrix and are involved in inducing the neovascularization process that accompanies disc degeneration (DD) and disc herniation (DH). In DH, newly formed blood vessels (1) contribute to resorption of the extruded disc tissue, which is variously composed of nucleus pulposus, annulus fibrosus, or endplate (2). Of clinical interest is the fact that of these tissues that may all or in various combinations form the herniated tissue, nucleus pulposus is the most leukotactic (3). In several studies (4,5), macrophages have been demonstrated in extruded disc tissue (Figs. 1, 2) to be instrumental in mediating tissue resorption and phagocytosis. Macrophages gain access to pathological disc tissue (DD or DH) by way of newly formed blood vessels (Fig. 3). Thus growth factors are also, at least indirectly, involved in the resorption process. At the moment, it is not yet known whether they may also have a more direct role. Of the growth factors we have screened, only one, namely transforming growth factor-beta (TGF-β), is present in normal disc (6,7). When the disc degenerates, and finally herniates, either into the nerve root canal or the spinal canal, an increasing number of growth factors become activated, creating a cascade that regulates tissue remodeling and neovascularization.

GROWTH FACTORS IN NORMAL AND PATHOLOGICAL DISC TISSUE (TABLES 1 AND 2)

The rationale for evaluating growth factors in intervertebral disc tissue is based on attempts at further understanding disc cell function. That function may be considered as one of the key elements in disc degenerative processes.

Insulin-like growth factor (IGF-I) receptor expression has been noted to decrease in disc cells with age (8). Furthermore, proteoglycan synthesis is reduced with age, and IGF-I-binding protein is more strongly expressed with age. In addition TGF-β expression has been demonstrated particularly in growing animals and its expression decreases with age (9,10).

In an experimental model comparing injured with intact annulus fibrosus, basic fibroblast growth factor (bFGF) and TGFβ were localized in blood vessels and annular cells near the lesion area (11). With time this expression was diminished. In normal control discs, the expression of bFGF and TGF-β was localized to sparsely distributed cells in the annulus fibrosus.

Painful degenerative human intervertebral discs showed neovascularization from adjacent intervertebral disc endplates. This is linked to nociceptive nerve ingrowth with the production of nerve growth factor (NGF) (12). Such NGF expression is noted only in discs painful at discography. Furthermore, significantly higher levels of interleukins (IL)-6 and IL-8 have been noted in discs operated for discogenic low back pain than for sciatica (13).

In extruded and sequestrated human intervertebral DHs, IL-1 and bFGF were localized especially in the granulation tissue area near the surface of the herniated disc (14). This expression was more intense in extruded and sequestrated discs than protruded ones. In addition, protruded discs have been demonstrated to express TGF-β1, IGF-I, IL-6, and IL-6R (15). mRNA for tumor necrosis factor-alpha (TNF-α), IL-8, IL-1α, IL-10, and TGF-β has been shown to be expressed in herniated lumbar intervertebral discs (16). In another

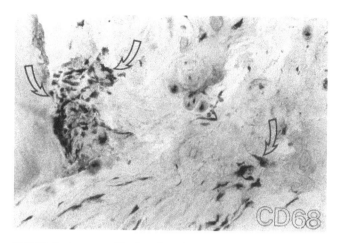

FIGURE 1 Low magnification view of macrophages (CD68, *open arrows*) in disc herniation tissue. Avidin-biotin-peroxidase complex staining with hematoxylin counterstaining.

study, mRNA coding TGF-α, EGF, TGF-β1, TGF-β3, EGF-R, and TGF-β type II receptor were found only occasionally in herniated human intervertebral discs.

In our own studies we have located bFGF, platelet-derived growth factor (PDGF) (Fig. 4A,B), vascular endothelial growth factor (VEGF), TGF-β1 (Fig. 5A), TGFβ2, and TGF-β type II receptor (Fig. 5B) in herniated human intervertebral discs (6,7,17,18). In normal control disc only TGF-β1 and 2, and TGF-β type II receptor were expressed (Fig. 4C). Furthermore, in degenerated discs bFGF and TGF-β1 and 2 and TGF-β type II receptor (Fig. 6B) were expressed, whereas degenerated but nonherniated discs did not express PDGF at all (Fig. 6A) (7). It could be concluded that growth factors are expressed in degenerated intervertebral disc, and in a different pattern compared with the normal nondegenerated disc (Fig. 7) (7). In degenerated intervertebral disc tissue chondrocyte-like disc cells of the nucleus pulposus express bFGF, TGF-β1, -2, and TGF-β receptor type II, but do not express PDGF (Fig. 7) (7). In the anterior annulus fibrosus of degenerated lumbar discs, the most prevalent growth factor expressed in chondrocyte-like disc cells seems to be bFGF, whereas TGF-β receptor type II is expressed both in fibroblast-like and in chondrocyte-like disc cells. Furthermore, in the posterior annulus fibrosus, the most prevalent growth factors expressed in chondrocyte-like disc cells seem to be bFGF and TGF-β2, together with TGF-β receptor type II (Fig. 7) (7).

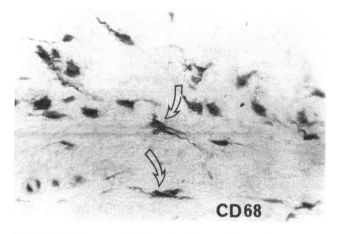

FIGURE 2 Higher magnification view of macrophages (CD68, *open arrows*) in disc herniation tissue. Avidin-biotin-peroxidase complex staining with hematoxylin counterstaining.

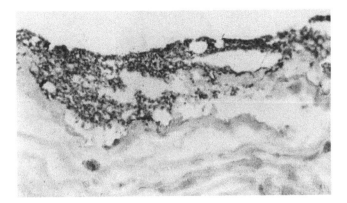

FIGURE 3 Newly formed blood vessels in disc herniation tissue.

Effect of Growth Factors on Disc Cells and Cartilage Cells

As is shown in Table 3, many growth factor effects on disc cells and cartilage cells are identical or similar. In the following, these effects are described in greater detail, first with respect to disc cells and then cartilage cells.

Effect of Growth Factors on Disc Cells

In cell cultures, TGF-β, FGF, IGF-I, and epidermal growth factor (EGF) have been demonstrated to be potent stimulators of cell proliferation (19). Especially cells from nucleus pulposus and from the transition zone were reactive. Furthermore, TGF-β1 and IGF-I decrease the level of active gelatinase A (MMP-2) in nucleus pulposus cells (20). In addition, IGF-I stimulates in a dose-dependent manner proteoglycan synthesis in nucleus pulposus cell cultures (21). This stimulation was especially noted in young nucleus pulposus.

In anulus fibrosus cell cultures, IGF-I and PDGF have been demonstrated to reduce apoptosis (22). Transforming growth factor-β1 initially enhances significantly the proliferation of annulus fibrosus cells (23); later on, it reduces the mitogenic response. Furthermore, TGF-β1 has been demonstrated to be a potent inducer of proteoglycan production both in annulus fibrosus and nucleus pulposus cell cultures (24).

In a rabbit experimental model that mimics the sequestration type of intervertebral DH, bFGF stimulated neovascularization and the proliferation of inflammatory cells (25). Furthermore, disc degradation was enhanced, and this effect was dose-dependent. Local application of the proinflammatory cytokine TNF-α on spinal nerve root reduces markedly nerve root conduction velocity (26), whereas epidural injection of bFGF facilitates the resorption of intervertebral disc tissue located in the epidural space (25).

Effect of Growth Factors on Cartilage Cells

In mature articular cartilage, extracellular matrix turnover is controlled particularly by IGF-1 (27). Other factors involved are the TGF-β superfamily (28) and chondrocyte-derived morphogenetic protein (29). Interestingly, inflammatory processes in cartilage seem to reduce its

TABLE 1 Occurrence of Growth Factors in Normal and Pathological Disc Tissues

	bFGF	PDGF	VEGF	TGF-β1	TGF-β2	TGF-βrec
ND	—	—	—	100%	100%	100%
DD	100%	—	NA	94%	94%	100%
DH	81%	78%	88%	100%	100%	100%

Abbreviations: bFGF, basic fibroblast growth factor; DD, degenerated disc; DH, disc herniation; NA, not analyzed; ND, normal disc; PDGF, platelet-derived growth factor; TGF-β, transforming growth factor-beta; TGF-βrec, transforming growth factor-beta receptor type II; VEGF, vascular endothelial growth factor.

TABLE 2 Occurrence of Growth Factors in Disc Cells and Blood Vessels in Normal and Pathological Disc Tissues

	bFGF	PDGF	VEGF	TGF-β1	TGF-β2	TGF-βrec
ND						
DC	—	—	—	100%	100%	100%
BV	—	—	—	—	—	—
DD						
DC	100%	—	—	94%	94%	100%
BV	Some	—	NA	Some	Some	Some
DH						
DC	67%	38%	—	100%	100%	97%
BV	48%	54%	88%	58%	37%	37%

Abbreviations: bFGF, basic fibroblast growth factor; BV, blood vessel; DC, chondrocyte-like disc cell; DD, degenerated disc; DH, disc herniation; NA, not analyzed; ND, normal disc; PDGF, platelet-derived growth factor; TGF-β, transforming growth factor-beta; TGF-βrec, transforming growth factor-beta receptor type II; VEGF, vascular endothelial growth factor.

responsiveness to IGF-1 (30). Furthermore, normal cartilage seems not to enhance proteoglycan synthesis after exposure to TGF-β1 (31). In addition, osteoarthritic cartilage chondrocytes seem to be sensitized to TGF-β1. The catabolic cytokine IL-1 does not suppress the anabolic effect of TGF-β, as it does to the otherwise more effective bone morphogenetic protein (BMP)-2 (31). Chondrocytes in human articular cartilage cell culture have shown a diminished sensitivity to TGF-β with age (32). Immature cartilage was the most reactive.

Significant levels of IGF-1, TGF-β, and BMPs (part of the TGF-β superfamily) are present in OA cartilage (33–36). Transforming growth factor-β1 has been shown to inhibit cartilage degradation (37). It also markedly upregulates the tissue inhibitor of matrix metalloproteinase (TIMP)-1 and TIMP-3 (38). Insulin-like growth factor-1 has been suggested to limit extracellular matrix degradation (39). In addition, together with IL-1 it increases IGF-binding

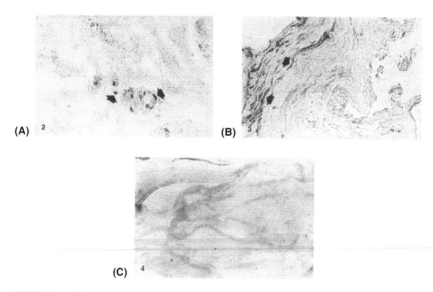

FIGURE 4 (**A**) An extrusion from a 40-year-old woman. *Note*: Platelet-derived growth factor (PDGF) immunopositivity in the nuclei of disc cells (*arrows*) [avidin biotin complex (ABC) immunostaining, hematoxylin counterstaining, original magnification ×370]. (**B**) PDGF immunopositive fibroblasts (*arrows*) in a sequester from a 52-year-old woman (operation level L5-S1, ABC immunostaining, hematoxylin counterstaining, original magnification ×370). (**C**) A normal control disc from a 50-year-old man. *Note*: Total lack of immunoreaction (level L4-5, PDGF antibody, ABC immunostaining, hematoxylin counterstaining, original magnification ×370). *Source*: Courtesy of Springer Science and Business Media, Berlin, Germany.

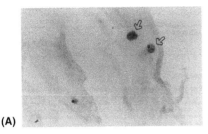 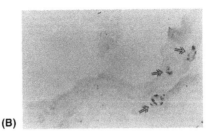

(A) **(B)**

FIGURE 5 **(A)** Transforming growth factor (TGF)-β1-immunopositive disc cells (*open arrows*) in nucleus pulposus of rapidly frozen herniated disc tissue from a 43-year-old male patient. *Note*: The intense cytoplasmic immunoreaction around counterstained nuclei. The operation level of the sequestered disc was L5-S1 [avidin biotin complex (ABC) peroxidase immunostaining (Vectastain); hematoxylin counterstaining; original magnification ×241]. **(B)** TGF-β receptor type II immunopositivity in nucleus pulposus disc cell groups (*open arrows*) in rapidly frozen herniated intervertebral disc from a 40-year-old male patient. The operation level of the disc protrusion was L4-L5 (immunostaining as in A; original magnification ×241). *Source*: Courtesy of Springer Science and Business Media, Berlin, Germany.

protein 5 synthesis (40). Insulin-like growth factor-1 also stimulates subchondral bony sclerosis in osteoarthritis (OA) (41).

Periosteal chondrogenesis is regulated by TGF-β1 in particular (42,43). In addition to TGF-β1, bFGF and IGF-1 have been shown to regulate proliferation and type II collagen expression in cultured periosteal tissue (44). In the growth plate, IGF-1, FGF, BMPs, and VEGF are considered as crucial regulators of chondrocyte proliferation and differentiation (45). In cell culture, chondrocyte apoptosis induced by collagenase may be inhibited by caspase inhibitors and IGF-1 (46).

Vascular endothelial growth factor is crucial for metaphyseal bone vascularization and is essential for establishing epiphyseal vascularization and regulating chondrocyte development and survival (47). It is produced by hypertrophic chondrocytes. Especially the soluble VEGF isoforms $VEGF_{120}$ and $VEGF_{164}$ are critical to diffuse to perichondrium and stimulate the epiphyseal vascular network. The insoluble isoform $VEGF_{188}$ is insufficient for these functions. Furthermore, in a *knock-out* study, VEGF was shown to be necessary for chondrocyte survival during bone development (48).

There has been an intense discussion regarding the effect of FGF in chondrocyte differentiation. It has been suggested by several investigators (49) that FGF inhibits chondrocyte differentiation. However, in a recent study (50) a clear promotion of chondrocyte differentiation was demonstrated. Furthermore there appears to be multiple pathways for FGF to affect chondrocyte cell cycle, cell growth arrest, and finally cellular differentiation. The effect of FGF-2 on

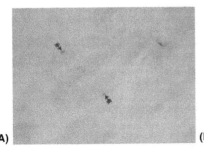 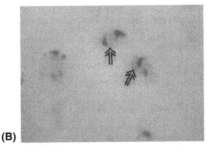

(A) **(B)**

FIGURE 6 **(A)** Platelet-derived growth factor (PDGF) immunostaining in posterior anulus fibrosus from a 40-year-old male patient. *Note*: The total lack of positive immunoreaction. *Arrows* mark pale nuclei of disc cells (avidin biotin complex peroxidase immunostaining method, original magnification ×370). **(B)** Transforming growth factor (TGF)-β receptor type II immunopositivity (*open arrows*) in a cluster of chondrocyte-like posterior anulus fibrosus disc cells from a 40-year-old male patient. The operation level was L4-5 (immunostaining as in A, original magnification ×370). *Source*: Courtesy of Springer Science and Business Media, Berlin, Germany.

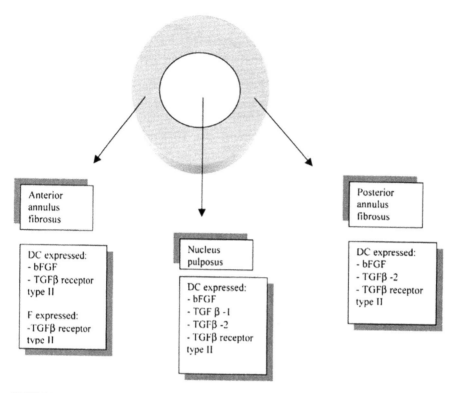

FIGURE 7 Expression of growth factors (bFGF, basic fibroblast growth factor, TGF-β1, -2, transforming growth factor-β1 and 2, receptor type II) in different disc regions. *Source*: Courtesy of Springer Science and Business Media, Berlin, Germany.

chondrogenesis in vitro has also been evaluated (51). It seemed to be most effective at low dosages. In addition, the study did not show any synergistic effect with IGF-I. The explanation for the lack of dose dependence may be the used dosage of FGF-2 (5 ng/ml and 25 ng/ml). Dose dependency to FGF-2 has been noted in another study (52). The investigators noted that FGF-2 significantly accelerated the appearance and increased the numbers of de novo repair cells at

TABLE 3 Comparison of Effect of Growth Factors on Disc Cells and Cartilage Cells

	Disc cells	Cartilage cells
TGFβ	Cell proliferation	Cell proliferation
	Proteoglycan synthesis/matrix turnover	Proteoglycan synthesis/matrix turnover
	MMP-2 $\downarrow$	TIMP-1 and TIMP-3 $\uparrow$
bFGF	Cell proliferation	Cell proliferation (varying effects by various FGF isoforms)
	Neovascularization	
	Disc degradation, extruded disc resorption	
IGF-1	Cell proliferation	Cell proliferation
	Proteoglycan synthesis/matrix turnover	Proteoglycan synthesis/matrix turnover
	MMP-2 $\downarrow$	
	Apoptosis $\downarrow$	Apoptosis $\downarrow$
EGF	Cell proliferation	
PDGF	Apoptosis $\downarrow$	Cell proliferation
VEGF	Neovascularization	Neovascularization, proliferation, differentiation, chondrocyte survival

Abbreviations: bFGF, basic fibroblast growth factor; EGF, epidermal growth factor; IGF-1, insulin-like growth factor 1; MMP, matrix metalloproteinase; PDGF, platelet-derived growth factor; TGF-β, transforming growth factor-β; TIMP, tissue inhibitor of matrix metalloproteinase; VEGF, vascular endothelial growth factor.

the cartilage surface in an intrinsic damage-repair model. The repair cells were shown to be chondrocytes. The dose-dependent effect of FGF-2 was attained only after a dosage of 50 ng/ml. It is interesting that also in this study a dosage of 25 ng/ml was less effective than a dosage of 12 ng/ml, but the effect was raised up to 10-fold at a growth factor level of 50 ng/ml. At the level of 100 ng/ml, the effect showed no further increase and with a longer period of exposure it was slightly reduced. This could by explained by receptor saturation.

In vitro effects of IGF, TGF-β, FGF, and BMP on chondrocyte proliferation have also been studied (53). Insulin-like growth factor-I-stimulated proliferation was dose- and time-dependent, whereas IGF-II was less effective. Furthermore, TGF-β2 and FGF-2 seemed to have a synergistic effect with IGF-I, whereas FGF-4, FGF-9, FGF-10, BMP-2, and BMP-4 had an antagonistic effect. The most potent proliferative effect was obtained by TGF-β, especially TGF-β2. Fibroblast growth factors had differing effects on chondrocyte proliferation; some of them (FGF-1, -2, -18) were stimulative, some of them (FGF-4, -9) were less effective, and some (FGF-10) suppressive. Bone morphogenetic proteins-2, -4, and -6 were all suppressive for chondrocyte proliferation, whereas platelet-derived growth factor (PDGF)-BB stimulated proliferation.

In cell culture, IGF-I has been noted to be inhibitive to nitric oxide (NO)-induced chondrocyte apoptosis (54). This inhibition was dose-dependent.

GROWTH FACTORS IN INTERVERTEBRAL DISC—HYPOTHESIS OF CELLULAR REMODELING (FIG. 8)

During development and growth, the intervertebral disc is a vascular tissue. Vascularity disappears during the second decade of life, at which time the disc obtains its "normal" avascular structure. In an animal model, intense TGF-β (9,10) and IGF-I (21) expression has been reported in young growing discs and interestingly, this expression decreased with age. Other growth factors have not been studied at this stage. At the adult stage, disc cell nutrition is mainly supplied to the disc through the endplates. Disc cells in different regions of the disc are modulated to the surrounding extracellular matrix. In annulus fibrosus, disc cells are spindle shaped, fibroblast-like cells. Nucleus pulposus cells are more rounded chondrocyte-like cells. In the adult disc, cells express TGF-β1 and -2, and TGF-β type II receptor. The disc cells maintain the extracellular matrix, and it can be postulated that disappearance of the vascularity may leave the disc cells with the capability to "remember" how to react to vascularity once again.

Mechanical trauma, overload, and genetic predisposition may produce susceptibility for the disruption of the circular collagen lamellae in the annulus fibrosus. This leads to neovascularization and activates disc cells. The essential area may be the border between nucleus pulposus and the inner zone of the posterior annulus fibrosus. Disc cells begin to express more growth factors. Furthermore, additional annular disc cells become more chondrocyte-like, and the disruption of the extracellular matrix proceeds, leading to more serious tissue damage. This cellular remodeling may spread from the initial starting area (the border between the nucleus pulposus and the posterior annulus fibrosus) to the entire intervertebral disc. There are different growth factors expressed at different time points during this process. At the same time, nerve ingrowth is coupled with neovascularization and this process may be painful.

Later on, because of more pronounced cellular remodeling and the progress of the collapse of the normal lamellar architecture of the collagen within the annulus fibrosus, the mechanical stress may be too intense especially in the posterior annulus fibrosus. This may lead to DH-producing sciatica. After herniation, the neovascularization and cellular remodeling still proceed. Furthermore, bulging of disc through the posterior longitudinal ligament exposes the disc tissue to the epidural space, where it can irritate the surrounding tissue, and itself be affected. The inflammatory cells, for example, macrophages, being present in the granulation tissue area, may deliver totally new growth factors to the intervertebral disc tissue. Growth factors may take part in a network consisting of cytokines, lymphokines, proteolytic enzymes, and their regulators. Nevertheless, the disc cells, and especially, the remodeling of

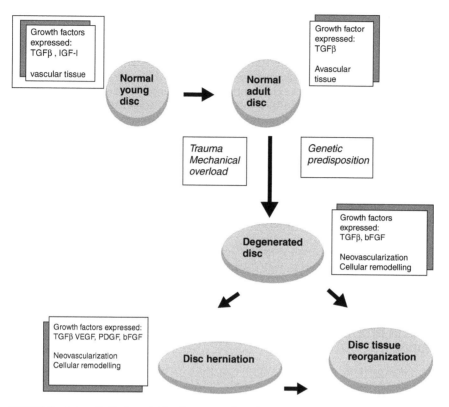

FIGURE 8 A hypothetical model for the expression of growth factors in intervertebral disc tissue during normal development and growth, and in pathological conditions starting from abnormal degeneration and ending in disc herniation followed by regenerative processes. The figure is discussed in greater detail in the text under the section "Growth Factors in Intervertebral Disc—Hypothesis for Cellular Remodeling." *Abbreviations*: bFGF, basic fibroblast growth factor; IGF-1, insulin-like growth factor 1; PDGF, platelet-derived growth factor; TGF-β, transforming growth factor-beta; VEGF, vascular endothelial growth factor.

the annular disc cells, may play an essential role in intervertebral disc metabolism and in the maintenance of the extracellular matrix of the disc.

With time, the size of the herniated disc becomes smaller. The cellular remodeling process continues over time in the prolapsed intervertebral disc tissue. The same process takes place in the remaining intervertebral disc tissue. This process may end in a steady-state situation, characterized possibly by a slow reorganization of the disc structure, or in reherniation. The DD process may also end directly in a reorganized end-stage.

REFERENCES

1. Virri J, Grönblad M, Savikko J, et al. Prevalence, morphology, and topography of blood vessels in herniated disc tissue. A comparative immunocytochemical study. Spine 1996; 21(16):1856–1863.
2. Moore RJ, Vernon-Roberts B, Fraser RD, et al. The origin and fate of herniated lumbar intervertebral disc tissue. Spine 1996; 21(18):2149–2155.
3. Grönblad M, Virri J, Habtemariam, et al. Comparison of the leukotactic properties of nucleus pulposus, anulus fibrosus, and cartilage following subcutaneous injection in pigs. In: Lewandrowski K.-U, Wise DL, Trantolo DJ, et al., eds. Advances in Spinal Fusion. Molecular Science, Biomechanics, and Clinical Management. New York, Basel: Marcel Dekker, Inc., 2004:217–224.
4. Grönblad M, Virri J, Tolonen J, et al. A controlled immunohistochemical study of inflammatory cells in disc herniation tissue. Spine 1994; 19(24):2744–2751.
5. Habtemariam A, Grönblad M, Virri J, et al. A comparative immunohistochemical study of inflammatory cells in acute-stage and chronic-stage disc herniations. Spine 1998; 23(20):2159–2166.

6. Tolonen J, Grönblad M, Virri J, et al. Transforming growth factor β receptor induction in herniated intervertebral disc tissue: an immunohistochemical study. Eur Spine J 2001; 10(2):172–176.
7. Tolonen J, Grönblad M, Vanharanta H, et al. Growth factor expression in degenerated intervertebral disc tissue. An immunohistochemical analysis of transforming growth factor β, fibroblast growth factor and platelet-derived growth factor. Eur Spine J 2006; 18:588–597.
8. Okuda S, Myougi A, Ariga K, et al. Mechanisms of age-related decline in insulin-like growth factor-I dependent proteoglycan synthesis in rat intervertebral disc cells. Spine 2001; 26(22):2421–2426.
9. Matsunaga S, Nagano S, Onishi T, et al. Age-related changes in expression of transforming growth factor beta and receptors in cells of intervertebral discs. J Neurosurg 2003; 98(suppl 1):63–67.
10. Nagano S, Matsunaga S, Takae R, et al. Immunolocalization of transforming growth factor betas and their receptors in intervertebral disc of senescence-accelerated mouse. Int J Oncol 2000; 17(3):461–466.
11. Melrose J, Smith S, Little CB, et al. Spatial and temporal localization of transforming growth factor beta, fibroblast growth factor-1, and osteonectin, and identification of cells expressing alpha-smooth muscle actin in injured annulus fibrosus: implications for extracellular matrix repair. Spine 2002; 27(16):1756–1764.
12. Freemont AJ, Watkins A, Le Maitre C, et al. Nerve growth factor expression and innervation of the painful intervertebral disc. J Pathol 2002; 197(3):286–292.
13. Burke JG, Watson RW, McCormack D, et al. Intervertebral discs which cause low back pain secrete high levels of proinflammatory mediators. J Bone Joint Surg Br 2002; 84(2):196–201.
14. Doita M, Kanatani T, Harada T, et al. Immunohistologic study of the ruptured intervertebral disc lumbar spine. Spine 1996; 21(2):235–241.
15. Specchia N, Pagnotta A, Toesca A, et al. Cytokines and growth factors in the protruded intervertebral disc of the lumbar spine. Eur Spine J 2002; 11(2):145–152.
16. Ahn SH, Cho YW, Ahn MW, et al. mRNA expression of cytokines and chemokines in herniated lumbar intervertebral discs. Spine 2002; 27(9):1–7.
17. Tolonen J, Grönblad M, Virri J, et al. Basic fibroblast growth factor immunoreactivity in blood vessels and cells of disc herniation. Spine 1995; 20(3):271–276.
18. Tolonen J, Grönblad M, Virri J, et al. Platelet-derived growth factor and vascular endothelial growth factor expression in disc herniation tissue: an immunohistochemical study. Eur Spine J 1997; 6(1):63–69.
19. Thompson JP, Oegema TR Jr, Bradford DS. Stimulation of mature canine intervertebral disc by growth factors. Spine 1991; 16(3):253–260.
20. Pattison ST, Melrose J, Ghosh P, et al. Regulation of gelatinase-A (MMP-2) production by ovine intervertebral disc nucleus pulposus grown in alginate bead culture by transforming growth factor-beta(1) and insulin-like growth factor-I. Cell Biol Int 2001; 25(7):679–689.
21. Osada R, Ohshima H, Ishihara H, et al. Autocrine/paracrine mechanism of insulin-like growth factor-1 on proteoglycan synthesis in bovine intervertebral discs. J Orthop Res 1996; 14(5):690–699.
22. Gruber HE, Norton HJ, Hanley, Jr. EN. Anti-apoptotic effects of IGF-1 and PDGF on human intervertebral disc cells in vitro. Spine 2000; 25(17):2153–2157.
23. Gruber HE, Fischer EC, Jr, Desai B, et al. Human intervertebral disc cells from the annulus: three-dimensional cultura in agarose or alginate and responsiveness to TGF-beta 1. Exp Cell Res 1997; 235(1):13–21.
24. Alini M, Li W, Markowic P, Aebi M, et al. The potential and the limimitations of a cell-seeded collagen/hyaluronan scaffold to engineer in intervertebral disc like matrix. Spine 2003; 28(5):446–454.
25. Minamide A, Hashizume H, Yoshida M, et al. Effects of basic fibroblast growth factor on spontaneous resorption of herniated intervertebral discs. An experimental study in the rabbit. Spine 1999; 24(10):940–945.
26. Aoki Y, Rydevik B, Kikuchi S, et al. Local application of disc-related cytokines on spinal nerve root. Spine 2002; 27(15):1614–1617.
27. Schalkwijk J, Joosten LAB, ban den Berg WB, et al. Insulin-like growth factor stimulation of chondrocyte osteoglycan synthesis by human synovial fluid. Arthritis Rheum 1989; 32(1):66–71.
28. Reddi AH. Cartilage-derived morphogenic proteins and cartilage morphogenesis. Microsc Res Tech 1998; 43(2):131–136.
29. Erlacher L, Ng CK, Ulrich R, et al. Presence of cartilage-derived morphogenic proteins in articular cartilage and enhancement of matrix replacement in vitro. Arthritis Rheum 1998; 41(2):263–273.
30. Schalkwijk J, Joosten LAB, van den Berg WB, et al. Chondrocyte nonresponsiviness to insulin-like growth factor I in experimental arthritis. Arthritis Rheum 1989; 32(7):894–900.
31. van Beuningen HM, van den Kraan PM, Arntz OJ, et al. Transforming growth factor beta-1 stimulates articular chondrocyte proteoglycan synthesis and induces osteophyte formation in the murine knee joint. Lab Invest 1994; 71(2):279–290.
32. Hickery MS, Bayliss MT, Dudhia J, et al. Age-related changes in the response of human articular cartilage to IL-1α and transforming growth factor beta (TGFβ). J Biol Chem 2003; 278(52):53063–53071.
33. Schlaak JF, Pfers I, Meyer zum Buschenfeld KH, et al. Different cytokine profiles in synovial fluid of patients with osteoarthritis, rheumatoid arthritis and seronegative spondylarthropathies. Clin Exp Rheumatol 1996; 14(2):155–162.

34. Martel-Pellletier J, DiBattista J, Lajaunesse D, et al. IGF/IGFBP axis in cartilage and bone in osteoarthritis pathogenesis. Inflamm Res 1998; 47(3):90–100.
35. Middleton JF, Tyler JA. Up-regulation of insulin-like growth factor I gene expression in the lesions of osteoarthritic human articular cartilage. Ann Rheum Dis 1992; 51(4):440–447.
36. Denko CW, Malemud CJ. Metabolic disturbances and synovial fluid responses in osteoarthritis. Front Biosci 1999; 4:D683–D693.
37. Chandrasekhar S, Harvey AK. Transforming growth factor beta is a potent inhibitor of IL-1 induced protease activity and cartilage proteoglycan degradation. Biochem Biophys Res Commun 1988; 157(3):1352–1359.
38. Hui W, Rowan AD, Cawston T. Modulation of the expression of matrix metalloproteinase and tissue inhibitors of metalloproteinases by TGF beta-1 and IGF-1 in primary human and bovine nasal chondrocytes stimulated with TNF-alpha. Cytokine 2001; 16(1):31–35.
39. Im HJ, Pacione C, Chubinskaya S, et al. Inhibitory effect of insulin like growth factor 1 and osteogenic protein-1 on fibronectin fragment and interleukin 1β stimulated matrix metalloproteinase 13 expression in human chondrocytes. J Biol Chem 2003; 278(28):25386–25394.
40. Sunic D, McNeil JD, Rayner TE, et al. Regulation of insulin like growth factor binding protein-5 by insulin like growth factor and interleukin 1α in bovine articular chondrocytes. Endocrinology 1998; 139(5):2356–2362.
41. Hilal G, Martel-Pelletier J, Pelletier JP, et al. Abnormal regulation of urokinase plasminogen activator by insulin like growth factor I in human osteoarthritic subchondral osteoblasts. Arthritis Rheum 1999; 42(10):2112–2122.
42. Lippiello L, Kaye C, Neumata T, et al. In vitro metabolic response of articular cartilage segments to low levels of hydrostatic pressure. Connect Tissue Res 1985; 13(2):99–107.
43. Miura Y, Fitzsimmons JS, Commissaro CN, et al. Enhancement of periosteal chondrogenesis in vitro: dose response to transforming growth factor beta-1 (TGFβ1). Clin Orthop 1994; 301:271–280.
44. Fukumoto T, Sanyal A, Fitzsimmons JS, et al. Differential effects of IGF-I, bFGF and TGFβ on proliferation and type II collagen mRNA expression during periosteal chondrogenesis. Trans Orthop Res Soc 2000; 25:1056.
45. van der Eerden BCJ, Karperien M, Wit JM. Systemic and local regulation of the growth plate. Endocrine Rev 2003; 24(6):782–801.
46. Lo My, Kim HT. Chondrocyte apoptosis induced by collagen degradation: inhibition by caspase inhibitors and IGF-I. J Orthop Res 2004; 22(1):140–144.
47. Maes C, Stockmans I, Moermans K, et al. Soluble VEGF isoforms are essential for establishing epiphyseal vascularization and regulating chondrocyte development and survival. J Clin Invest 2004; 113(2):188–199.
48. Zelzer E, Mamluk R, Ferrara N, et al. VEGFA is necessary for chondrocyte survival during bone development. Development 2004; 131(9):2161–2171.
49. Ornitz DM, Marie PJ. FGF signalling pathways in endochondral and intramembranous bone development and human genetic disease. Genes Dev 2002; 16(12):1446–1465.
50. Dailey L, Laplantine E, Priore R, Basilico C. A network of transcriptional and signalling events is activated by FGF to induce chondrocyte growth arrest and differentiation. J Cell Biol 2003; 161(6):1053–1066.
51. Veilleux N, Spector M. Effects of FGF-2 and IGF-I on adult canine articular chondrocytes in type II collagen-glycosaminoglycan scaffolds in vitro. Osteoarthritis Cartilage 2005; 13(3):278–286.
52. Henson FM, Bowe EA, Davies ME. Promotion of the intrinsic damage-repair response in articular cartilage by fibroblast growth factor-2. Osteoarthritis Cartilage 2005; 13(6):537–544.
53. Olney RC, Wanf J, Sylvester JE, et al. Growth factor regulation of human growth plate chondrocyte proliferation in vitro. Biochem Biophys Res Commun 2004; 317(4):1171–1182.
54. Allen RT, Robertson CM, Harwood FL, et al. Characterization of mature vs aged rabbit articular cartilage: analysis of cell density, apoptosis-related gene expression and mechanisms controlling chondrocyte apoptosis. Osteoarthritis Cartilage 2004; 12(11):917–923.

17 Biological Manipulation for Degenerative Disc Disease Utilizing Intradiscal Osteogenic Protein-1 (OP-1/BMP-7) Injection—An Animal Study

Mamoru Kawakami, Takuji Matsumoto, Hiroshi Hashizume, and Munehito Yoshida
Department of Orthopaedic Surgery, Wakayama Medical University, Wakayama City, Wakayama, Japan

Koichi Kuribayashi
Department of Immunology and Pathology, Kansai College of Oriental Medicine, Kumatori-Cho, Osaka, Japan

Susan Chubinskaya
Department of Biochemistry and Section of Rheumatology, Rush University Medical Center, Chicago, Illinois, U.S.A.

INTRODUCTION

Back pain is the most prevalent cause of disability in our society and has a huge socioeconomic impact because of explicit cost for the treatments and implicit costs, such as loss of productivity. There are two mechanisms of intervertebral disc degeneration that may contribute to back pain: loss of disc structure and mechanical properties, and a release of mediators that may sensitize nerve endings (1). Conventional and current treatments for disc degenerative disease include medication, physical therapy, intradiscal electrothermal therapy, and surgeries such as artificial nucleus pulposus replacement, intervertebral disc prostheses, and spinal fusion. These treatments may reduce pain; however, they cannot physically repair the affected intervertebral disc. An ideal treatment for degenerative disc disease, therefore, is to biologically repair the affected intervertebral disc and reduce pain. The biochemistry of the intervertebral disc plays an important role in its mechanical properties (2). Imbalance in organ homeostasis leads to intervertebral disc degeneration. It is thought that repair or regeneration of the degenerated intervertebral disc with the suppression of pain is a key for biological manipulation in a future treatment option.

In order to biologically intervene in disc degeneration and pain, it is necessary to develop an animal model of disc degeneration, which would allow to measure the pain and would make possible the application of the anabolic factors able to overcome degeneration processes induced in intervertebral disc.

Growth factors, such as fibroblast growth factor and transforming growth factor-β (TGF-β), have been shown to stimulate cell proliferation and matrix synthesis of intervertebral discs in vitro (3). A member of the TGF-β superfamily, osteogenic protein-1 (OP-1) or bone morphogenetic protein-7 (BMP-7), stimulates proteoglycan and collagen synthesis in rabbit intervertebral disc cells cultured in alginate beads (4). It has been also reported that the intradiscal injection of OP-1 stimulates synthesis of proteoglycan and collagen in normal intervertebral discs (5,6), and the injection of OP-1 following chondroitinase avidin-biotin-peroxidase complex (ABC)-induced chemonucleolysis results in the recovery of disc height in the rabbit (6,7).

Furthermore, several studies have identified inflammatory mediators and autoimmune reactions in lumbar disc herniation. As inflammatory mediators, biologically active substances in the arachidonic acid cascade, such as phospholipase A_2 (PLA$_2$) (8–11), and inflammatory cytokines, such as interleukin-1β (IL-1β) (8,10–13) and tumor necrosis factor-α (TNF-α)

(14–16), are related to pathophysiological mechanisms of painful radiculopathy in lumbar disc herniation. One appealing hypothesis is that leakage of these agents may produce excitation of the nociceptors, direct neural injury, nerve inflammation, or enhancement of sensitization to other pain-producing substances, leading to nerve root pain (17). We have evaluated these inflammatory mediators in our experimental animal models (8,11).

In this Chapter, an animal model is introduced, which was developed and utilized in our laboratories for research of pain associated with degenerated disc. In this model, we demonstrated the therapeutic efficacy of intradiscal injection of OP-1 in the reduction of degeneration and associated pain. Furthermore, we will also discuss the physiological mechanism of OP-1 in degenerative disc disease here.

AN ANIMAL MODEL

In order to evaluate the direct relationship between disc degeneration and back pain, it is necessary to develop an animal model of disc degeneration, in which pain could be measured. A number of experimental animal models of disc degeneration has been developed: the anterior part of the annulus fibrosus of a lumbar disc has been pierced with a scalpel blade in pigs (18,19); coil springs have been stretched and attached to produce a compressive force across the lumbar intervertebral discs of dogs (20,21); mouse tail discs have been loaded in vivo with an external compression device (22,23); and an Ilizarov-type apparatus has been applied to the tails of rats (24,25). These models have been used to assess the biomechanical behavior, biochemical composition, and biological changes in the intervertebral discs. Furthermore, a rabbit animal model of intervertebral disc degeneration has been recently developed, in which a needle puncture of the intervertebral disc resulted in a slowly progressive and reproducible degeneration of the intervertebral disc (26,27). However, in all these models the injury was done directly to the intervertebral disc. As low back pain in degenerative disc disease has been defined as nontraumatic pain, the traumatic or injured disc may not be suitable for pain research in degenerative disc disease. Thus, we have developed and utilized a rat model of disc degeneration, in which two tail intervertebral discs were immobilized and chronically compressed with an Ilizarov-type apparatus (28) based on the method of Iatridis et al. (24) and Mente et al. (25).

ASSESSMENT OF PAIN-RELATED BEHAVIOR

It has been reported that pain-related behaviors could be measured in experimental rat models of lumbar nerve root irritation (8,28–33). For the assessment of pain-related behaviors (34), hyperalgesia and the hypersensitivity to noxious stimuli were measured. As it is very difficult to evaluate axial pain or discogenic pain secondary to disc degeneration in the rat applying behavioral measurements, we have evaluated radicular pain of the hindpaw induced by the application of nucleus pulposus on the lumbar nerve roots. Nucleus pulposus tissues were harvested from the chronically compressed discs and applied to lumbar nerve roots. We demonstrated that the induction of hyperalgesia was greater and of a longer duration in those animals exposed to the compressed nucleus pulposus tissue as compared with control animals (normal nucleus pulposus tissue) (28).

OSTEOGENIC PROTEIN-1 INJECTION MODEL

Utilizing the animal model with degenerative coccygeal intervertebral disc described earlier (Fig. 1), we evaluated if intradiscal injection of OP-1 into the degenerated disc can preserve the motion of the affected disc and reduce pain-related behavior (35). Changes in the extracellular matrix and proinflammatory cytokines, such as PLA_2, IL-1β, and TNF-α in the disc were observed by Safranin-O staining and immunohistochemistry, respectively.

Surgical Protocol

All surgical procedures were performed with the rats anesthetized by an intraperitoneal injection of sodium pentobarbital (50 mg/kg). In order to make intervertebral disc degeneration,

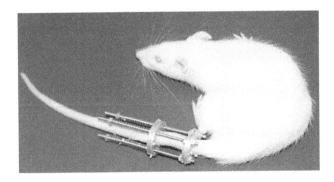

FIGURE 1 An animal model of disc degeneration, in which two tail intervertebral discs were immobilized and chronically compressed using an Ilizarov-type apparatus. This was used to evaluate relationships between disc degeneration and pain-related behavior. *Source*: From Refs. 28, 35.

two 0.8-mm diameter Kirschner's wires were inserted percutaneously through the third and fifth coccygeal vertebrae. Each wire was fixed separately to a specially designed aluminum ring, consisting of two 30-mm diameter external rings. The two rings were linked with four rods to immobilize and chronically apply compression on the Kirschner's wires until the tail exhibited maximum angular deformity. Four weeks after surgery, 1 µl of 0.2 µg/1 µl of OP-1 (provided by Stryker Biotech, Hopkinton, Massachusetts, U.S.A.) was injected into the nucleus pulposus of the instrumented vertebrae. The injection of OP-1 was performed with a Hamilton microliter™ syringe (Hamilton Company, Reno, Nevada, U.S.A.). Compression was continuously applied to the tail after OP-1 treatment (the OP-1 group). The tails were amputated eight weeks after primary treatment. In the sham group, an Ilizarov-type apparatus was applied to the tail without any compression. In the saline group, 1 µl of physiological saline was injected into the intervertebral discs of the instrumented vertebrae instead of OP-1. For histological examination and immunohistochemistry described next, two rats were used as naïve controls.

Mobility in the Fixed Vertebrae

Eight weeks after fixation of the tail with an Ilizarov-type apparatus, the mobility of the fixed vertebrae was manually evaluated in the saline and OP-1 groups. Manual palpation of the fixed tail after removal of the Ilizarov-type apparatus revealed that the instrumented vertebrae in the saline group were fixed and did not show any mobility of the vertebrae. However, the instrumented vertebrae in the OP-1 group had mobility motion after removal of the apparatus (35).

Pain Evaluation

To evaluate pain, tissue was retrieved from treated nucleus pulposus after amputation of the tail. The nucleus pulposus tissue was applied to the left L4 and L5 nerve roots after partial laminectomy. After surgery, all wounds were irrigated and washed with preservative-free sterile saline. The operative fields were closed in layers with 4-0 nylon sutures. Radicular pain was assessed by behavioral measurements as shown next.

Behavioral Observations

Motor function and reflex responses to mechanical noxious stimuli applied to both hindpaws were measured in all rats preoperatively, and up to three weeks postoperatively. Behavioral observations were made at the same time during the day. The same examiner performed all observations and was blinded to the treatment group being observed.

Motor Function

Rats were placed on the floor in an open field and their gait patterns were observed. All rats in the sham, saline, and OP-1 groups exhibited normal gait during the experimental period.

Mechanical Withdrawal Threshold

Using methods reported previously (8,29), reflex responses to noxious mechanical stimuli to both hindpaws were assessed quantitatively for all rats. Briefly, for the measurement of mechanical withdrawal threshold, rats were allowed to crawl freely under a piece of cloth. Once the rat had settled, the mechanical withdrawal threshold was measured on the dorsal surface of the hindpaw, between the fourth and the fifth metatarsal bones, using a specially designed apparatus made from a 50-ml syringe, a needle with a 2-mm dull tip, and plumbs. The threshold at which the hindpaw was withdrawn was expressed in grams. The placement of the stimuli was varied slightly from one trial to the next to avoid sensitizing the skin. Each trial was repeated three times at least five minutes apart, and the average of the results was determined. The percentage difference in withdrawal threshold from noxious stimuli between the ipsilateral and contralateral hindpaws was calculated using the appropriate formula:

$$\frac{(\text{Ipsilateral threshold} - \text{Contralateral threshold})}{\text{Contralateral threshold}} \times 100.$$

All values are presented as percentage differences. Negative percentages reflect hyperalgesia, whereas positive percentages reflect hypoalgesia.

Rats in the sham group exhibited evidence of mechanical hyperalgesia in the ipsilateral hindpaws for four days postoperatively. However, rats in the saline group showed evidence of mechanical hyperalgesia from two days to two weeks postoperatively. The mechanical hyperalgesia observed in the saline group was greater and of longer duration than that in the sham group. On the other hand, in the OP-1 groups, there were no significant differences in responses to noxious mechanical stimuli between right and left hindpaws. Mechanical hyperalgesia was not observed in the rats exposed to the nucleus pulposus treated with OP-1. (Fig. 2) (35).

Histological Examination

Eight weeks after insertion of the Kirschner's wires, the tail was amputated and the instrumented vertebrae were resected. After fixation in 10% neutral-buffered formalin, the specimens were decalcified in 10% ethylene-diamino-tetraacetic acid (EDTA) solution and then embedded in paraffin wax. The specimens were sectioned longitudinally in the sagittal plane at 5 μm and processed for histology. Safranin-O/fast green (36) staining was used to evaluate changes in the extracellular matrix of the intervertebral discs. Evaluation of the results was done with

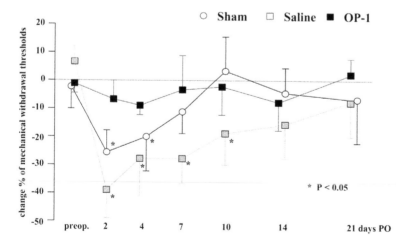

FIGURE 2 Rats in the sham group exhibited evidence of mechanical hyperalgesia in the ipsilateral hindpaws at four days postoperatively. However, the mechanical hyperalgesia observed in the saline group was greater and of longer duration than that in the sham group. On the other hand, in the osteogenic protein-1 groups, there were no significant differences in responses to noxious mechanical stimuli between right and left hindpaws. *Source*: From Ref. 35.

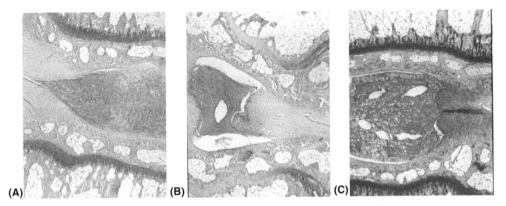

FIGURE 3 (**A**) The discs in the sham group. (**B**) The discs in the saline group displayed morphological and histological changes: loss of elongated shape and decrease in size of nucleus pulposus, displacement with regard to annulus fibrosis and substantial loss of proteoglycans in nucleus pulposus and end plate cartilage. (**C**) The discs treated with osteogenic protein-1 (OP-1). Treatment with OP-1 restored the morphology of the discs; the size of nucleus pulposus was significantly enlarged in comparison to control and compressed discs and represented normal oval shape. Safranin-O staining appeared very intense in the nucleus pulposus, end plate cartilage and annulus fibrosis. In the annulus fibrosis of the OP-1-treated discs, Safranin-O stain was increased indicating the accumulation of sulfated proteoglycans in this compartment. *Source*: From Ref. 35.

Nikon™ Eclipse 600 microscope (Nikon, Japan) with a Spot 2 camera and Metamorph® software (Universal Imaging Corporation, Pennsylvania, U.S.A.).

Untreated control discs exhibited normal morphology, elongated nucleus pulposus, and light Safranin-O stain within the nucleus pulposus. A few cells within annulus fibrosis were also stained with Safranin-O. The end-plate cartilage displayed normal Safranin-O staining. Sham-operated discs (Fig. 3A) morphologically looked similar to the control discs, but Safranin-O stain was more intense in the end-plate cartilage. The compressed discs in the saline group (Fig. 3B) displayed morphological and histological changes: a loss of elongated shape and a decrease in size of nucleus pulposus, a displacement with regard to annulus fibrosis, and a substantial loss of proteoglycans in nucleus pulposus and end-plate cartilage as detected by reduced Safranin-O staining. Treatment with OP-1 restored the morphology of the discs; the size of nucleus pulposus was significantly enlarged in comparison with the control and compressed discs and represented normal oval shape. Safranin-O staining appeared very intense in the nucleus pulposus, end-plate cartilage, and annulus fibrosis (Fig. 3C). In the annulus fibrosis of the OP-1-treated discs, Safranin-O stain was increased indicating the accumulation of sulfated proteoglycans in this compartment. The intensity of staining in all these areas was found to be much stronger than in the control discs (35).

Evaluation of Phospholipase A₂, Interleukin-1β, and Tumor Necrosis Factor-α

The specimens used for histological examination were also processed for immunohistochemistry with anti-PLA$_2$, IL-1β, and TNF-α antibodies. The distribution and localization of these proteins were evaluated in the intervertebral discs from the control, sham, and OP-1-treated groups.

Antibodies

Polyclonal antirabbit antibody for PLA$_2$ (Upstate Biotechnology, Waltham, Massachusetts, U.S.A.), polyclonal antirabbit IL-1β and rabbit antirat TNF-α antibodies (Chemicon International, Temecula, California, U.S.A.) were used for immunohistochemistry.

Immunohistochemistry

Prior to incubation with primarily antibodies, tissue sections were digested with keratanase [*Pseudomonas* sp; EC 3.2.1.103 (0.01 U/ml)], keratanase II [*Bacillus* sp; KS 36 (0.0001 U/ml)],

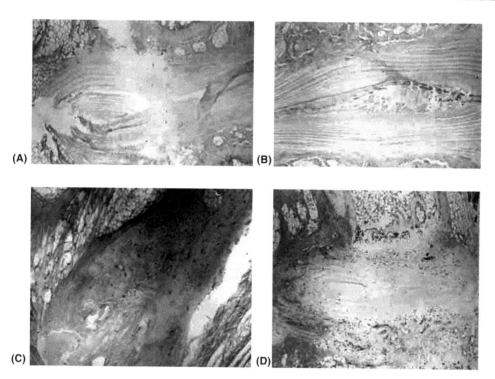

FIGURE 4 In the saline and osteogenic protein-1 (OP-1) groups, phospholipase A_2 (PLA_2) immunoreactivity was observed in the annulus fibrosus. OP-1 injection to the degenerative disc did not result in change of PLA_2 immunoreactivity. (**A**) The disc of the control, (**B**) the sham, (**C**) the saline, and (**D**) the OP-1 groups.

and chondroitinase ABC [*Proteus vulgaris*; EC 4.2.2.2 (0.01 U/ml)] in 100 mM Tris/50 mM Na-acetate buffer (pH 6.5) at 37°C for 90 minutes to increase the penetration of antibodies into cartilage. All three proteinases were obtained from Seikagaku (Tokyo, Japan). For negative controls, the primary antibodies were replaced with either normal serum or secondary antibody alone. Primary antibodies were applied at 1:100 dilution. To localize PLA_2, IL-1β, or TNF-α, horseradish peroxidase-conjugated rat immunoglobulin G (IgG) secondary antibody was used. Evaluation of the results was assessed with Nikon Eclipse 600 microscope with a Spot 2 camera; the images at 4× and 10× magnification were taken with the Metamorph software program (Universal Imaging Corporation, Pennsylvania, U.S.A.).

Phospholipase A_2 Immunoreactivity
In the saline and OP-1 groups, PLA_2 immunoreactivity was observed in the annulus fibrosus. Osteogenic protein-1 injection to the degenerated disc did not result in change of PLA_2 immunoreactivity (Fig. 4A–D).

Interleukin-1β Immunoreactivity
In normal untreated disc (Fig. 5A), utilization of anti-IL-1β antibody revealed a distinct cellular localization of IL-1β. Moderate stain was evident in the cells of nucleus pulposus, annulus fibrosus, and chondrocytes from end-plate. No matrix staining was found in the nucleus pulposus and annulus fibrosus, while in the end-plate light matrix stain was noticed. Sham operation induced an increase in autocrine IL-1β in the cells and the matrix of the nucleus pulposus (Fig. 5B). Matrices within other compartments remained negative for IL-1β protein. Intracellular staining of the annulus fibrosus and chondrocytes of the end-plate was reduced: fewer positive cells were detected in these areas and the intensity of staining was diminished. In the discs of the compressed saline-treated group, low levels of IL-1β were detected in the nucleus pulposus (Fig. 5C). However, very strong matrix and cellular stains were detected in the annulus fibrosus and end-plate. In the discs of the OP-1-treated group,

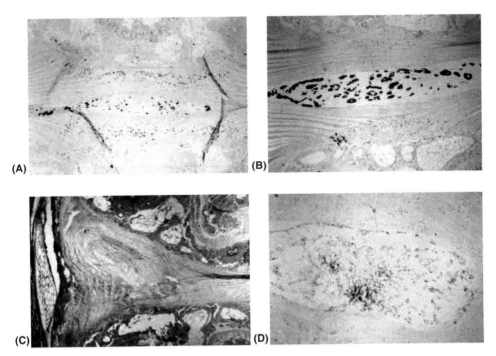

FIGURE 5 (**A**) In normal control disc, interleukin-1β (IL-1β) immunoreactivities were evident in the cells of nucleus pulposus, anulus fibrosus, and chondrocytes from end plate. No matrix staining was found in the nucleus pulposus and annulus fibrosus, while in the end plate light matrix stain was noticed. (**B**) Sham operation induced an increase in autocrine IL-1β in the cells and the matrix of the nucleus pulposus. Matrixes within other compartments remained negative for IL-1β. Intracellular staining of the anulus fibrosus and chondrocytes of the end plate was reduced: fewer positive cells were detected in these areas and the intensity of staining was diminished. (**C**) In the discs of the saline group, low levels of IL-1β were detected in the nucleus pulposus. However, very strong matrix and cellular stains were detected in the anulus fibrosus and end-plate. (**D**) In the discs of the osteogenic protein-1 group, a marked decrease in autocrine IL-1β was observed.

a marked decrease in autocrine IL-1(was observed (Fig. 5D). Light cellular and matrix stain for IL-1β was identified in the nucleus pulposus, annulus fibrosus, and chondrocytes, while the intensity of the stain was even lower than in the untreated disc.

Tumor Necrosis Factor-α Immunoreactivity

Similar effect of OP-1 injection was observed with TNF-α. Some background levels of TNF-α protein were detected in the untreated control disc (Fig. 6A). Tumor necrosis factor-α was identified in the cells and matrix of the nucleus pulposus and to a lesser extent in the annulus fibrosus. Relatively strong stain was found in the matrix of the end-plate. Cells in the end-plate were also positive for TNF-α. In the discs of the sham group, the pattern of staining was very similar to that of IL-1β in the same group with the increase of TNF-α in the matrix and cells of the nucleus pulposus (Fig. 6B). However, in other compartments of this disc (matrix of the annulus fibrosus and end-plate) the levels of TNF-α were decreased as compared with the untreated control. Light cellular staining was evident in the annulus fibrosus and end-plate. In the discs of the compressed saline-treated group, expression of autocrine TNF-α protein was clearly observed (Fig. 6C) and was higher than in all other experimental groups. Strong cellular and matrix staining was found in the nucleus pulposus, periphery of the annulus fibrosus, and end-plate. Chondrocytes and the matrix of end-plate were extremely strongly stained with the antibody against TNF-α. The pattern of TNF-α distribution in the end-plate was similar to that of IL-1β suggesting that mechanical compression to the discs induced the release of TNF-α into the matrix. In the discs of the OP-1-treated group (Fig. 6D), OP-1 primarily reduced the amount of TNF-α in the matrix of the nucleus pulposus and the end-plate.

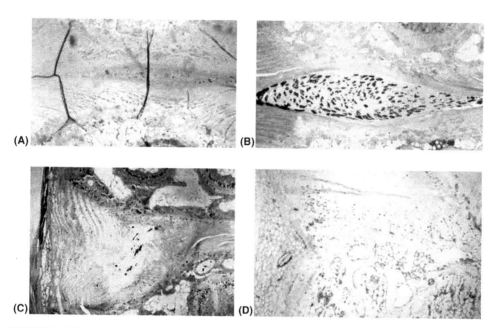

FIGURE 6 (**A**) Some background levels of tumor necrosis factor-α (TNF-α) protein were detected in the untreated control disc. It was identified in the cells and matrix of the nucleus pulposus and to a lesser extent in the annulus fibrosus. Relatively strong stain was found in the matrix of end plate. Cells in the end plate were also positive for TNF-α. (**B**) In the discs of the sham group, the increase of TNF-α in the matrix and cells of the nucleus pulposus were observed. (**C**) While, in the discs of the saline group, expression of autocrine TNF-α protein was clearly observed. Strong cellular and matrix staining was found in the nucleus pulposus, periphery of the annulus fibrosus and end plate. Chondrocytes and the matrix of end plate were extremely strongly stained with the antibody against TNF-α. (**D**) In the discs of the osteogenic protein-1 group, OP-1 primarily reduced the amount of TNF-α in the matrix of the nucleus pulposus and end-plate.

SUMMARY OF OSTEOGENIC PROTEIN-1 INJECTION IN DEGENERATED DISC

Chronic compression of the intervertebral discs results in disc degeneration, which may mimic degenerative disc disease in humans. Osteogenic protein-1 injection into the intervertebral disc, in which mechanical compression was applied to the tail, resulted in the inhibition of the mechanical hyperalgesia, induced by the nucleus pulposus. Intradiscal injection of OP-1 enhanced the replenishment of the extracellular matrix and downregulated the amount of IL-1β and TNF-α in all disc compartments including the nucleus pulposus, annulus fibrosus, and end-plate. All results described in this Chapter are summarized in Table 1.

PHYSIOLOGICAL MECHANISMS OF THE OSTEOGENIC PROTEIN-1 TREATMENT RELATED TO DEGENERATIVE DISC DISEASE AND PAIN

Anabolic and anticatabolic activities of OP-1 are related to the restoration of the disc mobility and morphology and abolishment of pain induced by the nucleus pulposus. These activities of OP-1 have been documented in different models of human and animal cartilage

TABLE 1 Summary of OP-1 Injection to the Degenerative Disc

| | Pain-related behavior | Mobility of the discs | Extracellular matrix | Immunohistochemistry | | |
				PLA$_2$	IL-1β	TNF-α
Sham	Pain	Mobile	Normal	$\pm$	$+$	$+$
Saline	Severe pain	Fixed	Decrease	$+$	$++$	$++$
OP-1	No pain	Mobile	Increase	$+$	$\pm$	$\pm$

Note: $\pm$, slightly positive immunoreactivity; $+$, positive immunoreactivity; $++$, marked positive immunoreactivity.

degeneration (37–41). These reports have clearly demonstrated that OP-1 can act as not only a potent cartilage anabolic factor, but also as an anticatabolic agent. Utilizing previously described animal model of disc degeneration, in which an Ilizarov-type apparatus was applied to the rat tail discs to generate injurious compression, we found that the intradiscal injection of OP-1 completely restored the morphology of the nucleus pulposus and the annulus fibrosus and stimulated the synthesis of the extracellular matrix in the intervertebral discs. The data obtained from this study confirmed that a direct injection of recombinant OP-1 into the chronically compressed intervertebral discs exhibits both anabolic and anticatabolic activities. Previously, an anabolic activity of OP-1 in adult articular cartilage has been reported, where OP-1 has been shown to stimulate the synthesis of the major extracellular matrix proteins including proteoglycans, hyaluronan, collagen type II with no induction of type I collagen, and cell proliferation (42). In the present study, the enlargement of the extracellular matrix in the vertebral discs treated with OP-1 observed by histology may be also because of an increase in proteoglycan and collagen synthesis.

The mechanisms of disc degeneration appear to be in the decrease of nutrition in the central disc, which causes a decline in pH levels. A lower pH is thought to be related to pain (43,44) and reduced pH of the nucleus pulposus tissue around the nerve root may lead to the enhancement of hyperalgesia. Therefore, intradiscal injection of OP-1 to the instrumented vertebrae, which resulted in an increase in the extracellular matrix, probably improved the supply of the nutrients to the disc and prevented a decline in pH levels.

On the other hand, OP-1 is thought to suppress IL-1 effect and thus reduce inflammation (42). With regard to intervertebral disc cells, Takegami et al. has reported that OP-1 enhances matrix replenishment by intervertebral disc cells previously exposed to IL-1 (45). Our current studies demonstrated that OP-1 injection to the degenerated disc downregulated IL-1β and TNF-α expression in the disc. This downregulation may be because of mechanisms of pain control after OP-1 injection.

The results of the current study indicate a role for OP-1 in pain reduction. Although it has been suggested that nucleus pulposus itself induces nerve injury, Lodslot et al. clearly demonstrated that nucleus pulposus had a toxic effect on the axons by blocking axonal outgrowth in vitro (46). There are also some reports that OP-1 induces or enhances dendritic formation or neuron growth (47,48). Collectively, these findings suggest that OP-1 may stimulate neural protection and regeneration after nerve injury. Based on our studies, OP-1 may also have antitoxic effect on the nerve root injury, which is induced by degenerated discs. We found that neither the nucleus pulposus nor gel form soaked with OP-1 did induce pain and neural damages (unpublished data). This result suggests that the leakage of OP-1 to the epidural space is safe for the neural tissues. However, we need to conduct further studies regarding not only biological and biomechanical assessment of OP-1-injected discs, but also precise mechanisms of OP-1 to the intervertebral disc.

CONCLUSION

Osteogenic protein-1 injection to the intervertebral disc, in which mechanical compression was applied in the tail, resulted in the inhibition of the mechanical hyperalgesia, induced by the nucleus pulposus. It enhanced the replenishment of the extracellular matrix by the nucleus pulposus cells. Not only was the activation of the nucleus pulposus cells after intradiscal injection of OP-1, but also the effect of OP-1 itself may be associated with the inhibition of pain-related behavior. Furthermore, OP-1 injection downregulated IL-1β and TNF-α production, which may be also a possible mechanism for attenuation of hyperalgesia after OP-1 injection into degenerated discs. An ideal treatment for degenerative disc disease is to biologically repair the affected intervertebral disc and reduce pain. From a clinical perspective, it is important to activate or regenerate intervertebral disc cells with no pain induction in order to treat disc degeneration. Anabolic and anti-inflammatory effect and positive effects for neural tissues of OP-1 are important for safety in clinical use as a novel drug therapy for degenerative disc disorders. Our current results suggest that intradiscal injection of OP-1 has a potential as a therapy for the treatment of discogenic pain.

ACKNOWLEDGMENTS

We are grateful to Stryker Biotech for providing OP-1 and to Ms. Nami Migita [Hopkinton, Massachusetts, U.S.A (Stryker Biotech)] for preparation of this Chapter.

REFERENCES

1. Buckwalter JA, Martin J. Intervertebral disk degeneration and back pain. In: Weinstein JN, Gordon SL, eds. Low Back Pain: A Scientific and Clinical Overview. Rosemont, IL: American Academy of Orthopaedic Surgeons, 1996:607–623.
2. Urban JP, McMullin JF. Swelling pressure of the lumbar intervertebral discs: influence of age, spinal level, composition, and degeneration. Spine 1988; 13:179–187.
3. Gruber HE, Fisher EC, Jr, Desai B, et al. Human intervertebral disc cells from the annulus: three-dimensional culture in agarose or alginate and responsiveness to TGF-beta1. Exp Cell Res 1997; 235:13–21.
4. Masuda K, Takegami K, An H, et al. Recombinant osteogenic protein-1 upregulates extracellular matrix metabolism by rabbit annulus fibrosus and nucleus pulposus cells cultured in alginate beads. J Orthop Res 2003; 21:922–930.
5. Takegami K, Masuda K, An H, et al. In vivo administration of Osteogenic protein-1 increases proteoglycan content and disc height in rabbit intervertebral disc. Ortho Res Soc Trans 2000; 25:338.
6. An H, Eugene J-MAT, Masuda K. Biological repair of intervertebral disc. Spine 2003; 28:S86–S92.
7. Takegami K, Masuda K, Kumano F, et al. Osteogenic potein-1 is most effective in stimulating nucleus pulposus and annulus fibrosus cells to repair their matrix after chondroitinase ABC-induced chemonucleolysis. Ortho Res Soc Trans 1999; 24:201.
8. Kawakami M, Matsumoto T, Kuribayashi K, et al. mRNA expression of interleukins, phospholipase A2, and nitric oxide synthase in the nerve root and dorsal root ganglion induced by autologous nucleus pulposus in the rat. J Orthop Res 1999; 17:941–946.
9. Franson RC, Saal JS, Saal JF. Human phospholipase A2 is inflammatory. Spine 1992; 17:S129–S132.
10. Kang JD, Stefanovic-Racic M, McIntyre LA, et al. Toward a biochemical understanding of human intervertebral disc degeneration and herniation. Contributions of nitric oxide, interleukins, prostaglandin E2, and matrix metalloproteinases. Spine 1997; 22:1065–1073.
11. Saal JS, Franson RC, Dobrow R, et al. High levels of inflammatory phospholipase A2 activity in lumbar disc herniations. Spine 1990; 15:674–678.
12. Miyamoto H, Saura R, Harada T, et al. The role of cyclooxygenase-2 and inflammatory cytokines in pain induction of herniated lumbar intervertebral disc. Kobe J Med Sci 2000; 46:13–28.
13. Takahashi H, Suguro T, Okajima Y, et al. Inflammatory cytokines in the herniated disc of the lumbar spine. Spine 1996; 21:218–224.
14. Igarashi T, Kikuchi S, Shubayev V, et al. Exogenous tumor necrosis factor-alpha mimics nucleus pulposus-induced neuropathology. Molecular, histologic, and behavioral comparisons in rats. Spine 2000; 25:2975–2980.
15. Olmarker K, Rydevik B. Selective inhibition of tumor necrosis factor-alpha prevents nucleus pulposus-induced thrombus formation, intraneural edema, and reduction of nerve conduction velocity: possible implications for future pharmacologic treatment strategies of sciatica. Spine 2001; 26:863–869.
16. Olmarker K, Larsson K. Tumor necrosis factor alpha and nucleus-pulposus-induced nerve root injury. Spine 1998; 23:2538–2544.
17. Goupille P, Jayson MI, Valat JP, et al. The role of inflammation in disk herniation-associated radiculopathy. Semin Arthritis Rheum 1998; 28:60–71.
18. Kaapa E, Han X, Holm S, Peltonen J, Takala T, Vanharanta H. Collagen synthesis and types I, III, IV, and VI collagens in an animal model of disc degeneration. Spine 1995; 20:59–66.
19. Kaapa E, Holm S, Han X, Takala T, Kovanen V, Vanharanta H. Collagens in the injured porcine intervertebral disc. J Orthop Res 1994; 12:93–102.
20. Hutton WC, Toribatake Y, Elmer WA, Ganey TM, Tomita K, Whitesides TE. The effect of compressive force applied to the intervertebral disc in vivo. A study of proteoglycans and collagen. Spine 1998; 23:2524–2537.
21. Hutton WC, Ganey TM, Elmer WA, et al. Does long-term compressive loading on the intervertebral disc cause degeneration? Spine 2000; 25:2993–3004.
22. Lotz JC, Colliou OK, Chin JR, Duncan NA, Liebenberg E. Compression-induced degeneration of the intervertebral disc: an in vivo mouse model and finite-element study. Spine 1998; 23:2493–2506.
23. Lotz JC, Chin JR. Intervertebral disc cell death is dependent on the magnitude and duration of spinal loading. Spine 2000; 25:1477–1483.
24. Iatridis JC, Mente PL, Stokes IA, Aronsson DD, Alini M. Compression-induced changes in intervertebral disc properties in a rat tail model. Spine 1999; 24:996–1002.

25. Mente PL, Stokes IA, Spence H, et al. Progression of vertebral wedging in an asymmetrically loaded rat tail model. Spine 1997; 22:1292–1296.
26. Masuda K, Aota Y, Muehleman C, et al. A novel rabbit model of mild, reproducible disc degeneration by an anulus needle puncture: correlation between the degree of disc injury and radiological and histological appearances of disc degeneration. Spine 2005; 30(1):5–14.
27. Sobajima S, Kompel JF, Kim JS, et al. A slowly progressive and reproducible animal model of intervertebral disc degeneration characterized by MRI, X-ray, and histology. Spine 2005; 30(1):15–24.
28. Kawakami M, Hashizume H, Nishi H, et al. Comparison of neuropathic pain induced by the application of normal and mechanically compressed nucleus pulposus to lumbar nerve roots in the rat. J Orthop Res 2003; 21:535–539.
29. Kawakami M, Tamaki T, Hayashi N, et al. Possible mechanism of painful radiculopathy in lumbar disc herniation. Clin Orthop 1998; 351:241–251.
30. Kawakami M, Weinstein JN, Spratt KF, et al. Experimental lumbar radiculopathy. Immunohistochemical and quantitative demonstrations of pain induced by lumbar nerve root irritation of the rat. Spine 1994; 19:1780–1794.
31. Hashizume H, DeLeo JA, Colburn RW, et al. Spinal glial activation and cytokine expression after lumbar root injury in the rat. Spine 2000; 25:1206–1217.
32. Deleo TA, Hashizume H, Rutkowski MD, et al. Cyclooxygenase-2 inhibitor SC-236 attenuates mechanical allodynia following nerve root injury in rats. J Orthop Res 2000; 18:977–982.
33. Olmarker K, Storkson R, Berge OG. Pathogenesis of sciatic pain: a study of spontaneous behavior in rats exposed to experimental disc herniation. Spine 2002; 27:1312–1317.
34. Bennett GJ, Xie YK. A peripheral mononeuropathy in rat that produces disorders of pain sensation like those seen in man. Pain 1988; 33:87–107.
35. Kawakami M, Matsumoto T, Hashizume H, et al. Osteogenic protein-1 (osteogenic protein-1/bone morphogenetic protein-7) inhibits degeneration and pain-related behavior induced by chronically compressed nucleus pulposus in the rat. Spine 2005; 30(17):1933–1939.
36. Rosenberg L. Chemical basis for the histological use of Safranin-O in the study of articular cartilage. J Bone Joint Surg 1971; 53A:69–82.
37. Merrihew C, Soeder S, Rueger DC, Kuettner KE, Chubinskaya S. Differential response of endogenous osteogenic protein-1 to interleukin-1β. J Bone Joint Surg Am 2003; 85-A(suppl 3):67–74.
38. Muehleman C, Kuettner KE, Rueger DC, Dijke P, Chubinskaya S. Immunohistochemical localization of osteogenic protein-1 and its receptors in rabbit articular cartilage. J Histochem Cytochem 2002; 50:1341–1350.
39. Nishida Y, Knudson CB, Knudson W. Osteogenic protein-1 inhibits matrix depletion in a hyaluronan hexasaccharide-induced model of osteoarthritis. Osteoarthritis Cartilage 2004; 12(5):374–382.
40. Huch K, Wilbrink B, Flechtenmacher J, et al. Effects of recombinant human osteogenic protein 1 on the production of proteoglycan, prostaglandin E2, and interleukin-1 receptor antagonist by human articular chondrocytes cultured in the presence of interleukin-1β. Arthritis Rheum 1997; 40: 2157–2161.
41. Koepp HE, Sampath KT, Kuettner KE, Homandberg GA. Osteogenic protein-1 (OP-1) blocks cartilage damage caused by fibronectin fragments and promotes repair by enhancing proteoglycan synthesis. Inflamm Res 1997; 47:1–6.
42. Chubinskaya S, Kuettner KE. Regulation of osteogenic proteins by chondrocytes. Int J Biochem Cell Biol 2003; 35:1323–1340.
43. Maves TJ, Gebhart GF, Meller ST. Continuous infusion of acidified saline around the rat sciatic nerve produces thermal hyperalgesia. Neurosci Lett 1995; 194(1–2):45–48.
44. Nachemson A. Intradiscal measurements of pH in patients with lumbar rhizopathies. Acta Orthop Scand 1969; 40:23–42.
45. Takegami K, Thonar EJ, An HS, et al. Osteogenic protein-1 enhances matrix replenishment by intervertebral disc cells previously exposed to interleukin-1. Spine 2002; 15(27):1318–1325.
46. Lidslot L, Olmarker K, Kayama S, et al. Nucleus pulposus inhibits the axonal outgrowth of cultured dorsal root ganglion cells. Eur Spine J 2000; 9:8–13.
47. Lein P, Johnson M, Guo X, et al. Osteogenic protein-1 induces dendritic growth in rat sympathetic neurons. Neuron 1995; 15:597–605.
48. Le Roux P, Behar S, Higgins D, et al. OP-1 enhances dendritic growth from cerebral cortical neurons in vitro. Exp Neurol 1999; 160:151–163.

18 | Clinical Strategies for Delivery of Osteoinductive Growth Factors

Frank S. Hodges and Steven M. Theiss
University of Alabama at Birmingham, Birmingham, Alabama, U.S.A.

INTRODUCTION

Since Marshall Urist first described the discovery of osteogenic proteins (1), there has been an increasing interest in the application of osteoinductive cytokines to simulate de novo bone formation in orthopaedic applications. As spine fusion is the most common bone grafting procedure (2), significant work has been done investigating the utility of various osteoinductive proteins for this purpose (3–13). Chief among these proteins are the bone morphogenetic proteins (BMPs). These proteins have been produced either by extracting and purifying them from animal or human cortical bone, or through recombinant techniques (2). As researchers studied the ability of various BMP preparations to form bone at the site of experimental fractures, segmental defects, and ultimately spine fusions, it became clear that a critical component of osteoinduction was the method of delivery of these proteins. When applied to an experimental fracture site in a small animal model, BMP could effectively be delivered by simply injecting the growth factor at the site in formulation buffer (14,15). However, this was not the case when BMP was used either in a higher animal model or in a more challenging model such as healing a critical-sized cortical defect, or in spine fusion (15,16). In these instances, the delivery method of the BMP became more critical and complex. This was for a variety of reasons related to the local environment in which the protein was applied and the conditions necessary for successful bone formation and healing. As the clinical success of these cytokines is often predicated on successful delivery, much investigation has been done to evaluate different delivery systems or carriers (3–5,8,9,12,15–17). This Chapter will discuss the various characteristics required of an effective carrier as well as the specific carriers being evaluated both clinically and experimentally.

CHARACTERISTICS OF THE IDEAL BONE MORPHOGENETIC PROTEIN DELIVERY SYSTEM

Seeherman and Wozney have described four main characteristics of the ideal BMP delivery vehicle or carrier (15,18). First, the carrier must be able to retain the BMP at the site of application, at the appropriate dose, for a sufficient period of time to induce bone formation. For the purposes of spine fusion, the required dose of BMP is supraphysiologic (5,12,15,16). A dose-dependent response has been noted. Should adequate concentrations not be present, then bony healing will not be affected by the administration of BMP (16). Retention of the protein by the carrier is also critical and can be influenced by the local environment. This is particularly true when the carrier is placed posterolaterally in the lumbar spine. Here, compression of a carrier by the erector spinae musculature may result in diffusion of the BMP and failure of bone formation, despite an appropriate dose of BMP applied initially (3). The exact time that BMP needs to be present at the site to effectively induce bone formation is unknown. The period of time following application that BMP has been detected locally does vary significantly between different carriers but ranges from seven days to up to three weeks (15).

The second characteristic of an effective delivery system is that the carrier be biocompatible and preferably bioresorbable. Ideally, the carrier would degrade shortly after it has completed its function. The reasoning for this is twofold. First, bioresorption decreases prolonged host exposure to a potentially immunogenic foreign object. Second, as bone is a dynamic structure with the ability to remodel, any retained carrier within the fusion mass will theoretically weaken its structural and mechanical integrity. Nonstructural carriers, if not resorbed, would leave a structural void within the fusion mass that could compromise the strength of the fusion. Structural carriers do provide a matrix across which bony fusion can form. However, these carriers are typically only mechanically strong in compression and as they are not dynamic structures, if not resorbed, their fatigability with time could also affect mechanical strength of the fusion mass (18). Resorption of the carrier typically occurs by a white blood cell-mediated inflammatory response. It is important that this inflammatory reaction not affect the healing process within the fusion mass. Studies have also shown that the addition of BMP to a carrier affects the type of inflammatory reaction that removes the carrier. Addition of BMP to a collagen carrier changes the mechanism of resorption from a mixed cell-mediated phagocytic mechanism to a primarily phagocytic picture and also speeds up the rate of resorption as compared with controls (15,18–20). The clinical significance of this finding on the mechanical properties of the fusion mass is not thought to be clinically significant.

The structural properties of the carrier are another important characteristic. A delivery system can be as simple as injection of BMP percutaneously in a water soluble buffer or as advanced as its incorporation into a composite of natural and/or synthetic polymers with an inorganic material such as hydroxyapatite. In addition to just retaining the BMP, a carrier may need to be osteoconductive itself, in order to supply a matrix into which bony ingrowth can occur (3,21,22). To allow this to happen, the carrier must possess the appropriate permeability to allow for cell immigration without hindering the formation of a fusion mass. The permeability can be created in the manufacturing process or can be created by alteration of the carrier once within the host environment. Different types of carriers are used both experimentally and clinically according to the structural characteristics needed for a specific application. More discussion follows regarding the different carrier types. The structural properties of the delivery system used would prove to be one of the most critical factors in successfully using BMP in spinal fusion applications.

The last important characteristic that an ideal delivery system must possess is the ability to make it to market. The product must be economically feasible to produce with consistent, reproducible results. It must be in a stable form that can be stored for periods of time while maintaining its sterility. The stringent guidelines set forth by the Food and Drug Administration (FDA) for its use must be met and it must also be relatively easy for providers and support staff to prepare for implantation.

TYPES OF BONE MORPHOGENETIC PROTEIN CARRIERS

There are four main categories of materials currently being investigated as potential BMP carriers. The first category is the natural polymers, of which collagen is the most widely used. Collagen is a component of the extracellular matrix of connective tissues and bone. Collagen sponges possess all the characteristics necessary of a carrier: they can be modified to alter their BMP retention times, are resorbable, provide a matrix into which fusion mass may grow, and are readily available. Numerous studies have been performed showing the efficacy of utilizing BMP in a collagen sponge carrier in fracture and fusion models (5,9,19,21,22). In fact, the first and only FDA-approved carrier at this time is the absorbable type-1 collagen sponge that is packaged with rhBMP-2. The product is known as INFUSE® bone graft for use within a tapered lordotic titanium interbody cage (LT-CAGE® Medtronic Sofamor Danek, Memphis, Tennessee, U.S.A.) for anterior lumber interbody fusion. It is also available for use in open diaphyseal tibia fractures. The sponge is resorbed over a two- to four-week period by a cell-mediated immune response. Other carriers, including bovine-derived collagen sponges are being investigated for clinical use in humans under stringent FDA-approved clinical studies. Specifically, a bovine collagen carrier combined with rhBMP 7 [osteogenetic protein-1 (OP-1)] is being used under a humanitarian device exemption for recalcitrant long bone nonunions. There is concern of an immunogenic reaction following implantation of a bovine absorbable collagen sponge as many of the human BMP trials have noted positive antibody titers. The significance of this has yet to be determined (23,24). If this precludes a patient from receiving future exposure to bovine collagen because of concern for an immune response remains to be seen. Use of recombinant human collagen as a synthetic biologic polymer is currently being evaluated (25). Its use could remove the potential at disease transmission. It can be manufactured with a specific amino acid sequence and, thus, could theoretically prevent the associated immunogenicity created with implantation of bovine collagen carriers.

A second group of possible carriers are inorganic materials. These include calcium phosphate ceramics, like hydroxyapatite and tricalcium phosphate, as well as calcium-sulfated cements. These materials have been used extensively over the past decade as bone graft extenders for use in orthopaedic, spinal, and periodontal surgery. As with collagen carriers, these products also possess all four desired characteristics of a BMP delivery system. Many studies have evaluated the use of inorganic materials as structural osteoconductive matrices for implantation with osteoinductive proteins (26,27). Inorganic materials can be engineered with customized three-dimensional structures as compared with collagen, which lacks rigidity. As well, its inherent porosity, either a product of manufacturing or postimplantation modification, has been shown to allow for faster bony ingrowth in histologic specimens. This more quickly creates a mechanically rigid fusion mass as compared with collagen carriers (28). Inorganic materials have also been used as bulking agents to resist compression from soft tissues in anatomic regions where such compression can diffuse the implanted BMP, decreasing the dose and reducing effectiveness (3,29).

There have been many synthetic polymers created and used experimentally as carriers of osteogenic proteins. The most commonly utilized polymers are polylactic acid, polyglycolic acid, and polylactide/glycolide (30–33). None to date have been approved for use in human subjects as carriers for BMP in spinal applications. They do, however, have very desirable characteristics with regard to removal of any concern for disease transmission as well as having design flexibility. There remains concern that the mode of degradation could have a detrimental effect on formation of bone. However, design modification and material selection should be able to circumvent this concern making synthetics a very attractive choice of delivery system (15,18).

The final category of BMP carriers are composites of these three carrier types. As Seeherman and Wozney have pointed out, most fractures will heal spontaneously without the use of BMP, whereas achieving spinal fusion via an interbody or posterolateral intertransverse technique will not occur without osteoconductive supplementation (15). A spinal fusion bed is similar to a segmental bone defect in that there is no close apposition of bone as in closed long bone models. In this circumstance, fusion would not primarily occur without some osteoconductive matrix to provide the lattice work across which bone could form. To that point, delivery systems for spinal applications may ideally require a structural component that will provide an osteoconductive matrix across which bony fusion can occur. Perhaps, the most extensively tested composite carrier is compression-resistant matrix (CRM) (Mastergraft Matrix®, Medtronic Sofamor Danek). This is a ceramic/collagen composite consisting of 14% hydroxyapatite/85% beta-tricalcium phosphate. When used posterolaterally in a nonhuman primate model, it successfully resulted in experimental spine fusion. It is currently undergoing human clinical testing (3). Another composite carrier undergoing clinical testing is the collagen carboxymethylcellulose (CMC) composite used to deliver OP-1 putty for posterolateral lumbar fusions. This composite carrier is completed by combining the putty with autogenous bone graft in the posterolateral spine (12,34).

THE CURRENT USE OF BONE MORPHOGENETIC PROTEIN CARRIERS IN CLINICAL SPINAL APPLICATIONS

The bulk of published research describing BMP for spinal applications has involved primarily its use in cervical and lumbar degenerative conditions, namely anterior cervical fusion, lumbar interbody fusion, and posterolateral intertransverse lumbar fusion. Achieving anterior fusion using BMP is fundamentally different from achieving posterior fusion. Applications have been more thoroughly studied in the lumbar spine than in the cervical spine. Perhaps, this is because of the fact that the literature cites a significantly higher rate of pseudoarthrosis in lumbar fusions, particularly posterolateral fusions (35). This, combined with the associated morbidity of harvesting iliac crest bone graft, makes BMP use an attractive alternative for all regions of the spine (36,37). Yet, despite the significant research studying the numerous carriers and BMP preparations, routine clinical use of BMP is limited to only a few clinical applications in the spine. The specific applications where it is currently being used or clinically investigated are lumbar interbody fusion, cervical interbody fusion, and lumbar posterolateral fusion.

Perhaps, the least challenging clinical spine application of a carrier/osteogenic protein combination is an anterior lumbar interbody fusion. This is because of several reasons. First, the carrier itself, in this instance, does not need any structural integrity, as the BMP is routinely combined with an interbody graft, such as a cortical allograft or interbody fusion cage. Second, the anatomic region where the BMP is implanted is devoid of soft tissues that may interfere with the ability of the carrier to retain the protein. Finally, there are no critical anatomic structures closely adjacent to the area of implantation. Even the neurologic elements in an anterior lumbar interbody fusion are separated from the implant by the posterior annulus and posterior longitudinal ligament. Therefore, it is not surprising that this application has been the most extensively studied and clinically successful. The carrier in this application is typically a structural graft, such as a cortical dowel or metallic cage, filled with rhBMP-2 soaked on an absorbable collagen sponge. Several clinical studies led to the FDA approval of recombinant BMP-2 on an absorbable collagen sponge combined with an interbody cage for anterior lumbar interbody fusion. Other structural interbody devices have subsequently been combined with the collagen sponge/rhBMP-2 implant with similarly successful results (21,22,38). A natural extrapolation of this technique to posterior or transforaminal lumbar interbody applications has occurred. This utilizes the same absorbable collagen carrier/rhBMP-2 combination in an interbody cage. Care was taken to keep the osteoinductive implant away from the exposed dura mater. Limited clinical studies have shown this to be a safe and effective technique (39,40). These methods of achieving fusion using BMP possess the theoretical risk of causing heterotopic intraforaminal or intracanal bone formation owing to both the insertion of the BMP via a posterior or posterolateral approach and the violation of the annulus/posterior longitudinal ligament complex. Further study needs to be completed to examine both the efficacy of BMP in achieving fusion in these applications as well the frequency and clinical significance of heterotopic bone formation within the canal or foramen.

Use of BMP to achieve cervical interbody fusion has also been investigated. Again, as in lumbar interbody fusions, the carrier most extensively studied is an absorbable collagen sponge/rhBMP2 implant contained within a structural interbody graft. Currently, clinical evaluations are ongoing. A single study has been published to date. In this study, both the control and experimental arms underwent simultaneous anterior cervical interbody fusion with a fibular allograft ring and anterior plate. The control group had the ring filled with autograft, while the experimental group had the ring filled with rhBMP-2 on an absorbable sponge. Fusion results were roughly equivalent. The experimental group had a statistically better improvement in arm pain and neck disability. The authors, however, note that the small sample size "precludes concluding it (BMP) to be superior (to autograft)" (23). It appears that BMP is at least equivalent to autogenous iliac crest bone grafting in achieving fusion. However, there remains theoretical concern about the effect of BMP on the adjacent retropharyngeal space and the exposed epidural space.

Perhaps, the most challenging spine application currently undergoing human clinical testing is posterolateral intertransverse process lumbar fusions. Use of the absorbable collagen sponge as a carrier of osteogenic proteins in this application has failed to form clinically relevant amounts of bone in a nonhuman primate model (9). As previously mentioned, this was thought to be because of muscle compression of the sponge and diffusion of the protein locally. This has been overcome by delivering the rhBMP-2 with a ceramic/collagen composite carrier (3,29). Similarly, studies have investigated the ability of rhBMP-7 (OP-1) in a composite carrier to induce posterolateral intertransverse lumbar fusion. The composite carrier in this instance is putty made of CMC and type-I collagen, combined with autograft. Two-year results showed this technique to have an equivalent fusion rate compared with autograft, with no adverse events reported (12,34).

As osteoinductive proteins are used more routinely for a variety of orthopaedic applications, the method of delivery will become more critical. Each osteoinductive application in each anatomic location requires different delivery parameters to optimize their performance. Already, alternative delivery methods, such as gene therapy, are being tested in lower animal models in an attempt to even more efficiently deliver the required cytokines to the desired location (41–43). As these techniques become available clinically, it is imperative that the clinician understands the potential benefits and limitations of the technology. Only then will we be able to intelligently apply these new techniques clinically to get not only maximum benefit for our patients, but also avoid unnecessary cost and morbidity in applying them where they have little chance of clinical success.

REFERENCES

1. Urist MR. Bone: formation by autoinduction. Clin Orthop Relat Res 2002; 395:4–10.
2. Yoon ST, Boden SD. Spine fusion by gene therapy. Gene Ther 2004; 11:360–367.
3. Barnes B, Boden SD, Louis-Ugbo J, et al. Lower dose of rhBMP-2 achieves spine fusion when combined with an osteoconductive bulking agent in non-human primates. Spine 2005; 30:1127–1133.
4. Boden SD, Kang J, Sandhu H, et al. Use of recombinant human bone morphogenetic protein-2 to achieve posterolateral lumbar spine fusion in humans: a prospective, randomized clinical pilot trial: 2002 Volvo Award in clinical studies. Spine 2002; 27:2662–2673.
5. Hecht BP, Fischgrund JS, Herkowitz HN, et al. The use of recombinant human bone morphogenetic protein 2 (rhBMP-2) to promote spinal fusion in a nonhuman primate anterior interbody fusion model. Spine 1999; 24:629–636.
6. Hotz G, Herr G. Bone substitute with osteoinductive biomaterials—current and future clinical applications. Int J Oral Maxillofac Surg 1994; 23:413–417.
7. Lovell TP, Dawson EG, Nilsson OS, et al. Augmentation of spinal fusion with bone morphogenetic protein in dogs. Clin Orthop Relat Res 1989; 243:266–274.
8. Magin MN, Delling G. Improved lumbar vertebral interbody fusion using rhOP-1: a comparison of autogenous bone graft, bovine hydroxylapatite (Bio-Oss), and BMP-7 (rhOP-1) in sheep. Spine 2001; 26:469–478.
9. Martin GJ, Jr., Boden SD, Marone MA, et al. Posterolateral intertransverse process spinal arthrodesis with rhBMP-2 in a nonhuman primate: important lessons learned regarding dose, carrier, and safety. J Spinal Disord 1999; 12:179–186.
10. Riley EH, Lane JM, Urist MR, et al. Bone morphogenetic protein-2: biology and applications. Clin Orthop Relat Res 1996; 324:39–46.
11. Sandhu H. Spinal fusion using bone morphogenetic proteins. Orthopedics 2004; 27:717–718.
12. Vaccaro AR, Patel T, Fischgrund J, et al. A pilot safety and efficacy study of OP-1 putty (rhBMP-7) as an adjunct to iliac crest autograft in posterolateral lumbar fusions. Eur Spine J 2003; 12:495–500.
13. Zhang H, Sucato DJ, Welch RD. Recombinant human bone morphogenic protein-2-enhanced anterior spine fusion without bone encroachment into the spinal canal: a histomorphometric study in a thoracoscopically instrumented porcine model. Spine 2005; 30:512–518.
14. Einhorn TA, Majeska RJ, Mohaideen A, et al. A single percutaneous injection of recombinant human bone morphogenetic protein-2 accelerates fracture repair. J Bone Joint Surg Am 2003; 85-A:1425–1435.
15. Seeherman H, Wozney J, Li R. Bone morphogenetic protein delivery systems. Spine 2002; 27:S16–S23.
16. Boden SD, Schimandle JH, Hutton WC. 1995 Volvo Award in basic sciences. The use of an osteoinductive growth factor for lumbar spinal fusion. Part II: Study of dose, carrier, and species. Spine 1995; 20:2633–2644.
17. Lindholm TS, Gao TJ. Functional carriers for bone morphogenetic proteins. Ann Chir Gynaecol Suppl 1993; 207:3–12.
18. Seeherman H, Wozney JM. Delivery of bone morphogenetic proteins for orthopedic tissue regeneration. Cytokine Growth Factor Rev 2005; 16:329–345.
19. Bouxsein ML, Turek TJ, Blake CA, et al. Recombinant human bone morphogenetic protein-2 accelerates healing in a rabbit ulnar osteotomy model. J Bone Joint Surg Am 2001; 83-A:1219–1230.
20. Li RH, Bouxsein ML, Blake CA, et al. rhBMP-2 injected in a calcium phosphate paste (alpha-BSM) accelerates healing in the rabbit ulnar osteotomy model. J Orthop Res 2003; 21:997–1004.
21. Burkus JK, Gornet MF, Dickman CA, et al. Anterior lumbar interbody fusion using rhBMP-2 with tapered interbody cages. J Spinal Disord Tech 2002; 15:337–349.
22. Burkus JK, Sandhu HS, Gornet MF, et al. Use of rhBMP-2 in combination with structural cortical allografts: clinical and radiographic outcomes in anterior lumbar spinal surgery. J Bone Joint Surg Am 2005; 87:1205–1212.

23. Baskin DS, Ryan P, Sonntag V, et al. A prospective, randomized, controlled cervical fusion study using recombinant human bone morphogenetic protein-2 with the CORNERSTONE-SR allograft ring and the ATLANTIS anterior cervical plate. Spine 2003; 28:1219–1225.

24. Hyder P, Singh G, Adam S. Humoral responses to type I collagen after surgical curettage procedures employing bovine collagen implants. Biomaterials 1992; 13:693–696.

25. Yang C, Hillas PJ, Baez JA, et al. The application of recombinant human collagen in tissue engineering. BioDrugs 2004; 18:103–119.

26. den Boer FC, Wippermann BW, Blokhuis TJ, et al. Healing of segmental bone defects with granular porous hydroxyapatite augmented with recombinant human osteogenic protein-1 or autologous bone marrow. J Orthop Res 2003; 21:521–528.

27. Edwards RB, III, Seeherman HJ, Bogdanske JJ, et al. Percutaneous injection of recombinant human bone morphogenetic protein-2 in a calcium phosphate paste accelerates healing of a canine tibial osteotomy. J Bone Joint Surg Am 2004; 86-A:1425–1438.

28. Minamide A, Kawakami M, Hashizume H, et al. Evaluation of carriers of bone morphogenetic protein for spinal fusion. Spine 2001; 26:933–939.

29. Akamaru T, Suh D, Boden SD, et al. Simple carrier matrix modifications can enhance delivery of recombinant human bone morphogenetic protein-2 for posterolateral spine fusion. Spine 2003; 28:429–434.

30. Boyan BD, Lohmann CH, Somers A, et al. Potential of porous poly-D,L-lactide-co-glycolide particles as a carrier for recombinant human bone morphogenetic protein-2 during osteoinduction in vivo. J Biomed Mater Res 1999; 46:51–59.

31. Kenley R, Marden L, Turek T, et al. Osseous regeneration in the rat calvarium using novel delivery systems for recombinant human bone morphogenetic protein-2 (rhBMP-2). J Biomed Mater Res 1994; 28:1139–1147.

32. Saito N, Okada T, Toba S, et al. New synthetic absorbable polymers as BMP carriers: plastic properties of poly-D,L-lactic acid-polyethylene glycol block copolymers. J Biomed Mater Res 1999; 47:104–110.

33. Schrier JA, DeLuca PP. Recombinant human bone morphogenetic protein-2 binding and incorporation in PLGA microsphere delivery systems. Pharm Dev Technol 1999; 4:611–621.

34. Vaccaro AR, Patel T, Fischgrund J, et al. A 2-year follow-up pilot study evaluating the safety and efficacy of op-1 putty (rhbmp-7) as an adjunct to iliac crest autograft in posterolateral lumbar fusions. Eur Spine J 2005; 14:623–629.

35. Boden SD, Schimandle JH, Hutton WC, et al. 1995 Volvo Award in basic sciences. The use of an osteoinductive growth factor for lumbar spinal fusion. Part I: Biology of spinal fusion. Spine 1995; 20:2626–2632.

36. Arrington ED, Smith WJ, Chambers HG, et al. Complications of iliac crest bone graft harvesting. Clin Orthop Relat Res 1996; 329:300–309.

37. Banwart JC, Asher MA, Hassanein RS. Iliac crest bone graft harvest donor site morbidity. A statistical evaluation. Spine 1995; 20:1055–1060.

38. Boden SD, Zdeblick TA, Sandhu HS, et al. The use of rhBMP-2 in interbody fusion cages. Definitive evidence of osteoinduction in humans: a preliminary report. Spine 2000; 25:376–381.

39. Haid RW, Jr., Branch CL, Jr., Alexander JT, et al. Posterior lumbar interbody fusion using recombinant human bone morphogenetic protein type 2 with cylindrical interbody cages. Spine J 2004; 4:527–538.

40. Mummaneni PV, Pan J, Haid RW, et al. Contribution of recombinant human bone morphogenetic protein-2 to the rapid creation of interbody fusion when used in transforaminal lumbar interbody fusion: a preliminary report. Invited submission from the Joint Section Meeting on Disorders of the Spine and Peripheral Nerves, March 2004. J Neurosurg Spine 2004; 1:19–23.

41. Alden TD, Pittman DD, Beres EJ, et al. Percutaneous spinal fusion using bone morphogenetic protein-2 gene therapy. J Neurosurg 1999; 90:109–114.

42. Boden SD, Titus L, Hair G, et al. Lumbar spine fusion by local gene therapy with a cDNA encoding a novel osteoinductive protein (LMP-1). Spine 1998; 23:2486–2492.

43. Hidaka C, Goshi K, Rawlins B, et al. Enhancement of spine fusion using combined gene therapy and tissue engineering BMP-7-expressing bone marrow cells and allograft bone. Spine 2003; 28:2049–2057.

19 | New Adjunct in Spine Interbody Fusion: Designed Bioabsorbable Cage with Cell-Based Gene Therapy

Chia-Ying Lin
Department of Neurosurgery, University of Michigan, Ann Arbor, Michigan, U.S.A.

Scott J. Hollister
Department of Biomedical Engineering, University of Michigan, Ann Arbor, Michigan, U.S.A.

Paul H. Krebsbach
Department of Biologic and Materials Sciences, University of Michigan, Ann Arbor, Michigan, U.S.A.

Frank La Marca
Department of Neurosurgery, University of Michigan, Ann Arbor, Michigan, U.S.A.

TRENDS IN SPINE FUSION

Spine fusions have been performed worldwide for a variety of reasons mainly correlated to pathological spine disorders and vertebral instability. The number of procedures increases dramatically and it has been estimated that nearly one million are performed each year (1). A recent report in 2001 (2) revealed that in the United States alone, approximately 360,000 patients underwent certain types of spinal arthrodesis. Among all these, indications that refer to spine arthrodesis are mostly low back pain, spondylosis and spondylolisthesis, rheumatoid instabilities, postdiscectomy, unstable fractures, trauma, and other lesions. Each of the above spine abnormalities presents different challenges to surgeons in achieving solid constructs to immobilize the disturbed motion segments.

Enormous efforts have been devoted to invent various approaches to achieve successful fusion. These approaches primarily attempt to abolish the degrees of freedom of predetermined functional spine segments by permanently suppressing motion. While nearly one-third of these approaches involves applying bone grafting, the application of autogenous bone graft from different sites such as iliac crest (3–5) becomes the gold standard in spinal fusion. Implants with high load-bearing capacity, including screw fixation, transpedicular instrumentation, anterior or posterior metal implants, and the various fuion cages as adjuncts for spinal fusion, are also commonly recruited to provide rigidity to achieve primary stability and facilitate graft incorporation that further facilitates bone healing. However, current approaches are also associated with a considerable rate of failure that involves the essences of the mechanics and biology of spinal fusion. Device loosening because of disuse osteopenia, hardward failure, loss of correction, pseudarthrosis, or the combined adverse symptoms are reported in a volume on clinical investigations of spinal fusion (4,6–9). Conventional bone graft harvesting morbidity (10–17) with inconsistent bone quality (4,7,8) also brings resource burdens when applying bone grafting to obtain solid arthrodesis. All of these have driven the search for alternatives or advances for vertebral fusion.

Extensive work to cope with present problems is in a full swing to improve healing and decrease the morbidity associated with autologous bone harvesting. Emergence of new design and fabrication techniques and the persistent efforts in the development of compliant biocompatible or biodegradable materials have created less rigid but still mechanically sound systems and make these devices capable of scaffolding tissue regeneration and achieve specific biological interactions to enhance spinal fusion. Gene transfer, recombinant protein delivery, and therapeutic cell-based transplantation provide novel opportunities to replace conventional grafting strategies with these bone graft substitutes that allow better exploitation of advances in a number of tissue engineering technologies. Hence, the attempt to orchestrate these tenets to perform better integration of developed technologies in this tissue-engineering era becomes the heart of the work to pursue a new development of a hybrid system that facilitates successful spine arthrodesis.

LUMBAR INTERBODY FUSION WITH CAGE

As aforementioned, spinal fusion benefits patients by significantly releasing their suffering if the source of accumulated difficulties can be traced to spinal instability. As a primary approach to arrest disabling back pain resulting from degeneration of vertebral segments, fusion immobilizes vertebral segments to reduce or even eliminate the persistent back pain mainly from the apparent pathologic mobility. Various instrumentations based on the conceptual mechanisms to permanently cease the vertebral mobility essentially provided surgeons multiple options to achieve bony union between vertebral segments, by taking both surgical techniques and clinical symptoms into account. Among all these systems, one prominent device is the spinal cage widely adopted in lumbar intervertebral arthrodeses as an adjunct by the approach of both posterior lumbar interbody fusion (PLIF) and anterior lumbar interbody fusion (ALIF). Ever since Dr. Ralph Cloward developed the PLIF to define the problem as the treatment of a broken intervertebral joint damaged by a disc rupture (18–20), continuous efforts followed by this significant contribution of the interbody fusion operation procedures have been devoted to achieve immediate stability and prompt healing on approached spine segments.

Indications for PLIF are supposedly reducing motion within the lumbar spine, such as instability arising from spondylolisthesis, as well as removal of the decompression exerted on nerve roots (21–23).

The PLIF involves inserting bone graft with the cage to inner disc space to activate a biological response that results in bone ingrowth across the disc space by linking contiguous vertebral bodies and thereby cease the motion at the segment. The spine is approached followed by the laminectomy, which allows visualization of the nerve roots. The facet joints are directly over the nerve roots that they may then be trimmed to give the nerve roots more room and to achieve the decompression. Following this procedure, the nerve roots are then retracted to one side. The disc space is cleaned off the disc material so that a bone graft, or interbody cages with bone, is then inserted into the disc space and the bone grows from vertebral body to vertebral body.

Generally, because the large spinal muscles do not need to be dissected off the transverse processes the PLIF approach leaves less scarring of the muscle and associated pain for the patient. This is an advantage over the posterolateral gutter fusion. However, the PLIF also has some noticeable disadvantages such that significant traction can injure the nerve root and the traction has the potential to result in chronic leg pain and back pain because substantial retraction of the nerve roots is necessary for the surgeon to gain access to the disc space. Moreover, potential excessive blood loss may occur during the surgery in this area as there are numerous veins (epidural veins) over the disc space.

When conducting lumbar interbody fusion with cages, most of the cages, in general, are placed in the front of the spine that is denoted as ALIF (24–27). The cages can be inserted through a small incision (minilaparotomy) or with an endoscope. However, it has been recognized that the cages may not fix the spine well enough in certain situations. The use of standalone interbody fusion cage devices will work best in single level, particularly effective at L5-S1 where there is not a lot of motion on the set of the segment. When fusion is applied at L4-L5 and above, patients, especially for those with a tall disc space or an associated isthmic spondylolisthesis, cages do not provide sufficient fixation and thus supplemental posterior fixation such as posterior pedicle screw supplementation is required.

While the ALIF spine fusion technique is still widely available, the approach is often combined with a posterior approach (anterior/posterior fusions) for the need to provide more rigid fixation than an anterior approach alone provides. The ALIF is similar to the PLIF, except that in the ALIF the disc space is fused by approaching the spine through the abdomen instead of through the back. Unlike the PLIF described here and the posterolateral gutter approaches, the ALIF approach has the advantage that nerve and the back muscles remain undisturbed. In addition, interbody cage with bone graft is placed in the front of the spine where it is in compression, and the condition in compression tends to make fusion better. However, it should be noticed that the ALIF comes with a disadvantage of the close proximity to the large blood vessels that go to the legs. Damages on these vessels may result in excessive blood loss.

In the near decade, the insertion of the cage devices has been dramatically increased. The reason attributed to the highly increasing rate of performing lumbar interbody cages to facilitate arthrodesis is mainly for three factors: the high rate of failure associated with the use of bone graft alone (20,28–30), the high rate of failure associated with the use of posterior fixation instrumentation, and the high rate of success associated to the use of fusion cages with bone grafts arousing biological responses. Interbody fusion cages have been developed to maintain the stability of the approached level during bony fusion. They provide immediate strong column support that has been tested in several biomechanical tests. However, favorable and short-term results have been pervasively reported, yet long-term clinical effects of interbody cages still remain unclear.

COMPARISON AND CLINICAL PERFORMANCE OF CURRENT CAGES

The reconstruction stability remains controversial among different cage designs. Although an increasing number of interbody procedures have been performed, postoperative complication associated with the use of cages have been accordantly reported. Dislocation of the cage such as migration or retropulsion claims the revision procedure to resolve the complication (31). Insufficient stability of the mechanical environment to the interbody fusion cages increase high risks that the dislocated devices encroach on the spinal canal and damage the spinal cord and nerve roots. To investigate these factors in spinal cages, Kanayama et al. (32) designed a study to compare stability and stress-shielding effect of different lumbar interbody fusion devices. They concluded that threaded fusion cages provide equivalent support as the nonthreaded designs; thus, they guarantee the sufficient reconstruction stiffness. However, they provide more stress-shielded environment within the device and the stress-shielding effect is correlated to the largest pore size rather than to the total porous area.

McAfee (33) in 1999 reviewed the current concepts through various designs currently adopted in spinal arthrodeses, either on the market or for studies in developing alternative implants. This review illustrated the mechanical, biological, and physiological roles of fusion cages, as well as results of clinical series. In this review, a large clinical series of 947 patients in a prospective, multicenter trial as the Bagby and Kuslich (BAK) Investigational Device Exemption Study was reported by Yuan et al., Kuslich et al., and Alpert (34–36). After 24 months follow-up postoperatively, 85% satisfaction of decreasing pain was reported. In the Investigational Device Exemption Study of the Ray cage, 24 months follow-up presented radiographic evidence of fusion, defined as an absence of motion as seen on flexion and extension radiographs (30). Brantigan et al. (37) reported the outcome that a successful clinical result was achieved in patients managed with the Brantigan cage (carbon-fiber cage). Last, the use of Harms vertical titanium-mesh cage developed by Harms et al. in 1991 has been advocated (38,39). However, there is no Investigational Device Exemption Study of the design so far.

Clinical results have showed satisfactory performance of cage-instrumented lumbar interbody fusion as the treatment for severe back pain induced by disc hermiation, degenerative end plates and osteophyte. Above 90% patients demonstrated fusion with less than 1% complication after a couple of years follow-up evaluation (40). However, some researchers (41,42) asserted that these results were as "initial, favorable fusion outcomes and attributed clinical effectiveness" because the equally unfavorable results have been also reported by other investigators (35,42–47). Because concerns have been rising for the required revision procedures by consistently reported complications postoperatively, the long-term effects of cage devices on the spinal segments emerged as an appealing topic for upcoming studies and observations and will provide information for the improvement or the new design concepts for cages.

POTENTIAL MODIFICATIONS OF DESIGN VARIABLES FOR NEW CAGE DEVELOPMENTS

The primary goals with the use of interbody fusion cages are to afford immediate stability to the motion segment until arthrodesis is complete and to correct the existing mechanical deformation. Cage design itself contains external shape, surface geometry, anchorage mechanism as well as pore dimension and deployment, which in turn determine the afterward performance of segmental stability, mechanical integrity, and the integration of tissue ongrowth and ingrowth. Besides the design of the cage, the limitations of the cage material weigh another big concern. Stress-shielding, migration of the cage, and pseudoarthrosis of the motion segment lead to complications that result in problems in lumbar interbody fusion. One of the endeavors in the present work to develop the new cage design is to magnify the request of the rigidity and stability without sacrificing essential compliance as the favorable stimulation for tissue regeneration. Further task is to create the whole device to be a porous-matrix-like structure that it can be qualified as a scaffold to increase osteoconduction and suitable for delivering biofactors as bone graft substitutes, such as genes, proteins, growth factors, and/or cells. In all, the goal herein is to develop a cage triplet as the pivot in spine arthrodesis to maintain segmental stability, deliver therapeutic biofactors, and therefore enhance spinal fusion.

Motion, Ingrowth, and Stability

Functional osseointegration is highly related to the local mechanical environment around the interface between bone and implants. Indeed, the way by which the induced motion performs will determine the patterns of the tissue formation. Cuillinane et al. (48) conducted a precisely controlled motion in an experimental mid-femoral defect and reported that the defect of mechanical treatment group failed to achieve union, but instead the neoarthroses formed. The architectural organization of molecular components within the newly formed tissue is influenced by their local mechanical environment, which has been investigated with a deep-to-superficial polarity on subcondral bone arcades and a flattened morphology in the midline. This pattern was directed by the applied symmetrical bending motion, which mimicked the mechanical environment in utero join development. Pilliar et al. and Simmons et al. (49–51) pioneered the limited movement between the implant and the surrounding tissue within as a necessary criterion for bone formation within porous-surfaced implants. Since then, they had studied the morphology of the tissue–porous-surfaced implant interface region from radiographic elucidation of their animal models to later numerical model.

An early report (49) from the group in 1981 showed that excessive movement prevents the calcification of the tissue within the pores and resulted in implant attachment by fibrous tissue only. However, they suggested that the implant fixation supported by fibrous tissue ingrowth could be adequate. In the recent studies (50,51), they developed computational analyses to justify their experimental tests. They concluded that different bone formation patterns corresponded to respective local mechanical environment. Appositional bone formation occurred when the strain components at the tissue–host bone interface were less than 8%, while localized, de novo bone formation occurred when the distortional tissue strain is approximately less than 3%. Thus, the evidences and studies illustrated here give the idea that controlled motion in devices with adjacent bone tissues provide some extent of manipulation of bone formation patterns and new construct stability.

Stress

Bone mechanical properties significantly depend on bone tissue structure. The milestone established by Julius Wolff (52) disserted that the bone structure could respond to alternations in stress. In Wolff's law, the structure will align along principal stress direction and the orientation could change if there is a change in mechanical stress direction. This discovery revealed the bone adaptation to mechanical environment and guided researches to proceed with profound studies on mechanically mediated bone adaptation. Essentially, Wolff's law implied that bone tissue keeps conducting optimization mechanism by remodeling process, aiming to obtain maximum mechanical efficiency with minimum mass.

During fracture healing, the tissue differentiation is related to mechanical stimulus accompanied through the fracture healing history. This theory was postulated by Carter and Blenman in 1988 (53). They sketched out the relation of mechanical stimulus to tissue growth, remodeling, and healing based on the level of vascularity. Earlier in 1987, Carter (54) also developed a osteogeneic index and applied the theory on the numerical models to judge the occurrence of bone, cartilage, and fibrous tissue. To some extent, the fusion process to achieve complete arthrodesis substantially resembles a process of fracture healing.

Followed by the healing, stress still plays an extremely determinant role in bone remodeling. Recall Wolff's law, the bone structure still undergoes an optimization to fit in the demand of mechanical requirement without redundancy in the intricate architecture. Guldberg et al. (55) set an in vivo model of hydraulic bone chamber in their canine metaphyseal trabecular bone and found solid evidence of microstructural adaptation during trabecular bone repair form microcomputed tomography images. The behavior of the microstructure adaptation within the bone chamber is somewhat reminiscent of one within the cage. Therefore, if the designed internal architecture could provide a controlled and predictable stimulation, more reliable construct strength would be acquired as proposed in the present work.

Implants shared the load previously imparted to the bone, and hence reduced the mechanical stimulation on bone. This phenomenon is known as stress-shielding. Again, in accordance with Wolff's law, bone would adapt itself by reducing its mass, either by becoming more porous (internal remodeling) or by making the structure thinner (external remodeling), to present the responsiveness to the reduction of stresses from the natural situation. It remains unclear whether the bone quality of the developing interbody fusion mass will be affected as a result of the shield-stress and how much the threshold of the shielding effect can be accepted for excess shielded stress may deteriorate the interbody fusion mass over the long period. One evidence provided by Cunningham et al. (56) in a more than eight years postoperative investigation shows the histological composition of cervical interbody fusion in thoroughbred horses and they discovered significant decrease in bone mineral density at the fusion site within the cage compared with the adjacent vertebral bodies. Although more investigations are required to find the answers in the case of spinal interbody fusion, numerous studies have been done in other applications in orthopedics, for instance, total hip joint replacement. A series of clinical reports showed resorption in a manner of reduced cortical thickness and increased porosity is seen in most patients who have received noncemented total hip arthroplasty. Recently, Dr. Martijn van Dijk and his group (42) published an observation of the effect of cage stiffness on the rate of lumbar interbody fusion. They selected the polymeric material poly(L-lactic acid) (PLLA) with an apparently lower elastic modulus (4.2 GPa) compared with titanium (110 GPa) and fabricated it into a conventional-wedged design. They found reduced stiffness of cages enhanced significantly by interbody fusion as compared with titanium cages after six months. The results from their large quadrupedal animal models showed significant improvement in the arthrodesis rate and the quality of trabecular bone in the new constructs (42,46,47). This result may indicate that reduced stiffness yields more compliance and compensates strain energy to the bone tissues.

The relationship between the change of bone density and strain energy was successfully quantified in a remodeling algorithm proposed by Huiskes et al. (57). The model included the idea of a lazy or homeostatic zone where a certain threshold interval exists. Bone mass increases when the strain energy density is above a certain level inferring the modeling from stress fractures. Below a certain threshold, there is excessive remodeling or absorption of bone; in between these levels is maintenance of bone structure. Therefore, the reduction of shielded stress would ensure bone tissue adjacent to the implant to acquire sufficient energy to maintain bone mineral density when the rigidity requirement is still first in priority.

Porosity

In tissue regeneration, porosity, pore size, and pore structure are important concerns that are critical for nutrient supply to transplanted cells. Large void volume implies that low volume fraction with a large surface ration is favorable for vascularization, extracellular matrix deposition, and maximal cell population. Internal pore connection increases diffusion rates to and from the center of the scaffold and enhances the vascularization that improves the mass transportation such as metabolic waste removal and nutrient supply. It has been postulated that bone tends to infiltrate into the pores of an inert porous system (58). Hence, by creating high porous scaffolding, progressive bone ingrowth can generate high bounding to stabilize the construct of bone and implants. Designing high porous structure for spinal cages may facilitate fusion rate and arthrodesis load bearing, especially when cell transplantation is conducted as an alternative biological component in the fusion system.

IMPLANTOLOGY AND OSTEOCONDUCTION
Influence of Implant Surface Geometry on Osseointegration

It has been shown earlier in a series of in vivo studies that implant surface geometry as a design variable significantly influences long-term implant performance (59–61). Early in 1979, Bobyn et al. examined the optimal pore size for the fixation of porous surfaced metal implants by the ingrowth of bone (62). The pore size was investigated to influence the rate of bone ingrowth and the retained maximum fixation strengths. They concluded that in the shortest period (eight weeks) a pore size range of approximately 50 to 400 μm ended up to provide the optimum or maximum fixation strength of 17 MPa. Almost near the same time, this group also showed that the surface configuration played another important role that influences the tensile strength of fixation of implants by bone ingrowth (63). The results indicated that implants with the multiple particle layer surface configurations develop a greater tensile strength of fixation than that provided by implants with the single particle layer surface configuration. Also, they suggested this fixation strength develops more quickly if the cortical bone is petaled prior to implantation. Recently, Simmons et al. (51) reported their study result as an integrated analysis to elucidate the differences in osseointegration caused by surface geometry and they found that all these influences from implant surface geometry can be attributed to the alteration of local tissue strains. In their computational model work, local tissue strain was predicted in two different designs of plasma-sprayed and porous-surfaced. The result indicated that porous surface structure provided with a larger secure region underwent low distortional and volumetric strains, whereas the plasma-sprayed implant provided little local strain protection to the healing tissue. Coincident with Pilliar's study, low distortional and volumetric strains are believed to favor osteogenesis.

In a more cellular-based study, Carter and Giori (60) suggested that proliferation and differentiation of the mesenchymal cells responsible for surrounding tissues formation of implants are regulated by the local mechanical environment. Recall Carter's theory of mechanical stimulus on tissue regeneration, the mesenchymal cells turn to be more osteogenic when experiencing low distortional strain and low compressive hydrostatic stress, provided under adequate vascularity.

Porous Materials

To regenerate tissues and organs with high vascularity, porous structure has been considered as a desirable geometry of scaffolds because of high void ratio and surface area. Many biomaterials have been fabricated into porous structures with defined global and local pore sizes as well as interconnected pore network. In 1972, Hulbert et al. (64) investigated the tissue reaction of porous ceramics versus nonporous ones. They found that tissue around discs of porous ceramics healed faster and presented a thinner fibrous encapsulation than the impervious implants. Blood vessel invasion was more rapid in those discs with pore size of 100 to 150 μm, indicating a richer blood supply.

Up to date, synthetic biodegradable polymers such as poly(propylene fumarate) and poly (latic-co-glycolic acid) have been pervasively used in tissue engineering. Peter et al. (65) reported some applications of polymer concepts in tissue engineering. They developed bone flaps with attached vascular pedicle to reconstruct defects and found blocks of vascularized bone were formed six weeks after implantation. Hacking et al. (66) have studied porous tantalum and their histological analysis showed complete tissue ingrowth throughout the porous tantalum implant. Tissue ingrowth and mature vascularity increased over time and the attachment strength was three- to sixfold greater compared with that reported in a similar study with porous beads.

MATERIALS FOR SPINAL CAGES
Metals

Metallic biocompatible materials created the metal age that has dominated the treatment of spine disorders in the most surgical scenarios over the last decades. Among these metals, stainless steel and titanium have been pervasively used in the development of new instrumentations. Anterior interbody cages are often titanium cylinders that are placed in the disc space. The cages made of titanium offer excellent fixation for the superior rigidity of titanium, and so in most cases with single level, additional instrumentation (e.g., pedicle screws) or postoperative back braces for support are not needed. Current popular cylindrical threaded titanium interbody cages used in interbody fusion include BAK® (Zimmer, Warsaw, IN), Harms Titanium-Mesh Cage™ (DePuySpine, Raynham, MA), Ray Threaded Fusion Cage™ (Stryker, Kalamazoo, MI), and Inter Fix™ (Medtronic Sofamor Danek, Memphis, TN).

Although metallic biocompatible materials provide excellent mechanical capacity for bearing high loads, several concerns from clinical follow-up have aroused attentions when using metal cages. One drawback of stainless steel and titanium cages is the potential for artifacts in the vicinity of the cage observed on medical imaging modalities, such as magnetic resonance imaging (MRI) and computed tomographic (CT) scanning. This could be relevant in the case of a neurological complication. Stainless steel implants are known to generate substantial metal artifact with MRI and CT (67,68). Titanium or titanium alloy consisting of titanium, aluminum, and vanadium (Ti-6Al-4V) show comparable amount of artifact on MRI, but appear as excellent images in the CT scan (69,70). Nevertheless, lesser field strength and the use of fast spin-echo techniques can reduce these artifacts (71–73).

The second concern could be the fact that solid fusion cannot be easily and definitely determined from simple radiographic analysis alone. The devices made of metals are not radiolucent and thus bring the difficulty to determine whether solid osseous fusion has occurred (osseous trabeculation, evidence of bone formation in and around the device) on radiographs. Complementary histological examinations of the tissue obtained in the hollow spaces from retrieved cages in the studies of Lange et al. (74) and Carvi et al. (75) confirmed sufficient bone growth in these areas. However, it is not feasible to be utilized as a determination for the outcome postoperatively.

The relatively high incidence of cage subsidence and complications related to considerable excessive stiffness of metallic cage devices also becomes a prominent point of criticism. This seems to be a common complication with the use of any metallic device. Stress-shielding in fusion segments applied with rigid spinal stabilization techniques with transpedicular screws has resulted in disuse osteopenia in fused vertebra in dog models (76–81). This osteopenia will likely lead to screw loosening and instrumentation failures (77). The stress-shielded environment provided by thick walls or cylindrical threads in conventional cage designs allow lower intracage pressure propagation (32), which leads to significant bone mineral density decrease in the long-term (56). Excessive cage rigidity may be associated with increased incidence of postoperative complications, such as stress-shielding, the migration or dislodgement of the cage, pseudarthrodesis, or the combined adverse symptoms (42).

Allograft

It remains common for the anterior approach to utilize allogeneous grafting materials corticocancellous blocks (82,83), corticocancellous dowels (84,85) such as, and femoral ring allografts (86). O'Brien (86) is credited with the concept of devising a hybrid interbody graft using a hybrid interbody graft consisting of a biological fusion cage (femoral cortical allograft ring) packed with autogenous cancellous bone graft. The concept introduced in this hybrid graft is that the femoral allograft ring provides the instant stability of the fusion construct, while the autogenous cancellous bone graft provides for long-term stability achieved by later complete arthrodesis. Femoral cortical dowels (87) are taken from cadaveric femurs and constructed in a dowel formation with a hollow intramedullary region for grafting bone. They are cut along the weight-bearing axis of the bone to provide structural stability. Current cylindrical threaded cortical bone dowels include MD[TM] II, MD[TM] III, MD[TM] IV (Medtronic Sofamor Danek, Memphis, Tennessee, U.S.A.) and Vertigraft® (DePuySpine, Raynham, Massachusetts, U.S.A.).

Because the femoral cortical dowels are not metallic, fusion can be assessed radiographically. They have also been shown to have osteoconductive properties. The intramedullary region can be filled with autogenous cancellous bone or bone morphogenetic protein (BMP) allowing the hybrid to be osteoinductive. These two properties fulfill the proper bone growth within the graft and the bone ongrowth along with a resorptive surface can be incorporated into the adjacent bone to form a bony union. The femoral cortical dowels provide adequate biomechanical stability that it has been shown that they can withstand forces of up to 25,000 N, therefore having the sufficient loading resistance required for an biomechanical stability to be an effective alternative to metallic implants. The disadvantage of a femoral dowel is that as it is an allograft, risks of pathogen propogation and disease transmission still remain concerned, although cases are extremely rare with current screening techniques.

Carbon Fiber-Reinforced Polymer

To overcome the major problems of image distortions in the postoperative assessment and stress-shielding-induced complications seen in metallic cages as described earlier, a family of implants made of a carbon fiber-reinforced polymer (CFRP), currently PEEK-Optima® (Invibio Inc., Greenville, South Carolina) from polyaryletherketones have been developed since the mid-1980s by Dr. John Brantigan (37). The (DePuyJAGUAR[TM] LUMBAR I/F CFRP CAGE® Spine, Raynham, Massachusetts, U.S.A.) is radiolucent, allowing postoperative visualization of the bone graft healing. The more compliant stiffness close to native bone properties decreases the incidence of complications related to high rigidity of devices, and favorable clinical series have been reported with successful outcomes (88,89). Generally, the device alone does not provide good fixation so that posterior pedicle screw supplementation is also necessary.

Biodegradable Polymers

Because of the deficiencies of imaging distortion, implant subsidence or migration, and stress-shielding associated with metallic implants, the use of biodegradable/bioabsorbable implants in spinal surgery has become prevalent. Biodegradable/bioabsorbable implants should possess several critical characteristics as advantages compared with conventional metallic implants. First, the immediate stability should be acquired to the spinal segment in which the device is implanted, and the stiffness should also be retained through degradation. Moreover, the implant should be radiolucent without postoperative image interference as presented in its metallic counterparts. The implant should also have the ability to aid transferring stress in the fusion process by the dynamic mechanism that as the implant degrades, its mechanical properties decline, and the degradation of the scaffold must be matched to the regeneration of tissue. This main advantage of a degradable/resorbable material confers initial and intermediate stability without long-term complications (e.g., stress-shielding or migration) of metallic spinal implants. The gradual degradation of bioabsorbable spinal implants allows progressive transfer of axial loads to bone, which are initially shared by the implant. Finally, the metabolites by implant breakdown should be able to be incorporated into normal cellular processes without inciting a metabolic derangement that possesses mutagenic or immunogenic properties of their host cells (90). However, reported complications associated with bioabsorbable implant use include synovitis, osteolysis, hypertrophic fibrous encapsulation, and sterile sinus tract formation (91–94). These brought concerns of the tendency of the bioabsorbable implant to incite aseptic inflammatory reactions during the resorption process.

The class of bioabsorbable material that has been most studied is the alpha-poly hydroxyl esters. Among them, two important compounds are poly(glycolic acid) (PGA) and poly(lactic acid) (PLA), which are based on the lactic acid monomer. Both materials have been shown to completely resorb within bone (95–97). However, different degradation products and inflammatory tissue reactions were found between these two polymers. Poly(glycolic acid) has been shown to propend to induce more inflammatory tissue reaction than PLA (98,99). In addition, degradation patterns and half-lives are also different for stereoisomers belonging to the same compound (97,100,101).

In clinical application, resorbable polymers used for surgical implants was first introduced by Kulkarni et al. (102), followed by various applications including sutures, repair of craniofacial defects, appendicular fracture fixation, and soft-tissue repair (93,95,96,101,103–107). The use of these materials in spinal surgery has only been advocated recently. Many current efforts have concentrated on using poly(α-hydroxy) acids with much lower stiffness than metallic materials to fabricate interbody fusion cages from designs previously used for titanium cages (42,108,109).

The use of bioabsorbable materials in spinal surgery is promising owing to the absence of many deficiencies associated with conventional metallic spinal implants, including image degradation and the incidence of stress-shielding and pseudarthrosis. The gradual degradation of bioabsorbable materials allows dynamization through resorption and may lead to higher fusion rates, further improving clinical outcomes in specific spinal applications. Clinical studies are underway to evaluate the viability of applying biodegradable/bioabsorbable materials in several fields of spinal surgery.

NEW DESIGN STRATEGY: TOPOLOGY OPTIMIZATION
Introduction of Topology Optimization and Homogenization

From this, the multiple roles played by fusion cages suggest that cage design can be optimized to concurrently enhance stability, biofactor delivery, and mechanical tissue stimulation to better integrate design variables reviewed for improved arthrodesis.

Modern structural optimization can be traced back to the development from the aerospace industries in the 1940s. In order to design with minimum weight and maximum stiffness for the aircraft structural components, the researchers developed plenty optimization solutions for columns, panels, and truss-like structure, based on analytical procedure to a specified type of geometry. Each analytical method was utilized toward a specific type of structural components, such as beams, plates, and columns. Until the 1960s when modern computers and finite element method (FEM) were developed, the structural analysis with mathematical programming embedded became possible. The structural optimization, however, was still limited to optimize the size and shape of the structure during the period. A more generalized and nonparametric optimization method which can simultaneously select the best geometric layout and topological configuration was not available until late 1980s. Such an optimization method is named "topology optimization" (or layout optimization), and it is reasonable to expect that structure resulting from topology optimization saves significant amount of materials to avoid redundancy over those designed by the size and the shape optimizations.

Topology Optimization

Structural topology optimization, which is a generous design method to find the optimal structural layouts in a nonparametric fashion, is truly a milestone for mechanic structural design. It involves the simultaneous optimization of the topology and the shape of internal boundaries in porous and composite continua. The topology optimization is based on the image-based representation and consists of a macroscopic variation of solid material and void in a fixed reference design domain. It is also called material distribution approach or black-and-white design as the density of structure is given by either 0 or 1 to present void or solid.

Ever since the epochal contribution by Bendsøe and Kikuchi (110) in 1988, the topology optimization method has progressed with a significant breakthrough from theory into practice. A FEM-based numerical topology optimization scheme was implemented to solve structural design problem with a homogenization-based method. Based on this implementation, many practical engineering problems have been successfully addressed over the last decade. Neves et al. (111) presented two computational models to design the periodic microstructure of cellular materials with optimal elastic properties. Kikuchi et al. (112) implemented this method to design the optimum layout of compliant mechanisms, and microstructure of composite materials. Topology optimization method is now leading to a fairly widespread acceptable methodology in industries.

Homogenization Theory

Homogenization theory allows the calculation of effective properties of periodic composite materials without enforcing limitation on the geometry of the given composite structure. The mathematical formulation assumes that the composite is composed of the periodic microstructures, and the microscopic scale is much smaller compared with the global dimension, named macroscopic. From the macroscopic point of view, the composite looks like a "homogeneous" material. The homogenization theory is the key technique within the topology optimization (110).

The homogenization theory was established by a school of French mathematicians in the 1970s (113). They cooporated the homogenization method with the G-convergence theory and solved many mechanics problems, such as linear elasticity, heat, and wave equations. In a monograph by Scachez-Palencia (114), the fluid flow in porous media, elasticity, electromagnetism, and vibration of solid mechanics were addressed. Later, a numerical homogenization method for elasticity was implemented by Guedes and Kikuchi (115) using an adaptive FEM. The homogenization-based topology optimization was considered to be a building block in structural optimization field, and was wildly implemented in different disciplines and applications.

New Biodegradable Cage Design Using Topology Optimization

Recent postoperative reports of complications requiring revision procedures aroused several major concerns with cage designs and cage materials (116); one in particular is the stress-shielding owing to the considerable excessive stiffness of metallic cage devices compared with the motion segments and vertebral bodies. Stress-shielding in fusion segments applied with rigid spinal stabilization techniques with transpedicular screws has resulted in disuse osteopenia in fused vertebra in dog models (76–81). This osteopenia will likely lead to screw loosening and instrumentation failures (77).

The stress-shielded environment provided by thick walls or cylindrical threads in conventional cage designs allow lower intracage pressure propagation (32), which leads to significant bone mineral density decrease in the long-term (56). Excessive cage rigidity may be associated with increased incidence of postoperative complications, such as stress-shielding, the migration or dislodgement of the cage, pseudarthrodesis, or the combined adverse symptoms (42). Many current efforts to reduce these complications have concentrated on using poly(α-hydroxy) acids with much lower stiffness than metallic materials to fabricate interbody fusion cages from designs previously used for titanium cages (42,108,109). The results from their large quadrupedal animal models showed significant improvement in the arthrodesis rate and the quality of trabecular bone in the new constructs (42,46,47,109). However, simply replacing the base material from the original design with biodegradable polymers may not be appropriate, especially for the development of load-bearing devices in spine arthrodesis, as degradable materials typically have less stiffness and strength than nondegradable materials. Furthermore, this stiffness and strength will degrade over time, further reducing the mechanical competency of the device.

Poly(α-hydroxy) acids such as polylactides and polygliycolides have been in great interest for extensive applications of orthopedic implants. Degradation induced by hydrolysis at this type of polymer is slower than diffusion and thus the bulk polymer matrix will be affected by erosion known as bulk erosion or homogeneous erosion. The progress of bulk erosion is complex and stochastic. However, the phenomenon indicates that a more generalized approach should be incorporated in the reinforcement of bulk erosion polymers to retain the mechanical demands through the degradation. According to Göpferich's model for bulk erosion (117), the lifetime of a polymer element (pixel in the model) is based on the assumption that the degradation of individual pixels is a Poisson process and can then be described by a first-order Erlang probability density function, $e(t) = \lambda e^{-\lambda t}$ where $e(t)$ is the probability that a pixel degrades at time t, λ is a degradation rate constant, and t is the random variable that designates the lifetime, namely the time between the start of experiment and the degradation of pixel. The degradation process is therefore considered as a randomized distribution and reinforcing specific features in an existing design against degradation becomes unpredictable. Nonetheless, the general concept of bulk degradation is that the polymer matrix will lose molecular weight and stiffness in a predictable average sense over time.

We proposed a new material density-weighting approach coupled with a developed integrated topology optimization technique (118) to create scaffold designs for bulk degrading materials that retain stiffness for longer time periods in our previous work (119). This approach creates scaffold designs de novo for specific anatomic regions and mechanical loading regimens. In the present Chapter, we demonstrate our previous work to apply this design approach to develop biodegradable spinal interbody fusion cages fabricated with an osteoconductive composite material of poly(propylene fumarate)/β-tricalcium phosphate (PPF/β-TCP) with low molecular weight (1200 Da). The results demonstrated that the new approach can create designs that retain superior integrity and greater stiffness for longer periods of time.

Design Concept Overview for Degradation Topology Optimization

We previously developed a topology optimization approach for designing biomaterial scaffold architecture that incorporates the degradation profile into the optimal design (119). Topology optimization (112,118,120–123) is a design technique that provides optimal distribution of material under applied force to satisfy the objective of maximal stiffness with desired porosity, under constraints of the design criteria. The macroscopic or first-scale topology optimization solution that provides the general density and location of material within the design domain is then discretized into finite elements, and each element will contain a predicted material density between 0 and 1. Zero indicates void space and 1 indicates complete material; values in between indicate partial material with the corresponding volume fraction. The effective modulus is thereby interpreted by the density method as: $E_{ijkl} = X_p E^0_{ijkl}$ to indicate the solid, porous, and void regions, where E_{ijkl} represents the effective modulus of each finite element, X_p is the fraction of the material, and the base material property is E^0_{ijkl}.

In the degradation design, the density in each element is weighted by the degradation profile. The proposed optimization method creates a density distribution map for selected time points during degradation. These different density distributions are then superposed using a time lasting and degrading modulus factor. The time lasting factor is defined as: $T_{wt} = (T_{total} - T_{current})/T_{total}$, where T_{total} is the total degradation duration and $T_{current}$ is the time at a selected point. This factor accounts for the influence of the time past implantation on reinforcement of the scaffold architecture. The degrading modulus factor is defined as: $E_{wt} = E^0_{ijkl}(T_{current})/E^0_{ijkl}(T_{initial})$. This factor indicates the weight percentage of the original material equivalent to the superposed material densities based on the degrading modulus at selected time points. The optimal global/macroscopic density distribution for degradation design is then interpreted as: $X_{pw} = \Sigma \, X_{pt} T_{wt} E_{wt}$, where X_{pw} is the final fraction of the base material and X_{pt} is the temporary fraction of the reduced/degraded modulus corresponding to a selected time point.

The resolution of the global degradation topology design is too coarse, however, to give the specific microstructure that will be located within that point of the scaffold. Furthermore, as we would like the microstructure to have specific elastic properties at a fixed porosity, homogenization-based topology optimization is used to design the microstructure (123,124). The microscopic or second-scale topology optimization approach gives the specific microstructure design that achieves a desired compliance while matching the predicted volume fraction of the macroscopic or first-level topology optimization. Note that this technique may be applied either to degradation design or only for designing the initial stiffness.

Spine Interbody Fusion Cage Design Using Degradation Topology Optimization

Conventional designs of spinal interbody fusion cage have mainly focused on providing immediate strength to maintain disc height. The geometrical features of these conventional designs show little distinction from each other and most of them fall into a category of a pipe shape with thick shells (32). However, this concept of providing immediate strength may not hold once degradable polymers replace metallic materials in the same design. The original designed architectures will only perform as they are proposed when these devices are made with permanent materials such as metallic alloys. The example of a biodegradable spine interbody fusion cage design using poly(propylene fumarate)/beta tricalcium phosphate demonstrates how the technique of the degradation topology optimization can create designs that meet critical requirements and objectives concurrently through the degradation. A global topology optimization algorithm (HyperMesh®; Altair Engineering, Troy, Michigan, U.S.A.) was used to predict a global layout density under the constraint that strain at the vertebral surface was less than 8%. Two rectangular block design domains were used to represent the location of the implanted cages and the multidirectional loads of the physiological range including compression, lateral bending, torsion, and flexion–extension were applied to these domains implanted between vertebrae. A FEM was then created to simulate the mechanical environment of the design domain within the disc space (Fig. 1). By using this approach, we developed the new cage design denoted as the optimal structure for degradation (OSDeg). In this Chapter, we also created a topology-optimized design targeted at the time 0 stiffness that did not account for degradation denoted as the optimal structure (OS) cage (119). We then compared the resulting stiffness versus time behavior for all three designs of optimal structure with degradation reinforcement (OSDeg), optimal structure without degradation reinforcement (OS), and conventional cylindrical threaded cage (CON), using both simulation and in vitro degradation experiments. The final density layouts of each selected time point are shown in Figure 2. For the PPF/β-TCP interbody fusion cage design in the present study, we selected time points at 0, 0.5, 0.65, and 0.85 T with corresponding base material moduli of 1000, 875, 780, and 250 MPa, respectively. More time points were selected in the latter half stage of degradation owing to the fact that significantly more mass is lost in the second half of the degradation period compared with the first half (117,125). Segmented density distributions that defined the total solid region, the low porous region (porosity = 35%), and the high porous region (porosity = 55%) are shown from the top to the bottom layers in Figure 3. Note that the specific regions that provide the major mechanical resistance against the external loads exhibited higher density levels in the degradation topology optimization approach compared with the standard, nondegrading topology optimization approach. The corresponding microstructures for porosities of 35% and 55% (Fig. 4) were further assigned to the density layouts and the final designs were completed.

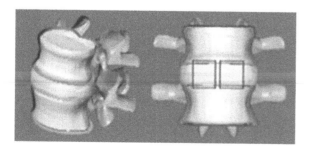

FIGURE 1 Two rectangular block design domains in the intervertebral disc space representing the location of the implanted cages are directly utilized to reflect a more realistic biomechanical environment under the multidirectional loads of the physiological range. A finite element model of the design domain is then created to further implement the integrated topology optimization of the design domain within the disc space.

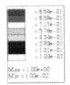

FIGURE 2 The corresponding density layouts of each selected time point through the degradation interpret the material density distribution derived from the topology optimization at the cage design domain in the disc space. Note that the *light gray* represents highest density level indicating total solid, while *dark gray* represents the lowest density level indicating void space. *Left to right:* the global density layout of poly(propylene fumarate)/β-tricalcium phosphate at the cage design domain at 0, 0.5, 0.65, and 0.85 *T* (*T* = total degradation period), with corresponding base material moduli of 1000, 875, 780, and 250 MPa, respectively.

DESIGNED DEGRADABLE SCAFFOLD (SCALED-DOWN CAGE) WITH CELL-BASED GENE THERAPY

Gene therapy is the process that one or more specific genes (also known as transgenes) are inserted into target somatic cells to synthesize specific proteins encoded by transgenes (126). According to the vectors that accomplish the insertion and enhance the access and the expression of a given DNA sequence in a host cell, two modalities of transferring genetic materials are distinguished (127). Transfection is the process of DNA uptake accomplished by a cell from the environment, while transduction refers to the insertion of genetic material into a host cell via a viral vector. Cell-based therapy includes various strategies based on the properties of mesenchymal stem cells to respond to appropriate environmental milieu to differentiate toward the osteogenic lineage. It has been widely known that postnatal bone marrow is one of the tissues harboring multipotent stem cells as the osteoprogenitor cells of skeletal tissues (128).

Effective tissue engineering of a load-bearing tissue such as bone requires a scaffold with appropriate mechanical properties that endure until the regenerated bone can carry load. In an ideal system, cells would differentiate into the desired tissue within a porous

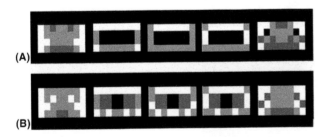

(A)

(B)

FIGURE 3 Segmented density distributions that define the total solid region, the low porous region (porosity = 35%), and the high porous region (porosity = 55%) from the top to the bottom layers of cage design domain in Fig. 2. *White regions* stand for the total solid region, *light gray* ones are for the low porous region, *dark gray* ones are for the high porous region, and *black ones* indicate the total void region. **(A)** Layers for optimal structure design from integrated topology optimization, which are segmented from the density layout at 0 *T* with initial poly(propylene fumarate)/β-tricalcium phosphate base modulus. **(B)** Layers for optimal structure degradation design from degradation topology optimization where the global density is created by weighting all the densities from each degradation time point with two weighting factors. The specific regions that provide the major mechanical resistance are upgraded to the higher density levels of the segmentation in the layout topology after they are applied with the density weighting approach.

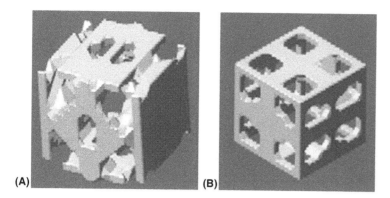

FIGURE 4 (**A**) The microstructure design for porosity of 35%. (**B**) The microstructure design for porosity of 55%.

scaffold and, as growth continued, the degrading scaffold would bear less of the mechanical load as the nascent bone bore an increasing amount. The authors have demonstrated a system that has the potential to achieve these goals (129). Scaffolds were computationally designed to be optimal for bearing load and allowing tissue ingrowth by the degradation topology optimization technique as aforementioned, and then manufactured from a degradable polymer, PPF, reinforced with a ceramic, β-TCP (Fig. 5). When these scaffolds were seeded with fibroblasts transduced to express BMP-7 and implanted subcutaneously, organized bone with marrow was formed in and around the scaffold (Fig. 6). Over increasing implantation times, both the amount of bone and its compressive modulus increased as the scaffold degraded. The apposition of new bone increased progressively along the designed contours

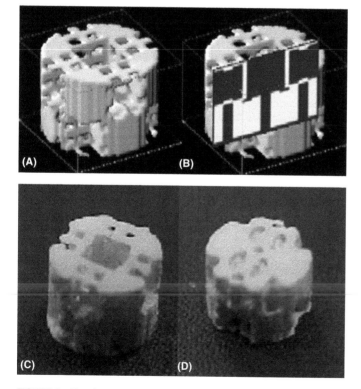

FIGURE 5 Topology optimization was used to design the scaffold (**A**) and its internal architecture (**B**). This design was faithfully produced in the fabricated poly(propylene fumarate)/β-tricalcium phosphate (**C**) and (**D**).

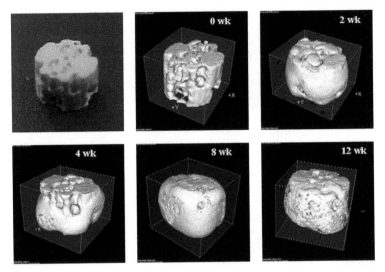

FIGURE 6 The μCT data was used to create three-dimensional surface renderings. A photograph of the scaffold (*top left*) and a scan of a scaffold that was not implanted (zero week) are provided for comparison. The renderings show an increase in bone volume at two weeks, followed by a slight decrease at four weeks. Full coverage of the scaffold by bone was observed at eight weeks. Somewhat less bone appeared covering the scaffold after 12 weeks than after eight weeks.

as implantation time lengthened. Interestingly, the bone localized on the scaffold contours became thicker and appeared brighter in the CT images. The data from the μCT scans were used to calculate bone volume and showed little change in bone volume (Table 1). Changes in bone formation after long implantation times were reflected largely in the geometry of the bone and the overall amount of the bone. Key in achieving these results was combination of the advantages of topology optimization, free form fabrication of a ceramic-reinforced degradable polymer, and ex vivo gene therapy.

Topology optimization allows great flexibility in altering hierarchical pores for different purposes, such as creating wide open channels in the macrostructure to allow initial mass exchange and small pores in microstructural architecture to maintain required porosity for blood vessel invasion, but still retain mechanical integrity. Reconstructions from our μCT data, validate that the design does perform as expected, in that we observed, a "bone formation front" that moved with increasing implantation times (Fig. 7). The "front" moved from the top of the center well until it coalesced with the infiltration of bone tissue from small pores to complete the full bone ingrowth. It is possible that concentric-like patterns were to allow the invasion of blood vessels (Fig. 6). It is also possible, however, that these channels were created by bone resorption triggered by lack of mechanical stimulation in the subcutaneous site. Whether these patterns will be affected by the design or they will be rather dominated by the loading milieu is not yet known.

The second key component of the approach used in the study was the use of the composite PPF/β-TCP material. This highly osteoconductive material led to bone formation along the

TABLE 1 Bone Volume in New Constructs at Predetermined Time Points

	Time (weeks)/volume (mm^3)				
	0	**2**	**4**	**8**	**12**
Bone-scaffold construct	45.80 ± 1.51[a]	55.28 ± 5.23	53.88 ± 2.91	55.33 ± 4.12	52.66 ± 3.40
Effective bone[b]		11.21 ± 5.23	8.08 ± 2.91	9.53 ± 4.12	6.86 ± 3.40

[a]The average volume of empty scaffolds.
[b]For each specimen, effective bone volume is defined as (the volume bone-scaffold construct) − (the average volume of empty scaffolds).

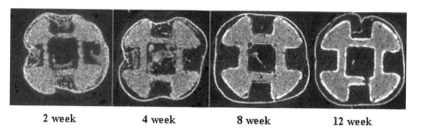

2 week   4 week   8 week   12 week

FIGURE 7   Cross-sections of the μCT data reveal increased bone apposition after 2-, 4-, 8-, and 12-weeks implantation. As implantation time increased, bone was more highly localized closely following the scaffold contours.

designed contours (Figs. 6 and 7). Manipulating tissue-material affinity though the addition of particles, such as the ceramic used here, helped direct bone ingrowth into pores as small as 400 μm in diameter. The combination of topology-optimized designs with osteoconductive biodegradable polymer composite can fulfill the goal of load bearing at the initial stage as a suitable tissue-engineering strategy.

Finally, the use of ex vivo gene therapy enabled the production of large amounts of biologically and mechanically functional tissue without the use of specific progenitor cells. Further, the use of transduced fibroblasts allowed osteogenesis to commence quickly and fill the designed void space with organized bone tissue and marrow. Therapeutically, autologous fibroblasts represent an easily biopsied source of immunocompatible cells that can be manipulated in vitro to express the desired transgene. When combined with a optimally designed scaffold of appropriate material composition, the transduced primary cells can combine with host cells to generate large amounts of functional tissue (130).

This combined approach has brought us a step closer in realizing the theoretical goal for using scaffolds in tissue engineering: a degradable biomaterial that allows functional tissue regeneration while retaining the overall mechanical properties as the scaffold degrades with reduced support resistance. This theoretical profile postulates that scaffold providing initial function in the tissue defect, followed by scaffold material and functional degradation that is compensated by bone regeneration that compensates for the degrading scaffold stiffness to maintain plateau stiffness within the range of normal tissue (131). The designed topology-optimized PPF/β-TCP scaffolds degraded with the stiffness dropping close to 60 MPa, but the declining stiffness was thereafter reinforced by the growing bone tissue and the stiffness of the construct remained at a plateau level between 60 and 70 MPa that is within the range of human trabecular bone (132), until the bone resorption occurred at 12 weeks owing to the lack of sufficient mechanical stimulation in the subcutaneous site.

CONCLUSION

By integrating advantages of topology-optimized design, biodegradable osteoconductive composite, and ex vivo gene therapy, we can achieve rapid osteogenesis and retain the stiffness of constructs to perform mechanical functions through the degradation time, even for ectopic implantations. These results show that this approach has potential for application in orthotopic sites with load-bearing demands, such as segmental fracture healing and spine arthrodesis.

In brief, techniques from modern molecular biology and bioengineering span tremendous applications to produce unique materials that have potent osteogenic activities, encompassing recombinant human osteogenic growth factors, such as BMP, transforming growth factor-β, and platelet-derived growth factors. Biological and nonbiological scaffolding materials also construct osteoconductive matrices to stimulate bone deposition directly. The delivery of pluripotent mesenchymal stem cells to induce osteogenesis also reaches the remarkable achievement to generate bone. These therapeutic approaches successfully bring the advent of the biotechnology era for the use in clinical setting.

Advances in computational structure engineering, biomaterial science, and bone biology bring novel opportunities to move the treatments for spine disorders beyond simple bone tissue fixation into the realm of spinal tissue engineering. The interdisciplinary principles form the foundation of spinal tissue engineering, and by the sophisticated integration of these bases, spinal fusion approaches can be foreseen to progress to a new era to give spine clinicians greater flexibilities to restore spine functions.

REFERENCES

1. Liberman JR, Daluiski A, Einhorn TA. The role of growth factors in the repair of bone. Biology and clinical application. J Bone Joint Surg Am 2002; 84-A:1032–1044.
2. Sanhu HS. Anterior lumbar interbody fusion with osteoinductive growth factors. Clin Orthop 2000; 371:56–60.
3. Cunningham BW, Kanayama M, Parker L, et al. Osteogenic protein (rhOP-1) versus autologous fusion in the sheep thoracic spine. A comparative endoscopic study using the BAK interbody fusion device. Spine 1999; 24:509–518.
4. Knop C, Fabian HF, Bastian L, et al. Late results of thoracolumbar fractures after posterior instrumentation and transpedicular bone grafting. Spine 2001; 26:88–99.
5. Wood GW, Boyd RJ, Carothers TA. The effect of pedicle screw/plate fixation of lumbar/lumbosacral autogenous bone graft fusions in patients with degenerative disc disease. Spine 1995; 20:819–830.
6. Crawford RJ, Askin GN. Fixation of thoracolumbar fractures with the Dick fixator: the influence of transpedicular bone grafting. Eur Spine J 1994; 3:45–51.
7. Katz JN. Lumbar spinal fusion. Surgical rates, costs, and complications. Spine 1995; 24S:78S–83S.
8. Kim CW, Abrams R, Lee G, et al. Use of vascularized fibular grafts as a salvage procedure for previously failed spinal arthrodesis. Spine 2001; 26:2171–2175.
9. Steinmann JC, Herkowitz N. Pseudoarthrodesis of the spine. Clin Orthop 1992; 284:80–90.
10. Arrington ED, Smit WJ, Chambers HG, et al. Complications of iliac crest bone graft harvesting. Clin Orthop 1996; 329:300–309.
11. Banwart JC, Asher MA, Hassanein RS. Iliac crest bone graft harvest donor site morbidity. Spine 1995; 20:1055–1060.
12. Kurz LT, Garfin SR, Booth RE. Harvesting autogenous iliac bone grafts: a review of complications and techniques. Spine 1989; 14:1324–1331.
13. Massey EW. Meralgia paresthetica secondary to trauma of bone graft. J Trauma 1980; 20:342–343.
14. Robertson PA, Wray AJ. Natural history of posterior iliac crest bone graft donation for spinal surgery. A prospective analysis of morbidity. Spine 2001; 26:1473–1476.
15. Summers BN, Eissenstein SM. Donor site pain from the ilium. A complication of lumbar spine fusion. J Bone Joint Surg Am 1989; 71-A:677–680.
16. Weikel AM, Habal MB. Meralgia paresthetica: a complication of iliac bone procurement. Plast Reconstr Surg 1977; 60:572–574.
17. Younger EM, Chapman MW. Morbidity at bone graft donor site. J Orthop Trauma 1989; 3:192–195.
18. Cloward RB. The treatment of ruptured lumbar intervertebral discs by vertebral body fusion. J Neurosurg 1953; 10:154.
19. Cloward RB. Spondylolisthesis: treatment by laminectomy and posterior lumbar interbody fusion. Clin Orthop 1981; 154:74–82.
20. Cloward RB. Posterior lumbar interbody fusion updated. Clin Orthop 1985; 193:16–19.
21. Herkowitz HN, Kurz LT. Degenerative lumbar spondylolisthesis with spinal stenosis: a prospective study comparing decompression with decompression and intertransverse process arthrodesis. J Bone Joint Surg Am 1991; 73A:802–808.
22. Mardjetko SM, Connoly PJ, Shott S. Degenerative lumbar spondylolisthesis: a meta-analysis of literature 1970–1993. Spine 1993; 19(suppl 20):S2256–S2265.
23. Stauffer AD, Coventry MB. Posteolateral lumbar spine fusion. J Bone Joint Surg Am 1972; 54A:1195–1204.
24. Blumenthal SL, Baker J, Dossett A, et al. The role of anterior lumbar fusion for internal disc disruption. Spine 1988; 13:566–569.
25. Chow SP, Leong J, Ma A, et al. Anterior spinal fusion for deranged lumbar intervertebral disc. Spine 1980; 5:452–458.
26. Leong JCY, Chun SY, Grange WJ, et al. Long-term results of lumbar intervertebral disc prolapse. Spine 1983; 8:793–799.
27. Loguidice VA, Johnson RG, Guyer RD, et al. Anterior lumbar interbody fusion. Spine 1988; 13:366–369.
28. Blume HG. Unilateral posterior lumbar interbody fusion: simplified dowel technique. Clin Orthop 1985; 193:75–84.
29. Crock HV. Observations on the management of failed spinal operations. J Bone Joint Surg Am 1976; 58-B:193–199.
30. Hutter CG. Posterior intervertebral body fusion. A 25-year study. Clin Orthop 1983; 179:86–96.

31. Uzi EA, Dabby D, Tolessa E, et al. Early retropulsion of titanium-threaded cages after posterior lumbar interbody fusion. Spine 2001; 26:1073–1075.
32. Kanayama M, Cunningham BW, Haggerty CJ, et al. In vitro biomechanical investigation of the stability and stress-shielding effect of lumbar interbody fusion devices. J Neurosurg 2000; 93:259–265.
33. McAfee PC. Current concepts review: interbody fusion cages in reconstructive operations on the spine. J Bone Joint Surg Am 1999; 81-A:859–880.
34. Alpert S. Summary of safety and effectiveness-BAK interbody fusion system. Presented at Report in PMA Document Mail Center, Washington, DC, September 20, 1996.
35. Kuslich SD, Ulstrom CL, Griffith SL, et al. The Bagby and Kuslich method of lumbar interbody fusion. History, techniques, and 2-year follow-up results of a United States prospective, multicenter trial. Spine 1998; 23:1267–1279.
36. Yuan HA, Kuslich SD, Dowdle JA Jr, et al. Prospective multicenter clinical trial of the BAK interbody fusion system. Presented at the Annual Meeting of the North American Spine Society, New York, October 22, 1997.
37. Brantigan JW, Steffee AD, Lewis ML, et al. Lumbar interbody fusion using the Brantigan I/F cage for PLIF and the VSP pedicle screw system: two year results of a Food and Drug Administration IDE clinical trial. Intersomatique du Rachis Lumbaire 1996.
38. Harms J. Screw-threaded rod system in spinal fusion surgery. Spine 1992; 6:541–575.
39. Harms J, Jeszenszky D, Stoltze D, et al. True spondylolisthesis reduction and monosegmental fusion in spondylolisthesis. Textbook Spinal Surg 1997; 2:1337–1347.
40. Greennough CG, Taylor LJ, Fraser RD. Anterior lumbar fusion: results, assessment techniques, and prognostic factors. Eur Spine J 1994; 3:225–230.
41. McAfee PC, Cunningham BW, Lee GA, et al. Revision strategies for salvaging or improving failed cylindrical cages. Spine 1999; 24:2147–2153.
42. van Dijk M, Smit TH, Sugihara S, et al. The effect of cage stiffness on the rate of lumbar interbody fusion: an in vivo model using poly(L-lactic acid) and titanium cages. Spine 2002; 27:682–688.
43. Brantigan JW, Steffee AD. A carbon fiber implant to aid interbody lumbar fusion. Two-year clinical results in the first 26 patients. Spine 1993; 18:2106–2107.
44. McAfee PC, Regan JJ, Geis WP, et al. Minimally invasive anterior retroperitoneal approach to the lumbar spine. Emphasis on the lateral BAK. Spine 1998; 23:1476–1484.
45. Ray CD. Threaded titanium cages for lumbar interbody fusions. Spine 1997; 22:667–679; discussion, 79–80.
46. van Dijk M, Smit TH, Burger EH, et al. Bioabsorbable poly-L-lactic acid cages for lumbar interbody fusion: three-year follow-up radiographic, histologic, and histomorphometric analysis in goats. Spine 2002; 27:2706–2714.
47. van Dijk M, Tunc DC, Smit TH, et al. In vitro and in vivo degradation of bioabsorbable PLLA spinal fusion cages. J Biomed Mater Res 2002; 63:752–759.
48. Cullinane DM, Fredrick A, Eisenberg SR, et al. Induction of a neoarthrosis by precisely controlled motion in an experimental mid-femoral defect. J Orthop Res 2001; 20:579–586.
49. Pilliar RM, Cameron HU, Welsh RP, et al. Radiographic and morphologic studies of load-bearing porous-surfaced structured implants. Clin Orthop 1981; 156:249–257.
50. Simmons CA, Meguid SA, Pilliar RM. Mechanical regulation of localized and appositional bone formation around bone-interfacing implants. J Biomed Mater Res 2001; 55:63–71.
51. Simmons CA, Meguid SA, Pilliar RM. Differences in osseointegration rate due to implant surface geometry can be explained by local tissue strains. J Orthop Res 2001; 19:187–194.
52. Wolff J. Das gaesetz der transformation der knochen. Berlin, German: A. Hirchwild, 1982.
53. Carter DR, Blenman PR, Beaupre GS. Correlations between mechanical stress history and tissue differentiation in initial fracture healing. J Orthop Res 1988; 6:734–748.
54. Carter DR. Mechanical loading history and skeletal biology. J Biomech 1987; 20:1095–1109.
55. Guldberg RE, Caldwell NJ, Guo XE, et al. Mechanical stimulation of tissue repair in the hydraulic bone chamber. J Bone Miner Res 1997; 12:1295–1302.
56. Cunningham BW, Haggerty CJ, McAfee PC. A quantitative densitometric study investigating the stress-shiedling effects of interbody spinal fusion devices: emphasis on long-term fusions in thoroughbred racehorses. Presented at the Annual Meeting of the Orthopaedic Research Society, New Orleans, Louisiana, March 9, 1998.
57. Huiskes R, Weinan H, Grootenboer HJ, et al. Adaptive bone-remodeling theory applied to prosthetic-design analysis. J Biomech 1987; 20:1135–1150.
58. Smith L. Ceramic plastic material as a bone substitute. Arch Surg 1963; 87:653.
59. Buser D, Schenk RK, Steinemann S, et al. Influence of surface characteristics on bone integration of titanium implants. A histomorphometric study in miniature pigs. J Biomed Mater Res 1991; 25:889–902.
60. Carter DR, Giori NJ. Effect of mechanical stress on tissue differentiation in the bony implant bed. In: Davies JE, ed. The Bone-Biomaterial Interface. Toronto, Canada: U. Toronto Press, 1989.
61. Maniatopoulos C, Pilliar RM, Smith DC. Threaded versus porous-surfaced designs for implant stabilization in bone-endodontic implant model. J Biomed Mater Res 1986; 20:1309–1333.

62. Bobyn J, Pilliar R, Cameron H, et al. The effect of porous surface configuration on the tensile strength of fixation of implants by bone ingrowth. Clin Orthop 1980; 149:291–298.

63. Bobyn JD, Pilliar RM, Cameron HU, et al. The optimum pore size for the fixation of porous-surfaced metal implants by the ingrowth of bone. Clin Orthop 1980; 150:263–270.

64. Hulbert SF, Morrison SJ, Klawitter JJ. Tissue reaction to three ceramics of porous and non-porous structures. J Biomed Mater Res 1972; 6:347–374.

65. Peter SJ, Miller MJ, Yasko AW, et al. Polymer concepts in tissue engineering. J Biomed Mater Res 1998; 43:442–447.

66. Hacking SA, Bobyn JD, Toh KK, et al. Fibrous tissue ingrowth and attachment to porous tantalum. J Biomed Mater Res 2000; 52:631–638.

67. Laakman RW, Kaufman B, Han JS. MRI imaging in patients with metallic implants. Radiology 1985; 157:711–714.

68. Mechlin M, Thickman D, Kressel HY, et al. Magnetic resonance imaging of postoperative-patients with metallic implants. Am J Roentgenol 1984; 143;1218–1284.

69. Levi AD, Choi WG, Keller PJ, et al. The radiographic and imaging characteristics of porous tantalum implants within the human cervical spine. Spine 1998; 23:1245–1250, discussion 51.

70. Wang JC, Yu WD, Sandhu HS, et al. A comparison of magnetic resonance and computed tomographic image quality after the implantation of tantalum and titanium spinal instrumentation. Spine 1998; 23:1684–1688.

71. Farahani K, Sinha U, Sinha S. Effect of field strength onsusceptibility artifacts in magnetic resonance imaging. Comput Med Imag Graph 1990; 14:409–413.

72. Ortiz O, Pait TG, McAllister P. Postoperative magneticresonance imaging with titanium implants of the thoracic and lumbar spine. Neurosurgery 1996; 38:741–745.

73. Tartaglino LM, Flanders AE, Vinitski S. Metallic artifactson MR images of the postoperative spine: reduction with fastspin-echo techniques. Radiology 1994; 190:565–569.

74. Lange M, Philipp A, Fink U. Anterior cervical spine fusion using RABEA-Titan-Cages avoiding iliac crest spongiosa: first experiences and results. Neurol Neurochir Pol 2000; 34(suppl 6):64–69.

75. Carvi y Nievas MN, Pollath A, Haas E. Cervical discectomy: bone graft or cage fusion? In: Brock M, Schwarz W, Wille C, eds. First Interdisciplinary World Congress on Spinal Surgery and Related Disciplines. Bologna: Monduzzi Editore, 2000:123–128.

76. Craven TG, Carson WL, Asher MA, et al. The effects of implant stiffness on the bypassed bone mineral density and facet fusion stiffness of the canine spine. Spine 1994; 19:1664–1673.

77. Dalenberg DD, Asher MA, Robinson RG, et al. The effect of a stiff spinal implant and its loosening on bone mineral content in canines. Spine 1993; 18:1862–1866.

78. Farey ID, McAfee PC, Gurr KR, et al. Quantitative histologic study of the influence of spinal instrumentation on lumbar fusions: a canine model. J Orthop Res 1989; 7:709–722.

79. Kandziora F, Kerschbaumer F, Starker M, et al. Biomechanical assessment of transoral plate fixation for atlantoaxial instability. Spine 2000; 25:1555–1561.

80. McAfee PC, Farey ID, Sutterlin CE, et al. The effect of spinal implant rigidity on vertebral bone density. A canine model. Spine 1991; 16:S190–S197.

81. Shirado O, Zdeblick TA, McAfee PC, et al. Quantitative histologic study of the influence of anterior spinal instrumentation and biodegradable polymer on lumbar interbody fusion after corpectomy. A canine model. Spine 1992; 17:795–803.

82. Hodgson AR, Stock FE. Anterior spinal fusion. Br J Surg 1956; 44:226–275.

83. Hodgson AR, Stock FE. Anterior spine fusion for the treatment of tuberculosis of the spine. J Bone Joint Surg Am 1960; 42:295–310.

84. Harmon PH. Anterior excision and vertebral body fusion operation for intervertebral disc syndromes of the lower lumbar spine. Clin Orthop 1963; 26:107–127.

85. Sacks S. Anterior interbody fusion of the lumbar spine. J Bone Joint Surg Am 1965; 47B:211–223.

86. O'Brien JP, Dawson MH, Heard CW. Simultaneous combined anterior and posterior fusion. Clin Orthop 1986; 203:191–195.

87. Lowery G, Kulkarni S, Pennisi AE. Use of autologous growth factors in lumbar spinal fusion. Bone 1999; 25:S47–S50.

88. Hashimoto T, Shigenobu K, Kanayama M, et al. Clinical results of single-level posterior lumbar interbody fusion using the Brantigan I/F carbon cage filled with a mixture of local morselized bone and bioactive ceramic granules. Spine 2002; 27:258–262.

89. Molinari RW, Gerlinger T. Functional outcomes of instrumented posterior lumbar interbody fusion in active-duty US servicemen: a comparison with nonoperative management. Spine J 2001; 1:215–224.

90. Ciccone WJ, Motz C, Bentley C, et al. Bioabsorbable implants in orthopaedics: new developments and clinical applications. J Am Acad Orthop Surg 2001; 9:280–288.

91. Bergsma JE, de Bruijn WC, Rozema FR, et al. Late degradation tissue response to poly(L-lactide) bone plates and screws. Biomaterials 1995; 16:25–31.

92. Bergsma JE, Rozema FR, Bos RRM, et al. Foreign body reactions to resorbable poly(L-lactide) bone plates and screws used for the fixation of unstable zygomatic fractures. J Oral Maxillofac Surg 1993; 51:666–670.

93. Bostman O, Hirvensalo E, Makinen J, et al. Foreign-body reactions to fracture fixation implants of biodegradable synthetic polymers. J Bone Joint Surg Am 1990; 72:592–596.

94. Tegnander A, Engebretsen L, Bergh K, et al. Activation of the complement system and adverse effects of biodegradable pins of polylactic acid (Biofix) in osteochondritis dissecans. Acta Orthop Scand 1994; 65:472–475.

95. Christel P, Chabot F, Leray JL, et al. Biodegradable composites for internal fixation. Biomaterials 1980:271–280.

96. Cutright DE, Hunsuck EE. The repair of fractures of the orbital floor using biodegradable polylactic acid. Oral Surg 1972; 33:28–34.

97. Miller RA, Brady JM, Cutright DE. Degradation rates of oral resorbable implants: rate modification with changes in PLA/PGA copolymer ratios. J Biomed Mater Res 1977; 11:711–719.

98. Cutright DE, Hunsuck EE. Tissue reaction to the biodegradable polylactic acid suture. Oral Surg Oral Med Oral Pathol 1971; 31:134.

99. Van der Elst M, Klein CP, Blieck-Hogervorst JM, et al. Bone tissue response to biodegradable polymers used for intramedullary fracture fixation: a long-term in vivo study in sheep femora. Biomaterials 1999; 20:121.

100. Hollinger JO, Battistone GC. Biodegradable bone repair materials. Synthetic polymers and ceramics. Clin Orthop 1986; 207:290.

101. Vert M, Christel P, Chabot F, et al. Bioresorbable plastic materials for bone surgery. In: Hastings GW, Ducheyne P, eds. Macromolecular Biomaterials. Boca Raton, FL: CRC Press, 1984:119–142.

102. Kulkarni RK, Pani KC, Neuman C, et al. Polylactic acid for surgical implants. Arch Surg 1966; 93:839.

103. Bucholz RW, Henry S, Henley MB. Fixation with bioabsorbable screws for the treatment of fractures of the ankle. J Bone Joint Surg Am 1994; 76:319–324.

104. Caborn DNM, Coen M, Neef R, et al. Quadrupled semitendinous-gracilis autograft fixation in the femoral tunnel: a comparison between a metal and a bioabsorbable interference screw. Arthroscopy 1998; 14:241–245.

105. Cohen B, Tasto J. Meniscal arrow. Tech Orthop 1998; 13:164–169.

106. Cordewener FW, Bos RR, Rozema FR, et al. Poly(L-lactide) implants for repair of human orbital floor defects: clinical and magnetic resonance imaging evaluation of long-term results. J Oral Maxillofac Surg 1996; 54:9–13.

107. Warme WJ, Arciero RA, Savoie FHI, et al. Nonabsorbable versus absorbable suture anchors for open Bankart repair: a prospective, randomized comparison. Am J Sports Med 1999; 27:742–746.

108. Kandziora F, Pflugmacher R, Kleemann R, et al. Biomechanical analysis of biodegradable interbody fusion cages augmented With poly(propylene glycol-co-fumaric acid). Spine 2002; 27:1644–1651.

109. Toth JM, Estes BT, Wang M, et al. Evaluation of 70/30 poly (L-lactide-co-D,L-lactide) for use as a resorbable interbody fusion cage. J Neurosurg 2002; 97:423–432.

110. Bendsoe MP, Kikuchi N. Generating optimal yopologies in structural design using a homogenization method. Comp Meth Appl Mech Eng 1988; 71:197.

111. Neves M, Rodrigues H, Guedes J. Optimal design of periodic linear elastic microstructures. Comput Struct 2000; 76:421.

112. Kikuchi N. Design optimization method for compliant mechanisms and material microstructure. Comp Math Appl Mech Eng 1998; 151:401.

113. Cioranescu D, Donato P. An Introduction to Homogenization. (Oxford, U.K.) Oxford University Press, 1999.

114. Scachez-Palencia E, Zaoui A. Homogenization Techniques for Composite Media. Springer-Verlag, 1987.

115. Guedes JM, Kikuchi N. Preprocess and postprocess for material based on the homogenization method with adaptive finite element methods. Comp Meth Appl Mech Eng 1989; 83:143.

116. Steffen T, Tsantrizos A, Fruth I, et al. Cages: designs and concepts. Eur Spine J 2000; 9(suppl 1):S89–S94.

117. Gopferich A. Polymer Bulk Erosion. Macromolecules 1997; 30:2598–2604.

118. Lin CY, Hsiao CC, Chen PQ, et al. Interbody fusion cage design using integrated global layout and local microstructure topology optimization. Spine 2004; 26:1747–1754.

119. Lin CY, Lin C, Hollister SJ. A new approach for designing biodegradable bone tissue augmentation devices by using degradation topology optimization. Presented at the 8th World Multiconference on Systemics, Cybernetics and Informatics, Orlando, FL, July 18, 2004.

120. Bendsoe MP. Optimization of Structural Topology, Shape, and Material. New York: Springer, 1995.

121. Bendsoe MP. Topology design of structures, materials and mechanisms—status and perspectives. In: Powell M, Scholtes S, eds. System Modeling and Optimization Methods, Theory and Applications. Boston: Kluwer Academic Publishers Group, 2000.

122. Kikuchi N, Suzuki K. A homogenization method for shape and topology optimization. Comp Math Appl Mech Eng 1991; 93:291–318.

123. Lin C, Kikuchi N, Hollister SJ. A novel method for internal architecture design to match bone elastic properties with desired porosity. J Biomech 2004; 37:623–636.
124. Hollister SJ, Maddox RD, Taboas JM. Optimal design and fabrication of scaffolds to mimic tissue properties and satisfy biological constraints. Biomaterials 2002; 23:4095–4103.
125. Yaszemski MJ, Payne RG, Haynes WC, et al. In vitro degradation of a poly(propylene fumarate)-based composite material. Biomaterials 1996; 17:2127–2130.
126. Alden TD, Varady P, Kallmes DF, et al. Bone morphogenetic protein gene therapy. Spine 2002; 27:S87–S93.
127. Hannallah D, Peterson B, Lieberman JR, et al. Gene therapy in orthopaedic surgery. J Bone Joint Surg Am 2002; 84-A:1046–1061.
128. Bianco P, Riminucci M, Gronthos S, et al. Bone marrow stromal cells: Nature, biology, and potential applications. Stem Cells 2001; 19:180–192.
129. Lin CY, Schek RM, Mistry AS, et al. Functional bone engineering using ex vivo gene therapy and topology-optimized, biodegradable polymer composite scaffolds. Tissue Eng 2005; 11:1589–1598.
130. Krebsbach PH, Gu K, Franceschi RT, et al. Gene therapy-directed osteogenesis: BMP-7-transduced human fibroblasts form bone in vivo. Hum Gene Ther 2000; 11:1201–1210.
131. Hutmacher DW. Scaffold design and fabrication technologies for engineering tissues—state of the art and future perspectives. J Biomater Sci Polym Ed 2001; 12:107–124.
132. Goulet RW, Goldstein SA, Ciarelli MJ, et al. The relationship between the structural and orthogonal compressive properties of trabecular bone. J Biomech 1994; 27:375–389.

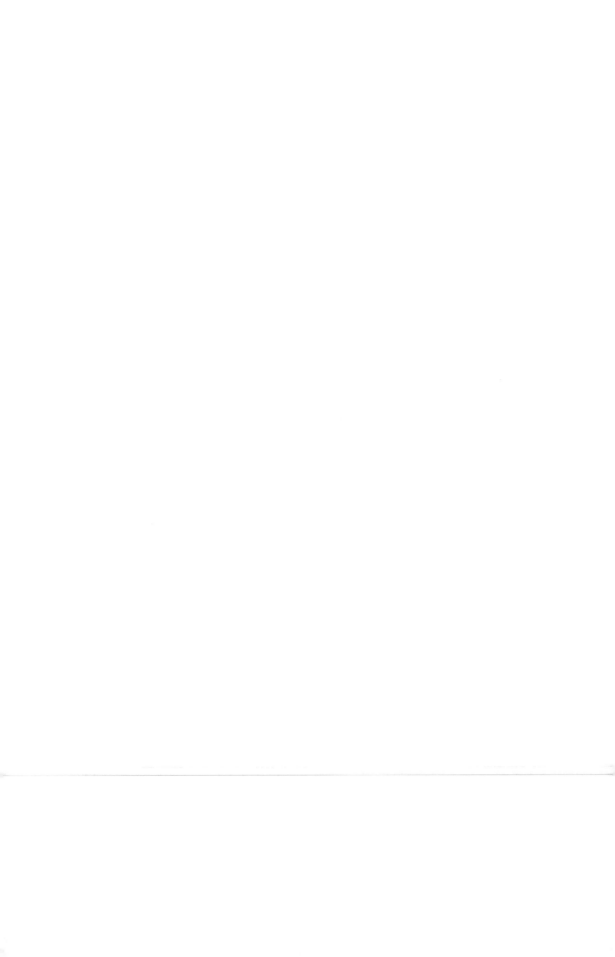

20 | Scientific Basis of Interventional Therapies for Discogenic Pain: Neural Mechanisms of Discogenic Pain

Yasuchika Aoki
Department of Orthopedic Surgery, Graduate School of Medicine, Chiba University, Chiba City, and Chiba Rosai Hospital Ichihara, Chiba, Japan

Kazuhisa Takahashi, Seiji Ohtori, and Hideshige Moriya
Department of Orthopedic Surgery, Graduate School of Medicine, Chiba University, Chiba City, Chiba, Japan

INTRODUCTION

Disorders of the lumbar intervertebral disc generate discogenic pain, which is considered to be a major source of low back pain (1,2). At the present time, there is little data regarding the pathophysiological mechanisms underlying the pathogenesis of low back pain. Clinically, the natural course of low back pain is usually favorable; acute low back pain frequently disappears within one to two weeks. In some cases, however, acute low back pain may become chronic, which is quite difficult to treat and has major socio-economic impacts. Although any of the spinal structures, such as intervertebral discs, facet joints, vertebral bodies, ligaments or muscles, can be a source of low back pain, the most common etiology of low back pain is a damaged lumbar intervertebral disc (1,3,4). The sensation of pain is transmitted by primary afferents from the disc to the dorsal horn of the spinal cord.

In order to understand the mechanism of pain, it is important to know normal sensory nerve transmission and to know how it is altered in the pathological state. For example, tissues that do not contain nerve fibers cannot be the origin of the pain sensation. This Chapter will focus on the characteristics of pain transmission from a disc, suggested pathomechanisms of discogenic pain, and the evaluation of current interventional therapies. While nonphysiological factors, such as social and psychological factors, may affect the extent and intensity of symptoms, treatments for discogenic pain should be based on a scientific knowledge of the pain mechanism. A better understanding of the scientific basis of discogenic pain is advantageous for both the surgeon and the patient.

SENSORY TRANSMISSION BY DORSAL ROOT GANGLION NEURONS

Primary afferents in peripheral nerves have a cell body in a dorsal root ganglion (DRG). In physiological conditions, nociceptive information is perceived via the peripheral terminals of the axons of DRG neurons. The axons of DRG neurons may be myelinated or unmyelinated, and are further classified into three major groups: A, B, and C. Group A is further subclassified into A-α, A-β, A-γ, and A-δ according to more precise specifications (Table 1). Group A and B axons are myelinated, whereas group C axons are unmyelinated. As described in Table 1, nociceptive information is normally transmitted by A-δ or C fibers. Of the two types of nociceptive fibers, A-δ fibers are larger; they are thinly myelinated and conduct impulses relatively quickly (5–15 m/sec). Some A-δ fibers respond only to noxious mechanical stimuli and are known as mechanonociceptors. Others respond to noxious chemical or thermal stimuli and are known as thermal mechanonociceptors. C fibers, which are the smaller of the two types of nociceptive fibers, are unmyelinated and conduct impulses slowly (0.2–1.5 m/sec). These fibers respond to noxious mechanical, chemical and thermal stimuli, and, under normal conditions, are activated only by tissue destruction. However, under certain conditions, such as tissue inflammation, these nociceptive fibers can be sensitized and respond to innocuous stimuli.

TABLE 1 Characteristics of Fibers in Peripheral Nerves

Fiber group	Innervation	Mean diameter μm (range)	Transmission (m/sec)	Threshold
A-α	Primary muscle spindle (afferents)	15 (12–20)	Rapid (70–120)	Low
A-β	Cutaneous touch and pressure afferents	8 (5–15)	Rapid (40–70)	Low
A-γ	Muscle spindle (afferents)	6 (6–8)	Rapid (20–40)	Low
A-δ	Mechanonociceptors, thermal mechanoceptors	<3 (1–4)	Slow (5–15)	High
B	Sympathetic preganglionic	3 (1–3)	Slow (5–15)	High
C	Mechanonociceptors, thermal mechano nociceptors, sympathetic postganglionic	1 (0.5–1.5)	Slow (0.2–1.5)	High

Based on the classification of their axons, DRG neurons are divided into two main subpopulations; small and large neurons. The large DRG neurons are thought to be mainly involved in proprioception, while most small DRG neurons are involved in nociception. A-δ and C fibers are the axons of the small, nociceptive neurons. Small DRG neurons are further subclassified into nerve growth factor (NGF)-sensitive neurons and glial cell line-derived neurotrophic factor (GDNF)-sensitive neurons. These express the high-affinity NGF receptor tyrosine kinase A (trkA) and the GDNF receptor, ret, respectively (5,6). NGF-sensitive neurons contain neuropeptides, such as substance P (SP) and calcitonin gene-related peptide (CGRP) (7), whereas GDNF-sensitive neurons lack neuropeptides, but bind isolectin B4 (IB4) derived from Griffonia simplicifolia (8,9). Previous studies indicate that NGF-sensitive neurons are critical to hyperalgesic responses induced by inflammation (10–12), whereas GDNF-sensitive neurons are important in neuropathic pain (13).

INNERVATION OF THE LUMBAR INTERVERTEBRAL DISC

The presence of sensory fibers in the lumbar intervertebral disc of humans (14–19), rats (20–22), and other animals (23,24) has been described. It has also been reported that SP and CGRP-immunoreaicitve (IR) nerve fibers are present in the disc (Fig. 1) (15,17,22,24–27). Because SP and CGRP are both expressed in nociceptive neurons and their axons (28,29), these SP- and CGRP-IR nerve fibers are thought to be involved in transmitting nociceptive information from the disc. Therefore, the presence of SP- and CGRP-IR nerve fibers suggests that the disc itself could be a source of pain.

To understand the nature of disc innervation, we should be aware of important findings that are closely related to the generation of discogenic low back pain. Generally, it is recognized that the innervation of the disc is very sparse (17) and restricted to the outermost part of the annulus fibrosus (16,18,19,30,31) and endplate (32,33). Bogduk et al. (16) reported that nerve fibers were present only within the outer one-third of the annulus fibrosus. More recently, the normal disc was described as being innervated only to a depth of up to 3.5 mm (18).

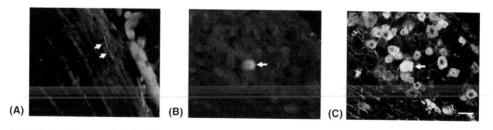

(A) **(B)** **(C)**

FIGURE 1 Fluorescent photomicrographs showing calcitonin gene-related peptide (CGRP)-positive nerve fibers in the **(A)** outer annulus of the rat L5-L6 disc, **(B)** dorsal root ganglion (DRG) neurons labeled following Fluoro-Gold application to the rat L5–L6 disc, and **(C)** CGRP-positive DRG neurons. Panels B and C are from the same section of the L1 DRG. Arrows indicate examples of a Fluoro-Gold-labeled neuron that is CGRP-positive. This DRG neuron is thought to be a CGRP-positive, nerve growth factor (NGF)-sensitive nociceptive neuron innervating the L5–L6 disc. The scale bar is 50 μm.

Autonomic fibers seem to extend deeper into the annulus fibrosus than nociceptive fibers (18). If nerve fibers are present only in the outermost part of the annulus, an annular tear confined to the inner annulus would not cause low back pain. Conversely, the disc can be the origin of pain only when an annular tear reaches the outermost part of the annulus fibrosus.

PAIN TRANSMISSION FROM THE LUMBAR INTERVERTEBRAL DISC
Pathway of Nerve Fibers Supplying the Lumbar Intervertebral Disc

It is important to know the pathways of nerve fibers from the disc when we attempt to block pain transmission. Bogduk et al. precisely reported the nerve supply to human lumbar discs. In this study, they described that there is a different nerve supply to each region of the disc (16). In the anterior portion of the disc, nerve fibers are derived from rami communicants or directly from paravertebral sympathetic trunks. In the lateral portion of the disc, nerve fibers are derived from rami communicants or directly from ventral primary rami. In the posterior portion of the disc, nerve fibers are derived from the sinuvertebral nerve, which arises from ventral primary rami or rami communicants (16).

To elucidate the nerve fiber pathway from the disc to DRGs, Nakamura et al. (34) investigated the effects of resection of the nerve fiber pathways on the nerve network of the posterior portion of rat lumbar intervertebral discs. They found that resection of sympathetic trunks decreased the density of nerve fibers of the posterior portion of rat L5–L6 discs. However, bilateral resection of the sympathetic trunks from L2 to L6 was necessary to eradicate the nerve bundles on the rat L5–L6 disc, suggesting that the posterior portion of lumbar intervertebral discs was innervated, at least in part, through the sympathetic trunks multisegmentally and bilaterally. Using the retrograde tracing method, Ohtori et al. (35) demonstrated that T13–L2 DRG neurons innervate the dorsal portion of the rat L5–L6 disc through the paravertebral sympathetic trunks, whereas L3–L6 DRG neurons innervate the L5–L6 disc through the sinuvertebral nerves.

Origin of Nerve Fibers in the Lumbar Intervertebral Disc

Since Luschka's report in 1850 (36), it had been believed that the lumbar intervertebral disc is innervated segmentally by DRG neurons via sinuvertebral nerves. However, recent studies suggested the possibility that the lower (L5–L6) disc was innervated mainly by upper (L2) DRG neurons in the rat (37,38). Using the retrograde tracing method, Morinaga et al. (39) demonstrated that the ventral portion of the rat L5–L6 disc is innervated by neurons in L1 and L2 DRGs. Following the study, it was demonstrated that DRG neurons innervating the lateral and dorsal portion of the rat L5–L6 disc are present in T13–L6 DRGs, but are mainly in the L1 and L2 DRGs as well as the ventral portion of the disc (35,40). In clinical practice, disc lesions most frequently occur in the L4–L5 and L5–S1 intervertebral discs (41). Because the rat L5–L6 disc corresponds to the human L4–L5 disc (42), nociceptive information from the human L4–L5 disc may be transmitted mainly by L1 and L2 DRG neurons if a similar innervation pattern is present in humans.

In addition, studies using rats have revealed that DRG neurons innervating other spinal structures, such as facet joints (43), spinous processes (44), back muscles (44) and sacroiliac joints (45,46), are also distributed in multilevel DRGs. These observations suggest that dorsal elements of the lumbar spine are innervated by more rostral DRGs because they are more distant from the DRGs in transverse section (distance from DRG: back skin > back muscle, spinous process > facet joint). Thus, it is suggested that the innervation territory of each DRG is conical in shape with the apex at the DRG and each territory is stacked with adjacent territories (44).

Characteristics of Disc-Innervating Neurons

Yamashita et al. used electrophysiological techniques to demonstrate that disc-innervating neurons have higher thresholds than neurons innervating other spinal structures, such as paravertebral muscles and facet joints (47,48). This indicates that disc-innervating neurons rarely

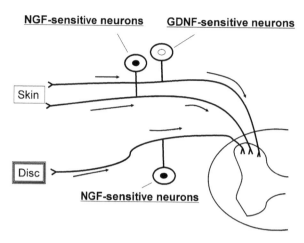

NGF-sensitive neurons   **GDNF-sensitive neurons**

Skin

Disc

NGF-sensitive neurons

FIGURE 2 Schematic representation of characteristics of skin- and disc-innervating neurons. Cutaneous tissue is innervated by nerve growth factor (NGF) and glial cell line-derived neurotrophic factor (GDNF)-sensitive neurons. The intervertebral disc is only innervated by NGF-sensitive neurons.

respond to mechanical stimuli under physiological conditions. However, there is a possibility that the threshold might be lowered in pathological conditions.

Recently, our study using a combination of a retrograde neurotracing and immunohistochemistry revealed that a large majority of nociceptive neurons innervating the disc belongs to the NGF-sensitive subtype that contains neuropeptides (Fig. 1) (49,50). Almost none of the nociceptive neurons innervating the disc belong to the GDNF-sensitive subtype (1.0%), whereas cutaneous tissue is innervated by both NGF- (41%) and GDNF-sensitive (20%) subtypes (Fig. 2) (27). Because these two neuron subtypes have different physiological and pharmaceutical characteristics (6), these findings provide critical information to understand the neuropathology of the painful disc. Gaining knowledge about the characteristics of NGF-sensitive neurons may help us understand the nature of discogenic pain.

It is well known that NGF contributes to inflammatory hyperalgesia via trkA expressed in small DRG neurons (10). In inflammatory states, NGF is synthesized in the inflamed tissue (51) and acts to sensitize the primary afferent neurons and produce hyperalgesia (52–56). Moreover, NGF regulates the expression of SP, CGRP, ATP-gated purinergic receptor (P2X$_3$), Transient Receptor Potential Vanilloid 1 (TRPV1) and other pain-related molecules in DRG neurons (57,58). From these observations, it is possible to speculate that the threshold of disc-innervating neurons may be lowered by the NGF induced in inflamed discs. The high sensitivity of disc-innervating neurons to NGF may help us to understand the neural mechanisms of discogenic pain.

PATHOMECHANISMS OF DISCOGENIC PAIN
Nerve Ingrowth

In 1970, Shinohara (59), using a silver impregnation technique, described the presence of nerve fibers in the inner annulus and nucleus pulposus obtained from patients with discogenic disorders. He hypothesized that scar tissue is formed in degenerated discs and nerve fibers accompany the scar tissues into the disc. Using immunohistochemistry, Coppes et al. (30,60) described the presence of SP-IR nerve fibers in the inner layers of the annulus fibrosus and nucleus pulposus. Because SP is implicated in pain sensation (28,29), the presence of SP-IR nerve fibers indicates that the disc can be the source of pain. Importantly, innervation of the inner disc was observed only in painful discs, but not in control discs. However, in these studies, there appears to be an inadequate number of control discs.

Following these studies, Freemont et al. (31) examined the innervation of the inner disc using 46 biopsy samples (30 from levels with pain and 16 with no pain). In this study, innervation of the inner disc was observed more frequently in painful discs than in asymptomatic discs. These authors further demonstrated the presence of growth-associated protein-43

(GAP-43)-IR fibers in inner painful discs. Because GAP-43 is recognized to be a marker of axonal growth, these findings strongly suggest that nociceptive nerve fibers were growing into the painful disc. From these observations, nerve ingrowth into the inner disc would seem to be a cause of chronic discogenic low back pain. If nerve fibers are distributed more extensively in the disc, the perception of nociceptive information may be facilitated.

Chemical Sensitization

Tumor necrosis factor-α (TNF-α) is expressed in the nucleus pulposus (61,62) and plays a role in generating sciatic pain in patients with disc herniation (63). Interleukin-1β (IL-1β), which is thought to be produced in tissues at disc herniation (64), has the capacity to produce hyperalgesia (52). NGF, which is up-regulated by such mediators, also has a sensitizing effect on nerve fibers (Fig. 3) (51,52). Previous reports indicate that the levels of inflammatory mediators and NGF are higher in painful discs than in asymptomatic discs (65,66), suggesting that they may play a role in sensitizing the painful disc.

Our recent studies revealed that most DRG neurons innervating the disc are NGF-sensitive neurons, which are closely related to the inflammatory pain state (49,50). In inflammatory states, NGF, which is synthesized in inflamed tissue, acts to upregulate the expression of various pain-related molecules in primary afferent neurons and sensitizes them (57,58), consequently producing hyperalgesia (Fig. 3) (52–56). From these observations, disc inflammation is critical for sensitizing neurons innervating the disc. However, sensitization would not occur without the exposure of annular nerve endings to chemical irritants. If nerve fibers

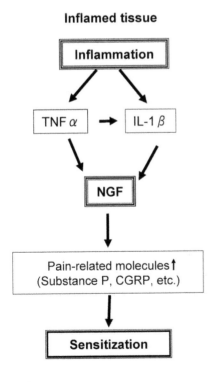

FIGURE 3 Schematic representation of the nerve growth factor (NGF)-mediated pain state. NGF is synthesized in inflamed tissue, through the action of tumor necrosis factor-α (TNF-α) and interleukin-1β (IL-1β). Locally synthesized NGF may act on dorsal root ganglion (DRG) neurons that have NGF-sensitivities to upregulate the production of pain-related molecules, such as substance P, calcitonin gene-related peptide (CGRP), and so on. Finally, NGF-sensitive DRG neurons are sensitized, so that they are easily excited by mechanical stimuli.

extend into the disc, it is more likely that the inflammatory mediators reach the nerve ending and sensitize them.

The intervertebral disc is under constant mechanical stress; increased intervertebral motion is related to the generation of discogenic pain (67). If "sensitization of the disc" occurs, increased mechanical stress is likely to play a role in activating the sensitized nerve endings. However, if the disc is not sensitized, it is possible that increased mechanical stress does not of itself cause discogenic pain.

EFFECTS OF DISC DEGENERATION ON PAIN GENERATION

Intervertebral discs undergo changes during the aging process. Disc degeneration, one of the age-related changes of the disc structure, is thought to be a cause of chronic discogenic low back pain (68). However, disc degeneration is commonly observed in patients in the absence of low back pain, suggesting that the correlation between disc degeneration and pain is not clear cut (69–71). Actually, a previous study revealed that 35% of subjects between 20- and 39-years old have signs of disc degeneration on MRI scans although they do not suffer low back pain symptoms (69). Thus, it is important to note that disc degeneration is part of the natural aging process and we should pay attention to the differences between a degenerated disc and the painful disc.

As reviewed by Urban et al. (72), the morphology of disc tissues becomes more disorganized in the degenerated disc. During the degeneration process, the annular layers become irregular and scar tissue is formed in the disc (73). The disruption of the tight collagen fiber network of the annulus gives nerve fibers and blood vessels a pathway to extend into the inner disc. Degenerated discs also exhibit multiple changes, such as loss of proteoglycan content (74), failure of nutrient supply (75,76), stress concentration of the annulus and endplate (77), and so on. These changes may affect the generation of discogenic pain, although disc degeneration alone is not necessarily a cause of discogenic pain.

Loss of Proteoglycan

A previous report proposed that proteoglycans are implicated in the regulation of neurite growth in the central nervous system (78). Although the details, at the molecular level, of the effects of proteoglycans on axonal growth are still unknown, proteoglycans could bind to a neuronal surface receptor or to a membrane component near the receptor, resulting in the inhibition of axonal growth (78).

Using a sheep annular lesion model, Melrose et al. (79) showed that the degree of nerve ingrowth into the disc was inversely correlated with proteoglycan levels, suggesting the inhibitory effect of proteoglycans on nerve ingrowth into the disc. Johnson et al. (80) demonstrated that aggrecan, a proteoglycan that is found in the disc, inhibits nerve fiber growth in vitro. These authors also reported that disc aggrecan has inhibitory effects on endothelial cell adhesion and cell migration in vitro (81), which suggests that it also inhibits vascularization of the disc. Neovascularization of the degenerated disc is closely related to nerve ingrowth (82,83); suggesting that the loss of proteoglycan is, at least in part, associated with the generation of discogenic pain by providing nerve fibers the opportunity to extend more deeply into the disc.

Failure of the Nutrient Supply

The lumbar intervertebral disc is the largest avascular tissue in the body; nutrients, such as glucose, and oxygen are supplied mainly by diffusion through the cartilaginous endplate from capillaries that originate in the vertebral bodies (84,85). The metabolism of the lumbar intervertebral disc is mainly anaerobic, even at high oxygen tensions (86). During the process of disc degeneration, the nutrient supply to the disc is likely to decrease, resulting in a lowered oxygen tension and production of lactic acid; pH values in the disc can fall to below pH 6.0 in some cases (85). Under these conditions, the production of the extracellular matrix by disc cells would decrease and the degeneration of the disc would progress (87).

Also, under low extracellular pH, a condition that frequently occurs in inflamed tissues, nerve fibers could be sensitized. For example, acidic conditions decrease the temperature threshold for TRPV1 activation (88,89). TRPV1 normally responds to heat stimuli in the noxious range ($>43°C$), but can even be activated at room temperature in acidic conditions (pH ≤ 5.9). TRPV1-positive nerve fibers are thought to be present in lumbar intervertebral discs of rats (27,90).

To summarize, changes in nutrient supply to the disc are associated with disc degeneration and might, to an as yet unknown extent, be associated with discogenic pain.

Stress Concentration in the Annulus

Lumbar intervertebral discs receive loads that constantly vary depending on posture (91,92). When changing posture, intervertebral discs provide the motion segment with both flexibility and strength, and function as a shock absorber. It is believed that the normal disc is able to spread the load evenly over the vertebral endplate, resulting in a relatively constant pattern of stress distribution.

McNally et al. (93) performed measurements of the distribution of compressive stress within loaded cadaveric intervertebral discs and found that the stress profiles measured across each disc varied considerably among discs and were highly dependent on the severity of degenerative changes. When stress profiles in the discs of patients were examined, several characteristic features of the pattern of stress distribution were found. These authors also examined the association between the stress pattern and pain provocation on discography (77). The results indicated that increased stress concentrations in the posterolateral annulus were most strongly associated with pain provocation. It seems reasonable that the nociceptors in the outer annulus respond to concentrated stress. This study also found that depressurization of the nucleus predicted pain provocation (77). McNally et al. (77) revealed that the patterns of stress distribution vary even in discs showing the same degree of degeneration. This finding may be an explanation for the difference between the degenerated disc and the painful disc.

EFFECTS OF DISC INFLAMMATION ON PAIN GENERATION

It has been reported that an inflammatory response was induced in the epidural space by inserting autogenous nucleus pulposus, but not by the injection of normal saline (94). Following this study, the effect of the nucleus pulposus on the nerve root was investigated further. Olmarker et al. (95,96) found that the nucleus pulposus has the capacity to cause nerve root pain and that the phenomenon was due to the action of TNF-α. Inflammatory mediators, such as TNF (62), IL1 (97), IL6 (64), IL-8 (65), phospholipase A2 (98), and prostaglandin (99), have been found in the intervertebral disc. It is recognized that these molecules affect the sensitivity of DRG neurons, resulting in the generation of the sensation of pain (51,52,100). Recently, Burke et al. (65) examined the production of inflammatory mediators in lumbar intervertebral discs and found that levels of inflammatory mediators were higher in painful discs than in asymptomatic discs. These results indicate that disc inflammation may persist in those patients with discogenic pain. As previously mentioned, these inflammatory mediators have sensitizing effects on disc afferents, indicating that disc inflammation induces sensitization of disc-innervating neurons.

Our previous study revealed that disc inflammation has the potential to promote axonal growth of DRG neurons into the disc (101). Olmarker et al. (102) demonstrated that nucleus pulposus placed in the subcutaneous space induced an ingrowth of nerve fibers and blood vessels into the nucleus and that such ingrowth can be reduced by TNF-α inhibitor. These results suggest that inflammatory mediators in the disc cause not only sensitization, but also nerve ingrowth into the disc. Moreover, our most recent results suggest that disc inflammation also induces axonal growth into the dorsal horn of spinal cord (103). It had previously been reported that reorganization of the sensory network in the dorsal horn could cause chronic pain (104); therefore, these results lead us to believe that disc inflammation may play an important role in the generation of discogenic pain.

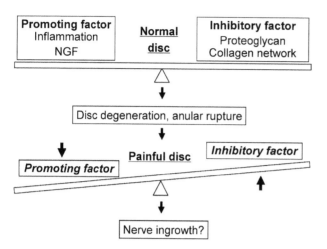

FIGURE 4 Nerve ingrowth into the disc may be regulated by a balance between promoting factors and inhibitory factors. In the normal disc, proteoglycans have inhibitory effects on nerve ingrowth. Also, tight collagen networks of the annulus fibrosus can represent a barrier to nerve ingrowth. In painful discs, the level of inflammatory mediators, including nerve growth factor (NGF), is thought to be higher than that in normal discs. If a lesion occurs in the disc, the level of inflammatory mediators, including NGF, may increase and the collagen network may be destroyed. Also, during the degeneration process, the level of proteoglycan would decrease. Thus, disruption of the balance between promoting and inhibitory factors may induce nerve ingrowth into the disc.

In contrast, proteoglycans have an inhibitory effect on nerve ingrowth into the disc (See the section "Effects of Disc Degeneration on Pain Generation"). Some factors, including pro-inflammatory mediators, may promote nerve ingrowth while other factors, such as proteoglycans, may inhibit nerve ingrowth. It is possible that nerve ingrowth may not occur in the lumbar intervertebral disc if a balance between these opposing factors is maintained (Fig. 4).

On the other hand, Freemont et al. (66) demonstrated that NGF is present in painful discs, but not in asymptomatic discs. Because NGF is induced by inflammatory mediators, such as TNF-α and IL-1β (51,52), NGF expression in the painful disc might be associated with disc inflammation. The high-affinity NGF receptor trk-A-expressing nerve fibers were also shown to be present in painful discs, but not in asymptomatic discs; this suggests that NGF has sensitizing effects on trk-A-expressing fibers. In addition, our recent study suggested that almost all of the nociceptive DRG neurons innervating the rat disc belong to a subgroup of neurons that are sensitive to NGF (49,50). Accordingly, nociceptive information in the disc is mainly transmitted by NGF-sensitive neurons, but not by GDNF-sensitive neurons (Fig. 2) see the section "Characteristics of Disc-Innervating Neurons").

Thus, in order to understand the mechanism of discogenic pain, it is important to understand NGF-mediated pain (Fig. 3). In addition to its sensitizing effects, NGF has neurotrophic activity and may promote nerve ingrowth into the disc. These observations suggest that NGF plays a key role in the generation of discogenic pain (Fig. 5).

SCIENTIFIC BASIS FOR THE DIAGNOSIS OF DISCOGENIC PAIN
Discography

Clinically, discography is used as a diagnostic tool for patients with discogenic pain. The criterion for a positive discogram is a concordant pain response during the disc injection (105). Painful discs produce intense pain even with a low pressure injection, whereas asymptomatic discs do not produce pain with a high pressure injection.

As reviewed by Cohen et al. (106), the concept of chemical sensitization may explain the different responses to discography between painful and asymptomatic discs. We conjecture that sensitized nerve fibers in the disc may even respond to a low-pressure injection, and induce a concordant pain, whereas nonsensitized fibers may not even respond to a high

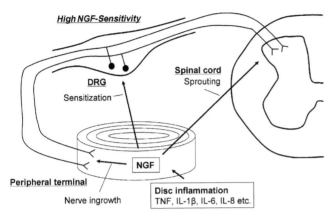

FIGURE 5 Schematic representation of the suggested mechanism for discogenic pain. The level of inflammatory mediators is high in painful discs. If disc inflammation occurs, nerve growth factor (NGF) may be induced by inflammatory mediators in the disc to act on dorsal root ganglion (DRG) neurons via peripheral terminals in the disc. Most of the small nociceptive DRG neurons innervating the disc are NGF-sensitive and project to the dorsal horn of spinal cord, suggesting their high NGF-sensitivity. NGF has a role in promoting nerve ingrowth into the disc, sensitization of DRG neurons, and sprouting in the dorsal horn; therefore, NGF may play a key role in the generation of discogenic pain.

pressure injection. Because of the relatively high incidence of false-positive results, the validity of discography is currently arguable (107,108). However, from the neuropathological point of view, discography seems to be a reasonable diagnostic tool for sensitized discs.

Magnetic Resonance Imaging

In recent years, the diagnosis of spinal abnormalities, such as tumors, infections, and disc herniation, has become much easier by the emergence of magnetic resonance imaging (MRI). Although many previously undetectable abnormalities can be visualized non-invasively by MRI, it is still difficult to distinguish painful discs from asymptomatic discs. Several studies revealed that many people without back pain have abnormal MRI findings, such as degeneration or bulging of a disc (69–71). Many attempts have been made to use MRI to determine a specific finding correlated with discogenic pain. As a result, a high-intensity zone (HIZ) (109,110), loss of signal intensity in T2-weighted images (68,111), and changes in adjacent vertebral body marrow (111,112) were weakly or moderately associated with low back pain. At present, the diagnostic value of these findings seems inadequate for clinical use (111,113,114). Because pathological changes in the painful disc, such as nerve growth, sensitization and stress concentration of disc afferents, are not detectable by MRI, painful discs cannot be diagnosed by MRI alone. Thus, MRI findings are not the best predictors of chronic discogenic low back pain; MRI should be used as a diagnostic adjunct to discography. Technological advances may offer increased diagnostic value for MRI; therefore, further investigations are expected.

SCIENTIFIC BASIS OF THERAPIES FOR DISCOGENIC PAIN

In summary, we think that nerve ingrowth into the disc and sensitization of the disc afferents could be two major neuropathological mechanisms for chronic discogenic pain (Fig. 5) (115). If so, treatments for chronic discogenic pain should be targeted to these neuropathological changes. Lumbar interbody fusion may completely improve these neuropathological changes, because the operated discs will not undergo mechanical stress after complete bone union is achieved. Other interventional therapies may have limited value for improving the neuropathological changes.

Blockade

Blocking the transmission of nociceptive information from the disc is one of the therapeutic regimens for patients with discogenic low back pain. Local analgesia can be applied to the epidural space, nerve root, or paravertebral sympathetic trunks to interrupt the nociceptive information from the disc. Because the aim of these treatments is to block the sensation from the disc, it is essential to understand the sensory pathway from the disc to the dorsal horn of spinal cord. As previously mentioned (see section "Pain Transmission from Lumbar Intervertebral Disc"), the lower lumbar intervertebral discs are thought to be innervated multisegmentally by two distinct pathways. One is via adjacent sinuvertebral nerves, and another is via sympathetic trunks (35). DRG neurons innervating the lower discs are mainly located in L2 DRG; their main pathway from the disc is via paraveretebral sympathetic trunks (34,39,116).

These findings may explain why the blockade of paravertebral sympathetic trunks is effective for some patients with discogenic disorders (117,118). Based on this evidence, Nakamura et al. (116) performed L2 spinal nerve blocks in a series of patients with chronic discogenic low back pain with very good effect. There was no definitive proof, but blocking the spinal nerve at the corresponding level seems to be less effective than the L2 spinal nerve block.

However, these treatments have a limitation in that the analgesic effects may be short-lasting. Clinically, the long-term effects are controversial even if steroids are used with the local anesthesia (119). To obtain long-lasting effects, neurolytic agents, which destroy nerve fibers, are used in some cases.

Anti-inflammatory Drugs

Nonsteroidal anti-inflammatory drugs (NSAIDs), which have analgesic and anti-inflammatory effects, are usually used to treat patients with discogenic pain. The analgesic action is due to cyclo-oxygenase inhibition with decreased prostaglandin production. Some patients obtain significant pain relief with a NSAID. However, if symptoms do not improve, the clinician should try another treatment.

Corticosteroids, which have been presumed to have anti-inflammatory effects are widely used for the treatment of patients with chronic discogenic pain, although their efficacy remains controversial (120–124). Khot et al. (122) performed a prospective randomized study to examine the therapeutic effect of intradiscal steroid injection, and concluded that intradiscal steroid injections, compared with a saline placebo, do not improve the clinical outcome in patients with discogenic back pain. On the other hand, Butterman et al. (124) demonstrated that spinal steroid injections are effective in patients with MRI findings of discogenic inflammation, specifically adjacent inflammatory end-plate changes. These results suggest that it is appropriate to use anti-inflammatory drugs when the symptom of pain is thought to result mainly from disc inflammation.

Recently, it was reported that the application of TNF-α inhibitors and IL-1-receptor antagonist protein into the disc was effective for the treatment of discogenic pain (125,126). TNF-α and IL-1β have the capacity to reduce mechanical nociceptive thresholds and induce inflammatory hyperalgesia (127,128). Because these inflammatory mediators are thought to be major factors causing pain in the inflammatory state, neutralizing these mediators is expected to be an effective future treatment for discogenic pain.

Previous studies suggested that neutralizing NGF using anti-NGF or a trkA-IgG fusion molecule may prevent the hyperalgesia induced by inflammation and nerve injury (10,12,129–131). Our studies revealed that the lumbar intervertebral disc is more sensitive to NGF than other tissues (27,50,115); this suggests that NGF may be a key factor generating discogenic pain (Fig. 5). In addition, it was reported that anti-NGF reduced nerve fiber growth in cutaneous tissues (132). Thus, neutralizing NGF may affect both "sensitization" and "nerve ingrowth," which are thought to be pathomechanisms of discogenic pain (see "Pathomechanisms of Discogenic Pain"). At present, the effects of neutralizing NGF therapy have not been examined clinically. However, neutralizing NGF therapy might be more effective for discogenic low back pain than for other pain states, because the disc is more sensitive to NGF than other tissues (see the section "Characteristics of Disc-Innervating Neurons").

Antibodies against TNF-α are now in clinical use for the treatment of arthritis, and have been shown to reduce pain. Because TNF-α has the potential to upregulate NGF production, NGF production may be suppressed by the anti-TNF-α antibodies. Thus, in the future, neutralizing TNF-α is expected to be an effective treatment for discogenic pain.

These anti-inflammatory drugs may reduce sensitization of the disc afferents. However, the drugs may not improve the extensive innervation that already exists in the painful disc. Moreover, it is unclear how long the effects of these treatments continue in the discs.

Intradiscal Electrothermal Therapy

Recently, the minimally invasive intradiscal electrothermal therapy (IDET), a procedure that involves placing a thermal catheter into the disc and heating the tissue, has been used to treat discogenic pain (133). Although there are numerous reports evaluating the therapeutic effects of IDET for chronic discogenic low back pain, the efficacy of IDET remains controversial at this time (134–138).

The aim of this procedure is to shrink collagen fibrils and coagulate nociceptive fibers in the discs (133). Thermal energy should be effective to achieve these goals. Generally, the temperature of the catheter is increased to 90°C, according to a uniform protocol. During this procedure, the disc temperature is thought to reach approximately 55°C, resulting in the shrinkage of collagen fibrils and the coagulation of nerve fibers (139). Also, a recent in vitro study suggested that stress concentration in the annulus, which is thought to be a cause of discogenic pain, is improved after IDET (140). IDET would seem to be an effective treatment for discogenic pain if it can achieve these beneficial effects on the pathomechanisms of discogenic pain, such as nerve ingrowth and stress concentration. However, whether IDET can achieve or not these beneficial effects remain controversial.

Kleinstueck et al. (141) reported that the disc did not reach the effective temperature range except for a very limited margin (1–2 mm) around the catheter. Using sheep, Freeman et al. (142) examined whether IDET can coagulate nerve fibers in experimentally degenerated discs induced by stab incision. They showed that there was no difference in the number of nerve fibers in the outer annulus between the discs that had undergone IDET and the discs that had not. Therefore, we are not able to exclude the possibility that nerve fibers can not be completely coagulated. It is possible that disc inflammation occurs following this procedure and induces nerve ingrowth and sensitization again. Considering these problems, further investigations are needed to determine whether IDET can be an effective treatment for discogenic pain.

Surgery

Interbody fusion, via either an anterior or posterior approach, is considered to be the most widely used treatment for discogenic pain. The aims of this treatment are to remove the pain generators and to stabilize the spinal segment. During the surgical procedure, part of the pain generators, such as nerve fibers and inflammatory mediators, should be removed. Also, remaining nerve fibers should not be subjected to mechanical stresses if the spinal segment is completely stabilized. Thus it would seem that interbody fusion is an effective treatment for patients with discogenic pain.

Posterolateral fusion is sometimes used to treat patients with discogenic pain. The aim of this treatment is to stabilize the anterior spinal column by stabilizing the posterior column. Because the intervertebral disc itself is not treated with this procedure, nerve fibers and inflammatory mediators may remain in the disc. If a small degree of motion remains after the procedure, pain does not disappear entirely. Clinically, it is known that the discs at the level of prior posterolateral fusion can be a source of discogenic pain. Barrick et al. (143) described cases in which anterior interbody fusion at the level of prior posterolateral fusion provided significant improvements in pain and function. This suggests that, in some cases, posterolateral fusion might be insufficient treatment. Fritzell et al. (144) performed a multicenter randomized study to examine the therapeutic effects of three surgical techniques on chronic low back pain. They compared posterolateral fusion, posterolateral fusion with instrumentation, and poster-olateral fusion with instrumentation and interbody fusion. The study showed that all three surgical techniques were effective for patients with chronic low back pain, with no significant difference between the three. The data from this study suggests that the effects on discogenic pain are similar between posterolateral fusion alone and posterolateral fusion with instrumentation and interbody fusion in most cases. However, from the neuropathological view point, interbody fusion is more reasonable for treating discogenic pain than posterolateral fusion. It should be emphasized that there is a possibility that posterolateral fusion is less effective in some cases.

Based on the concept that abnormal loading rather than motion could be the cause of pain, dynamic stabilization devices were developed. One of these devices is the Graf ligament system. Grevitt et al. (145) reported that 72% of patients showed "excellent" or "good" results at the average 24-months follow-up period. They recently reported the results of a seven-year follow-up of patients with the device, and concluded that the device has proved as successful as fusion in the majority of patients (146). However, this system has the same limitations as posterolateral fusion in the nerve fibers, inflammatory mediators and small degrees of motion may remain in the disc.

Total disc replacement has been developed to allow motion of the operated segment and to avoid the adjacent disc problem due to increased stresses. As reviewed by German et al. (147), disc replacement provided clinical results similar to fusion. With this procedure, the origins of discogenic pain would be removed and the mechanical load would be transmitted by the device. However, it is possible that preserved motion can be a mechanical stimulus if the nerve fibers remain in the treated disc.

Disc Repair

Disc repair is expected to be a future treatment for discogenic pain. It would seem to be the ideal treatment for disc degeneration because it increases proteoglycan and collagen synthesis, and normalizes the intradiscal environment (148–150). The limitation to this treatment is that this approach cannot restore the endplate dysfunction that accompanies disc degeneration; none-theless, researchers have been fascinated by the prospect of regenerating a degenerated disc.

However, disc degeneration is usually not painful, which indicates that, in most cases, regeneration of a degenerated disc is not necessary. To ascertain the clinical significance of disc repair, the potential effects on the suggested causes of disc pain need to be examined. We will look first at the effects of disc repair on nerve ingrowth into the disc. Because aggrecan has suppressive effects on nerve fiber growth (80), an increase of proteoglycan content might suppress the nerve ingrowth into the disc. Also, if the tight collagen network was reconstructed by disc repair, it could serve as a physical barrier to nerve ingrowth. However, there is a poten-tial limitation in that nerve fibers already extending into the disc might not disappear when the disc is regenerated. A combination of disc repair with IDET might solve the problem. Second, we will consider the effects of disc repair on sensitization of the afferent neurons. Unfortu-nately, there is no clear evidence for the therapeutic effects of disc repair on sensitization. If the levels of inflammatory mediators are decreased by the treatment, the threshold of the affer-ent neurons should be raised. Third, if the degenerated disc is biomechanically restored by disc repair, stress distribution in the disc might be normalized.

Clinicians are anticipating that disc regeneration will become an optional treatment for discogenic pain. However, to elucidate the therapeutic effects of this treatment, further investigation is needed.

CONCLUSIONS

The treatment of discogenic pain will likely continue to evolve through the appearance of new strategies, such as novel anti-inflammatory drugs, IDET, newly designed materials and instru-ments and disc repair, among others. Clinically, the origin of pain felt by patients with back pain cannot be limited to the intervertebral disc. Particularly, facet joint osteoarthrosis usually accompanies disc degeneration (151–153). In this Chapter, we focused only on the pathology of the intervertebral disc. However, we must be aware of other factors, such as facet joints, ligaments, muscles and veretebral bodies, all of which contribute to back pain.

The accuracy of diagnosis of discogenic pain is not yet satisfactory. As previously mentioned, discography is the gold-standard diagnostic tool, but it has a relatively high incidence of false-positive and false-negative results. Consequently, data of clinical trials should be interpreted based on the premise that the data might include some low back pain patients with non-discogenic pain origin. The development of diagnostic tools and improvement of treatment decision-making processes are also important for improving the clinical results of interventional therapies for discogenic pain.

In this Chapter, we evaluated the treatments for discogenic pain using basic scientific knowledge. However, our current knowledge about the pathogenesis of discogenic pain is imperfect. Progress in basic research is certain to increase our understanding of the pathomechanisms of discogenic pain. To make appropriate treatment choices for discogenic pain, decisions should be based on currently available clinical evidence and scientific studies regarding the efficacy of different therapies for discogenic pain.

REFERENCES

1. Nachemson A. The lumbar spine an orthopedic challenge. Spine 1976; 1:59–71.
2. Andersson GB. Epidemiological features of chronic low back pain. Lancet 1999; 354:581–585.
3. Mooney V. Presidential address. International Society for the Study of the Lumbar Spine. Dallas, 1986. Where is the pain coming from? Spine 1987; 12:754–759.
4. Deyo RA, Weinstein JN. Low back pain. N Engl J Med 2001; 344:363–370.
5. Silverman JD, Kruger L. Selective neuronal glycoconjugate expression in sensory and autonomic ganglia: relation of lectin reactivity to peptide and enzyme markers. J Neurocytol 1990; 19:789–801.
6. Snider WD, McMahon SB. Tackling pain at the source: new ideas about nociceptors. Neuron 1998; 20:629–632.
7. Averill S, McMahon SB, Clary DO, et al. Immunocytochemical localization of trkA receptors in chemically identified subgroups of adult rat sensory neurons. Eur J Neurosci 1995; 7:1484–1494.
8. Molliver DC, Wright DE, Leitner ML, et al. IB4-binding DRG neurons switch from NGF to GDNF dependence in early postnatal life. Neuron 1997; 19:849–861.
9. Bennett DL, Michael GJ, Ramachandran N, et al. A distinct subgroup of small DRG cells express GDNF receptor components and GDNF is protective for these neurons after nerve injury. J Neurosci 1998; 18:3059–3072.
10. Woolf CJ, Safieh-Garabedian B, Ma QP, et al. Nerve growth factor contributes to the generation of inflammatory sensory hypersensitivity. Neuroscience 1994; 62:327–331.
11. Mantyh PW, Rogers SD, Honore P, et al. Inhibition of hyperalgesia by ablation of lamina I spinal neurons expressing the substance P receptor. Science 1997; 278:275–279.
12. Koltzenburg M, Bennett DL, Shelton DL, et al. Neutralization of endogenous NGF prevents the sensitization of nociceptors supplying inflamed skin. Eur J Neurosci 1999; 11:1698–1704.
13. Malmberg AB, Chen C, Tonegawa S, et al. Preserved acute pain and reduced neuropathic pain in mice lacking PKCgamma. Science 1997; 278:279–283.
14. Antonacci MD, Mody DR, Heggeness MH. Innervation of the human vertebral body: a histologic study. J Spinal Disord 1998; 11:526–531.
15. Ashton IK, Roberts S, Jaffray DC, et al. Neuropeptides in the human intervertebral disc. J Orthop Res 1994; 12:186–192.
16. Bogduk N, Tynan W, Wilson AS. The nerve supply to the human lumbar intervertebral discs. J Anat 1981; 132:39–56.
17. Konttinen YT, Gronblad M, Antti-Poika I, et al. Neuroimmunohistochemical analysis of peridiscal nociceptive neural elements. Spine 1990; 15:383–386.
18. Palmgren T, Gronblad M, Virri J, et al. An immunohistochemical study of nerve structures in the anulus fibrosus of human normal lumbar intervertebral discs. Spine 1999; 24:2075–2079.
19. Roberts S, Eisenstein SM, Menage J, et al. Mechanoreceptors in intervertebral discs. Morphology, distribution, and neuropeptides. Spine 1995; 20:2645–2651.
20. Kojima Y, Maeda T, Arai R, et al. Nerve supply to the posterior longitudinal ligament and the intervertebral disc of the rat vertebral column as studied by acetylcholinesterase histochemistry. II. Regional differences in the distribution of the nerve fibers and their origins. J Anat 1990; 169: 247–255.
21. Kojima Y, Maeda T, Arai R, et al. Nerve supply to the posterior longitudinal ligament and the intervertebral disc of the rat vertebral column as studied by acetylcholinesterase histochemistry. I. Distribution in the lumbar region. J Anat 1990; 169:237–246.

22. McCarthy PW, Carruthers B, Martin D, et al. Immunohistochemical demonstration of sensory nerve fibers and endings in lumbar intervertebral discs of the rat. Spine 1991; 16:653–655.

23. Cavanaugh JM, Kallakuri S, Ozaktay AC. Innervation of the rabbit lumbar intervertebral disc and posterior longitudinal ligament. Spine 1995; 20:2080–2085.

24. Gronblad M, Weinstein JN, Santavirta S. Immunohistochemical observations on spinal tissue innervation. A review of hypothetical mechanisms of back pain. Acta Orthop Scand 1991; 62:614–622.

25. Imai S, Konttinen YT, Tokunaga Y, et al. An ultrastructural study of calcitonin gene-related peptide-immunoreactive nerve fibers innervating the rat posterior longitudinal ligament. A morphologic basis for their possible efferent actions. Spine 1997; 22:1941–1947.

26. Korkala O, Gronblad M, Liesi P, et al. Immunohistochemical demonstration of nociceptors in the ligamentous structures of the lumbar spine. Spine 1985; 10:156–157.

27. Aoki Y, Ohtori S, Takahashi K, et al. Expression and co-expression of VR1, CGRP, and IB4-binding glycoprotein in dorsal root ganglion neurons in rats: differences between the disc afferents and the cutaneous afferents. Spine 2005; 30:1496–1500.

28. Hokfelt T, Kellerth JO, Nilsson G, et al. Substance p: localization in the central nervous system and in some primary sensory neurons. Science 1975; 190:889–890.

29. Kuraishi Y, Hirota N, Sato Y, et al. Evidence that substance P and somatostatin transmit separate information related to pain in the spinal dorsal horn. Brain Res 1985; 325:294–298.

30. Coppes MH, Marani E, Thomeer RT, et al. Innervation of annulus fibrosis in low back pain. Lancet 1990; 336:189–190.

31. Freemont AJ, Peacock TE, Goupille P, et al. Nerve ingrowth into diseased intervertebral disc in chronic back pain. Lancet 1997; 350:178–181.

32. Brown MF, Hukkanen MVJ, McCarthy ID, et al. Sensory and sympathetic innervation of the vertebral endplate in patients with degenerated disc disease. J Bone Joint Surg Br 1997; 84:147–153.

33. Fagan A, Moore R, Vernon Roberts B, et al. ISSLS prize winner: The innervation of the intervertebral disc: a quantitative analysis. Spine 2003; 28:2570–2576.

34. Nakamura S, Takahashi K, Takahashi Y, et al. Origin of nerves supplying the posterior portion of lumbar intervertebral discs in rats. Spine 1996; 21:917–924.

35. Ohtori S, Takahashi Y, Takahashi K, et al. Sensory innervation of the dorsal portion of the lumbar intervertebral disc in rats. Spine 1999; 24:2295–2299.

36. Luschka HV. Die Nerven des menschlichen Wirbelkanales. Tubingen: Laupp, 1850.

37. Takahashi Y, Nakajima Y, Sakamoto T, et al. Capsaicin applied to rat lumbar intervertebral disc causes extravasations in the groin skin: a possible mechanism of referred pain of the intervertebral disc. Neurosci Lett 1993; 161:1–3.

38. Takahashi Y, Morinaga T, Nakamura S, et al. Neural connection between the ventral portion of the lumbar intervertebral disc and the groin skin. J Neurosurg 1996; 85:323–328.

39. Morinaga T, Takahashi K, Yamagata M, et al. Sensory innervation to the anterior portion of lumbar intervertebral disc. Spine 1996; 21:1848–1851.

40. Aoki Y, Takahashi Y, Takahashi K, et al. Sensory innervation of the lateral portion of the lumbar intervertebral disc in rats. Spine J 2004; 4:275–280.

41. Moneta GB, Videman T, Kaivanto K, et al. Reported pain during lumbar discography as a function of annular ruptures and disc degeneration. A re-analysis of 833 discograms. Spine 1994; 19: 1968–1974.

42. Greene EC. Anatomy of the Rat. New York: Hafner Publishing Company, 1963:5–6.

43. Suseki K, Takahashi Y, Takahashi K, et al. Innervation of the lumbar facet joints. Origins and functions. Spine 1997; 22:477–485.

44. Takahashi Y, Chiba T, Kurokawa M, et al. Stereoscopic structure of sensory nerve fibers in the lumbar spine and related tissues. Spine 2003; 28:871–880.

45. Murata Y, Takahashi K, Yamagata M, et al. Sensory innervation of the sacroiliac joint in rats. Spine 2000; 25:2015–2019.

46. Murata Y, Takahashi K, Yamagata M, et al. Origin and pathway of sensory nerve fibers to the ventral and dorsal sides of the sacroiliac joint in rats. J Orthop Res 2001; 19:379–383.

47. Yamashita T, Cavanaugh JM, el-Bohy AA, et al. Mechanosensitive afferent units in the lumbar facet joint. J Bone Joint Surg Am 1990; 72:865–870.

48. Yamashita T, Minaki Y, Oota I, et al. Mechanosensitive afferent units in the lumbar intervertebral disc and adjacent muscle. Spine 1993; 18:2252–2256.

49. Ozawa T, Aoki Y, Ohtori S, et al. The dorsal portion of the lumbar intervertebral disc is innervated primarily by small peptide-containing dorsal root ganglion neurons in rats. Neurosci Lett 2003; 344:65–67.

50. Aoki Y, Ohtori S, Takahashi K, et al. Innervation of the lumbar intervertebral disc by nerve growth factor-dependent neurons related to inflammatory pain. Spine 2004; 29:1077–1081.

51. Woolf CJ, Allchorne A, Safieh-Garabedian B, et al. Cytokines, nerve growth factor and inflammatory hyperalgesia: the contribution of tumour necrosis factor alpha. Br J Pharmacol 1997; 121:417–424.

52. Safieh-Garabedian B, Poole S, Allchorne A, et al. Contribution of interleukin-1 beta to the inflammation-induced increase in nerve growth factor levels and inflammatory hyperalgesia. Br J Pharmacol 1995; 115:1265–1275.
53. Dmitrieva N, McMahon SB. Sensitisation of visceral afferents by nerve growth factor in the adult rat. Pain 1996; 66:87–97.
54. Rueff A, Dawson AJ, Mendell LM. Characteristics of nerve growth factor induced hyperalgesia in adult rats: dependence on enhanced bradykinin-1 receptor activity but not neurokinin-1 receptor activation. Pain 1996; 66:359–372.
55. Kasai M, Mizumura K. Endogenous nerve growth factor increases the sensitivity to bradykinin in small dorsal root ganglion neurons of adjuvant inflamed rats. Neurosci Lett 1999; 272:41–44.
56. Shu X, Mendell LM. Nerve growth factor acutely sensitizes the response of adult rat sensory neurons to capsaicin. Neurosci Lett 1999; 274:159–162.
57. Priestley JV, Michael GJ, Averill S, et al. Regulation of nociceptive neurons by nerve growth factor and glial cell line derived neurotrophic factor. Can J Physiol Pharmacol 2002; 80:495–505.
58. Ramer MS, Bradbury EJ, McMahon SB. Nerve growth factor induces P2X(3) expression in sensory neurons. J Neurochem 2001; 77:864–875.
59. Shinohara H. A study on lumbar disc lesion. Significance of histology of free nerve endings in lumbar discs. J Japan Orthop Assoc 1970; 44:553–570.
60. Coppes MH, Marani E, Thomeer RT, et al. Innervation of "painful" lumbar discs. Spine 1997; 22: 2342–2349; discussion 2349–2350.
61. Olmarker K, Larsson K. Tumor necrosis factor alpha and nucleus-pulposus-induced nerve root injury. Spine 1998; 23:2538–2544.
62. Weiler C, Nerlich AG, Bachmeier BE, et al. Expression and distribution of tumor necrosis factor alpha in human lumbar intervertebral discs: a study in surgical specimen and autopsy controls. Spine 2005; 30:44–53; discussion 54.
63. Karppinen J, Korhonen T, Malmivaara A, et al. Tumor necrosis factor-alpha monoclonal antibody, infliximab, used to manage severe sciatica. Spine 2003; 28:750–753; discussion 753–754.
64. Takahashi H, Suguro T, Okazima Y, et al. Inflammatory cytokines in the herniated disc of the lumbar spine. Spine 1996; 21:218–224.
65. Burke JG, Watson RW, McCormack D, et al. Intervertebral discs which cause low back pain secrete high levels of proinflammatory mediators. J Bone Joint Surg Br 2002; 84:196–201.
66. Freemont AJ, Watkins A, Le Maitre C, et al. Nerve growth factor expression and innervation of the painful intervertebral disc. J Pathol 2002; 197:286–292.
67. Panjabi MM. Low back pain and spinal instability. In: Weinstein JN ed. Low Back Pain: A Scientific and Clinical Overview. American Academy of Orthopaedic Surgeons, 1996:367–384.
68. Luoma K, Riihimaki H, Luukkonen R, et al. Low back pain in relation to lumbar disc degeneration. Spine 2000; 25:487–492.
69. Boden SD, Davis DO, Dina TS, et al. Abnormal magnetic-resonance scans of the lumbar spine in asymptomatic subjects. A prospective investigation. J Bone Joint Surg Am 1990; 72:403–408.
70. Powell MC, Wilson M, Szypryt P, et al. Prevalence of lumbar disc degeneration observed by magnetic resonance in symptomless women. Lancet 1986; 2:1366–1367.
71. Jensen MC, Brant-Zawadzki MN, Obuchowski N, et al. Magnetic resonance imaging of the lumbar spine in people without back pain. N Engl J Med 1994; 331:69–73.
72. Urban JP, Roberts S. Degeneration of the intervertebral disc. Arthritis Res Ther 2003; 5:120–130.
73. Boos N, Weissbach S, Rohrbach H, et al. Classification of age-related changes in lumbar intervertebral discs: 2002 Volvo Award in basic science. Spine 2002; 27:2631–2644.
74. Lyons G, Eisenstein SM, Sweet MB. Biochemical changes in intervertebral disc degeneration. Biochim Biophys Acta 1981; 673:443–453.
75. Nachemson A, Lewin T, Maroudas A, et al. In vitro diffusion of dye through the end-plates and the annulus fibrosus of human lumbar inter-vertebral discs. Acta Orthop Scand 1970; 41:589–607.
76. Roberts S, Urban JP, Evans H, et al. Transport properties of the human cartilage endplate in relation to its composition and calcification. Spine 1996; 21:415–420.
77. McNally DS, Shackleford IM, Goodship AE, et al. In vivo stress measurement can predict pain on discography. Spine 1996; 21:2580–2587.
78. Bovolenta P, Fernaud-Espinosa I. Nervous system proteoglycans as modulators of neurite outgrowth. Prog Neurobiol 2000; 61:113–132.
79. Melrose J, Roberts S, Smith S, et al. Increased nerve and blood vessel ingrowth associated with proteoglycan depletion in an ovine annular lesion model of experimental disc degeneration. Spine 2002; 27:1278–1285.
80. Johnson WE, Caterson B, Eisenstein SM, et al. Human intervertebral disc aggrecan inhibits nerve growth in vitro. Arthritis Rheum 2002; 46:2658–2664.
81. Johnson WE, Caterson B, Eisenstein SM, et al. Human intervertebral disc aggrecan inhibits endothelial cell adhesion and cell migration in vitro. Spine 2005; 30:1139–1147.

82. Kauppila LI. Ingrowth of blood vessels in disc degeneration. Angiographic and histological studies of cadaveric spines. J Bone Joint Surg Am 1995; 77:26–31.
83. Johnson WE, Evans H, Menage J, et al. Immunohistochemical detection of Schwann cells in innervated and vascularized human intervertebral discs. Spine 2001; 26:2550–2557.
84. Urban JP, Holm S, Maroudas A. Diffusion of small solutes into the intervertebral disc: as in vivo study. Biorheology 1978; 15:203–221.
85. Urban JP. The role of the physicochemical environment in determining disc cell behaviour. Biochem Soc Trans 2002; 30:858–864.
86. Holm S, Maroudas A, Urban JP, et al. Nutrition of the intervertebral disc: solute transport and metabolism. Connect Tissue Res 1981; 8:101–119.
87. Ishihara H, Urban JP. Effects of low oxygen concentrations and metabolic inhibitors on proteoglycan and protein synthesis rates in the intervertebral disc. J Orthop Res 1999; 17:829–835.
88. Caterina MJ, Schumacher MA, Tominaga M, et al. The capsaicin receptor: a heat-activated ion channel in the pain pathway. Nature 1997; 389:816–824.
89. Tominaga M, Caterina MJ, Malmberg AB, et al. The cloned capsaicin receptor integrates multiple pain-producing stimuli. Neuron 1998; 21:531–543.
90. Ohtori S, Takahashi K, Moriya H. Existence of brain-derived neurotrophic factor and vanilloid receptor subtype 1 immunoreactive sensory DRG neurons innervating L5/6 intervertebral discs in rats. J Orthop Sci 2003; 8:84–87.
91. Nachemson A, Morris JM. In vivo measurements of intradiscal pressure. Discometry, a method for the determination of pressure in the lower lumbar discs. J Bone Joint Surg Am 1964; 46:1077–1092.
92. Nachemson A, Elfstrom G. Intravital dynamic pressure measurements in lumbar discs. A study of common movements, maneuvers and exercises. Scand J Rehabil Med Suppl 1970; 1:1–40.
93. McNally DS, Adams MA. Internal intervertebral disc mechanics as revealed by stress profilometry. Spine 1992; 17:66–73.
94. McCarron RF, Wimpee MW, Hudkins PG, et al. The inflammatory effect of nucleus pulposus. A possible element in the pathogenesis of low-back pain. Spine 1987; 12:760–764.
95. Olmarker K, Rydevik B, Nordborg C. Autologous nucleus pulposus induces neurophysiologic and histologic changes in porcine cauda equina nerve roots. Spine 1993; 18:1425–1432.
96. Olmarker K, Nutu M, Storkson R. Changes in spontaneous behavior in rats exposed to experimental disc herniation are blocked by selective TNF-alpha inhibition. Spine 2003; 28:1635–1641; discussion 1642.
97. Le Maitre CL, Freemont AJ, Hoyland JA. The role of interleukin-1 in the pathogenesis of human intervertebral disc degeneration. Arthritis Res Ther 2005; 7:R732–R745.
98. Saal JS, Franson RC, Dobrow R, et al. High levels of inflammatory phospholipase A2 activity in lumbar disc herniations. Spine 1990; 15:674–678.
99. Kang JD, Georgescu HI, McIntyre-Larkin L, et al. Herniated lumbar intervertebral discs spontaneously produce matrix metalloproteinases, nitric oxide, interleukin-6, and prostaglandin E2. Spine 1996; 21:271–277.
100. Sommer C, Kress M. Recent findings on how proinflammatory cytokines cause pain: peripheral mechanisms in inflammatory and neuropathic hyperalgesia. Neurosci Lett 2004; 361:184–187.
101. Aoki Y, Ohtori S, Ino H, et al. Disc inflammation potentially promotes axonal regeneration of dorsal root ganglion neurons innervating lumbar intervertebral disc in rats. Spine 2004; 29:2621–2626.
102. Olmarker K. Neovascularization and neoinnervation of subcutaneously placed nucleus pulposus and the inhibitory effects of certain drugs. Spine 2005; 30:1501–1504.
103. Aoki Y, Takahashi K, Ohtori S, et al. Neuropathology of discogenic low back pain: A review. Internet J Spine Surg 2005; 2(1), http://www.ispub.com/ostia/index.php?xmlFilePath=journals/ijss/vol2n1/pain.xml
104. Woolf CJ, Shortland P, Coggeshall RE. Peripheral nerve injury triggers central sprouting of myelinated afferents. Nature 1992; 355:75–78.
105. Carragee EJ, Alamin TF. Discography. A review. Spine J 2001; 1:364–372.
106. Cohen SP, Larkin TM, Barna SA, et al. Lumbar discography: A comprehensive review of outcome studies, diagnostic accuracy, and principles. Reg Anaesth Pain Med 2005; 30:163–183.
107. Holt EP Jr. The question of lumbar discography. J Bone Joint Surg Am 1968; 50:720–726.
108. Carragee EJ, Tanner CM, Yang B, et al. False-positive findings on lumbar discography. Reliability of subjective concordance assessment during provocative disc injection. Spine 1999; 24:2542–2547.
109. Aprill C, Bogduk N. High-intensity zone: a diagnostic sign of painful lumbar disc on magnetic resonance imaging. Br J Radiol 1992; 65:361–369.
110. Carragee EJ, Barcohana B, Alamin T, et al. Prospective controlled study of the development of lower back pain in previously asymptomatic subjects undergoing experimental discography. Spine 2004; 29:1112–1117.
111. Kjaer P, Leboeuf-Yde C, Korsholm L, et al. Magnetic resonance imaging and low back pain in adults: a diagnostic imaging study of 40-year-old men and women. Spine 2005; 30:1173–1180.
112. Toyone T, Takahashi K, Kitahara H, et al. Vertebral bone-marrow changes in degenerative lumbar disc disease. An MRI study of 74 patients with low back pain. J Bone Joint Surg Br 1994; 76:757–764.

113. Videman T, Battie MC, Gibbons LE, et al. Associations between back pain history and lumbar MRI findings. Spine 2003; 28:582–588.
114. Jarvik JG, Hollingworth W, Heagerty PJ, et al. Three-year incidence of low back pain in an initially asymptomatic cohort: clinical and imaging risk factors. Spine 2005; 30:1541–1548; discussion 1549.
115. Aoki Y, Takahashi Y, Ohtori S, et al. Distribution and immunocytochemical characterization of dorsal root ganglion neurons innervating the lumbar intervertebral disc in rats: a review. Life Sci 2004; 74:2627–2642.
116. Nakamura SI, Takahashi K, Takahashi Y, et al. The afferent pathways of discogenic low-back pain. Evaluation of L2 spinal nerve infiltration. J Bone Joint Surg Br 1996; 78:606–612.
117. El-Mahdi MA, Abdel Latif FY, Janko M. The spinal nerve root "innervation," and a new concept of the clinicopathological interrelations in back pain and sciatica. Neurochirurgia (Stuttg) 1981; 24:137–141.
118. Connally GH, Sanders SH. Predicting low back pain patients' response to lumbar sympathetic nerve blocks and interdisciplinary rehabilitation: the role of pretreatment overt pain behavior and cognitive coping strategies. Pain 1991; 44:139–146.
119. Gajraj NM. Selective nerve root blocks for low back pain and radiculopathy. Reg Anesth Pain Med 2004; 29:243–256.
120. Simmons JW, McMillin JN, Emery SF, et al. Intradiscal steroids. A prospective double-blind clinical trial. Spine 1992; 17:S172–S175.
121. Fanciullo GJ, Hanscom B, Seville J, et al. An observational study of the frequency and pattern of use of epidural steroid injection in 25,479 patients with spinal and radicular pain. Reg Anaesth Pain Med 2001; 26:5–11.
122. Khot A, Bowditch M, Powell J, et al. The use of intradiscal steroid therapy for lumbar spinal discogenic pain: a randomized controlled trial. Spine 2004; 29:833–836; discussion 837.
123. Woodward AH. Re Khot A, Bowditch M, Powell J, et al. The use of intradiscal steroid therapy for lumbar spinal discogenic pain: a randomized controlled trial. Spine 2004; 29:833–837, 2474–2475.
124. Buttermann GR. The effect of spinal steroid injections for degenerative disc disease. Spine J 2004; 4:495–505.
125. Wehling P. The use of combination of IL-1ra/IGF-1/PDGF in the treatment of lumbar disc pain: pathophysiological background, safety, and 6 month clinical experience. 29th International Society for the Study of the Lumbar Spine. Cleveland, OH, May 14–18, 2002.
126. Tobinick EL, Britschgi-Davoodifar S. Perispinal TNF-alpha inhibition for discogenic pain. Swiss Med Wkly 2003; 133:170–177.
127. Cunha FQ, Poole S, Lorenzetti BB, et al. The pivotal role of tumour necrosis factor alpha in the development of inflammatory hyperalgesia. Br J Pharmacol 1992; 107:660–664.
128. Ferreira SH, Lorenzetti BB, Bristow AF, et al. Interleukin-1 beta as a potent hyperalgesic agent antagonized by a tripeptide analogue. Nature 1988; 334:698–700.
129. McMahon SB, Bennett DL, Priestley JV, et al. The biological effects of endogenous nerve growth factor on adult sensory neurons revealed by a trkA-IgG fusion molecule. Nat Med 1995; 1:774–780.
130. Bennett DL, Koltzenburg M, Priestley JV, et al. Endogenous nerve growth factor regulates the sensitivity of nociceptors in the adult rat. Eur J Neurosci 1998; 10:1282–1291.
131. Ro LS, Chen ST, Tang LM, et al. Effect of NGF and anti-NGF on neuropathic pain in rats following chronic constriction injury of the sciatic nerve. Pain 1999; 79:265–274.
132. Diamond J, Holmes M, Coughlin M. Endogenous NGF and nerve impulses regulate the collateral sprouting of sensory axons in the skin of the adult rat. J Neurosci 1992; 12:1454–1466.
133. Saal JS, Saal JA. Management of chronic discogenic low back pain with a thermal intradiscal catheter. A preliminary report. Spine 2000; 25:382–388.
134. Saal JA, Saal JS. Intradiscal electrothermal treatment for chronic discogenic low back pain: a prospective outcome study with minimum 1-year follow-up. Spine 2000; 25:2622–2627.
135. Saal JA, Saal JS. Intradiscal electrothermal treatment for chronic discogenic low back pain: prospective outcome study with a minimum 2-year follow-up. Spine 2002; 27:966–973; discussion 973–964.
136. Wetzel FT, McNally TA, Phillips FM. Intradiscal electrothermal therapy used to manage chronic discogenic low back pain: new directions and interventions. Spine 2002; 27:2621–2626.
137. Biyani A, Andersson GB, Chaudhary H, et al. Intradiscal electrothermal therapy: a treatment option in patients with internal disc disruption. Spine 2003; 28:S8–S14.
138. Pauza KJ, Howell S, Dreyfuss P, et al. A randomized, placebo-controlled trial of intradiscal electrothermal therapy for the treatment of discogenic low back pain. Spine J 2004; 4:27–35.
139. Shah RV, Lutz GE, Lee J, et al. Intradiskal electrothermal therapy: a preliminary histologic study. Arch Phys Med Rehabil 2001; 82:1230–1237.
140. Pollintine P, Findlay G, Adams MA. Intradiscal electrothermal therapy can alter compressive stress distributions inside degenerated intervertebral discs. Spine 2005; 30:E134–E139.

141. Kleinstueck FS, Diederich CJ, Nau WH, et al. Temperature and thermal dose distributions during intradiscal electrothermal therapy in the cadaveric lumbar spine. Spine 2003; 28: 1700–1708; discussion 1709.

142. Freeman BJ, Walters RM, Moore RJ, et al. Does intradiscal electrothermal therapy denervate and repair experimentally induced posterolateral annular tears in an animal model? Spine 2003; 28:2602–2608.

143. Barrick WT, Schofferman JA, Reynolds JB, et al. Anterior lumbar fusion improves discogenic pain at levels of prior posterolateral fusion. Spine 2000; 25:853–857.

144. Fritzell P, Hagg O, Wessberg P, et al. Chronic low back pain and fusion: a comparison of three surgical techniques: a prospective multicenter randomized study from the Swedish lumbar spine study group. Spine 2002; 27:1131–1141.

145. Grevitt MP, Gardner AD, Spilsbury J, et al. The Graf stabilisation system: early results in 50 patients. Eur Spine J 1995; 4:169–175; discussion 135.

146. Gardner A, Pande KC. Graf ligamentoplasty: a 7-year follow-up. Eur Spine J 2002; 11(suppl 2): S157–S163.

147. German JW, Foley KT. Disc arthroplasty in the management of the painful lumbar motion segment. Spine 2005; 30:S60–S67.

148. Sakai D, Mochida J, Yamamoto Y, et al. Transplantation of mesenchymal stem cells embedded in Atelocollagen gel to the intervertebral disc: a potential therapeutic model for disc degeneration. Biomaterials 2003; 24:3531–3541.

149. An HS, Takegami K, Kamada H, et al. Intradiscal administration of osteogenic protein-1 increases intervertebral disc height and proteoglycan content in the nucleus pulposus in normal adolescent rabbits. Spine 2005; 30:25–31; discussion 31–22.

150. Yoon ST, Park JS, Kim KS, et al. ISSLS prize winner: LMP-1 upregulates intervertebral disc cell production of proteoglycans and BMPs in vitro and in vivo. Spine 2004; 29:2603–2611.

151. Butler D, Trafimow JH, Andersson GB, et al. Discs degenerate before facets. Spine 1990; 15:111–113.

152. Swanepoel MW, Adams LM, Smeathers JE. Human lumbar apophyseal joint damage and intervertebral disc degeneration. Ann Rheum Dis 1995; 54:182–188.

153. Moore RJ, Crotti TN, Osti OL, et al. Osteoarthrosis of the facet joints resulting from anular rim lesions in sheep lumbar discs. Spine 1999; 24:519–525.

21 | Molecular Diagnosis of Spinal Infection

Naomi Kobayashi
Department of Anatomic Pathology and Orthopaedic Surgery, The Cleveland Clinic Foundation, Cleveland, Ohio, U.S.A.

Gary W. Procop
Clinical Microbiology, The Cleveland Clinic Foundation, Cleveland, Ohio, U.S.A.

Hiroshige Sakai
Department of Anatomic Pathology and Orthopaedic Surgery, The Cleveland Clinic Foundation, Cleveland, Ohio, U.S.A.

Daisuke Togawa and Thomas W. Bauer
Department of Anatomic Pathology and Orthopaedic Surgery and The Spine Institute, The Cleveland Clinic Foundation, Cleveland, Ohio, U.S.A.

INTRODUCTION

Infectious diseases, including infection after surgery, are troublesome problems for orthopedic surgeons. Vertebral osteomyelitis or diskitis is the most common spinal infectious disease, and the most frequent etiologic agent is *Staphylococcus aureus* (1). Less commonly, organisms such as *Eikenella* (2), *Candida* sp. (3), and *Bacteroides* sp. (4), amongst others may also cause vertebral osteomyelitis. *Mycobacterium tuberculosis* (*Tb*) is also an important cause of spinal infection (i.e., Pott's Disease), especially in developing parts of the world. Nontuberculosis mycobacteria may also cause vertebral osteomyelitis (5). Thus, like most orthopedic infections, a wide variety of organisms can be important pathogens, but most infections are due to *S. aureus* (6).

More rapid and accurate identification of the causative organisms of infectious diseases have direct implications for successful treatment. The basis of bacterial identification continues to utilize the Gram stain, conventional culture, and biochemical identification. Histologic identification of microorganisms in tissue, and noting the acute inflammation that accompanies an infection can also be helpful for diagnosis (7). In most hospitals, these conventional methods continue to be the first and only choice. However, sensitivity, and specificity are ongoing problems, with some cases of osteomyelitis remaining culture negative (8). The identification of *Tb* takes a very long time by culture, and Ziehl-Nielsen staining of direct clinical specimens lacks sensitivity (9). With recent developments in molecular biological technology, several new methods to diagnose infection have emerged. The basis for most new assays is the polymerase chain reaction (PCR), a test that can detect bacteria at the molecular level.

In this Chapter, we describe several recently developed assays using molecular methods to diagnose spinal infections.

CONVENTIONAL POLYMERASE CHAIN REACTION

PCR technology has been developed during the past two decades and has been applied as a diagnostic method for a variety of infectious diseases (10–13). The basic principle of PCR consists of three steps. Briefly, the first step is denaturation of double-stranded DNA. As a second step, primers (forward and reverse) anneal to each target sequence. The final step is the extension of primers through the action of DNA polymerase. These three steps in effect copy the target DNA, and repeating these steps amplifies the target DNA exponentially. This PCR technology makes it possible to identify bacterial DNA with much higher sensitivity compared with culture methods, and may be superior to culture in some situations, particularly for the detection of fastidious microorganisms.

Mariani et al. were the first to apply PCR for the detection of bacterial DNA in orthopedic infections (14). They showed higher sensitivity of PCR comparing with standard culture for detecting of bacteria from synovial fluid, and suggested the importance of molecular assays. Following this, several investigators (15–19) have applied PCR for detecting bacterial DNA from orthopedic specimens, especially joint implants. The important point of detecting adherent bacteria on implants and instruments, is that many of these bacteria form a biofilm (20,21) that makes it difficult to isolate the organism using conventional microbiologic techniques. Ha et al. (22) investigated biofilm formation on various types of spinal implants, and noted that it is important to dislodge the biofilm by some mechanical method, such as ultrasound (23,24) or scraping (25). Tunney et al. (18) applied PCR combined with ultrasonication for hip implants, and suggested that occult infections have not been detected by conventional culture. However, Ince et al. (16) reported that PCR was not superior to routine bacteriologic culture for detection of low-grade infections associated with implants and concluded that aseptic loosening of implants might not be related to low-grade infection. The differences of results between these PCR studies might be due to the several factors, including differences in the sites from which specimens were collected, patient category, and the sensitivity of each PCR assay itself, and the traditional microbiologic methods used. Thus, the interpretation of PCR results related to bacteria that are adherent to implants has been controversial.

Most of these studies have employed a universal PCR that targets a portion of the 16S rRNA gene, which codes for ribosomal RNA. Ribosomal RNA is an essential constituent for all organisms, so using PCR to target conserved regions in the 16S rRNA gene allows detection of a wide variety of bacteria and has been used in various infectious diseases (26–29). One significant limitation of this approach is that contaminating bacteria or even bacterial DNA may be detected thereby producing false-positive results.

REAL-TIME POLYMERASE CHAIN REACTION

Recently, so-called "real-time PCR" has been developed and has been broadly applied for clinical use (30). This is a new format of PCR, more formally known as homogeneous PCR, wherein both amplification and detection of target DNA occurs simultaneously and within the same reaction vessel, using a variety of fluorescently-labelled detector molecules. In addition, the "time-to-positivity," as determined by the crossing threshold (Ct) can be used to quantify the amount of DNA present (i.e., real-time PCR is innately a quantitative reaction). In other words, we can see the amplification of target DNA early in the PCR reaction, representing a higher concentration of target DNA. Therefore, it is possible to quantify the concentration of target DNA by comparing the Ct of the test specimen with quantitative standards. Another useful feature of real-time PCR is "melt-curve analysis," which may be performed following the amplification reaction. These features of real-time PCR are based on the binding of the fluorescently-labeled probes to the amplified product. Oligonucleotide detector probes termed fluorescence resonance energy transfer (FRET) probes provide some of the most useful melting curves, and can even differentiate single nucleotide polymorphisms (SNPs). Briefly, these two probes bind adjacent to one another at a specific site of the amplified DNA. When these probes are hybridized, they generate specific fluorescence that is detected by a charge-coupled device (CCD) camera. When thermal energy is incrementally introduced into the system while fluorescence is monitored, then a melting curve analysis is performed. As the thermal energy breaks the hydrogen bonds that hold the oligonucleotide FRET probes in place, the specific fluorescence will be lost. The peak temperature at which the probes are dissociated depends on the binding affinity of the probes to amplified product (amplicon), which in turn is directly related to the oligonucleotide sequence. Based on these technologies, we have developed several real-time PCR assays, optimized these for use in detecting orthopedic infection, and have validated the reliability of these methods on specimens from patients with clinical spinal infections, as described subsequently.

GENUS OR SPECIES-SPECIFIC POLYMERASE CHAIN REACTION

One persistent problem with PCR is the occurrence of false positive results related to its high sensitivity (31–34). Prior to the advent of real-time PCR, contamination was often secondary to the inadvertent introduction of amplicon into the laboratory. Amplicons, the small amplified products of the PCR reaction, are high-efficiency templates that are responsible for false-positive reactions if they are introduced into clinical specimens. Another cause of false-positive reactions that is unique to "broad-range" bacterial PCR is the presence of *Escherichia coli* DNA that is naturally associated with DNA polymerase reagent, since thermostable DNA polymerase is obtained from recombinant *E. coli*.

One strategy to avoid this contamination issue is to use "species-specific PCR," that does not detect *E. coli* DNA. Species-specific real-time PCR assays have been developed for many kinds of bacterial organisms (35–39), and from an orthopedic perspective would be best applied when a particular organism is expected based on the clinical setting or radiographic findings, for example a typical case of spinal tuberculosis (40–42). Naturally a limitation of a species-specific PCR assay, however, is that it will not detect other organisms.

An alternative, perhaps intermediate, solution is the development of "genus" specific PCR, to detect a group of important bacteria that does not include *E. coli*. For example, we designed a genus-specific primer and probe set for the LightCycler® (Roche Applied Science, Indianapolis, Indiana, U.S.A.) based on the *tuf* gene (36), which encodes for the elongation factor Tu, an essential constituent of the bacterial genome. The *tuf* gene has been used for several genus specific assays previously (43,44). In our assay, the target was *Staphylococcus* species which includes *S. aureus* and *S. epidermidis*, the most frequent bacteria causing orthopedic infections (1,45–47). One of the advantages of this assay is that we have been able to get negative results for negative controls, that is, the *E. coli* DNA associated with DNA polymerase is not detected and therefore does not cause a false-positive reaction. This assay detects all *Staphylococcus* species, but the negative control (nuclease-free water), which contains DNA polymerase, is negative (Fig. 1).

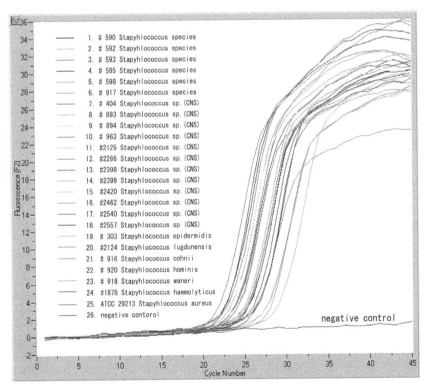

FIGURE 1 *Staphylococcus* species-specific real-time polymerase chain reaction. All test samples DNA of *Staphylococcus* species were positive, while the negative control was negative.

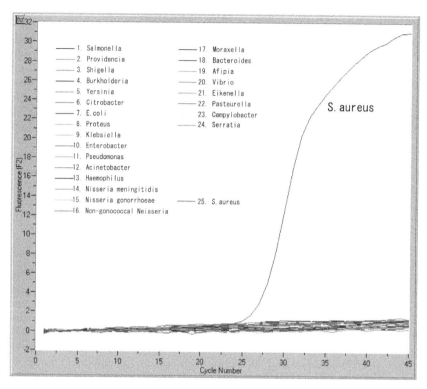

FIGURE 2 Specificity test for *Staphylococcus* species-specific real-time polymerase chain reaction. A sample of *S. aureus* was positive, while all other bacteria were negative.

Furthermore, most bacteria except *Staphylococcus* species were negative (Fig. 2). We showed extremely high specificity and sensitivity for blood cultures with this assay (36). This specificity may be very useful for diagnosis of typical pyogenic osteomyelitis caused by *Staphylococcus* species, but it is insufficient to detect occasional infections caused by gram-negative bacteria or *M. tuberculosis*. Shrestha et al. (37) described a broad-range real-time PCR that detects mycobacteria and differentiates *M. tuberculosis* from nontuberculosis mycobacteria. We have used this assay numerous times on clinical specimens in whom disease caused by mycobacteria was suspected; this assay proved useful to identify *M. tuberculosis* more rapidly than traditional culture (48). One patient had skeletal tuberculosis, not of the spine, but rather of the femoral condyle. In this case, the infection was not suspected before surgery, but when necrotizing granulomas were discovered the mycobacteria PCR was ordered, which proved positive. Thus, real-time PCR, especially an assay that may provide species level information, can be useful for rapid, definite diagnosis in clinical use.

BROAD-RANGE UNIVERSAL POLYMERASE CHAIN REACTION

When screening a bacterial infection, wherein any of the numerous clinically-important bacteria may be the cause of disease, a broad-range "universal" bacterial PCR is desirable. As described earlier, most universal PCR assays target the 16S rRNA gene. We also have evaluated a primer set of our design for the 16S rRNA gene, which was optimized to detect the most common causes of orthopedic infections. These primers were designed to ensure the detection of the six gram-positive species and five gram-negative species that are most frequently associated with orthopedic infections (Table 1), and to exclude common contaminants such as *Propionibacterium acne* (*P. acne*). Figure 3 shows that all samples of cultured bacterial strains were positive with this PCR, including the negative control. The amplification of nuclease free water and *P. acne* were almost the same, and later than 30 cycles, which was

TABLE 1   The Target Bacteria of Universal Polymerase Chain Reaction
Optimized for Orthopedic Infections

Gram-positive bacteria	Gram-negative bacteria
Staphylococcus aureus	*Escherichia coli*
Staphylococcus epidermidis	*Enterobacter* sp.
Viridans streptococci	*Klebsiella pneumoniae*
Streptococcus pneumoniae	*Proteus mirabilis*
Streptococcus pyogenes	*Pseudomonas aeruginosa*
Enterococcus sp.	

definitely later than other bacteria. Because of the issue of DNA polymerase containing *E. coli* DNA from the recombinant *E. coli* strain from which it was derived, we defined as true positives as those specimens wherein the amplification occurred prior to the cycle at which nuclease free water demonstrated amplification. Adherence to this definition would result in the classification of the *P. acne* as negative, which was our intention (Fig. 3). The FRET hybridization probes used with this assay were designed to distinguish gram-positive and gram-negative species by postamplification melt-curve analysis (Fig. 4). The FRET hybridization probes were 100% homologous with the target hybridization site in gram-positive bacteria, which results in a higher melting peak temperature, compared with the lower melting peak temperature of the gram-negative bacteria wherein there is incomplete homology between the FRET probes and the hybridization site (i.e., nucleotide mismatches). To further differentiate these bacteria, we explored another technology, DNA sequencing by synthesis.

SEQUENCING ASSAY

A truly broad-range universal bacterial PCR targets numerous bacterial species that include gram-positive and gram-negative bacteria, as well as mycobacteria and nocardiae. Although conceivably every possible bacterial species that demonstrated amplification with such an assay could be identified with a specific hybridization probe, this approach is labor-intense and cost-ineffective. An alternative, cost-effective approach for the determination of the identity of the bacterium is by postamplification DNA sequencing. The traditional sequencing by termination (i.e., Sanger sequencing) approach has been used successfully by many groups for the sequence-based identification of bacteria, mycobacteria, and fungi (49–51).

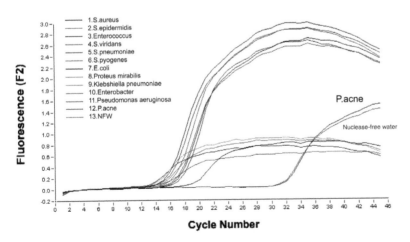

FIGURE 3   Broad-range universal real-time polymerase chain reaction optimized for the detection of bacterial pathogens associated with orthopedic infections. All samples were positive, but the amplification of *Prepionibacterium acnes* and nuclease-free water occurred after 30 cycles, which was obviously later than other samples.

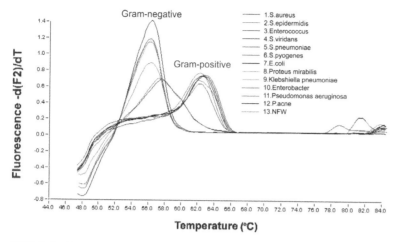

FIGURE 4 Melting peak analysis of universal real-time polymerase chain reaction. All gram-negative species had lower melting peaks than all gram-positive species except for *Propionibacterium acnes*.

A relatively new method of DNA sequencing, sequencing-by-synthesis or pyrosequencing, is now available. Pyrosequencing is relatively new light-generating sequencing technology (52–54) that could be described as "real-time" sequencing (55,56), and is based on a different principle than Sanger sequencing. We have used a Pyrosequencing® (Biotage, Inc., Massachusetts) assay (57) to differentiate gram-positive from gram-negative bacteria species based on an SNP. The third nucleotide position generated from our sequencing primer differentiated the vast majority of gram-positive from gram-negative bacterial species (57). In addition to the Gram stain information, additional downstream sequence information was useful for subclassification of many of the gram-negative bacilli. For example, we described a clinical situation of a spinal infection wherein the assay correctly characterized the etiologic agent as a gram-negative bacillus, but also further subclassified it into a subset of the Enterobacteriacieae that contained *Proteus mirabilis*, which the culture confirmed as the causative agent (Fig. 5) (57). In this case, the sequence generated was GGTCGATTTAACGCGTTA. The presence of a "T" in the third nucleotide position (GGT) classified the bacteria present as a gram-negative organism. Prior to testing, this had been confirmed by analyzing numerous GenBank database (58) sequences, as well as testing and validation battery of well characterized bacterial isolates (57). Furthermore, downstream sequences made it possible to categorize the organism in a group of Enterobacteriaceae that contained *P. mirabilis*. A comparison with the 16S rRNA partial gene of *P. mirabilis* obtained from GenBank demonstrates a perfect match with the sequence that we obtained from pyrosequencing. We have subsequently specimens from 13 patients with clinical spinal infections, which included deep wound infection, epidural abscess, osteomyelitis, and diskitis. With conventional culture, six cases were negative, six were gram-positive species, and one was gram-negative species. The PCR result and molecular gram stain classification by pyrosequencing were all compatible with culture results. Figure 6 is another example of pyrosequencing for a case of deep wound infection

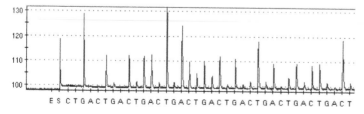

FIGURE 5 Pyrosequencing for a clinical sample. The sequences were read as GGTCGATTTAACGCGTTA ... that was identified as gram-negative species and *Proteus mirabilis* group. *Source*: From Ref. 57.

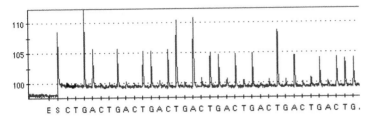

FIGURE 6 Pyrosequencing for another clinical sample. The sequences were read as GGAGTGCTTAATGC ... that was categorized as gram-positive, *Staphylococcus aureus* group.

after spinal reconstruction. These sequences were read as GGAGTGCTTAATGC ... , which was compatible with the expected sequences of *S. aureus* by GenBank database (Fig. 7). The culture result was also *S. aureus*. Thus, the combination of real-time PCR and pyrosequencing may represent a powerful tool for rapid identification and characterization of bacteria causing spinal infections and other orthopedic infections.

OTHER MOLECULAR ASSAYS

DNA microarray is relatively new technology (59), which can detect numerous gene expressions simultaneously, and has also been applied to infectious diseases (60–63). It can be useful also for identification of biofilm-formative strain (64). Fluorescent in situ hybridization (FISH) is a technique that can be used to localize some specific DNA sequences, and also can be applied bacterial identification (65–67). This assay is useful to identify a species in relatively large number of bacteria such as cultured blood specimens. Though each of these technologies has its own advantages, they have not been applied to orthopedic infections at present and need more experiments for clinical use.

PROBLEMS AND LIMITATIONS

We have described the usefulness, and potential advantages of molecular assays for diagnosing infection, but assays of this type are not yet in routine clinical use for several reasons. The first problem is cost effectiveness. Although PCR has been recognized as having adequate cost effectiveness (68,69), other emerging assays such as Pyrosequencing may still be too expensive for clinical routine use. Another factor that needs improvement is the DNA extraction. Manual extraction methods take about two hours, which is substantially longer than real-time PCR and Pyrosequening itself. Recently, automated DNA extraction methods such as MagNA Pure (Roche Diagnostics, Indiana, U.S.A.) have become available and are expected to improve turnaround time (70). We are investigating a direct real-time PCR without prior

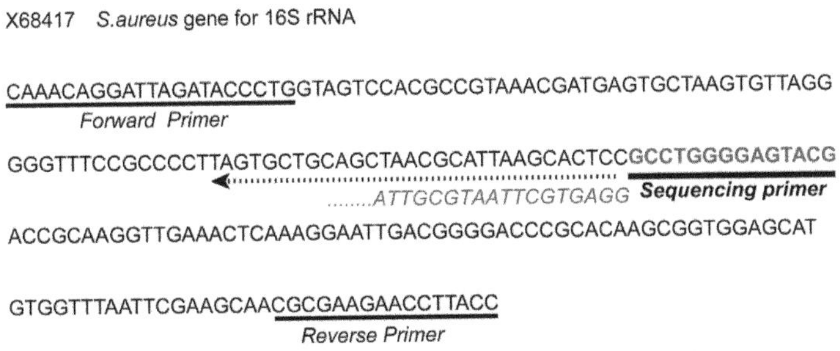

X68417   *S.aureus* gene for 16S rRNA

CAAACAGGATTAGATACCCTGGTAGTCCACGCCGTAAACGATGAGTGCTAAGTGTTAGG
          Forward Primer

GGGTTTCCGCCCCTTAGTGCTGCAGCTAACGCATTAAGCACTCCGCCTGGGGAGTACG
          ◄···
                 ....*ATTGCGTAATTCGTGAGG* **Sequencing primer**
ACCGCAAGGTTGAAACTCAAAGGAATTGACGGGGACCCGCACAAGCGGTGGAGCAT

GTGGTTTAATTCGAAGCAACGCGAAGAACCTTACC
          Reverse Primer

FIGURE 7 16S rRNA gene of *Staphylococcus aureus* obtained from GenBank database, which will be amplified by universal polymerase chain reaction. The expected sequence next to the sequencing primer is GGAGTGCTTAATGC ... , a match to the sequence that was obtained.

DNA extraction for joint implants, in which ultrasonication is used for both biofilm dislodgement and DNA release (71,72).

One of the most important limitations of the 16S rRNA universal PCR based assay is the presence of native bacterial DNA in the recombinant DNA Polymerase reagent (31–34) as described above. Corless et al. (32) have investigated several methods to eliminate contamination in the Taq reagent, and showed it was difficult without loss of sensitivity. The use of ultra pure Taq reagent in the future should allow much greater sensitivity of universal PCR assays, without the problem of false-positive reactions. The use of combinations of several assays might be necessary to screen samples, and to then identify organisms with enough specificity to guide antibiotic use.

CONCLUSION

Clinical judgment should always been used when interpreting laboratory test results, including PCR results. This is especially when there is a discrepancy between PCR and culture results, or a discrepancy between any laboratory test and the clinical findings. The presence of a positive PCR result in the presence of a negative culture may be due to (*i*) a true positive PCR result indicating an infection that was not detectable by culture, (*ii*) PCR detection of nonviable bacteria, and (*iii*) a false positive PCR result due to contamination of the sample or of a reagent. It may be difficult to resolve these possibilities using laboratory data alone. In such instances, correlation with histology, radiographic findings, and clinical symptoms may be more important than ever. Molecular technology will continue to make steady progress in the future, will gradually be implemented as a routine method for the detection of more and more infectious agents, and will, hopefully, enhance our ability to more aptly diagnose infectious diseases. It is therefore important for all surgeons to understand the basic principles, advantages, disadvantages, limitations, and clinical importance of these tests as they become available.

REFERENCES

1. Carragee EJ. Pyogenic vertebral osteomyelitis. J Bone Joint Surg Am 1997; 79(6):874–880.
2. Lehman CR, Deckey JE, Hu SS. *Eikenella corrodens* vertebral osteomyelitis secondary to direct inoculation: a case report. Spine 2000; 25(9):1185–1187.
3. Garbino J, Schnyder I, Lew D, et al. An unusual cause of vertebral osteomyelitis: Candida species. Scand J Infect Dis 2003; 35(4):288–291.
4. Mukhopadhyay S, Rose F, Frechette V. Vertebral osteomyelitis caused by Prevotella (Bacteroides) melaninogenicus. South Med J 2005; 98(2):226–228.
5. Petitjean G, Fluckiger U, Scharen S, et al. Vertebral osteomyelitis caused by non-tuberculous mycobacteria. Clin Microbiol Infect 2004; 10(11):951–953.
6. Weisz RD, Errico TJ. Spinal infections. Diagnosis and treatment. Bull Hosp Jt Dis 2000; 59(1):40–46.
7. Bauer TW, Brooks PJ, Sakai H, et al. A diagnostic algorithm for detecting an infected hip arthroplasty. Orthopedics 2003; 26(9):929–930.
8. Floyed RL, Steele RW. Culture-negative osteomyelitis. Pediatr Infect Dis J 2003; 22(8):731–736.
9. Kivihya-Ndugga L, van Cleeff M, Juma E, et al. Comparison of PCR with the routine procedure for diagnosis of tuberculosis in a population with high prevalences of tuberculosis and human immunodeficiency virus. J Clin Microbiol 2004; 42(3):1012–1015.
10. Eisenstein BI. The polymerase chain reaction. A new method of using molecular genetics for medical diagnosis. N Engl J Med 1990; 322(3):178–183.
11. Eisenstein BI. New molecular techniques for microbial epidemiology and the diagnosis of infectious diseases. J Infect Dis 1990; 161(4):595–602.
12. Tang YW, Procop GW, Persing DH. Molecular diagnostics of infectious diseases. Clin Chem 1997; 43(11):2021–2038.
13. Yang S, Rothman RE. PCR-based diagnostics for infectious diseases: uses, limitations, and future applications in acute-care settings. Lancet Infect Dis 2004; 4(6):337–348.
14. Mariani BD, Martin DS, Levine MJ, et al. The Coventry Award. Polymerase chain reaction detection of bacterial infection in total knee arthroplasty. Clin Orthop 1996; 331:11–22.
15. Clarke MT, Roberts CP, Lee PT, et al. Polymerase chain reaction can detect bacterial DNA in aseptically loose total hip arthroplasties. Clin Orthop Relat Res 2004; 427:132–137.
16. Ince A, Rupp J, Frommelt L, et al. Is "aseptic" loosening of the prosthetic cup after total hip replacement due to nonculturable bacterial pathogens in patients with low-grade infection? Clin Infect Dis 2004; 39(11):1599–1603.

17. Tunney MM, Patrick S, Curran MD, et al. Detection of prosthetic joint biofilm infection using immunological and molecular techniques. Methods Enzymol 1999; 310:566–576.
18. Tunney MM, Patrick S, Curran MD, et al. Detection of prosthetic hip infection at revision arthroplasty by immunofluorescence microscopy and PCR amplification of the bacterial 16S rRNA gene. J Clin Microbiol 1999; 37(10):3281–3290.
19. Tarkin IS, Henry TJ, Fey PI, et al. PCR rapidly detects methicillin-resistant staphylococci periprosthetic infection. Clin Orthop Relat Res 2003; 414:89–94.
20. Donlan RM. Biofilm formation: a clinically relevant microbiological process. Clin Infect Dis 2001; 33(8):1387–1392.
21. Dunne WM, Jr. Bacterial adhesion: seen any good biofilms lately? Clin Microbiol Rev 2002; 15(2):155–166.
22. Ha KY, Chung YG, Ryoo SJ. Adherence and biofilm formation of Staphylococcus epidermidis and Mycobacterium tuberculosis on various spinal implants. Spine 2005; 30(1):38–43.
23. Nguyen LL, Nelson CL, Saccente M, et al. Detecting bacterial colonization of implanted orthopaedic devices by ultrasonication. Clin Orthop Relat Res 2002; 403:29–37.
24. Tunney MM, Patrick S, Gorman SP, et al. Improved detection of infection in hip replacements. A currently underestimated problem. J Bone Joint Surg Br 1998; 80(4):568–572.
25. Neut D, van Horn JR, van Kooten TG, et al. Detection of biomaterial-associated infections in orthopaedic joint implants. Clin Orthop 2003; 413:261–268.
26. Goldenberger D, Kunzli A, Vogt P, et al. Molecular diagnosis of bacterial endocarditis by broad-range PCR amplification and direct sequencing. J Clin Microbiol 1997; 35(11):2733–2739.
27. Greisen K, Loeffelholz M, Purohit A, et al. PCR primers and probes for the 16S rRNA gene of most species of pathogenic bacteria, including bacteria found in cerebrospinal fluid. J Clin Microbiol 1994; 32(2):335–351.
28. Monstein HJ, Kihlstrom E, Tiveljung A. Detection and identification of bacteria using in-house broad range 16S rDNA PCR amplification and genus-specific DNA hybridization probes, located within variable regions of 16S rRNA genes. Apmis 1996; 104(6):451–458.
29. Lang S, Watkin RW, Lambert PA, et al. Evaluation of PCR in the molecular diagnosis of endocarditis. J Infect 2004; 48(3):269–275.
30. Mackay IM. Real-time PCR in the microbiology laboratory. Clin Microbiol Infect 2004; 10(3):190–212.
31. Meier A, Persing DH, Finken M, et al. Elimination of contaminating DNA within polymerase chain reaction reagents: implications for a general approach to detection of uncultured pathogens. J Clin Microbiol 1993; 31(3):646–652.
32. Corless CE, Guiver M, Borrow R, et al. Contamination and sensitivity issues with a real-time universal 16S rRNA PCR. J Clin Microbiol 2000; 38(5):1747–1752.
33. Trampuz A, Osmon DR, Hanssen AD, et al. Molecular and antibiofilm approaches to prosthetic joint infection. Clin Orthop 2003; (414):69–88.
34. Newsome T, Li BJ, Zou N, et al. Presence of bacterial phage-like DNA sequences in commercial Taq DNA polymerase reagents. J Clin Microbiol 2004; 42(5):2264–2267.
35. Farrell JJ, Doyle LJ, Addison RM, et al. Broad-range (pan) Salmonella and Salmonella serotype typhi-specific real-time PCR assays: potential tools for the clinical microbiologist. Am J Clin Pathol 2005; 123(3):339–345.
36. Sakai H, Procop GW, Kobayashi N, et al. Simultaneous detection of Staphylococcus aureus and coagulase-negative staphylococci in positive blood cultures by real-time PCR with two fluorescence resonance energy transfer probe sets. J Clin Microbiol 2004; 42(12):5739–5744.
37. Shrestha NK, Tuohy MJ, Hall GS, et al. Detection and differentiation of Mycobacterium tuberculosis and nontuberculous mycobacterial isolates by real-time PCR. J Clin Microbiol 2003; 41(11):5121–5126.
38. Wilson DA, Yen-Lieberman B, Reischl U, et al. Detection of Legionella pneumophila by real-time PCR for the mip gene. J Clin Microbiol 2003; 41(7):3327–3330.
39. Shrestha NK, Tuohy MJ, Hall GS, et al. Rapid identification of Staphylococcus aureus and the mecA gene from BacT/ALERT blood culture bottles by using the LightCycler system. J Clin Microbiol 2002; 40(7):2659–2661.
40. Joseffer SS, Cooper PR. Modern imaging of spinal tuberculosis. J Neurosurg Spine 2005; 2(2):145–150.
41. De Vuyst D, Vanhoenacker F, Gielen J, et al. Imaging features of musculoskeletal tuberculosis. Eur Radiol 2003; 13(8):1809–1819.
42. Griffith JF, Kumta SM, Leung PC, et al. Imaging of musculoskeletal tuberculosis: a new look at an old disease. Clin Orthop Relat Res 2002; (398):32–39.
43. Ke D, Picard FJ, Martineau F, et al. Development of a PCR assay for rapid detection of enterococci. J Clin Microbiol 1999; 37(11):3497–3503.
44. Martineau F, Picard FJ, Ke D, et al. Development of a PCR assay for identification of staphylococci at genus and species levels. J Clin Microbiol 2001; 39(7):2541–2547.
45. Haddad FS, Masri BA, Campbell D, et al. The PROSTALAC functional spacer in two-stage revision for infected knee replacements. Prosthesis of antibiotic-loaded acrylic cement. J Bone Joint Surg Br 2000; 82(6):807–812.

46. Dietz FR, Koontz FP, Found EM, et al. The importance of positive bacterial cultures of specimens obtained during clean orthopaedic operations. J Bone Joint Surg Am 1991; 73(8):1200–1207.
47. Sanderson PJ. Infection in orthopaedic implants. J Hosp Infect 1991; 18(Suppl A):367–375.
48. Kobayashi N, Fraser T, Bauer TW, et al. The use of real-time PCR for rapid diagnosis of skeletal tuberculosis. A Case Report. Arch Pathol Lab Med 2006; 130(7):1053–1056.
49. Woo PC, Tsoi HW, Leung KW, et al. Identification of Mycobacterium neoaurum isolated from a neutropenic patient with catheter-related bacteremia by 16S rRNA sequencing. J Clin Microbiol 2000; 38(9):3515–3517.
50. Clarridge JE 3rd. Impact of 16S rRNA gene sequence analysis for identification of bacteria on clinical microbiology and infectious diseases. Clin Microbiol Rev 2004; 17(4):840–862.
51. Patel JB. 16S rRNA gene sequencing for bacterial pathogen identification in the clinical laboratory. Mol Diagn 2001; 6(4):313–321.
52. Grahn N, Olofsson M, Ellnebo-Svedlund K, et al. Identification of mixed bacterial DNA contamination in broad-range PCR amplification of 16S rDNA V1 and V3 variable regions by pyrosequencing of cloned amplicons. FEMS Microbiol Lett 2003; 219(1):87–91.
53. Tuohy MJ, Hall GS, Sholtis M, et al. Pyrosequencing as a tool for the identification of common isolates of Mycobacterium sp. Diagn Microbiol Infect Dis 2005; 51(4):245–250.
54. Jordan JA, Butchko AR, Durso MB. Use of pyrosequencing of 16S rRNA fragments to differentiate between bacteria responsible for neonatal sepsis. J Mol Diagn 2005; 7(1):105–110.
55. Ronaghi M, Karamohamed S, Pettersson B, et al. Real-time DNA sequencing using detection of pyrophosphate release. Anal Biochem 1996; 242(1):84–89.
56. Ronaghi M, Uhlen M, Nyren P. A sequencing method based on real-time pyrophosphate. Science 1998; 281(5375):363, 365.
57. Kobayashi N, Bauer TW, Togawa D, et al. A molecular gram stain using broad range PCR and pyrosequencing technology: a potentially useful tool for diagnosing orthopaedic infections. Diagn Mol Pathol 2005; 14(2):83–89.
58. http://www.ncbi.nlm.nih.gov/
59. Schena M, Shalon D, Davis RW, et al. Quantitative monitoring of gene expression patterns with a complementary DNA microarray. Science 1995; 270(5235):467–470.
60. Bryant PA, Venter D, Robins-Browne R, et al. Chips with everything: DNA microarrays in infectious diseases. Lancet Infect Dis 2004; 4(2):100–111.
61. Call DR. Challenges and opportunities for pathogen detection using DNA microarrays. Crit Rev Microbiol 2005; 31(2):91–99.
62. Campbell CJ, Ghazal P. Molecular signatures for diagnosis of infection: application of microarray technology. J Appl Microbiol 2004; 96(1):18–23.
63. Piersanti S, Martina Y, Cherubini G, et al. Use of DNA microarrays to monitor host response to virus and virus-derived gene therapy vectors. Am J Pharmacogen 2004; 4(6):345–356.
64. Lazazzera BA. Lessons from DNA microarray analysis: the gene expression profile of biofilms. Curr Opin Microbiol 2005; 8(2):222–227.
65. Gonzalez V, Padilla E, Gimenez M, et al. Rapid diagnosis of Staphylococcus aureus bacteremia using S. aureus PNA FISH. Eur J Clin Microbiol Infect Dis 2004; 23(5):396–398.
66. Moter A, Gobel UB. Fluorescence in situ hybridization (FISH) for direct visualization of microorganisms. J Microbiol Methods 2000; 41(2):85–112.
67. Wilson DA, Joyce MJ, Hall LS, et al. Multicenter evaluation of a Candida albicans peptide nucleic acid fluorescent in situ hybridization probe for characterization of yeast isolates from blood cultures. J Clin Microbiol 2005; 43(6):2909–2912.
68. van Cleeff M, Kivihya-Ndugga L, Githui W, et al. Cost-effectiveness of polymerase chain reaction versus Ziehl-Neelsen smear microscopy for diagnosis of tuberculosis in Kenya. Int J Tuberc Lung Dis 2005; 9(8):877–883.
69. Shrestha NK, Shermock KM, Gordon SM, et al. Predictive value and cost-effectiveness analysis of a rapid polymerase chain reaction for preoperative detection of nasal carriage of Staphylococcus aureus. Infect Control Hosp Epidemiol 2003; 24(5):327–333.
70. Wilson D, Yen-Lieberman B, Reischl U, et al. Comparison of five methods for extraction of Legionella pneumophila from respiratory specimens. J Clin Microbiol 2004; 42(12):5913–5916.
71. Belgrader P, Hansford D, Kovacs GT, et al. A minisonicator to rapidly disrupt bacterial spores for DNA analysis. Anal Chem 1999; 71(19):4232–4236.
72. Fykse EM, Olsen JS, Skogan G. Application of sonication to release DNA from Bacillus cereus for quantitative detection by real-time PCR. J Microbiol Methods 2003; 55(1):1–10.

22 | Review of the Effect of COX-II Agents on the Healing of a Lumbar Spine Arthrodesis

Mark R. Foster
Department of Orthopaedic Surgery, University of Pittsburgh School of Medicine, Pittsburgh, Pennsylvania, U.S.A.

MOTIVATION

Lumbar spine fusion is a major but common surgical procedure, which involves significant tissue dissection, with attendant blood loss and pain. Nonsteroidal anti-inflammatories must be stopped before surgery because of the antiplatelet activity which would increase the surgical bleeding, but the cyclooxygenase-II (COX-II)-specific inhibitors have reduced the gastrointestinal (GI) side effects and low antiplatelet activity (1,2) and further, they play an important role as a potential adjunct to other analgesics after surgery (3). A long convalescence follows, as bone healing is expected optimistically to occur in six to 12 months, and the bone fusion to mature after about two years. Following this major procedure is a prolonged convalescence, during which analgesics are required and chronic narcotic usage is common. Patients undergoing these procedures are often unable to work, deliberately stressed by the adversarial legal system, to either force them back to work expeditiously or to settle. Depression often occurs during the stress of the situation, and the depressing effect of narcotic drugs, and diminished self-image from loss of productivity. Many of these patients have unrelieved severe pain, motivating consideration of surgery and requiting significant doses of narcotics. The surgical procedure is scheduled after a sufficient duration to qualify as an exhaustion of conservation therapy, and often also delayed by insurance denials or litigation, resulting in some degree of tolerance and dependence on opioids before surgery. Inactivity during this disability and recovery may lead to weight gain, further prolonging of the subsequent rehabilitation to restore muscle tone and conditioning, and contribution to the possibility of developing a chronic dependence on opioids.

NONSTEROIDAL ANTI-INFLAMMATORY DRUGS (NSAIDs)

NSAIDs are preferred for many orthopedic injuries, such as muscular sprains and strains, to avoid narcotic habituation, and this preference is often extended to bone fractures. This common usage has not been widely recognized as a particular problem for bone healing, perhaps due to lack of awareness of the literature that might cause concern, and adequate forces driving fracture healing to overcome these potential impediments. NSAIDs are known principally to inhibit prostaglandin production, but are also understood to affect leukotriene synthesis, superoxide generation, lysosomal enzyme release, neutrophil release, and neutrophil aggregation and adhesion. Certain cell-membrane functions are also affected as enzyme activity of nicotinamide adenine dinucleotide phosphate (NADPH) oxidase in neutrophils, the activity of phospholipase C in macrophases, transmembrane anion transport, oxidative phosphorylation, and uptake of arachidonate (4). Further, leukocyte function is impaired and rheumatoid factor production is decreased. Finally, cartilage metabolism has been extensively studied as being effected by NSAIDs. Although, concern has been expressed about steroid injections in joints as toxic to the cartilage, NSAIDs may have a similar deleterious effect on chondrocyte function (5). In fact, deterioration of joints was suggested to be faster in patients with a potent inhibitor of prostaglandin synthetase (diclofenac) as opposed to a relatively mild prostaglandin inhibitor (azapropazone) (6). As cartilage is damaged in osteoarthritis, a treatment for osteoarthritis would be preferred when further toxicity on the cartilage metabolism was not at issue; however, bone healing has not had similar scrutiny.

The extensive list of effects of NSAIDs given in a "drug therapy" review (4) does not include consideration of an adverse affect on osteogenesis, or bone healing.

BONE EFFECTS OF PROSTAGLANDINS

Prostaglandins have been shown to be active in the regulation of bone metabolism (7). Prostaglandin E_2 (PGE_2) was shown to increase cyclic 3', 5', adenosinemonophosphate (AMP) to stimulate bone resorption in cultured fetal rat long bones (8). Prostaglandins are multifunctional regulators with stimulatory and inhibitory affects on bone formation and resorption. The major product of most bone cell and organ culture systems appears to be PGE_2, but there are others, such as $PGF_{2\alpha}$ and prostocyclin PG_2, also produced by skeletal tissues. Early work focused on stimulation of bone resorption, and prostaglandins were thought responsible for the hypercalcemia that occurs with malignancy (9), the inflammatory bone loss of periodontal disease (10,11), and rheumatoid arthritis (12), and a mechanism for the loosening of joint replacements (13,14).

Isolated osteoclasts showed inhibition at high concentrations of prostaglandin (15,16). This inhibition is rapid but transient as opposed to stimulation of resorption by recruitment of new osteoclasts or exogenous prostaglandins increasing their production of osteoclast—like multinuclear cells (17). The response to stimuli that activates osteoclast formation can be inhibited by nonsteroidal anti-inflammatory drugs (NSAIDs), such as indomethacin, suggesting a role for endogenous prostaglandins (18). The concept has been promoted that prostaglandins act as facilitators or enhancers of resorptive responses to cytokines and growth factors. One exception is transforming growth factor-beta (TGF-β), as TGF-β inhibits osteoclasts directly, but stimulates prostaglandin production (19). At low concentrations, TGF-β can enhance osteoclast formation for marrow cells by prostaglandin-dependent mechanism (20).

Prostaglandins have a complex role in bone remodeling, which may lead to either bone resorption or formation (21,22). Prostaglandins are produced for bone homeostasis, and regulated by mechanical forces, cytokines, growth factors, and hormones. They are involved in remodeling, produced by osteoblasts from adjacent marrow, vascular structures, and from connective tissue. Bone cells produce prostaglandins in varying amounts, particularly in bone PGE_2, which is also the most potent bone absorber. Increased PGE_2 is associated with osteoclasts, and may be responsible for erosion of cartilage, and injects the articular bone in chronic arthritic disease (23).

Stimulatory and inhibitory effects of prostaglandins in collagen synthesis were initially reported in bone organ cultures (24). At low concentrations, in the presence of glucocorticoids, PGE_2 increased collagen synthesis; whereas, at high concentrations or in the presence of insulin-like growth factor-I (IGF-1), the major effect was inhibitory. Inhibition of collagen synthesis by prostaglandins is found in cultured synovial cells and fibroblasts treated with interleukin (IL-1), and may be an important mechanism for the loss of bone and connective tissue in inflammation (25). The stimulatory or anabolic effect of cortisol in organ culture probably involves an increase in replication and differentiation with osteoblast precursors. Mitogenic and differentiation effects may be independent; cultures treated with aphidicoline (blocks DNA synthesis) still show an increase in collagen synthesis in response to PGE_2. Prostaglandins increase the differentiation of cultured bone cells, and accelerate the formation of mineralized bone nodules in vitro (26).

Prostaglandin E_2 at low concentrations stimulates alkaline phosphatase activity through cyclic AMP production (27). In cell cultures, PGE_2 and $PGF_{2\alpha}$ can stimulate DNA synthesis by cyclic AMP-independent mechanism, probably by activating protein kinase C (28). The anabolic effects of PGE_2 may be mediated by IGF-1 or $PGF_{2\alpha}$, but not PGE_2, and was found to stimulate the expression of IGF-1 receptor and IGF BP-2, but not IGF-1 production through a protein kinase C pathway (29). Prostaglandins have been shown to increase the amount of active TGF-β in the medium of cultured fetal rat long bones (30). Prostaglandins, when administered, appear to stimulate bone formation (31–34). In fracture repair, prostaglandins stimulate (35) and inhibit (36) callous formation, suggesting an important role of prostaglandins. This is less evident for the anabolic effect of endogenous prostaglandins, but the fact that heterotopic ossification occurs after hip replacement in humans (37) or demineralized bone implantation in rats (38). As this can be prevented by NSAIDs, it is suggested that endogenous prostaglandins do play a role in new bone formation.

Fracture healing in a rat model has been shown to be adversely effected by indomethacin (39,40), as have also aspirin (36) and other nonsteroidal anti-inflammatories (41). Further, bone ingrowth has been effected by indomethacin (42), in addition to aspirin and ibuprofen (43). The biological fixation of porous-coated implants (44) has also been affected. Specifically, nonsteroidal anti-inflammatories have an adverse effect on the posterior spine fusion in the rat (45). Cyclooxygenase-I is the constitutive or the "housekeeping" enzyme that regulates the homeostasis of all cells, while the COX-II enzyme is the rapidly inducible form which responds to systemic or local stress, and is inhibited by the COX-II selective inhibitors. The COX-II selective nonsteroidal anti-inflammatories have been shown to inhibit fracture healing (46), in addition to the nonselective forms (46–48) and COX-II as an enzyme appears to regulate the mesenchymal cell differentiate toward the osteoblastic line (49), and is in fact a crucial part of bone repair (50,51).

HETEROTOPIC OSSIFICATION

Patients at risk of heterotopic ossification, for example, revision of total hip surgery, have been treated with anti-inflammatories, which are recognized to be helpful in delaying mineralization (52), or inhibiting heterotopic ossification (53–55) as an alternative to radiation and other treatment for those conditions. The use of indomethacins for heterotopic ossification may result in nonunion (56) elsewhere, which may result in a relative preference in some cases for radiation prophylaxis. Unfortunately, a single dose of torodol in the recovery room, an anti-inflammatory preferred because of its lack of respiratory depression when used as an analgesic in this setting, has been shown to inhibit bone formation with actually a statistically significantly diminished result from this major lumbar procedure (57). Despite the prolonged convalescence and time for bone to heal, this result has to be considered as catastrophic with the significant risks and pain, which is undergone as part of this procedure.

The mechanism beyond the complexity of bone formation is not understood (58), but various investigations have attempted to uncover the biological process involved. The potential for using an analgesic of the COX-II category, which was approved for pain in the postoperative period, and avoiding narcotics during the prolonged convalescence of a lumbar spine fusion, would be vastly preferred to the customary situation where opioids are used for significant periods, and dependence is a substantial risk, almost presumed. This alternative would certainly be very quickly accepted into the armentariam, and would represent a very significant advantage for those patients who are otherwise customarily perpetuated indefinitely on opioids, and this represents a very substantial number of patients.

MECHANICAL FORCES

Beyond the complexity of bone formation mechanisms and regulation to balance formation and removal (osteoporosis is the lack of balance or specifically less formation than removal), we cannot presume that heterotopic bone formation has identical mechanisms. That is, bone which is formed in the intertransverse process space with posterior lumbar spine fusion or in the intervertebral disc space for an anterior lumbar spine fusion is heterotopic, and may have unique characteristics for remodeling, hemostatis, and osteogenesis. Finally, bone, which is not stressed on a regular basis, will undergo excessive remodeling or "disuse osteoporosis," as muscle contraction forces in addition to bearing weight are necessary to maintain bone integrity. For example, an ankle fracture in a cast for a prolonged period will have evident loss of bone in a spotty fashion on X-rays. For this reason, fractures are treated functionally or by weight bearing when possible. This functional treatment may also be effective in fractures, which have failed to heal. For example, tibial nonunion, where the failure of a fracture in the tibia, to heal over a customary period of time, may beneficially be treated with weight bearing forces in a cast or "functional" brace. After fracture, a medullary rod may maintain an alignment, and is preferred over a plate, as the rod stabilizes without sharing weight-bearing stresses, but if the fibular heals prematurely, a resection may be indicated to allow weight-bearing stress on the tibia. As a structural mechanical member of the body's skeleton, bone is expected to support and form a superstructure upon which muscles act and other tissues are suspended or protected.

This clinical behavior has been confirmed in vitro where bone cells have been shown to proliferate in response to mechanical stimulation (59,60). This intracellular response of cell proliferation (61), which results from the conversion of an extracellular signal—mechanical forces, is referred to as signal transduction (62). A conformational change in a receptor protein is thought to occur as a result of a ligand binding to a cell-surface receptor, and thus converting the extracellular signal into an intracellular response (63). One biochemical pathway involved in signal transduction is the inositol phosphate cascade (64). The binding of a ligand to the cell surface receptor activates C-phospholipase, a membrane-bound enzyme that hydrolyzes phosphatidyl inositol 4,5 biphosphate. This then activates two intracellular messengers inositol 1,4,5 triphosphate and diacylglyceral. The inositol 1,4,5 triphosphate causes a rapid release of calcium (65) from intracellular stores of calcium, and the increased concentration of cytosolic calcium triggers many intracellular processes. In turn, inositol 1,4,5 triphosphate is phosphorylated into inositol 1,3,4,5 tetraphosphate that further increases the concentration of cytosolic calcium by transiently opening calcium channels into the cell membrane (66). The second messenger diacylglyceral activates protein kinase C, which phosphorylates many proteins, activates many enzymes (67), and is important in controlling cellular processes and proliferation (68), and protein kinase C also results in the synthesis of prostaglandins (69).

CYCLOOXYGENASE-II

The COX-II agents have a mechanism distinguishable from prostaglandin inhibition, the customary and common nonsteroidal anti-inflammatory mechanism of action, which inhibits mineralization. Whereas the effects of prostaglandins (COX-I pathway) are involved in the fluid balance through the kidneys, and the beneficial protective mechanism of the stomach, these are differentially less effective with COX-II agents. Thus, fluid retention problems and particularly the dyspepsia, in addition to GI bleeding, are dramatically reduced as compared with prior prostaglandin-mediated nonsteroidal anti-inflammatories. In fact, patients on coumadin may use COX-II agents, and not have disturbance of their protime when degenerative conditions require an anti-inflammatory.

Many factors have been demonstrated to regulate bone and cartilage homeostasis, and prostaglandin production has been demonstrated to regulate COX-II expression, with minimal effects on COX-1 (70). In cultured human osteoblasts, an upregulation of PGE_2, through COX-II isoenzyme, has been demonstrated from the parathyroid hormone (71). The relationship between prostaglandins, which are inhibited and studied extensively from a pharmaceutical standpoint, and other bioactive proteins, such as TGF-β and the family of bone morphogenic proteins (BMP), have been approached more from a macroscopic level, as substances which may be used adjunctively in surgery to enhance the results for example, of a lumbar spine fusion. Recombinant human BMP-2 has been considered and demonstrated a reversal of the inhibitory effect of Ketorolac on lumbar spine fusion (72), because of its availability through genetic engineering; mediation of this effect, which may include prostaglandins and other substances, has not been investigated.

Mechanical perturbation results in an increased concentration of cytosolic calcium (64), which can be in response to shear stress, or indentation of cell membranes in endothelial cells with muscle cells, cardiac muscle cells, and glial cells. Mechanical compression of articular cartilage explants causes a significantly increased COX-II protein expression and PGE_2 production from porcine articular cartilage. Several authors have found increased cellular proliferation and production of PGE_2 after mechanical stimulation of bone cells by various means (73–75). Inhibition of COX-II was associated with decreased nitric oxide (NO) production, whereas inhibition of nitric oxide synthase (NOS) activity increased PGE_2 production (76).

Mechanical stresses, which are part of bone homeostasis, have been shown to induce COX-II mRNA expression in bone cells, which have been harvested from elderly women, from the iliac crest, with increased production of prostaglandins and upregulation of the COX-II mRNA (77).

In an effort to consider the effect of COX-II agents during the healing phase of a lumbar fusion, the customary rabbit model suggested that healing was not prevented with the COX-II agent, while inhibited by customary nonsteroidal anti-inflammatory (78). Further confirmation in the rabbit model was obtained by comparing a control of saline against indomethacin and celebrex, a COX-II selective inhibitor. It was observed that there was a statistically significant diminution of fusion with indomethacin, but not with the celebrex, at least not to a level of statistical significance (39,42,45). The mechanism was considered as inhibition of bone-forming cells on endosteal bone surfaces; reduction of immune and inflammatory responses; and inhibition of prostaglandin synthesis. The COX-II inhibitors are shown to reduce the cartilage in the fractured callus in a rat model, but they do not alter the hard callus, which is reduced with indomethacin (79). This delay in mineralization is the therapeutic advantage of a nonsteroidal in reducing heterotopic bone formation in multiply operated hip replacement or other clinical situations. Concern exists with regard to ligament healing, a collagen restructuring, where a COX-II inhibitor has been reported to impair ligament healing in rats (80), whereas indomethacin caused a 42% increase in the strength of the medial collateral ligament in rats, 32% decrease in strength was reported with COX-II agents. Clearly, the mechanisms are not understood; hence, these results remain unexplained; cartilage is inhibited in bone healing and collagen model bone is not, whereas in ligaments, which are collagen, healing COX-II agents are inhibitory. This study would seek to characterize those mechanisms, and establish a role for these agents as analgesics, but also perhaps therapeutic in these clinical situations.

SUMMARY

The selective COX-II inhibitors have been under scrutiny for cardiac toxicity, but Celebrex appears to have survived. It has no antiplatelet effect; has been shown that it does not cause GI bleeding; is effective for pain; and may be helpful in potentiating opioid analgesia. Nonnarcotic analgesics would be an advantage, strongly preferred both during and after a lumbar spine fusion, owing to the risk of habituation or even addiction over the customarily prolonged course of convalescence, and the subsequent administration after bone healing for chronic pain. Unfortunately, prostaglandin inhibitors have been shown to have a marked inhibitory effect on bone graft consolidation and new bone formation, particularly mineralization. The mechanism of action is unknown with regard to bone healing, but would be mediated through the prostaglandin mechanism, which is how these drugs are understood and reviewed here. Evidence is accumulating that the COX-II inhibitors have a less profound effect on bone healing than NSAIDs, and which may be reversible, if their use is limited to approximately two weeks.

CONCLUSIONS

Cyclooxygenase-II selective inhibitors have been shown to reduce both intermembranous bone formation and endochondral ossification (50), but the osteogenesis appeared restored by the addition of PGE_2 to the cultures and BMP-2, which demonstrates the central, critical role of COX-II enzymes in bone formation. Further, this illustrates a convergence of the use of the PGE_2, where prostaglandins have been studied and understood from a pharmaceutical's standpoint, to the clinical use of BMP-2, which has been used experimentally to form bone. However, the connection between BMPs and the prostaglandins has not been elucidated, or perhaps significantly considered. This specific application of spinal fusion represents a challenging clinical situation, and thus even a modest reduction in bone formation may be highly significant. The question has been raised (81) whether the advantage of the COX-II in terms of analgesia (82), without respiratory depression, risk of enhancing bleeding and potentiation of opiates, is actually safe, as there may be some reduction if the COX-II medications are continued on a prolonged, indefinite basis. Further study is required, but as indicated here, the availability of these drugs may be synergistic in converging extensive areas of investigation, as we evaluate relative risks against very substantial advantages in clinical applications.

REFERENCES

1. Gilron I, Milne B, Hong M. Cyclooxygenase-2 inhibitors in postoperative pain management: current evidence and future directions. Anesthesiology 2003; 99:1198–1208.
2. Sinatra R. Role of COX-2 inhibitors in the evolution of acute pain management. J Pain Symptom Manage 2002; 24(1 suppl):S18–S27.
3. Dahl JB, Kehlet H. Non-steroidal anti-inflammatory drugs: rationale for use in severe postoperative pain. Br J Anaesth 1991; 66:703–712.
4. Brooks PM, Day, RO. Non steroidal anti-inflammatory drugs—differences and similarities. N Engl J Med 1991; 324(24):1716–1725.
5. Ghosh P. Anti-rheumatic drugs and cartilage. Bailliers Clin Rheumatol 1998; 2:309–338.
6. Rashad S, Revell P, Hemmingway A, Low F, Rainsford K, Walker, F. Effect of non-steroidal anti-inflammatory drugs on the course of osteoarthritis. Lancet 1989; 2:519–522.
7. Poznanski AK, Ferpach SK, Berry TE. Bone changes from prostaglandin therapy. Skelet Radiol 1985; 14:20–25.
8. Kline DC, Raisz LG. Prostaglandins: stimulation of bone resorption and tissue culture. Endocrinology 1970; 86:1436–1440.
9. Minkan C, Fredricks RS, Pokress S, et al. Bone resorption and humeral hypercalcemia of malignancy-stimulation of bone resorption in vitro by tumor extracts is inhibited by prostaglandin synthesis inhibitors. J Clin Endocrinol Metab 1981; 53:941–947.
10. Harris M, Jenkins MV, Bennett A, Wills MR. Prostaglandin production in bone resorption by dental cysts. Nature 1993; 45:213–215.
11. Harvey W, Guat-Chen F, Gordon D, et al. Evidence for fibroblasts as the major source of prostocyclin and prostaglandin synthesis in dental cyst in man. Arch Oral Biol 1984; 29:223–229.
12. Robinson DR, Tasjian AH Jr, Levine L. Prostaglandin—stimulated bone resorption by rheumatoid synovia—possible mechanism for bone destruction in rheumatoid arthritis. J Clin Invest 1975; 56:1181–1187.
13. Horowitz SM, Rapuano BP, Lane JM, Burstein AH. The interaction of the macrophage and the osteoblast in the pathophysiology of aseptic loosening of joints. Calcif Tissue Int 1994; 54:320–324.
14. Goldring SR, Schiller AL, Roelake M, Rourke CM, O'Neil DA. The Synovial—like membrane at the bone—cement interface and loose total hip replacements and his proposed role in bone lysis. JBJS 1994; 64A:575–584.
15. Conaway HH, Diez LF, Raisz LG. Effects of prostocycline and prostaglandin E_1 on bone formation in the presence and absence of parathyroid hormone. Calcif Tissue Int 1986; 38:130–134.
16. Fuller K, Chambers TJ. Effects of arachadonic acid metabolites on bone resorption by isolated rat osteoclasts. J Bone Miner Res 1989; 4:209–215.
17. Collins DA, Chambers TJ. The effects of prostaglandins E_1, E_2 and F_2 Alpha Osteoclast formation in most bone marrow cultures. J Bone Miner Res 1991; 6:157–164.
18. Akatsu T, Takahasi N, Debaki K, et al. Prostaglandin promotes osteoclast-like cell formation by a mechanism involving cyclic adenocene $3',5'$ monophosphate in mouse bone marrow cell cultures. J Bone Miner Res 1989; 4:29–35.
19. Marcelli C, Yates AJ, Monday JR. In vitro effects of human recombinant transforming growth factor beta on bone turn over in normal mice. J Bone Miner Res 1990; 5:1087–1092.
20. Shinar G, Rodan GA. Biphasic effects of transforming growth factor- beta on the production of osteoclast-like cells in mouse bone marrow cultures: the role of prostaglandins and the generation of these cells. Endocrinology 1990; 126:3153–3158.
21. Kawaguchi H, Pilbeam CC, Harrison JR, Raisz, LG. The role of prostaglandins in the regulation of bone metabolism. Clin Orthop Rel Res 1998; 313:36–46.
22. Dubois RN, et al. Cyclooxygenase Biol Dis 1998; 2:1063–1073.
23. Robinson DR, et al. Prostaglandin-stimulated bone resorption by rheumatoid synovia: a possible mechanism for bone destruction in rheumatoid arthritis. J Clin Invest 1975; 56:1181–1188.
24. Blumenkrantz N, Sondergaard J. Effective prostaglandin E1 and F2 alpha on biosynthesis of collagen. Nat New Biol 1972; 239:246–251.
25. Goldring MB, Krane, SM. Modulation by recombinant interleukin-1 of synthesis of type I and III collagens and associated procollagen mRNA levels in cultured human cells. J Bio Chem 1987; 262:16724–16729.
26. Flanagan AM, Chambers TJ. Stimulation of bone nodule formation in vitro by prostaglandin E1 and prostaglandin E2. Endocrinology 1992; 130:443–448.

27. Hakeda Y, Ikeda E, Kurihara N et al. Induction of osteoblasts excel differentiation by Forskolin stimulation of sicklic AMP production in Alkoline phosphatase activity. Biochem Biophys Res Commun 1985; 838:49–53.

28. Hakeda Y, Hotta T, Kurihara N et al . Prostaglandin E2 and F2 alpha stimulate differentiation and proliferation, respectively of clonal osteoblastic MC3 T3-E1 cells by different second messengers in vitro. Endocrinology 1987; 121:1966–1974.

29. Hakeda Y, Harada S, Matsumoto T et al. Prostaglandin F2 alpha stimulates proliferation of clonal osteoblastic MC3, T3-E1 cells by up regulation of insulin-like growth factor-1 receptor. J Biol Chem 1991; 266:21044–21050.

30. Dallas SL, Park-Snyder S, Mayazono K, et al. Characterization and autoregulation of latent transforming growth factor beta (TGF-B) in osteoblastic—like cell lines: Production of a latent complex lacking the latent TGF- binding protein. J Biol Chem 1994; 269:6815–6822.

31. Akamine T, Jee WSS, Kee, HZ, Li XJ, Lin BY. Prostaglandin E2 prevents bone loss and adds extra bone to immobilized distal femoral metaphases in female rats. Bone 1992; 13:11–22.

32. Drvaric DM, Park WJ, Wyly JB et al. Prostaglandin-induced hyperostosis. A case study. Clin Orthop 1989; 246:300–304.

33. Jee WSS, Ueno K, Deng YP, Woodbury DM. The effects of prostaglandin E2 in growing rats increased metaphaseal hard tissue and corticoendosteal bone formation. Calcif Tissue Int 1985; 37:138–156.

34. Poznanski AK, Ferpach SK, Berry TE. Bone changes from prostaglandin therapy. Skelet Radiol 1985; 14:20–25.

35. Keller J, Kilmar A, Bak B, Sudder P. Effects of local prostaglandin E2 on fracture callus in rabbits. Acta Orthop Scand 1993; 64:59–63.

36. Allen HL, Wase A, Bear WT. Indomethacin and aspirin: effect of nonsteroidal anti-inflammatory agents on the rate of fracture repair in the rat. Acta Orthop Scand 1980; 51(4):595–600.

37. Kjaersgaarddandersen P, Nafei A, Teichert G et al. Indomethacin for prevention of heterotopic ossification—a randomized controlled study in 41 hip arthroplasties. Acta Orthop Scand 1993; 64:639–642.

38. DiCesare PE, Nimni ME, Peng L, Yazd M, Cheung DT. Effects of indomethacin on mineralized bone—induced heterotopic ossification in the rats. J Orthop Res 1991; 9:855–861.

39. Bo J, Sudmann E, Marton P. Effect of indomethacin on fracture healing in rats. Acta Orthop Scand 1976; 17(6):588–599.

40. Sudmann E, Dregelid E, Besses A, Morland J. Inhibition of fracture healing by indomethacin in rats. Eur J Clin Invest 1979; 9(5):333–339.

41. Altman RD, Latta LL, Keer R, Renfree K, Hornicek F, Banovac K. Effect of nonsteroidal anti-inflammatory drugs on fracture healing: a laboratory study in rats. J Orthop Trauma 1994; 9(5): 392–400.

42. Keller J, Trancik TM, Young FA, St. Mary E. Effects of indomethacin on bone ingrowth. J Orthop Res 1989; 7(1):28–34.

43. Trancik T, Mills W, Vinson N. The effect of indomethacin, aspirin, and ibuprofen on bone ingrowth into a porous-coated implant. Clin Orthop 1989; 249:113–121.

44. Cook SD, Barrack RI, Dalton JE, Thomas KA, Brown TD. Effects of indomethacin on biologic fixation of porous-coated titanium implants. J Arthroplasty 1995; 10(3):351–358.

45. Dimar JR, Ante WA, Zhang YP, Glassman SD. The effects of non-steroidal anti-inflammatory drugs on posterior spinal fusions in the rat. Spine 1996; 21(16):1870–1876.

46. Gerstenfeld LC, Thiede M, Seibert K. et al. Differential inhibition of fracture healing by non-selective and cyclooxygenase-2 selective non-steroidal anti-inflammatory drugs. J Orthop Res 2003; 21(4): 670–675.

47. Simon AM, Manigrasso MB, O'Connor JP. Cyclo-oxygenase 2 function is essential for bone fracture healing. J Bone Miner Res 2002; 17(6):963–976.

48. Endo K, Salryo K, Komatsubara S et al. Cyclooxygenase-2 inhibitor inhibits the fracture healing. J Physiol Anthropol Appl Hum Sci 2002; 21(5):235–238.

49. Brown KM, Saunders MM, Kirsch T, Honahue HJ, Reid JS. Effect of COX-2-specific inhibition on fracture healing in the rat femur. J Bone Joint Surg Am 2004; 860a(1):116–123.

50. Zhang X, Schwartz EM, Young DA, Puzas JE, Rosier RN, O'Keefe RJ. Cyclooxygenase-2 regulates mesenchymal cell differentiation into the osteoblast lineage and is critically involved in bone repair. J Clin Invest 2002; 109(11):1405–1415.

51. Simon AM, O'Connor JP. Acute inhibition of cyclooxygenase-2 impairs fracture healing. Transactions of the 49th Annual Orthopaedic Research Society 2003; 29:314.

52. Lindholm TS, Tornkvist H. Inhibitory effect on bone formation and calcification exerted by the anti-inflammatory drug Ibuprofen. Scand J Rheumatol 1981; 10:38–41.

53. Gebur P, Soelperg M, Orsnes T, Wilbek H. Naproxen prevention of heterotopic ossification after hip arthroplasty: a prospective controlled study of 55 patients. Acta Orthop Scand 1991; 62:226–229.

54. Elmstedt E, Lindholm TS, Nilsson OS, Tornkvist H. Effect of ibuprofen on heterotopic ossification after hip replacement. Acta Orthop Scand 1985; 56:25–27.

55. Solheim E, Pinholt EM, Bang G, Sudmann E. Inhibition of heterotopic osteogenesis in rats by a new bioerodible system for local delivery of indomethacin. J Bone Joint Surg 1992; 74A:705–712.
56. Burd TA, Hughes MS, Anglen JO. Heterotopic ossification prophylaxis with indomethacin increases the risk of long bone nonunion. J Bone Joint Surg Br 2003; 85(5):700–705.
57. Glassman SD, Rose SM, Dimar JR, Puno RM, Campbell MJ, Johnson JR. The effect of postoperative nonsteroidal anti-inflammatory drug administration on spinal fusion. Spine 1998; 23(7): 834–838.
58. Sudmann E, Bang G. Indomethacin—induced inhibition of haversian remodeling in rabbits. Acta Orthop Scand 1979; 50:621–627.
59. Brighton CT, Stafford B, Gross SB, Leatherwood DE, Williams JL, Pollack SR. The proliferation and synthetic response of isolated calverial bone cells of rats to cyclical biaxial mechanical strain. JBJS 1991; 73A:320–331.
60. Buckley MJ, Banes AJ, Levine LG, et al. Osteoblasts increase their rate of division in a line in response to a Cyclic, mechanical tension in vitro. Bone and Mineral 1998; 4:225–236.
61. Hasegawa S, Sato S, Saito S, Suzuki Y, Brunette DM. Mechanical stretching increases the number of cultured bone cells synthesizing DNA and alters their pattern of protein synthesis. Calcif Tissue Int 1985; 37:431–436.
62. Jones DB, Bingmann D. How do osteoblasts respond to mechanical stimulation. Cells Mater 1991; 1:329–340.
63. Jones DB, Molte H, Scholubbers JG, Turner E, Veltel D. Biochemical signal transduction of mechanical strain on osteoblasts like cells. Biomaterials 1991; 12:101–110.
64. Berridge J. Inositol triphosphate and diacylglycerol as second messengers. Biochem J 1984; 220: 345–360.
65. Vergara J, Tsien RY, Delay M. Inositol 1,4,5 triphosphate: the impossible chemical leak in exitation – contraction coupling in muscle. Proc Natl Acad Sci USA 1985; 82:6352–6356.
66. Williamson JR, Hansen CA. Formation and metabolism of ositol phosphate, the inositol trise/tretroki-sphosphate pathway. Advances in Experimental Medicine. New York, Plenum Press, 1988:183–195.
67. Binderman I, Shimshoni Z, Somjen D. Biochemical pathways involved in the translation of physical stimulus into biological message. Calcif Tissue Int 1984; 36(Suppl 1):S82–S85.
68. Binderman I, Zor U, Kaye AM, Shimshoni Z, Harell A, Somjen D. The transduction of mechanical force into biochemical events in bone cells may involve activation of phospholipase A_2. Calcif Tissue Int 1988; 42:261–266.
69. Sekar MC, Hokin LE. The role of phosphoinositides in signal transduction. J Membr Biol 1986; 89:193–210.
70. Morrisset S, et al. Regulation of cyclooxygenase-2 expression in bovine condrocytes in culture by interleukin-1 alpha, tumor necrosis factor – alpha cortiocords, and 17 beta-estradiol. J Rheumatol 1998; 25:1143–1146.
71. Maciel FM. Induction of cyclooxygenase-2 by parathyroid hormone in human osteoblasts culture. J Rheumatol 1997; 24:2429–2435.
72. Martin GJ, Boden SD. rhBMP-2 Reverses the inhibitory effect of Ketorolac (Torodol) in posterolateral spine fusion. Proceedings of the 13th Annual North American Spine Society, San Francisco, CA. October 28–31, 1998: 136.
73. Harell A, Dekel S, Binderman I. Biochemical effect of mechanical stress on cultured bone cells. Calcif Tissue Res 1977; 22(suppl):202–207.
74. Sandy JR, Meghji S, Farndal RW, Meikle MC. Dual elevation of cyclic AMP and inositol phosphates in response to mechanical deformation of murine osteoblasts. Biochem Biophys Acta 1989; 1010:265–269.
75. Somjen D, Binderman I, Berger E, Harell A. Bone remodeling induced by physical stress is prosta-glandin E_2 mediated. Biochem Biophys Acta 1980; 627:91–100.
76. Yeh CK, Rodan GA. Tensile forces enhance prostaglandin E synthesis in osteoblastic cells grown on collagen ribbons. Calcif Tissue Int 1984; 36(suppl 1):S67–S71.
77. Fermor B, Weinberg JB, Pisetsky D, Fink C, Misukonis M, Guilak F. Interaction of cyclooxygenase 2 (COX2) and nitric oxide synthase 2 (NOS 2) pathways in response to mechanical compression of articular cartilage explants. Orthopaedic Research Society. 47 Annual Meeting,. Paper #. 173, San Francisco, CA, February 25–28, 2001.
78. Joldersma M, Burger EH, Semeins CM, Klein-Nulend J. Mechanical stress induces COX-2 mRNA expression in bone cells from elderly women. J Biomech January 2000; 33(1):53–61.
79. Lewis SJ, Long J, Kuklo TR et al. The effect of COX II inhibitors on spinal fusion. North Am Spine Soc Oct 2000:64–65.
80. Simon AM, Sabatino CT, O'Conner JP. The effects of cyclooxygenase II inhibitors in fracture healing. Orthopaedic Research Society. 47th Annual Meeting. Paper # 205, San Francisco, CA, February 25–28, 2001.
81. Elder C, Dahners L, Weinhold P. A COX II inhibitor impairs ligament healing in the rat. Orthopaedic Research Society. 47th Annual Meeting. Poster # 750, San Francisco, CA, February 25–28, 2001.
82. Einhorn T. Use of COX-2 inhibitors in patients with fractures. Is there a trade off between pain relief and healing? AAOS Bull 2002; 50(5):43–44.

23 | Motion Preservation Instead of Spinal Fusion

Aditya V. Ingalhalikar
Department of Neurosurgery, University of Iowa, Iowa City, Iowa, U.S.A.

Patrick W. Hitchon
Department of Neurosurgery, University of Iowa, Carver College of Medicine, Iowa City, Iowa, U.S.A.

Tae-Hong Lim
Department of Biomedical Engineering, University of Iowa, Iowa City, Iowa, U.S.A.

INTRODUCTION

Approximately one percent of the U.S. population is chronically disabled because of back pain and an additional one percent is temporarily disabled (1,2). More than 20 million working days are lost each year because of back pain, resulting in financial losses estimated as high as $100 billion per year (1,2). Disorders of the intervertebral disc are a major contributor to these statistics. The conventional treatment for lumbar degenerative disc disease (DDD) involves disc excision with or without fusion. However, fusion techniques do not guarantee satisfactory results. Clinical and biomechanical studies indicate that fusion results in altered kinematics and clinical problems at the adjacent motion segments. To overcome the perceived drawbacks of fusion (static instrumentation), dynamic spinal implants has been developed and used that maintain the natural kinematics of the spine, reestablish clinical stability, and maintain the caliber of neural foramina while avoiding the development of adjacent level degenerative changes.

The aim of the present Chapter is to review the biomechanics of fusion and draw a detailed comparison with the concept of motion preservation in the light of mechanical principles and biomechanical studies. Light will also be shed on the basic biomechanical design criteria that are involved in designing the artificial disc.

A REVIEW OF SPINE FUSION

The conventional treatment for DDD involves disc excision with or without fusion. Spine fusion was introduced for the first time by Hibbs and Albee in 1911 (3). It involves removal of the degenerated segment (4) and fusion of the vertebrae so that motion is eliminated.

Though fusion stands as the most common spine surgery performed for the management of severe low back pain, it is controversial in terms of the conflict it presents between immediate relief and long term consequences. Spinal fusion procedures have been reported to have various adverse effects, which in addition to loss of motion include bone graft donor site pain, pseudoarthrosis, spinal stenosis, spondylolysis acquisita and accelerated degeneration of the adjacent unfused segments (5–11).

Clinical Studies

Clinical studies indicate that fusion results in altered kinematics and clinical problems at the adjacent motion segments. Frymoyer et al. (12) reported roentgenographic evaluation of accelerated degeneration at the free segment above the lumbosacral fusion. Hypertrophic degenerative arthritis of facet joints, spinal stenosis, and severe disc degeneration are the major pathologic conditions observed at the level adjacent to fusion (11). According to an investigation of 58 patients Schlegel et al. (13) suggested that incorrect sagittal and coronal alignments caused degeneration at the adjacent level by inducing too much motion at that level. Gillet (14) analyzed the fate of the transitional segment in a homogenous group of patients who were operated upon during a 14 year period for degenerative conditions of the lumbar spine. These patients had proven resistant to conservative treatment, and were followed for a period of 2 to 15 years. They observed that 41% of the patients developed transitional segment alterations and 20% needed a secondary operation for extension of the fusion. Similar observations have been made about fusion in the cervical spine. Hilibrand et al. (15) studied the radiculopathy and myelopathy referable to the motion segment adjacent to the site of previous anterior arthrodesis of the cervical spine. They observed that symptomatic adjacent—segment disease may affect more than one-fourth of all patients within ten years after anterior fusion. They also observed that a single level fusion involving fifth and sixth cervical vertebra and preexisting radiographic evidence of degeneration at adjacent levels are likely to be the indicators for new disease.

Biomechanical Studies

From a biomechanical point of view, elimination of motion at the operated level increases motion and stresses/loads at the adjacent level as the patient tries to maintain his/her preoperative physiologic range of motion. It is hypothesized that these increased loads and motion may be the reason for the observed adjacent motion segment pathologies. Intradiscal pressure (IDP) is the only parameter, which offers a direct way to determine the loading conditions in spine (16–18).

Biomechanical studies confirm these clinical observations through a study of IDP (as a measure of stress) and motion at the levels adjacent to fusion. Biomechanical studies have shown that addition of instrumentation significantly affects the IDP in the levels above fusion. Dekutoski et al. (19) compared motion changes in segments adjacent to fusion for in vitro and in vivo tests on canine specimens. They found that the in vivo facet motion at L2–3 increased post instrumentation of L3–7. They also found that under load control (in vitro), the facet motion at L2–3 did not increase significantly post instrumentation, however, under motion controlled set-up, facet motion increased significantly post instrumentation and also was similar to the in vivo facet motion. Weinhoffer et al. (20), Chow et al. (21), and Cunningham et al. (22) studied the effect of spinal destabilization and instrumentation on lumbar IDP. They concluded that the addition of instrumentation significantly affected the IDP in the levels above a simulated fusion and the rise in pressure was more prominent with multiple levels of fusion. Also, application of segmental instrumentation changes the motion pattern of the residual intact motion segments, and the changes in the motion pattern become more distinct as the fixation range becomes more extensive and the rigidity of the construct increases (23). A number of studies point towards the same issue in cervical spine. Eck et al. (24) and DiAngelo et al. (25) reported a significant increase in motion and pressure at the level adjacent to a simulated fusion in the cervical spine. Phillips et al. (26) carried out lumbar fusion surgeries in rabbits and then observed the change in histology of adjacent level discs at three, six, and nine months, respectively. They observed an initial loss of normal parallel arrangement in collagen fibers in annulus, disorganization and loss of distinction between annular lamellae and finally disorganized annulus tissue and annular tears. Also, they observed an initial proliferative response followed by loss of chondrocytes and notochordal cells in the nucleus pulposus. Narrowing of disc space, endplate sclerosis and the formation of osteophytes at adjacent disc spaces was observed radiographically.

In view of the above stated studies it becomes imperative that the motion at the affected segment be retained to maintain the natural biomechanics of the spine and hence avoid future complications and degeneration at the adjacent motion segment due to fusion. To overcome limitations of fusion (static instrumentation), it is necessary to investigate the effects of dynamic spinal instrumentation which would retain motion at the diseased segment and thereby aim to maintain the natural kinematics of the spine, reestablish clinical stability and maintain the caliber of neural foramina while avoiding the development of adjacent degenerative changes. To serve this end, Artificial Disc implants were developed and many have a fairly long track record in Europe, a few of them have recently started to gain approval in the United States.

MOTION PRESERVATION—TOTAL DISC REPLACEMENT

Total Disc Replacement Arthroplasty involves replacement of the degenerated disc with an artificial joint. From a biomechanical and clinical perspective implantation of the artificial disc at the site of a diseased disc aims to theoretically

1. restore motion to the spine,
2. reestablish stability,
3. maintain the caliber of the neural foramina, while avoiding the development of adjacent degenerative changes,
4. avoid complications from instrumentation or postoperative immobilization, and
5. allow an early return to function.

Design Criteria

In order to satisfy its clinical objective and mimic the biomechanical functionality of a natural intervertebral disc the artificial disc should meet certain design criteria.

Geometry and Placement

The Functional Spinal Unit is a complex 3 joint structure with the spinal cord and nerves exiting through the neural foramina. Stability and flexibility of the unit depends on maintaining the inter-relationship between various anatomical structures in such as the ligaments and various spinal muscles. The artificial disc should be contained inside the intervertebral space, exceptions being for any attachment points. The height of the disc should be such that it does not exert any excessive preloading of the facet joints or the ligamentous structures. Excessive local preloading may result in increased stiffness of the motion segment which may prove detrimental to the overall biomechanics of the spine. In terms of angulations, the artificial disc should maintain the wedge shaped structure of the natural intervertebral disc so as to maintain the lordotic angle in the sagittal plane, be it the cervical or lumbar spine. This would confirm that the spinal muscles do not have to work overtime to maintain the quiet standing posture. Placement in the transverse plane should be such that the loading on the facet joints and adjoining muscles is not asymmetric. It has been shown through finite element studies (27) that antero-posterior positioning of the artificial disc affects the motion segment flexural stiffness and posterior element loading. A posteriorly placed artificial disc, predicted no facet loads in compression, whereas an anteriorly placed disc increased the facet loads 2.5 times compared to the intact. Hence it is suggested that during surgical intervention, the artificial disc be placed in such a way that the posterior margin of the disc is aligned with the posterior margin of the verterbral body.

Kinematics

The artificial disc should be capable of simulating the physiologic motion of the natural joint, for example, a typical healthy lumbar L4–L5 joint experiences 13° of flexion, 3° of extension, 3° of lateral bending and 0–1° of axial rotation (4). In addition to this it is also essential that the center of rotation of the artificial disc fall on the same loci as that of the natural healthy joint, which is located in the posterior half (4) of the disc space. These factors are critical in physiologic motion preservation.

Dynamics

Effective load transmission remains a critical design criterion towards objective functioning of the artificial disc. The material and stiffness of the artificial disc should be such that it allows physiologic load transmission through all the adjacent spinal structures. Too much or little load transmission through the artificial disc would be detrimental. For example, too much of load transmission through the disc might lead to bone resorption as against too little load transmission will reduce stability of the construct and might lead to bone deposition, for example, in the form of osteophytes at the bone, implant interface.

Types of Artificial Discs

A number of artificial intervertebral discs were developed and used in Europe in the last two decades (22,29–40). Certain artificial disc designs are just recently getting approved for clinical applications in the United States.

The AcroFlex lumbar artificial disc was designed by Steffee and Fraser in the 1990s. This disc used HP-100 silicon elastomer cushion attached to two titanium endplates (41). The most prominent lumbar disc prostheses include the ProDisc® II (Synthes Spine, Paoli, Pennsylvania, U.S.A.), Charite® (DePuy Spine, Inc, Raynham, Massachusetts) and Maverick™ (Medtronic Sofamor Danek, Memphis, Tennessee) artificial discs. The ProDisc is an articulating disc with polyethylene core. The metal endplates are plasma sprayed with titanium and have two vertical fins for fixation in the endplates. The Charite® was introduced in 1987 and is the first artificial disc design to be approved by the FDA for clinical application in the United States. It consists of a biconvex ultra-high-molecular-weight polyethylene nucleus. It interfaces with two endplates of cobalt-chromium-molybdenum alloy coated with titanium and hydroxiapatite. The endplates are primarily fixed through dorsal and ventral teeth. One of the most significant features of this design is the mobile sliding core. This allows adjustment of the two adjacent vertebral bodies to each other and avoids stress risers in the facet joints. The Maverick prosthesis was conceived by Mathews and Le Huec. It is a metal on metal (cobalt–chromium) type implant with posterior rotation axis. It allows normal motion in the sagittal and frontal planes.

Biomechanical Evaluation

Though theoretically sound, the efficacy and safety of the artificial disc needs to be carefully evaluated through biomechanical studies and long term clinical evaluations.

We would like to present here the few biomechanical studies done till date documenting the evaluation of the biomechanics of the artificial disc.

Cunningham et al. (22) compared the total disc replacement arthroplasty to conventional stabilization techniques and the intact spine using the SB Charite disc, by applying pure moments. They observed that the artificial disc restored motion to the level of the intact segment in flexion—extension and lateral bending, and increased motion in the axial rotation. The authors also report that the artificial disc restores motion at the adjacent level as compared to the increased motion in the fusion techniques, in all three degrees of freedom.

Hitchon et al. (42) compared the AD implanted cadaveric spine motion at L4–5, with the intact and discectomy state using pure moments of 1.5, 3, 4.5, and 6 Nm. Implantation of the AD was associated with a decrease in motion in all directions compared to the discectomy state, and with an increase in motion compared to the intact spine. This increase in motion was however was not significantly different from the intact motion.

Ingalhalikar (43) performed a study wherein they compared the segmental motion and IDP with the Maverick ball and socket (Fig. 1) artificial disc (AD) implanted in the human cadaveric spine at L4–5. Rotation at L3–4, L4–5, and L5–S1 was measured using a displacement controlled setup. The objective (Fig. 2) of the study was to evaluate the biomechanics of the AD implanted spine against the intact (control) and the subsequent addition of pedicle screws (PS) at L4–5 with the AD left in place. In flexion the AD showed a decrease in flexion compared to the intact condition ($p > 0.05$), whereas the pedicle screw instrumentation decreased the flexion motion when compared with the intact and AD states ($p < 0.05$) (Fig. 3). At the rostral adjacent level (L3–L4), the AD revealed a minor increase in flexion motion compared to the intact condition ($p > 0.05$). The increase in flexion with pedicle screw was significant when compared with the intact spine ($p < 0.05$), but insignificant when compared to the AD state ($p > 0.05$) (Fig. 3). The AD produced a small increase in flexion of the caudal adjacent segment (L5–S1) compared to the intact ($p > 0.05$). The addition of pedicle screws resulted in an increase in flexion at L5–S1 that was significant compared to the intact state ($p < 0.05$), but insignificant ($p > 0.05$) when compared to the AD implanted spine (Fig. 3).

With flexion, the AD showed a minor decrease in disc pressure compared to the intact condition, whereas pedicle score (PS) produced a minor increase in IDP compared with the

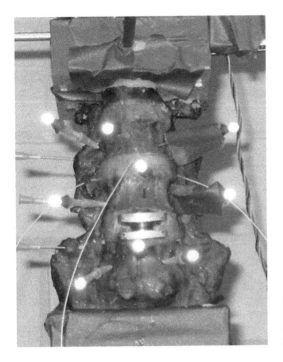

FIGURE 1 Photograph of the ball and cup design–Maverick™ Total Disc Replacement (Medtronic Sofamor Danek, Memphis, Tennessee, U.S.A.) artificial disc implanted at L45 in the lumbo-sacral spine.

intact and AD implanted state. These changes in intradisc pressure (IDP) were not however significant ($p > 0.05$).

Similar studies have been carried out on the cervical spine. DiAngelo et al. (25) used displacement controlled setup to compare the motion pattern of single level cervical artificial disc against the intact spine and single level anterior plating. They observed that use of an artificial disc did not alter the motion patterns at either the instrumented level or the adjacent segments compared with the intact segment for all modes of testing.

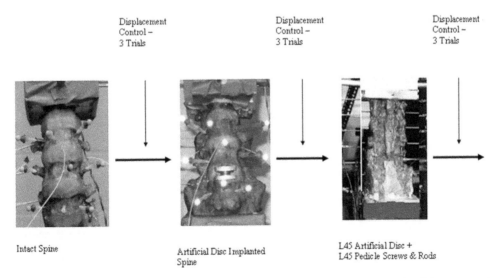

FIGURE 2 Experimental paradigm: comparison of the intact, artificial disc implanted and pedicle screws and rods with AD spine using displacement control setup. *Abbreviation*: AD, artificial disc.

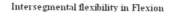

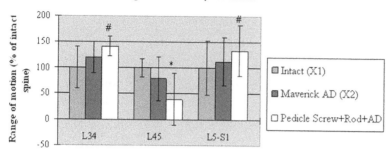

Intersegmental flexibility in Flexion

FIGURE 3 Graph demonstrating mean flexion motion at L3–4, L4–5 and L5–S1 in response to L4–5 AD implantation and L4–5 pedicle screws and rods with AD left in place. Motion of intact segment is considered as 100%. *Note*: #, indicates statistical significance ($p < 0.05$) compared to the intact; *, indicates statistical significance ($p < 0.05$) compared to all cases. *Abbreviation*: AD, artificial disc.

Important Considerations for Study Design
The Testing Modality
The testing modality plays a critical role in determining the results for the biomechanical evaluation of spine arthroplasty. Displacement controlled loading is the preferred method of testing (13) and is proved experimentally to closely resemble the in vivo conditions (25), as against the pure moment loading.

In terms of mechanical engineering principles, Figure 4 shows a diagrammatic illustration comparing load controlled using pure moments and displacement controlled loading mechanics. It is known that a pure moment applied to a column at one end distributes the same moment throughout its length. Assuming that the ligamentous cadaveric spine is a column made up of multiple segments it should be understood that implantation of an artificial disc would not reproduce its effect at the adjacent level, when applying a pure moment. The adjacent motion segment would be responding to the same moment load and not the manipulation at the implanted level. This has been corroborated experimentally (42). As against this a displacement controlled setup applying a predetermined displacement to the spine would reproduce the contribution of each motion segment as a part of the overall displacement. Any manipulation at the implanted level would result in a change in the adjacent segment

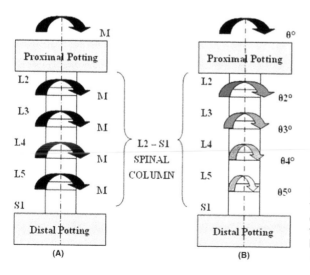

FIGURE 4 Diagrammatic illustration comparing the mechanics of: (**A**) pure moments and (**B**) displacement control testing modalities. Observe that in pure moment setup, $M = M2 = M3 = M4 = M5$ and in displacement control setup, $\theta° = \theta2° + \theta3° + \theta4° + \theta5°$.

mechanics as each motion segment tries to accommodate its kinematics to suit the overall applied displacement.

ASTM Standards
Recently the ASTM—American Society for Testing and Materials has introduced Standard F2346-05 (Copyright 2005 ASTM International) for the Standardization of Test Methods for Static and Dynamic Characterization of Spinal Artificial Discs.

CONCLUSION

At present, total disc arthroplasty seems to be one of the potential methods of maintaining mobility in place of the degenerated lumbar disc. The potential benefits would be established through long term clinical evaluations. Also, more biomechanical studies need to be done to analyze the effect of the artificial disc on the posterior elements under physiologic loads. It may be suggested that the artificial disc should also be studied once computational models are available which incorporate the effect of spinal muscles.

ACKNOWLEDGMENT

The authors acknowledge the support of Medtronic Sofamor Danek (Memphis, Tennessee, U.S.A.) in making this study possible.

REFERENCES

1. Andersson GB. Epidemiological features of chronic low-back pain. Lancet 1999; 354(9178):581–585.
2. Andersson HI, Ejlertsson G, Leden I, et al. Musculoskeletal chronic pain in general practice. Studies of health care utilisation in comparison with pain prevalence. Scand J Prim Health Care 1999; 17(2):87–92.
3. Albee FH. Transplantation of a portion of the tibia into the spine for Potts disease. A preliminary report. JAMA 1911; 57:885.
4. Panjabi W. Clinical Biomechcanics of the Spine. 1978:78–81.
5. Froning EC, Frohman B. Motion of the lumbosacral spine after laminectomy and spine fusion. Correlation of motion with the result. J Bone Joint Surg Am 1968; 50(5):897–918.
6. Harris RI, Wiley JJ. Acquired spondylolysis as a sequel to spine fusion. J Bone Joint Surg Am 1963; 45:1159–1170.
7. Anderson CE. Spondyloschisis following spine fusion. J Bone Joint Surg Am 1956; 38-A(5):1142–1146.
8. Rombold C. Spondylolysis: A complication of spine fusion. JBJS Am 1965; 47:1237–1242.
9. Bitan F, Bex M, Kapoff AJ, et al. Success factors in posterolateral arthrodesis of the lumbosacral spine. Rev Chir Orthop Reparatrice Appar Mot 1984; 70(6):465–471.
10. Lee CK, NAL. Lumbosacral spinal fusion. A biomechanical study. Spine 1984; 9(6):574–581.
11. Lee CK. Accelerated degeneration of the segment adjacent to a lumbar fusion. Spine 1988; 13(3):375–377.
12. Frymoyer JW, Matteri RE, Hanley EN, et al. Disc excision and spine fusion in the management of lumbar disc disease. A minimum ten-year follow-up. Spine 1978; 3(1):1–6.
13. Schlegel JD, Smith JA, Schleusener RL. Lumbar motion segment pathology adjacent to thoracolumbar, lumbar, and lumbosacral fusions. Spine 1996; 21(8):970–981.
14. Gillet P. The fate of the adjacent motion segments after lumbar fusion. J Spinal Disord Tech 2003; 16(4):338–345.
15. Hilibrand AS, Carlson GD, Palumbo MA, et al. Radiculopathy and myelopathy at segments adjacent to the site of a previous anterior cervical arthrodesis. J Bone Joint Surg Am 1999; 81(4):519–528.
16. Nachemson A. Measurement of intradiscal pressure. Acta Orthop Scand 1959; 28:269–289.
17. Nachemson AL. Disc pressure measurements. Spine 1981; 6(1):93–97.
18. Sato K, Kikuchi S, Yonezawa T. In vivo intradiscal pressure measurement in healthy individuals and in patients with ongoing back problems. Spine 1999; 24(23):2468–2474.
19. Dekutoski MB, Schendel MJ, Ogilvie JW, et al. Comparison of in vivo and in vitro adjacent segment motion after lumbar fusion. Spine 1994; 19(15):1745–1751.
20. Weinhoffer SL, Guyer RD, Herbert M, Griffith SL. Intradiscal pressure measurements above an instrumented fusion. A cadaveric study. Spine 1995; 20(5):526–531.
21. Chow DH, Luk KD, Evans JH, et al. Effects of short anterior lumbar interbody fusion on biomechanics of neighboring unfused segments. Spine 1996; 21(5):549–555.

22. Cunningham BW, Kotani Y, McNulty PS, et al. The effect of spinal destabilization and instrumentation on lumbar intradiscal pressure: an in vitro biomechanical analysis. Spine 1997; 22(22):2655–2663.
23. Shono Y, Kaneda K, Abumi K, et al. Stability of posterior spinal instrumentation and its effects on adjacent motion segments in the lumbosacral spine. Spine 1998; 23(14):1550–1558.
24. Eck JC, Humphreys SC, Lim TH, et al. Biomechanical study on the effect of cervical spine fusion on adjacent-level intradiscal pressure and segmental motion. Spine 2002; 27(22):2431–2434.
25. DiAngelo DJ, Robertson JT, Metcalf NH, et al. Biomechanical testing of an artificial cervical joint and an anterior cervical plate. J Spinal Disord Tech 2003; 16(4):314–323.
26. Phillips FM, Reuben J, Wetzel FT. Intervertebral disc degeneration adjacent to a lumbar fusion. An experimental rabbit model. J Bone Joint Surg Br 2002; 84(2):289–294.
27. Dooris AP, Goel VK, Grosland NM, et al. Load-sharing between anterior and posterior elements in a lumbar motion segment implanted with an artificial disc. Spine 2001; 26(6):E122–E129.
28. Pearcy MJ. Stereo radiography of lumbar spine motion. Acta Orthop Scand 1985; 212:1–41.
29. DiAngelo DJ, Foley KT, Morrow BR, et al. In vitro biomechanics of cervical disc arthroplasty with the ProDisc-C total disc implant. Neurosurg Focus 2004; 17(3):E7.
30. McAfee PC, Fedder IL, Saiedy S, et al. SB Charite disc replacement: report of 60 prospective randomized cases in a US center. J Spinal Disord Tech 2003; 16(4):424–433.
31. de Kleuver M, Oner FC, Jacobs WC. Total disc replacement for chronic low back pain: background and a systematic review of the literature. Eur Spine J 2003; 12(2):108–116.
32. Hochschuler SH, Ohnmeiss DD, Guyer RD, et al. Artificial disc: preliminary results of a prospective study in the United States. Eur Spine J 2002; 11(Suppl 2):S106–S110.
33. Enker P, Steffee A, Mcmillin C, et al. Artificial disc replacement. Preliminary report with a 3-year minimum follow-up. Spine 1993; 18(8):1061–1070.
34. Griffith SL, Shelokov AP, Buttner-Janz, et al. A multicenter retrospective study of the clinical results of the LINK SB Charite intervertebral prosthesis. The initial European experience. Spine 1994; 19(16):1842–1849.
35. Ray CD. The PDN prosthetic disc-nucleus device. Eur Spine J 2002; 11(Suppl 2):S137–S142.
36. Delamarter RB, Fribourg DM, Kanim LE, et al. ProDisc artificial total lumbar disc replacement: introduction and early results from the United States clinical trial. Spine 2003; 28(20):S167–S175.
37. McAfee PC, Polly DW Jr, Cunningham B, et al. Clinical summary statement. Spine 2003; 28(20):S196–S198.
38. Zigler JE. Clinical results with ProDisc: European experience and U.S. investigation device exemption study. Spine 2003; 28(20):S163–S166.
39. Szpalski M, Gunzburg R, Mayer M. Spine arthroplasty: a historical review. Eur Spine J 2002; 11(Suppl 2):S65–S84.
40. Ahren N. j.m.i.m.w.a.a.d.p.I., 1998.
41. Szpalski M, Gunzburg R, Mayer M. Spine arthroplasty: a historical review. Eur Spine J 2002; 11(Suppl 2):S65–S84.
42. Hitchon PW, Eichholz K, Barry C, et al. Biomechanical studies of an artificial disc implant in the human cadaveric spine. J Neurosurg Spine 2005; 2(3):339–343.
43. Ingalhalikar AV. Effect of Lumbar Total Disc Arthroplasty on the Segmental Motion and Intradiscal Pressure at Adjacent Level: An In Vitro Biomechanical Study. MS Thesis, 2005.

24 | Intervertebral Disc Arthroplasty as an Alternative to Spinal Fusion: Rationale and Biomechanical and Design Considerations

Andrew P. White
Department of Orthopaedic and Neurological Surgery, Thomas Jefferson University Hospital, Philadelphia, Pennsylvania, U.S.A.

James P. Lawrence and Jonathan N. Grauer
Department of Orthopaedics and Rehabilitation, Yale University, New Haven, Connecticut, U.S.A.

INTRODUCTION

The majority of patients with degenerative disc disease are treated nonoperatively. If conservative treatment fails, surgical intervention may be considered for the appropriate patient. Arthrodesis, or fusion, is an accepted surgical option for the patient with isolated degenerative disc disease in the cervical or lumbar spine. While successful fusion eliminates motion at a potentially painful level and offers the ability to restore intervertebral height and alignment, it does have significant limitations. For example, successfully achieving a surgical fusion is not always correlated with relief of pain. Further, there is the risk of pseudarthrosis, and potential morbidity associated with bone graft harvest, as well as concern of adjacent segment disease. Intervertebral disc arthroplasty is evolving as a surgical alternative to fusion.

Disc arthroplasty aims to eliminate a potentially painful disc while restoring and/or maintaining motion. The development of such motion preserving implants has relied upon an understanding of the normal, native functional spinal unit. The complex relationship between two vertebrae, including the intervening disc, paired facet joints, and related ligaments dictate the anatomic goals of disc replacement. It is implicit that the biomechanical properties of a disc arthroplasty device should closely mimic the normal intervertebral disc. Since the functional requirements for an arthroplasty device is dictated by the anatomy it strives to replace, different factors may be at play in the cervical and lumbar spine. Additionally, to preserve and maintain motion, the materials used for these devices must withstand the test of time.

RATIONALE FOR MOTION PRESERVING IMPLANTS

Arthroplasty has developed as an alternative to spinal fusion secondary to the real and perceived shortcomings of spinal fusion. The results of lumbar spine fusion for the treatment of degenerative disc disease are not universally satisfactory. The problems of adjacent segment disease, pseudarthrosis, and the potential morbidity of bone graft harvest continue to be limitations. And, importantly, there is a poor correlation between successful fusion and good clinical outcome; despite achieving a high rate of spinal fusion by modern techniques (>90 to 95%), clinical outcomes of the same magnitude have not been achieved (1). Inappropriate indications, imprecise diagnoses, and psychosocial factors have each been blamed for this variability in pain reduction following spinal arthrodesis.

There are additionally morbidities specific to posterior lumbar approaches. Disruption of posterior ligaments and paraspinal muscles, particularly at the boundaries of the fused segment, may increase the likelihood of postoperative pain, and can be considered a risk factor for the development of adjacent motion abnormalities and possible adjacent level disc degeneration. Anterior-alone arthroplasty procedures may circumvent some of the complications related to posterior surgery.

Spinal fusion is typically augmented by autograft. Although autologous bone is the material most likely to promote fusion, pseudarthrosis rates range from 5% to 35% (2). Donor bone may be limited in amount because of poor bone quality or due to previous graft harvest. Additionally, the harvest of autograft may be associated with chronic donor site pain, infection, fracture, herniation, and injury to surrounding structures (3). There is good evidence, however, that lumbar fusion can be performed without autograft; allograft with recombinant human bone morphogenetic protein (BMP) have been used to augment fusion, with good results, thus circumventing the typical morbidities of autograft harvest.

Adjacent Segment Degeneration: Cervical

The term "adjacent segment degeneration" is used to describe the arthrosis of the vertebral joints caudal or cranial to a fused segment; this phrase is used to describe the pathophysiologic and radiographic changes that may be observed. The term "adjacent segment disease" refers to the syndrome of symptoms that may be associated with the arthrosis. From a biomechanical standpoint, it has been argued that since a segmental fusion creates a longer moment arm, it may contribute to adjacent level degeneration by increasing adjacent level moments. Biomechanical studies have demonstrated that cervical fusion alters the kinematics of the adjacent segments when compared with intact specimens and cervical arthroplasty devices. DiAngelo et al. (4) have demonstrated that the motion lost at the fusion level is compensated by an increase in motion at the adjacent levels. Measuring this effect at the level of the disc, Eck et al. (5) demonstrated that an increase in the intradiscal pressure occurs both cephalad and caudad to the fusion level.

When considering the clinical data examining adjacent segment degeneration following cervical arthrodesis, it is important to consider the high incidence of spondylosis in the normal population. Degenerative changes occur in at least one cervical level in a vast majority of the population (6,7). Gore and Sepic (8) observed the onset of adjacent segment degeneration in 25% of 121 patients as well as the progression of existent disease in 25% of patients who had prior anterior cervical discectomy and fusion (ACDF) with a mean follow-up of five years. Interestingly, they found no correlation between the radiographic findings and clinical symptoms. It was hypothesized that this degeneration may be related to natural history alone. These authors published an additional report on 50 patients that revealed that 14% of patients had additional surgery for adjacent level disease after (ACDF) (9).

Hilibrand et al. (10) reported on 409 cases of anterior cervical decompression and fusion performed for radiculopathy or myelopathy. They reported a similar rate of additional surgery (14%) and an annual adjacent segment degeneration incidence of 3%. Using Kaplan–Meier survivorship curves, they concluded that the study population did have a significant risk of developing adjacent segment disease (13.6% at five years and 25.6% at 10 years of follow-up). The authors noted, however, that fusions of longer length had a lower risk of adjacent segment disease. This inverse relationship between length of moment arm and risk of degeneration suggested that longer fusions may have circumvented the natural progression of degeneration at these levels by including them in the fusion, rather than allowing degeneration at these levels adjacent to the fusion. Overall, this paper suggested that adjacent segment disease may be related to the natural history of cervical spondylosis.

Adjacent Segment Degeneration: Lumbar

Even for those patients that undergo an uncomplicated lumbar arthrodesis and enjoy an excellent reduction of pain, many surgeons remain concerned about the potential for development of radiographic and clinically symptomatic adjacent level disease.

The influence of lumbar segment fusion on adjacent levels remains a topic of controversy. Cadaveric studies have demonstrated that lumbosacral fusions increase motion at the non-fused adjacent levels and that this transfer of motion appears to be greatest with the use of instrumentation (11). It has also been reported that lumbar fusion increases the intradiscal pressure at adjacent levels and that elevated pressures correlate with the number of levels fused (12). In canine specimens, spinal fusion has been associated with alterations in proteoglycan synthesis in the adjacent disc (13).

Clinically, however, the consequences of fusion on the adjacent segment remain unclear. The relative risk of an adjacent fusion, as compared to the natural progression of degenerative changes, has undergone considerable debate. Many authors have presented cohort studies evaluating the relationship between lumbar arthrodesis and the rate of adjacent segment degeneration, with conflicting results. Rahm et al. reported a five year follow-up of 49 patients who underwent posterior instrumented lumbar fusion. The authors reported a 35% rate of adjacent segment degeneration and found that the degenerated patients had poorer clinical outcomes (14). In support of a causal relationship between fusion and adjacent segment disease, the authors reported that their patients who developed pseudarthrosis were less likely to develop adjacent segment degeneration. Lehmann et al. (15) presented a cohort of 62 lumbar arthrodesis patients with mean follow-up of 33 years. Although 45% of patients had developed radiographic degeneration at the segment caudal to the arthrodesis, and while there was a correlation between segmental degeneration and stenosis, there was no correlation between these radiographic findings and the patients' clinical symptoms.

Several other studies present data that does not support the proposed causal relationship between lumbar fusion and adjacent segment disease. Penta et al. (16) reported a 10 year follow-up on 52 patients that underwent interbody fusion at the lumbosacral junction; they found no difference in the rate of adjacent segment disease as compared to matched control patients who did not undergo surgery. Additionally, longer fusions were not associated with worse degeneration in their study. Throckmorton et al. (17) recently evaluated the association of adjacent level degeneration and outcomes of posterior lumbar fusion. Patients that were fused adjacent to a normal disc were compared to patients that were fused adjacent to a degenerative disc using the SF-36. Those patients fused adjacent to a degenerative disc scored better, and there was no difference between the two groups in the need for further surgery. These studies indicated that the risk of developing clinically symptomatic adjacent segment disease was not increased by a neighboring fusion.

The rate of clinically significant adjacent segment disease following lumbar arthrodesis has ranged from 41% (with 20% of patients requiring a second operation for extension of the fusion) (18) to 27% of patients requiring additional surgery in retrospective studies over varying periods of time (19). Although the majority of reported cases involve a segment directly adjacent to the arthrodesis, selection bias must still be considered. It is likely that a patient with one degenerative disc is more likely to develop another degenerative disc than a patient without degenerative disc disease, regardless of whether a fusion was performed. In fact, the recent study by Ghiselli et al. (20) found no correlation between the rate of adjacent segment disease and the length of fusion in 215 patients following posterior lumbar fusion. While there remains considerable controversy regarding the clinical significance of adjacent level degeneration, it is one issue to be considered when evaluating arthroplasty as an alternative to arthrodesis.

By maintaining motion, it is hypothesized that the longer moment arm and potential forces generated by fusion would be precluded by disc arthroplasty. Conceptually this is appealing. Nonetheless, the body of literature on disc degeneration adjacent to fusion is not without debate. Long term patient follow-up over many decades will be required to demonstrate if this affect is borne out by disc arthroplasty in the clinical setting.

GOALS OF INTERVERTEBRAL ARTHROPLASTY

Disc arthroplasty aims to eliminate a potentially painful disc while restoring and/or maintaining motion. This is often considered for treatment of pain related to symptomatic disc degeneration that has failed conservative measures. As described earlier, an artificial disc would ideally replicate the complex biomechanical properties of the native disc, resist wear, and provide long-term symptomatic relief.

It is presumed by many that surgical interventions utilizing a hypothetical "ideal" intervertebral arthroplasty implant to recreate the function of a normal disc would revolutionize the treatment of discogenic back pain. Compared to the experience with hip, knee, or other peripheral joint arthroplasty, the understanding of motion restoration for a degenerative spinal segment is a young science. The question of how closely an implant must mimic nature to achieve its goals, particularly in long-term treatment, remains outstanding. The function of a normal intervertebral anatomy and biomechanics is an important starting point for this discussion.

INTERVERTEBRAL DISC ANATOMY

The nucleus of the normal disc is a mucoid material. Its large fraction of water (70 to 90%) is retained by a matrix of glycosaminoglycans, proteoglycans, and collagen (predominantly Type II collagen). Proteoglycans are large macromolecules, and are particularly responsible for generating oncotic forces. In fact, the water component of a disc can constitute 250% of the weight of the gel-like material. Biomechanically, the nucleus can display properties of either a solid or liquid substance depending on the rate of applied loads; it is viscoelastic.

In the lumbar spine, the annulus fibrosis consists of concentric collagen layers surrounding the nucleus. The collagen is predominantly Type I in the lumbar annulus. Its layers are arranged in alternating orientation of parallel fibers approximately 65° from the vertical plane and are thinnest posterolaterally. The orientation of the annular fibers serves to restrain the functional spinal unit from extremes of motion.

The cervical intervertebral disc differs from the lumbar disc in that it lacks a concentric and circumferential annulus fibrosis. The cervical disc annulus is well developed anteriorly, but it tapers laterally and posterior towards the anterior edge of the uncinate process on each side. Additionally, the crossing arrangement of collagen fibers seen in the lumbar spinal unit is absent in the cervical spine.

The vertebral endplate is a thin layer of cartilage located between the vertebral body and the intervertebral disc. The normal endplate is composed of both hyaline and fibrocartilage. The intervertebral disc is dependent on diffusion across the endplate for nutrition and waste processing.

INTERVERTEBRAL DISC BIOMECHANICS

The intervertebral disc and the facet joints comprise a three-joint complex. These joints are subjected to complex loading conditions. Forces and rotations occur in the axial, sagittal, and coronal planes (Fig. 1). These motions include flexion-extension, lateral bending, axial rotation, translation, and compression and distraction. The intervertebral soft tissues, including the disc, allow for considerable dynamism in these motions, but also provide a certain degree of restraint. It is very important to note that combinations and coupled loads are the rule and not the exception. In the cervical spine, the facet joints are oriented in a relatively coronal plane, and provide limited resistance to flexion-extension and lateral bending. In the lumbar spine, however, the facet joints are oriented in a more sagittal plane and therefore primarily restrict rotational motion.

In the cervical spine, there is the additional relationship of the uncinate processes with the rest of the functional spinal unit. These articulations contribute to complex coupled motion in this region. For example, lateral bending results in rotation of the spinous processes away from the concave side of the direction of bending.

Differences are not only between the cervical and lumbar motion segments, but there are more subtle differences at each individual level. Level-specific motion properties are related to morphologic differences, anatomic position in relation to sagittal contour, and specific muscular and ligamentous attachments. For example, there is increased segmental motion as one progress caudally in the lumbar spine (21).

One method for describing vertebral motion is to define and follow its instantaneous center of rotation (COR). The instantaneous COR is the point in a moving rigid body (or extension outside the body) which does not translate during a given instantaneous movement of that

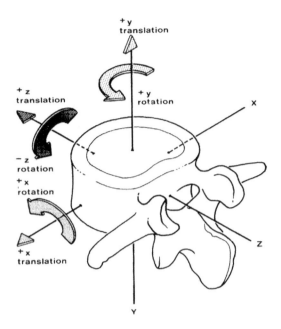

FIGURE 1 Orthogonal planes of motion in the lumbar spine. *Source*: From Ref. 36.

body. The path of the instantaneous COR can be used to describe intervertebral motion. This can facilitate description of complex motion patterns, particularly with regard to the coupled motions that are characteristic of the normal spine (22). For example, with a normal lumbar flexion-extension motion arc, the path of the instantaneous COR moves along an elliptical pathway (Fig. 2) since flexion-extension is necessarily coupled to translation (23). To contrast this with the cervical spine, the COR traces a different path and has been found to lie in the subjacent vertebral body (24).

It has been demonstrated that the path of the instantaneous COR is more variable and more anterior in degenerative cadaver discs as compared to normal controls (25). This highlights the fact that motion parameters change as the disc degenerates. In fact, it has been suggested that changes in the path of the instantaneous COR may be predictive of early disc

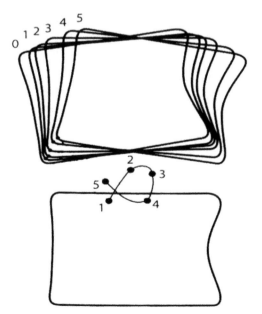

FIGURE 2 Changes in the instantaneous center of rotation (COR) with flexion and extension in the lumbar spine; in the normal disc, the path of the COR with flexion–extension traces an ellipse. *Source*: From Ref. 51.

degeneration. Reestablishing normal motion characteristics of the native disc, including the dynamic COR, is one goal of an ideal disc arthroplasty.

Loading in Normal Discs

As previously discussed, the human intervertebral disc is composed of collagen, proteogly-cans, and mucopolysaccharides. This tissue amalgam is viscoelastic, meaning that its mechanical properties change depending on load. Accordingly, it is important to consider the magnitude and duration of applied load in describing disc properties (26).

As the disc is compressed, the annular fibers tighten, and the nucleus develops increased hydrostatic pressure, which resists axial compression. This resistance to deformation is described by its modulus of elasticity (ratio of stress to strain). A material with a low modulus of elasticity easily deforms under a small load, while a material with a high modulus deforms less. For a given load applied to an intervertebral disc, the greater the modulus of elasticity, the less it deforms. Clinically, this means that there are complex scenarios seen by the disc with normal motion patterns. For example, with changes in posture, annular fibers become pre-tensioned and respond differently to applied loads.

Moreover, the relative distribution of the components of the three-joint complex is variable. In pure compression, approximately 80% of the load is borne by the intervertebral disc and approximately 20% is borne by the facets (27). Finite element modeling has been used to show that this distribution can vary with the disc seeing anywhere from 75% to 97% of the load, depending on the degree of flexion or extension. Disc loading is complex and dynamic; it related to the variable relationship with COR coupled motion, directed by the facets and other intervertebral tissues.

Loading in Abnormal Degenerative Discs

Degeneration of the intervertebral disc is characterized by early fissures, alterations in structure, and changes in mechanical properties. Overall, the disc becomes less viscous and more fibrotic during the degradation process (28). In addition, the degenerative disc has been shown to have lower intradiscal pressure and correspondingly carries less of the motion segment's load. This typically corresponds to a transfer in loads to the posterior elements (29).

Fujiwara et al. (30) conducted flexibility testing of MRI-graded degenerative discs in flexion, extension, lateral bending, and axial rotation. Their results showed that segmental flexibility increased with moderate disc degeneration and then decreased with more advanced disc degeneration (30). This is consistent with the three stages of degeneration defined by Kirkaldy-Willis (31).

In general, the normal intervertebral disc is a highly complex structure which allows for dynamic load bearing and motion. The components of the disc complex (the nucleus, annulus, and vertebral endplates) work in concert with the facets to allow physiologic motions with a dynamically changing COR while providing resistance against compressive and deforming loads. In the diseased state, these functions are observed to become compromised.

Fusion Biomechanics

Cervical fusions may be performed from anteriorly or posteriorly for degenerative changes, instability, or coupled with decompressive procedures. Lumbar fusions may be performed from anteriorly or posteriorly for back pain attributable to disc degeneration, instability, or deformity.

One of the benefits of spinal fusion is the control over alignment. An anatomic relationship is surgically determined and becomes permanent once the goal of bony fusion is met. Restoration of height and maintenance of lordosis are paramount. An important biomechanical consideration is that spinal fusion circumvents the dilemma of balancing the complex forces of the three-joint complex. Because fusion involves eliminating motion at the level being addressed, consideration of facet load at that level becomes immaterial.

Intervertebral Disc Arthroplasty Biomechanics

There have been many implant designs attempting to recreate the complex motions of the native disc. In fact, there is a more than 50 year history of patents for such devices (32). The majority of these prostheses are focused on the lumbar spine as compared to the cervical spine. Despite the many implant designs, very few have reached the stage of animal studies and even fewer have progressed to human clinical trials.

One method of classifying intervertebral arthroplasty devices, established by Errico (33), is to define the level of restraint that a device provides in each of the modes of motion. If a device allows hypermobility, beyond the range of the normal disc, it is classified as "unconstrained" in that mode of motion. If the device permits a range of motion that approximates the normal disc, it is classified as "semi-constrained" in that mode of motion. And if a device restricts range of motion to less than that of the normal disc, it is termed "constrained" in that mode of motion. The important attribute of this classification system is that it recognizes that an intervertebral disc replacement device should closely mimic the normal biomechanics of the intervertebral linkage and that each motion must be independently considered.

Each disc arthroplasty device has specific motion characteristics. Each possesses relative merits and limitations. However, it is important to note that none fully recreate the motion characteristics of the native disc. It is not known, how closely an arthroplasty implant must mimic normal motion mechanics to successfully achieve its goals in a lasting fashion.

As an example, the lumbar (Fig. 3) and cervical (Fig. 4) ProDisc® (Synthes, Inc., West Chester, Pennsylvania, U.S.A.) implants employ a concave superior endplate which articulates with a convex polyethylene insert that is fixed to the inferior endplate. Since this articulation cannot resist rotation, it is unconstrained for this mode of motion, relying on the facet joints and the remaining soft tissue linkages to resist rotation. This device does allow flexion, extension, and lateral bending in the normal range of motion that approximates the native disc and is thus semi-constrained in these modes. This device does not allow translation or compression and is therefore considered fully constrained in these modes of motion. From a biomechanical standpoint, it is also important to note that the fixed inferior component of the ProDisc® maintains a fixed instantaneous COR throughout the flexion-extension arc. This is also referred to as a "ball and socket" type design.

The Charité® (DePuy Spine, Raynham, Massachusetts, U.S.A.) lumbar arthroplasty (Fig. 5) is another example; it contains a bi-convex, sliding polyethylene core between two metal base plates, each with concave bearing surfaces. This device has no significant rotational resistance between the core and base plates, and is therefore unconstrained for this motion. The Charité implant approximates normal ranges of motion in flexion, extension, and lateral bending, and as such is semi-constrained in these modes. Due to the double articulation of the sliding core with the superior and inferior endplates, translation is also permitted in a

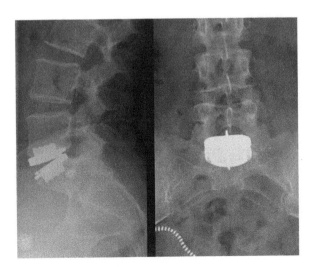

FIGURE 3 The ProDisc® (Synthes, Inc., West Chester, Pennsylvania, U.S.A.) II lumbar implant; a concave superior endplate articulates with a convex polyethylene insert that is fixed to the inferior endplate. Since this "ball and socket" articulation cannot resist rotation, it is unconstrained for the mode of motion, relying on the facet joints and the remaining soft tissue linkages to resist rotation.

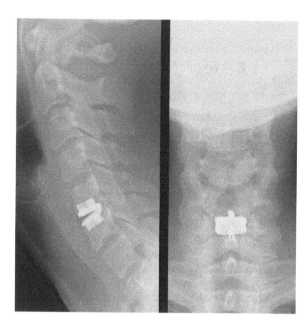

FIGURE 4 The ProDisc-C® (Synthes, Inc., West Chester, Pennsylvania, U.S.A.) cervical implant; a concave superior endplate articulates with a convex polyethylene insert that is fixed to the inferior endplate. Since this "ball and socket" articulation cannot resist rotation, it is unconstrained for the mode of motion, relying on the facet joints and the remaining soft tissue linkages to resist rotation.

semi-constrained fashion. It is suggested that, by translating with motions such as flexion and extension, it can better approximate normal disc motion coupling (34). Its design, however, permits no motion in pure compression; in this mode, and it has been suggested that the facets see more than normal loading patterns (35).

While many of the intervertebral disc arthroplasty designs are classified as "semi-constrained" for flexion and extension, lateral bending, and even axial rotation, none of the designs currently under investigation allow motion in the compression and distraction mode. This is in contrast to the native disc which allows between 0.5 mm and 1.5 mm of compression (36). This motion is critical to effectively allow certain coupled motions. For example, to achieve flexion with translation a certain degree of compression is required.

The Arcoflex, designed by Steffee as a series of lumbar implants in the 1990s consists of a pair of metal implants bound to an interposed elastic disc (Fig. 6). The first generation elastic material was abandoned secondary to concerns for potential carcinogenesis, and the implantation of the second halted when a discrepancy of longevity between in vivo and ex vivo

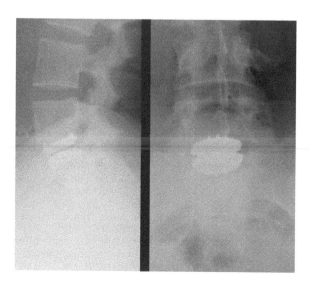

FIGURE 5 The SB Charité® III (DePuy Spine, Raynham, Massachusetts, U.S.A.) lumbar implant. The device features a bi-convex, sliding polyethylene core between two metal base plates, each with concave bearing surfaces. This device is unconstrained in rotation and semi-constrained in flexion, extension, and lateral bending. Due to the double articulation of the sliding core with the superior and inferior endplates, translation is also permitted in a semi-constrained fashion. The pathway of the center of rotation (COR) with this model is believed to mimic the elliptical path of the COR. Its design, however, permits no motion in pure compression.

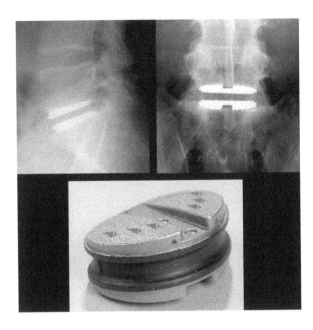

FIGURE 6 The second-generation Fraser/Steffee Acroflex implant (Synthes, Inc., West Chester, Pennsylvania, U.S.A.) featured two titanium endplates interposed by a polyolefin rubber core. A vulcanization process was used to secure the core and the endplates. *Source*: From Ref. 32.

testing was established by investigators. The biomechanical advantages of such an arthroplasty device, however, are clear; the ability to preserve disc height, allow semi-constrained motions in all modes including compression, and having the additional potential of recreating the proper functional relationship with the facet joints is advantageous. This type of design holds the potential to recreate coupled motions characterized by a normal COR path. Such an implant, however, will require the development of an elastic biomaterial that matches and maintains the material properties of the native disc for decades of use.

IMPLANT DESIGN AND MATERIAL CONSIDERATIONS
Bone-Implant Contact Area

Contact area is critical to the maintenance of the intended bone-implant interface. This was demonstrated early in the history of disc arthroplasty designs with observations of the Fernstrom ball (Fig. 7) prosthesis. This was a stainless steel ball placed between the vertebral bodies. Due to its spherical morphology, forces were focused upon a very small area of the central vertebral endplate; "point-loading" was thus induced. The Fernstrom (37) ball was

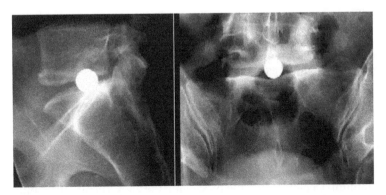

FIGURE 7 The Fernstrom prosthesis (inserted at L5-S1) demonstrating subsidence into the vertebral endplates. *Source*: From Ref. 32.

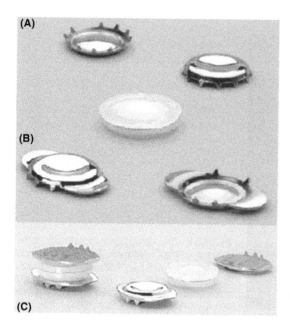

FIGURE 8 The evolution of the Charité® implant (DePuy Spine, Raynham, Massachusetts, U.S.A.) The first generation (**A**) featured stainless steel endplates and a smaller contact area. The second generation (**B**) added lateral fins to increase the contact area. The third generation (**C**) features cobalt-chromium endplates. *Source*: From Ref. 52.

implanted in about 250 patients. Intervertebral height was lost in 88% of cases in the four to seven year follow-up period as implants subsided through the vertebral endplates.

Subsequent disc arthroplasty designs have incorporated larger contact areas with the vertebral endplates to reduce the risk of subsidence. While the early Charité I device offered a much larger contact surface than Fernstrom's ball, subsidence was still observed in early clinical trials (38). This shortcoming appears to have been resolved by the third generation Charité implants which had a larger footplate and increased contact area over the peripheral endplate regions (Fig. 8). This modification dramatically decreased the rate of subsidence (39,40).

The cervical vertebral endplate differs from the lumbar endplate. Primarily, the uncinate processes limit lateral exposure of the endplate surfaces and may have to be contoured for implant placement. As with the lumbar discs, the benefits of endplate contouring must be balanced against weakening the endplate and facilitating subsidence.

Implant Endplate Materials

Materials chosen for the implant endplate must be durable enough to withstand repetitive physiologic loading. Further considerations include the reactivity, modulus of elasticity, ultimate strength, ductile behavior, imaging characteristics, ease of manufacture, and cost of the material (41,42). The three types of alloys that have been used for implant endplates include stainless steel, cobalt-chromium, and titanium.

Stainless steel is an amalgam of iron, carbon, chromium, nickel, and molybdenum. Implants made of stainless steel are the least expensive to fabricate, feature relatively low corrosion, and have a relatively high elastic modulus. The experience of the Charité implant's evolution highlights the use of stainless steel as an endplate material. The first generation featured stainless steel endplates with relatively low contact endplate areas. Subsidence occurred in many of these devices, in part due to the large difference in elastic modulus between the relatively rigid steel and the softer cancellous bone. Later versions of the Charité device have broader and flat endplates manufactured from a lower modulus cobalt-chromium-molybdenum (Co–Cr–Mo) alloy, which appears to have improved the issue of subsidence in clinical trials.

The cobalt–chromium alloys, commonly used in total joint prostheses, strike a balance between stainless steel and titanium. Depending on the processing the alloy, cobalt–chromium can achieve a useful range of strength and ductility, endowing it with great versatility for implants. However, such implants are significantly more expensive than stainless steel to manufacture (43). The Charité, ProDisc, Maverick, and FlexiCore implants all have endplates manufactured from cobalt–chromium alloys.

Titanium alloys are particularly attractive for use in medical applications, because they have high biocompatibility. They are also more resistant to corrosion than stainless steel or Co–Cr, and typically yield fewer artifacts on magnetic resonance imaging than other metallic implants. Titanium also boasts a lower elastic modulus than cobalt–chrome alloys or stainless steel (closer to that of bone), but has relatively higher susceptibility to notching and wear debris generation. The clinical experience with solid titanium arthroplasty implants is relatively limited. Titanium spray coatings however, such as with the Maverick implant, are being used.

Bone–Implant Interface

Immediate fixation of a disc arthroplasty implant to the endplate may be achieved via profile characteristics such as screws, serrations, or fins. These structural features may aid in the insertion of the device, serve to limit early displacement, and facilitate long term stability. As an example, the ProDisc implant features a single midline sagittal fin. A slot to accept this fin is crested in the vertebral body based on anatomic landmarks and performed under fluoroscopic guidance. The slot acts to guide the implant into proper alignment. Furthermore, the fin stabilizes the implant relative to the vertebral endplates.

Other patented designs have been proposed that feature spikes, fins, ramps, or ridges, or even screws to achieve bony fixation. For example, the Charité® has small teeth and the Maverick has fins.

Long-term fixation of a disc arthroplasty device may also be facilitated with microstructure surfaces features aimed at increasing bony ingrowth. This has been used in appendicular joints for some time with well-established clinical advantages. Options for inducing bony ingrowth include titanium spraying or mesh, calcium sulfate coating, and hydroxyapatite coating. For example, the ProDisc features titanium spraying of the cobalt–chromium endplates. Porous coated surfaces require approximately six weeks of little or no motion to establish bony ingrowth (which may be provided by macrostructural features).

Implant–Implant Interfaces

The majority of modern intervertebral arthroplasty implants are composed of multiple components. Several interfaces exist. One type of interface is the type between bearing surfaces—surfaces that are designed to articulate. The "fixed" type of interface, however, is between two surfaces that are held together. As with any material–material interface, this one is subject to forces, dislodgement, and wear due to micro motion. Although there is significantly less motion at non-articulating interfaces, micro-motion does occur between these materials of different elastic properties.

For example the ProDisc has a contact between the polyethylene and the inferior endplate into which it is snapped. Conversely, the Charité has no such fixed interface with its mobile core.

Bearing Surfaces

The materials used at the bearing surface of an arthroplasty have specific requirements. The articulation must allow low-friction motion, resist permanent deformation, and have limited wear. This interface is usually believed to be the defining variable for longevity of most well-fixed arthroplasty devices.

It has been proposed, in order to reduce the risk of revision surgery, that a lumbar intervertebral arthroplasty should maintain acceptable function for 50 years. Considering that a typical adult makes 125,000 lumbar flexion movements yearly (44), an acceptable prosthesis should endure over 100 million cycles without significant degeneration. Both the ability of the implant to resist fatigue, and the host response to particulate debris, including toxicity and implant related osteolysis, has been considered.

Ultrahigh molecular weight polyethylene is used as a bearing material for many intervertebral disc arthroplasty implants. This has been established from other joint arthroplasty experience for its favorably low creep, or gradual deformation under mechanical stress. However, polyethylene wear debris has been in issue in other joints. Nonetheless, metal-on-polyethylene intervertebral disc arthroplasty animal studies (45) and early clinical reports (46) suggest that wear debris is not an evident problem. Wear-related osteolysis and loosening has not been described. It has been suggested that since the intervertebral space is not enveloped by synovial tissue, there may be relative immunity to the macrophage cytokine response with intervertebral arthroplasty as compared to hip or knee arthroplasty. Additionally, it has been suggested that this discrepancy may be due to the relatively low ranges of motion and loads seen by the intervertebral arthroplasty compared to the hip or knee arthroplasty. Other possibilities include limited particle generation, benign particle size and shape, a safe particle release rate, or an insufficiently short length of clinical follow-up.

In general, metal-on-metal articulations offer a reduced wear rate as compared with polyethylene on metal bearings. With regard to total hip arthroplasty, simulator wear testing has demonstrated dramatically less particulate wear in comparison with metal-on-polyethylene articulations and cohort studies have reported minimal to no osteolysis at a mean follow-up of five years. While this reduced wear rate may eventually be demonstrated for intervertebral disc prostheses, no data have yet been established. Additionally, metal-on-metal bearing surfaces are associated with little to no load damping. The presence of elevated levels of metal ions in the blood and urine of patients with metal-on-metal devices has been reported. Postmortem studies have reported significant increases in metal ion concentrations in the liver, kidney, spleen, heart, and lymphatic tissue. While these reports have raised concern for toxicity or for inducing metal hypersensitivity, a causal relationship with adverse clinical sequelae has not been established.

OPERATIVE TECHNIQUES

The technique for implantation of disc arthroplasty devices is device-specific. Training is important. To this end the FDA has mandated that surgeons undergo a specific training course prior to implantation of the Charité device—the first lumbar disc arthroplasty device with FDA approval.

Cervical Surgical Approach and Techniques

Cervical arthroplasty makes use of the standard anterolateral Smith–Robinson–Southwick approach. Since most spinal surgeons are experienced with this exposure, an access surgeon is not typically required.

In younger patients with soft disc herniations, the cervical arthroplasty implantation is typically less difficult than in the older, degenerative population as releases is not necessary. In patients with cervical spondylotic radiculopathy or myelopathy, wider uncinate resection and spondylotic ridge removal may be required. While fusion obviates this aspect of surgical technique, procedures intending to preserve motion may lead to recurrence of spondylosis in this patient population (47). Considering this ongoing risk of spur formation with continued motion, inadequate technique may be associated with propagation of spondylosis. Particularly when this procedure is considered for patients with compression of the neural elements, extensive decompression is crucial. Fusion may limit the importance of this step as opening the disc space and foramen via graft placement may be sufficient.

The disc space is prepared by a complete discectomy. Any non-osseous tissue is removed from the vertebral endplates. Careful endplate preparation is critical to the proper placement and long term integration of the prosthesis and vertebral bone. The sizing and placement of each device is specific to that prosthesis, and should be tailored to the anatomic level.

Lumbar Surgical Approaches and Techniques

Lumbar disc arthroplasty is generally performed through the standard anterior retroperitoneal approach (48). There are several approach issues that are specific to arthroplasty, however. First and foremost, the disc space exposure and preparation must be wider and more complete than generally used for fusion procedures. The patient and table must be positioned such that biplanar fluoroscopy is readily accomplished intra-operatively. Additionally, maintaining midline reference is crucial for implant alignment. To accomplish this, some even advocate standing midline between the flexed and abducted legs.

An access surgeon is commonly consulted to perform the approach particularly in patients with previous abdominal procedures. Access to the L4–L5 disc space requires mobilization of the vena cava and left iliac vein as well as the aorta and left iliac artery. The iliolumbar vein must also be mobilized or and is regularly ligated. The sympathetic chain may require careful mobilization; it is found beneath the iliolumbar vein and is in close contact with the L4 and L5 vertebral bodies. Symptoms of sympathectomy or RSD may follow injury to the sympathetic chain. The L5–S1 disc space, however, is typically caudal to the aortic bifurcation. It can be exposed by blunt dissection and retraction of the left and right iliac arteries and veins. The use of bipolar electrocautery is recommended to reduce the risk or retrograde ejaculation. Hand held or table-integrated retractors maintain the exposure.

The surgical technique used for the implantation of lumbar arthroplasty prostheses can be compared with that of the anterior lumbar interbody fusion (ALIF). One important difference is the precision required to prepare the disc space to provide biomechanical stability of the arthroplasty device (49). Complete discectomy, including removal of the posterior annulus, is important to ensure parallel retraction of the disc space before implantation. Care must be taken to balance the intervertebral soft tissues. A limited retraction of the posterior endplates may result in increased risk of device migration as well as limited opening of the neuroforamen. The endplate cartilage is removed, with care to preserve the cortical bone for improved bony ingrowth potential. The resection of osteophytes and/or endplate flattening may be required to achieve a well balanced force distribution between vertebral body and prosthesis endplate.

While the above surgical techniques for cervical and lumbar disc arthroplasty is similar for each device, there are important variations as well. As the mid and long term results of intervertebral arthroplasty become clearer, evolution of surgical technique is likely to progress.

MECHANICAL EVALUATION OF MOTION PRESERVING IMPLANTS

The typical mechanical evaluation of spinal implants has been significantly altered by the increased interest in intervertebral arthroplasty. Historically, most spinal implants were designed to provide stability, focusing on the evaluation of rigidity and fatigability of the implant. Protocols based on the analysis of segmental movements resulting from the application of pure rotational moments were established. These methods were standardized for the testing of traditional rigid implants, and must be modified for the testing of motion-preserving implants (50).

There are categories of evaluation. First, one may evaluate how well a particular device achieves its functional biomechanical objectives. The definition of the functional objective, however, is not always well defined. For example, with regard to an intervertebral arthroplasty device, is the functional goal to restore the very complex motion of a normal disc? Or is it to provide some particular motion that is theorized to reduce the risk of adjacent segment disease? Perhaps the functional goal is pain relief; if so, what motion parameters are associated with pain? Once a mechanical functional goal is established, it can be tested.

A second category of assessment is the appraisal of how an implant might affect the surrounding tissues; does the device affect the vertebral elements in a way which is clinically acceptable? For example, does a device impart loads to other structures (such as the facet joints) which could be undesirable? Does the segmental transfer of loads through an implant impart forces to the interface between the device and the vertebral body that may cause dissociation, for example?

A third category of assessment is to evaluate the longevity of the implant; will the device withstand the number and type of loading cycles demanded by its use for an acceptable duration before fatigue? This is usually focused on the assessment of potential wear of the bearing surface.

Each of these categories of mechanical assessment is considered in the development of the arthroplasty implants. Typically, cadaver models of device implantation are used for evaluation of specimen loading and testing of functional biomechanical objectives. Cadaver models can also be used to evaluate the effect of an implant on surrounding tissue structures. Measurement of internal loads, measurement of internal deformation, and measurement of externally induced loads can be made. Longevity testing is typically carried out in machines, however, which simulate the motion parameters dictated by normal or cadaver anatomic structures, but still allow testing of many millions of cycles under continuous conditions.

CONCLUSIONS

While many of the disc arthroplasty designs currently under human investigation endeavor to mimic the natural linkage between vertebral bodies, none match the well defined motion characteristics of the elegantly complex natural disc. It is uncertain if current designs are biomechanically "good enough" to provide long term resolution of pain without device-related complications; well designed clinical trials are in progress. History suggests that further developments will be forthcoming, which many contemporary critics suggest are necessary if realistic facet preservation and device longevity are to be met.

SUMMARY

Intervertebral disc arthroplasty has been developed to address the shortcomings and complications associated with spinal arthrodesis. Pseudoarthrosis, infection, and bone graft morbidities often rank secondarily to the pervasive dilemma of arthrodesis: the poor predictability of pain relief. Furthermore, many surgeons remain concerned about the potential for clinically symptomatic adjacent level disease following successful fusion.

The progress that has been made in the development of the intervertebral disc arthroplasty stems from an understanding of normal intervertebral disc mechanics. The goals of an intervertebral disc replacement device include restoration of disc height and motion. It is implicit that an intervertebral disc replacement device should closely mimic a healthy, natural intervertebral linkage, complement the function of the facet joints, and resist wear to provide lasting function.

This Chapter reviews the rationale for intervertebral disc arthroplasty, including the speculative concerns and the evidence concerning adjacent segment disease. The biomechanics and material properties of both the natural and prosthetic disc will be examined as it relates to prosthesis design. Operative techniques including placement of the device will be reviewed. Finally, the methods of biomechanical evaluation of these implants will be considered.

REFERENCES

1. West JL III, Bradford DS, Ogilvie JW. Results of spinal arthrodesis with pedicle screw-plate fixation. J Bone Joint Surg Am 1991; 73:1179–1184.
2. Steinmann JC, Herkowitz N. Pseudoathrosis of the spine. Clin Orthop 1992; 284:80–90.
3. Banwart JA, Asher MA, Hassanein RS. Iliac crest bone graft harvest donor site morbidity. A statistical evaluation. Spine 1995; 20:1055–1060.
4. DiAngelo DJ, Roberston JT, Metcalf NH, et al. Biomechanical testing of an artificial cervical joint and an anterior cervical plate. J Spinal Disord Tech 2003; 16:314–323.
5. Eck JC, Humphreys SC, Lim TH, et al. Biomechanical study on the effect of cervical spine fusion on adjacent-level intradiscal pressure and segmental motion. Spine 2002; 27:2431–2434.
6. Boden SD, McCowin PR, Davis DO, et al. Abnormal magnetic-resonance scans of the cervical spine in asymptomatic subjects: a prospective investigation. J Bone Joint Surg Am 1990; 72:1178–1184.
7. Gore DR, Sepic SB, Gardner GM. Neck pain: a long-term follow-up of 205 patients. Spine 1987; 12:1–5.
8. Gore DR, Sepic SB. Anterior cervical fusion for degenerated or protruded discs: a review of one hundred forty-six patients. Spine 1984; 9:667–671.
9. Gore DR, Sepic SB. Anterior discectomy and fusion for painful cervical disc disease: a report of 50 patients with an average follow-up of 21 years. Spine 1998; 23:2047–2051.

10. Hilibrand AS, Carlson GD, Palumbo MA, Jones PK, Bohlman HH. Radiculopathy and myelopathy at segments adjacent to the site of a previous anterior cervical arthrodesis. J Bone Joint Surg Am 1999; 81:519–528.
11. Lee CK, Langrana NA. Lumbosacral spinal fusion: a biomechanical study. Spine 1984; 9:574–581.
12. Weinhoffer SL, Guyer RD, Herbert M, Griffith SL. Intradiscal pressure measurements above an instrumented fusion. Spine 1995; 20:526–531.
13. Bushell GR, Ghosh P, Taylor TF, et al. The effect of spinal fusion on the collagen and proteoglycans of the canine intervertebral disc. J Surg Res 1978; 25:61–69.
14. Rahm MD, Hall BB. Adjacent-segment degeneration after lumbar fusion with instrumentation: a retrospective study. J Spinal Dis 1996; 9:392–400.
15. Lehmann TR, Spratt KF, Tozzi JE, et al. Long-term follow-up of lower lumbar fusion patients. Spine 1987; 12:97–104.
16. Penta M, Sandhu A, Fraser RD. Magnetic resonance imaging assessment of disc degeneration 10 years after anterior lumbar interbody fusion. Spine 1995; 20:743–747.
17. Throckmorton TW, Hilibrand AS, Mencio GA, Hodge A, Spengler DM. The impact of adjacent level disc degeneration on health status outcomes following lumbar fusion. Spine 2003; 28:2546–2550.
18. Gillet P. The fate of the adjacent motion segments after lumbar fusion. J Spinal Disorders Tech 2003; 16:338–345.
19. Lee CK. Accelerated degeneration of the segment adjacent to a lumbar fusion. Spine 1988; 13:375–377.
20. Ghiselli G, Wang JC, Bhatia NN, Hsu WK, Dawson EG. Adjacent segment degeneration in the lumbar spine. J Bone Joint Surg Am 2004; 86:1497–1503.
21. White AA, Panjabi MM. The basic kinematics of the human spine. Spine 1978; 3:12–20.
22. Ogston NG, King GJ, Gertzbein SD, Tile M, Kapasouri A, Rubenstein JD. Centrode patterns in the lumbar spine; baseline studies in normal subjects. Spine 1986; 11:591–595.
23. Pearcy MJ, Bogduk N. Instantaneous axes of rotation of the lumbar vertebral joints. Spine 1988; 13:1033–1041.
24. Dvorak J, Panjabi MM, Novotny JE, Antinnes JA. In vivo flexion/extension of the normal cervical spine. J Orthop Res 1991; 9:828–834.
25. Gertzbein SD, Seligman J, Holtby R, et al. Centrode characteristics of the lumbar spine as a function of segmental instability. Clin Orthop 1986; 208:48–51.
26. Race A, Broom ND, Robertson P. Effect of loading rate and hydration on the mechanical properties of the disc. Spine 2000; 25:662–669.
27. Nachemson A. Lumbar intradiscal pressure. Acta Ortho Scand 1960; 43:1–104.
28. Horst M, Brinckmann P. Measurement of the distribution of axial stress on the end-plate of the vertebral body. Spine 1981; 6:217–232.
29. Yang KH, King AI. Mechanism of facet load transmission as a hypothesis for low-back pain. Spine 1984; 9:557–565.
30. Fujiwara A, Lim TH, An HS, et al. The effect of disc degeneration and facet joint osteoarthritis on the segmental flexibility of the lumbar spine. Spine 2000; 25:3036–3044.
31. Yong-Hing K, Kirkaldy-Willis WH. The pathophysiology of degenerative disease of the lumbar spine. Orthop Clin North Am 1983; 14:491–504.
32. Szpalski M, Gunzburg R, Mayer M. Spine arthroplasty: a historical review. Eur Spine J 2002; 11:S65–S84.
33. Errico TJ. Lumbar disc arthroplasty. Clin Orthop Rel Res 2005; 435:106–117.
34. Cunningham B, Gordon J, Dmitriev A, et al. Biomechanical evaluation of total disc replacement arthroplasty: an in vitro human cadaveric model. Spine 2003; 28:110–117.
35. Lemaire JP, Skalli W, Lavaste F, et al. Intervertebral disc prosthesis: results and prospects for the year 2000. Clin Orthop 1997; 337:64–76.
36. Panjabi MM, White AA III. Biomechanics in the Musculoskeletal System. 3rd ed. New York: Churchill Livingstone, 2001.
37. Fernstrom U. Arthroplasty with intracorporal endoprothesis in herniated disk and in painful disc. Acta Chir Scand 1966; 355:154–159.
38. Link H. History, design and biomechanics of the Link SB Charite artificial disc. Eur Spine J 2002; 11:98–105.
39. Cinotti G, David T, Postacchini F. Results of disc prosthesis after a minimum follow-up period of 2 years. Spine 1996; 15:995–1000.
40. Lemaire JP, Skalli W, Lavaste F, et al. Intervertebral disc prosthesis: results and prospects for the year 2000. Clin Orthop 1997; 337:64–76.
41. Bao QB, McCullen GM, Higham PA, et al. The artificial disk: theory, design, and materials. Biomaterials 1996; 17:1157–1167.
42. Hallab N, Link HD, McAfee PC. Biomaterial optimization in total disc arthroplasty. Spine 2003; 28:139–152.
43. Taksali S, Grauer JN, Vaccaro AR. Material considerations for intervertebral disc replacement implants. Spine J 2004; 4:231–238.

44. Kostuik JP. Intervertebral disc replacement. In: Bridwell KH, DeWald RL, eds. The textbook of Spinal Surgery. 2nd ed. Philadelphia: Lippincott–Raven, 1997:2257–2266.
45. Cunningham BW, Dmitriev AE, Hu N, McAfee PC. General principles of total disc replacement arthroplasty: seventeen cases in a nonhuman primate model. Spine 2003; 28:118–124.
46. Dooris AP. Experimental and theoretical investigations into the effects of artificial disc implantation on the lumbar spine. PhD Dissertation. Iowa University, 2001.
47. Sekhon LH. Cervical arthroplasty in the management of spondylotic myelopathy. J Spinal Disord Tech 2003; 16:307–313.
48. Gumbs AA, Shah RV, Yue JJ, Sumpio B. The open anterior paramedian approach for spine procedures. Arch Surg 2005; 140:339–343.
49. Mayer HM, Weichert K, Korge A, Qose I. Minimally invasive total disc replacement: surgical technique and preliminary clinical results. Eur Spine J 2002; 11:S124–S130.
50. McNally DS. The objectives for the mechanical evaluation of spinal instrumentation have changed. Eur Spine J 2002; 11: S179–S185.
51. Buckwalter JA, Einhorn TA, Simon SR (eds). Orthopaedic basic science: biology and biomechanics of the musculoskeletal system. American Academy of Orthopaedic Surgeons. Illinois: Rosemont, 2000.
52. Bono, G. History and evolution of disc replacement. The Spine J 2004; 4S:145–150.

25 Biomechanical Aspects of the Spine Motion Preservation Systems

Vijay K. Goel, Ahamed Faizan, Leonora Felon, and Ashok Biyani
Department of Bioengineering and Orthopedic Surgery, University of Toledo, Toledo, Ohio, U.S.A.

Dennis McGowan
Spine and Orthopedic Surgery Associates, Kearney, Nebraska, U.S.A.

Shih-Tien Wang
Department of Orthopedics and Traumatology, Taipei, Taiwan

INTRODUCTION

Fusion surgery is the current state of the art surgical treatment for most of the acquired or iatrogenic spine instabilities/disorders. The procedure restores spinal alignment, and reduces pain. With the recent advances in the fusion techniques, successful fusion rates have approached very high, but have failed to reflect a comparable increase in the successful clinical outcome. The clinical outcomes after fusion appear to be quite inconsistent; a systematic review of mainly retrospective case series suggest that satisfactory clinical outcomes may range from just 16% to as high as 95%, with an average of around 68% (2). In addition, an apprehension of adjacent segment disease in the long-term follow-up has always been a concern.

From a biomechanical point of view, rigid spinal fusion is inherently a nonphysiologic procedure. Furthermore, with the age group of the patients shifting to the younger population, fusion may not be the most appropriate procedure for this group. Consequently, nonfusion technologies are evolving to provide a more physiological solution to the problem at-hand. The nonfusion systems range from replacing the entire disc (artificial discs), nuclear replacements, or maintaining the disc with a controlled motion of the segment (Dynamic systems). Motion preservation is becoming one of the most important aspects of the spinal surgery today. The motion preservation systems restore the stability of the spinal column by providing physiological motion similar to the healthy spine. This Chapter briefly describes the biomechanical aspects of the motion preservation systems.

TOTAL DISC REPLACEMENT TECHNOLOGIES

The main goals of spinal arthrosis (artificial disc replacements) are to restore normal mobility for the degenerated spinal segment and its disc height. Currently, three devices, in the category of device primarily for motion (preservation), have been given investigational device exemptions (IDEs) by the FDA and are in different stages of the FDA's regulatory process: the Medtronic Sofamor Danek "Maverick®," the Spinecore "FlexiCore®," and the Synthes "ProDisc®," and a fourth device from DePuy-Spine "Charité®," has been approved by the FDA. The Charité disc (DePuy Spine, Inc., Raynham, Massachusetts, U.S.A.) has a mobile articulating core with two bearing surfaces. The Maverick lumbar disc (Medtronic Sofamor Danek, Memphis, Tennessee, U.S.A.) and ProDisc (Synthes, Paoli, Pennsylvania, U.S.A.), have a single ball-and-socket type articulating surface. The Charité artificial disc can be categorized as a bi-articular design, whereas the Maverick and ProDisc can be described as a uni-articular design. Obviously, these design features will influence the degree of similarities between an implant and the intact segment biomechanics (e.g., segments with mobile core disc implants versus no mobile core). Both the clinical and biomechanical issues are important in the design and development of artificial discs. For example, all of these designs must possess methods of attachment to the vertebral body endplates, and a strategy for revision surgery.

From a biomechanical perspective, issues such as the biocompatibility wear debris generation, compressive stiffness, and ranges of motion are important (1).

The hypothesis is that such a disc will inhibit the progression of spinal degeneration of the adjacent segments that is thought to accompany spinal fusion. Thus, an ideal design for a total disc prosthesis should mimic the healthy human disc in that it will provide a proper range of motion (quantity; e.g., typical lumbar region values are 12 to 17, 6.3 to 8. 6, 1 to 2 degrees in flexion plus extension, lateral bending and axial rotation respectively, and 1.2 mm of axial compression), proper patterns of motion (quality, nonlinear load-deformation behavior), proper stiffness (e.g., 50 to 3214 N/mm in axial compression, 0.9 to 1.9, 2.1 to 2.6, 1.1 to 2.3, and 2.0 to 2.7 Nm per degree, respectively in flexion, extension, lateral bending, and axial rotation), and stability. Depending on the design, presently available prosthetic discs provide different degrees of stiffness and freedom of motion. A limited number of finite element and cadaver studies delineating the biomechanical characteristics of total disc replacement (TDR) devices have been pursued, although with several limitations.

Buttner-Janz and Zippel reported on biomechanical tests on the SB Charite I and II (4). A servo hydraulic machine applied compressive loads in either slow cyclic (quasi-static) or dynamic conditions. Hysteresis was found in the polyethylene with compressive loads to 4.2 kN. Cold flow in the plastic was seen in loads between 6 and 8 kN and at 10.5 kN, and the height of the slip core was reduced by 10%. Dynamic testing included rotating the implant through $\pm 10°$ about the neutral position at 5 to 10 Hz under a compressive load of 700 N. The compressive load was increased with one "weekly maximum load of 8.0 kN" and several intermediate load levels. Testing was carried out to 20 million cycles. The authors found no significant alteration to the implants after the dynamic tests other than "slight track marks" on the plates and core. Ahrens et al. (5) reported the results of in vitro tests performed with the Link SB III. Five fresh/frozen L4–L5 motion segments were tested by applying pure moments in extension, flexion, left and right lateral bending and torsion. The rotational responses at the maximum moment for the intact and implanted disc specimens were measured. No significant difference between intact and implanted segment rotation in extension or lateral bending was observed. The implanted segments rotated more in flexion and torsion, as compared to the intact specimens.

Two significant design changes (larger contact surface area and different metal component of the endplates) have resulted in the SB III used today. Although the first two designs experienced a number of failures including metal plate failure (31%), anterior implant dislocation (22%), and subsidence (31%) (6), the Link SB III prosthesis has had a considerably better success rate. In one study no metal end plate failure was found and subsidence was reduced to 3% and anterior dislocation to 9% (7). Cinotti reported on 46 patients implanted with the SB Charite® III at an average follow-up time of 3.2 years. Dislocation occurred in 2% and subsidence in 9%. Average sagittal plane rotation range was 9° for the implanted level and 16° for the adjacent level. Placing the disc prosthesis posteriorly as opposed to anteriorly also increased the range of motion. Cinotti attributed a large portion of the unsatisfactory results to the surgical learning curve and proper patient selection (10).

Cunningham et al., quantified the multidirectional intervertebral kinematics (range of motion and centers of rotation) following TDR arthroplasty (Charité disc) compared to conventional stabilization techniques (fusion) in a cadaver model (8,9). When compared to the intact, at the instrumented level, Charité disc placement resulted in an increase of the range of motion (ROM) by 44% in axial rotation, 3% in flexion and extension, and 16% in lateral bending. The fusion reduced the motion by 80% in axial rotation, 93% in flexion and extension, and 83% in axial rotation. No significant changes were found at the adjacent levels. Based on flexion-extension radiographs, the intervertebral centers of rotation were calculated and it was found that disc replacement with Charité preserved the normal mapping of segmental motion (11).

An in vitro biomechanical test of Sofamor Danek Disc Prosthesis (ball and socket gliding surface type design) was performed on seven fresh human cadaveric lumbosacral spines (9). Pure bending moments, up to 6 Nm, were applied to L1. For each specimen, the intact spine was loaded in flexion and extension, and the three-dimensional displacements of each vertebral level were recorded simultaneously. Surgery was performed to excise the anterior longitudinal ligament at L4–L5, the anterior portion of the annulus, and the nucleus. The joint was distracted, and the ball and socket components of the artificial disc were inserted. The load–displacement characteristics then were recorded in flexion and extension to 6 Nm, as was done previously with the intact spine. The results demonstrated that the disc was effective in restoring the motion to intact values. However, amount of deviation from the intact varied with the location of the disc prosthesis within the specimen; and post-test dissection revealed that the disc location varied from specimen to specimen.

Finite element (FE) analyses have also been recruited in an effort to perturbate design to optimize the mechanical behavior of artificial discs. Dooris et al. (11) modified a previously validated intact finite element model to create models implanted with a ball-and-cup and slip core-type artificial discs via an anterior approach (Figs. 1A and B). To study surgical variables, small and large windows were cut into the annulus, and the implants were placed anteriorly and posteriorly within the disc space. The anterior longitudinal ligament was also restored. Models were subjected to either 800 N axial compression force alone or to a combination of 10 Nm flexion-extension moments and 400 N axial preload. Implanted model predictions were compared with those of the intact model. The predicted rotations for the two disc implanted models were in agreement with the experimental data.

For the ball and socket design, disc facet loads were more sensitive to the anteroposterior location of the artificial disc than to the amount of annulus removed. For 800 N axial compression, implanted models with an anteriorly placed artificial disc exhibited facet loads 2.5 times greater than loads observed with the intact model, whereas posteriorly implanted models predicted no facet loads in compression. Implanted models with a posteriorly placed disc exhibited greater flexibility than the intact and implanted models with anteriorly placed discs. Restoration of the anterior longitudinal ligament (ALL) reduced pedicle stresses, facet loads, and extension rotation to nearly intact levels. The models suggested that, by altering placement of the artificial disc in the anteroposterior direction, a surgeon can modulate motion-segment flexural stiffness and posterior load-sharing, even though the specific disc replacement design has no inherent rotational stiffness.

The motion data, as expected, differed between the two disc designs (ball and socket, and slip core) and as compared to the intact as well, (Fig. 1C). Similar changes were observed for the loads on the facets (Fig. 1D).

In summary, the results revealed that both of these devices do not restore motion and loads across facets back to the intact case. (These designs restore the intact biomechanics in a limited sense.) These differences are not only due to the size of the implants but the inherent design differences. Ball and socket design has a more "fixed" center of rotation as compared to the slip core design in which the center of rotation (COR) undergoes a wider variation. Further complicating factor is the location of the disc within the annular space itself, a parameter under the control of the surgeon. Thus, it will be difficult to restore biomechanics of the segment back to normal using such designs. Only clinical follow-up studies will provide the effects of such variations on the changes in spinal structures as a function of time.

The classic flexibility testing protocol is not appropriate for the understanding of the biomechanics of the construct at the adjacent levels (12,13). This protocol applies pure moments as loads and measures the resulting displacements, both for the intact and instrumented cases. However, constant pure moments are not appropriate for measuring effects of implants, like the TDRs, at adjacent levels (12–14). The net motion of a longer construct following alterations is not similar if only pure moments are applied—fusions will limit motion and other interventions may increase motion, a reflection of the change in stiffness of the segment. This testing protocol may have shortcomings for clinical applications. For example, with forward flexion, there are clinical demands to get to ones shoes to tie them, to reach a piece of paper fallen to the floor, etc. It would thus be advantageous to use a protocol that would achieve the same overall range of motion for the intact specimen and instrumented construct by applying pure moments that distribute evenly down the column. Goel et al. (15) carried out a finite element study, as a part of an on going larger investigation, that dealt with the use of such a protocol (termed Hybrid approach) to investigate the effects of the disc implantation at one

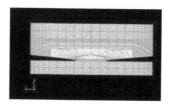

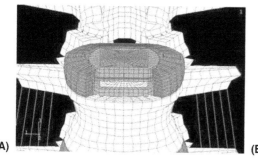

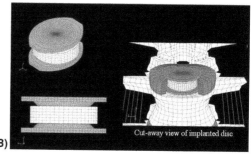

(A)

(B)

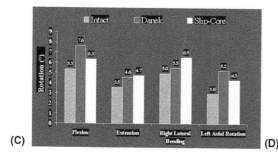

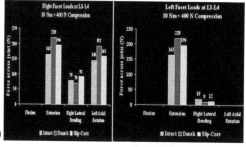

(C)

(D)

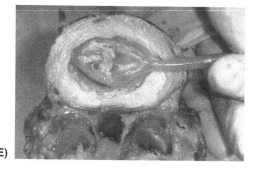

(E)

FIGURE 1 The intact finite element model of a ligamentous segment was modified to simulate (**A**) the ball and socket type artificial disc implant, (**B**) the slip core type artificial disc implant. (**C**) Predicted rotations for the two disc designs. (**D**) Predicted facet loads for the two disc designs. (**E**) In situ curable prosthetic inter vertebral nucleus. *Source*: Adapted from Ref. 21.

level on the kinematics, load sharing and stresses in various structures at the implanted and adjacent segments for a mobile articulating core type artificial disc design (Charité® Artificial Disc). Using this approach they found that the Charité® disc placement slightly increases motion at the implanted level with a resultant increase in facet loading when compared to the adjacent segments. The motions and loads decrease at the adjacent levels.

Dmitriev et al. (16) conducted an in vitro investigation of cervical adjacent level intradiscal pressures (IDPs) following a total disc replacement arthroplasty. They concluded that artificial disc replacement does not affect the adjacent segment IDPs.

Most of the current disc designs are of ball and socket design. These are placed, in the cervical region, using an anterior approach following the dissection of the anterior longitudinal ligament and annulus. In extension, the absence of the ALL with the ball and socket design can lead to an increase in motion, compared to the intact. In order to overcome such potential shortcomings of the ball and socket design, a new type of disc has been developed by Abbott Spine,

Inc, Austin, Texas, U.S.A. (17). The unique feature of the design is a flap attached to the anterior part of the spine to compensate for the lost ligaments. The material properties of the flap are very similar to that of the ligaments and hence it helps spine to replicate the natural biomechanics. The finite element studies suggest that such an artificial disc produced range of motion very similar to that of the intact spine and hence proving the efficacy of the device. More animal and cadaveric studies are required to validate the results obtained from finite element model (FEM).

Goffin et al. (18) studied the trials of Bryan® cervical disc prosthesis (Medtionic Sofamor Danek, Memphis, Tennessee, U.S.A.) in patients for treatment of single and two-level disc diseases. Patients with radiculopathy and/or myelopathy underwent implantation, and effectiveness of the device was evaluated in follow-ups. One year after the surgery flexion/extension motion per level averaged $7.9 \pm 5.3°$ in the single and $7.4 \pm 5.1°$ in bi-level placements. They concluded that device alleviates neurologic symptoms and signs similar to anterior cervical discectomy and fusion. The early randomized clinical trials for comparison of fusion with disc replacement showed that disc replacement patients reported significantly less pain and disability (19).

The long-term effect of wear debris in these designs is also a concern if implanted in a younger age group of patients. Hallab et al. (20) did a study that highlighted the association between the spinal implants particulate wear debris and the increased potential for osteolysis. Dooris investigated the wear characteristics of the Sofamor Danek Disc Prosthesis (21) by simultaneously compressing and oscillating the implant ball component over the implant socket component in a saline bath for $14.5°$ ($\pm 0.3°$) flexion and $4.5°$ ($\pm 0.3°$) extension with 700 N vertical load. Periodic mass measurements of the components determined the mass changes. Three pairs of artificial disc components were tested to 10 million cycles. The results demonstrated less than 3×10^{-3} mL of wear particles over no less than five years by most estimates. The gravimetric changes produced by the wear simulation indicated that this prosthesis showed good resistance to wear. Functional changes (e.g., range of motion, integrity) were negligible. The wear depth rate was less than 0.1 mm/10 million cycles, resulting in very small changes in implant dimensions or kinematics. Extremely low wear rates have also been reported for Charité® discs.

Additional work is needed to estimate the long-term effects of artificial discs, and newer disc designs being fabricated out of elastomers, and the artificial discs in the cervical region.

ARTIFICIAL NUCLEUS REPLACEMENT

As the name suggests, these devices replace the degenerated nucleus and leave the annulus intact. The current designs of the nucleus prosthesis have four different approaches to reproduce the biomechanical effect of incompressible hydrostatic pressure within the nucleus cavity:

1. Cavity filled with fluid, gel, oil, or soft polymer
2. Solid body in the disc space
3. Hydrophilic polymer in various shapes, sizes, and numbers
4. Injection of biomaterial into the nucleus cavity for in situ polymerization

The first design approach is to replace the nucleus pulposus by structures with impermeable cavity(s) (such as balloon or bladder) filled or inflated with fluids, gas, or other injectable materials after placing into the disc by a minimally invasive surgical technique (22). The second approach is inserting a solid body such as a metal ball in the nucleus cavity. The third is implanting dehydrated or partially hydrated hydrophilic materials in a permeable balloon or fibrous jacket, or rods/beads into the nucleus cavity where the implanted material becomes hydrated. The fourth approach is to inject biomaterials into the nucleus cavity where it will be polymerized into a shape.

Some designs of nucleus prosthesis have been evaluated by in vitro and in vivo animal studies and/or by clinical trial in human, and have demonstrated favorable results of restoring the disc function and clinical improvements.

Recent reports on biomechanical tests of the prosthetic disc nucleus (PDN) showed that it produced some degree of stabilization and distraction. Loads of 7.5 Nm and 200 N axial compressions were applied to six L4–L5 specimens. Nucleotomized spines increased rotations by 12% to 18% depending on load orientation, but implanted spines (implant placed transversely) showed a change of −12% to +2% from the intact with substantial reductions in neutral zone. Up to 2 mm of disc height was recovered by insertion. The device, however, was implanted and tested in its desiccated form. The biomechanics of the hydrated prosthesis may vary considerably from that of its desiccated form.

In vitro biomechanical testing of curable prosthetic intervertebral nucleus (PIN) was performed on five fresh-frozen osteo-ligamentous three-segment human lumbar spines (Fig. 1E). The spines were tested in four configurations: intact, denucleated, implanted, and fatigued. Cyclic loading from 250 to 750 N at 2 Hz for at least 100,000 cycles produced fatiguing. Nuclectomy was performed through a 5.5 mm trephine hole in the right middle lateral side of the annulus. The device was inserted into the nucleus cavity through a small hole in the annulus and liquid polymer injected into the balloon under controlled pressure inflating the balloon, filling the cavity, and distracting the intervertebral disc. The results revealed that PIN device could reverse the destabilizing effects of a nuclectomy and restored normal segment stiffness. Significant increase in disc height were also achieved. Adjacent motion segments had minimal kinematic changes after implantation of the nucleus prosthesis, suggesting a normal load-sharing relationship. After fatiguing, the implanted segment behaved similar to intact adjacent segments, further evidence of a normal load-sharing condition. No implant extrusion or endplate fracture was observed in any of implanted disc levels after the fatigue test.

The preliminary results for some of nucleus devices indicate problems of migration, extrusion, vertebral endplate changes and/or subsidence. Design criteria for nucleus prosthesis should include methods for proper load transfer from the vertebral body to the annulus fibrosus though the prosthetic nucleus and for stabilization of prosthesis within the disc (22).

Some aspects of nucleus prostheses designs may cause adverse effects on surrounding structures or prosthesis instability. A small contact surface area at the interface between nucleus prosthesis and the vertebral endplates produces abnormal stress concentration that may be the cause for changes in the vertebral body adjacent to the endplates and for subsidence. Uncontrolled and excessive lateral wall bulge of nucleus prostheses with thin-walled fluid filled balloon or cavity may be a contributing factor for prosthetic migration during compression bending. Another area of concern with nucleus prosthesis is postimplant stability within the disc. Implanted prosthesis should be stable throughout the range of motion during compression-bending and compression-torsion. Abnormal movement of the implanted prosthesis within the disc during the range of motion may cause harmful effects of the annulus. Proper "fitting" and/or interlocking at the interface between nucleus prosthesis and the annulus are desired to prevent this "loose fitting" problem.

Some designs have features to overcome these possible problems by minimizing lateral wall bulge, increasing the contact surface area and/or by self-contouring of prosthesis for congruous fit to the nucleus cavity (22). Nucleus prostheses with in situ polymerization may have, in general, better congruous fitting than other preformed prostheses.

ARTIFICIAL FACETS

To restore normal function at a diseased segment, artificial facets may be an alternative to other surgeries for treatment of severe facet tropism, facet hypertrophy, arthritic or degenerated facet joints, spinal stenosis, after laminectomy and facetectomy surgeries, and artificial facets may be used in conjunction with artificial discs. Facet replacements must restore normal motion in flexion, extension, lateral bending, and axial rotation and must perform well under shear and torsional loads. The prosthesis also should be easy to place in all patients and fix to the bone well to reduce the risk of loosening. The facet replacement market is miniscule at present and all implants are in research and design stages. However, this technology has potential.

Zhu et al. (23) carried out cadaver testing on seven lumbar spine segments to investigate the performance of the Total Facet Arthroplasty Systems™ (TFAS™) artificial facets (Archus Orthopedics, Redmond, Washington, U.S.A.). There was no significant difference between

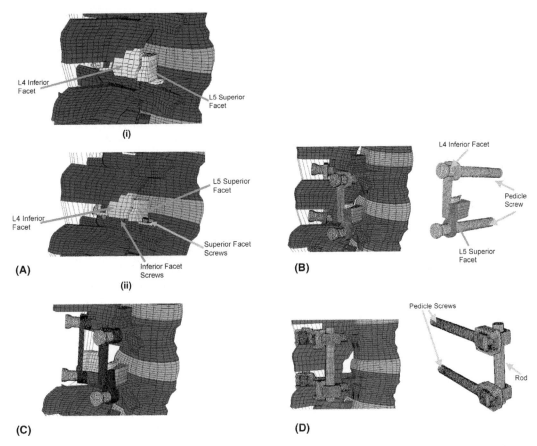

FIGURE 2 **(A)** (*i*) L3–S1 finite element model with artificial facet caps at L4–L5. (*ii*) L3–S1 finite element model with artificial facet caps secured with screws at L4–L5. **(B)** The pedicle screw based artificial facet design with a 3 mm thick stem connecting the metal facets to the pedicle screw. **(C)** The wide laminectomy model with the support pedicle screw based design at L4–L5. **(D)** A rigid screw and rod system across the L4–L5 motion segment. *Source*: Adapted from Ref. 24.

implanted and intact spine in flexion, extension, lateral bending and axial rotation. They showed that TFAS™ restored both the range and pattern of segmental motion to that of the intact spine and played a significant role in flexion, extension and axial rotation. The conclusion of the study was that TFAS™ system grossly reproduced the guiding and mechanical blocking roles of the natural lumbar facet joints.

Shaw and associates have done finite element studies to investigate the different artificial facet designs (24). Three different facet joint replacement systems were simulated in an FE spine model with laminectomy surgery. These were pedicle screw based artificial facets, facet caps replacement and pedicle screw based facet with additional support systems (Figs. 2A–D). For comparison, a rigid pedicle screw and rod system was also simulated. The motion increase was most likely due to partial removal of the ligamentum flavum and capsular ligaments. Stability to the lumbar spine was not restored when artificial facets were used across a wide laminectomy. Designs having a "capsular ligament" surrounding the joint may help to reduce the increased motion. Facet loads decreased in all loading modes with all implant designs at L4–L5 and adjacent levels. The decrease in facet loads may result in accelerated disc degeneration at the implanted and adjacent levels and future surgical intervention for young patients. All implant stresses were well below the actual yield strength of titanium; therefore, the implants are unlikely to mechanically fail.

Although the preliminary studies are encouraging; the facet replacement technology is relatively very new and hence considerable clinical trials and biomechanical studies is required before we confidently make any conclusion about their use in human.

Dynamic Stabilization Systems

Spinal fusion surgeries aim at limiting the motion of the segment and thus restoring its stability. Spinal arthroplasty (artificial disc and facets) devices restore motion by sharing the kinematics of the remaining joints of the spinal motion segment. Dynamic stabilization systems aim at altering favorably the movement and load transmission through the spinal motion segment (25). The hypothesis behind dynamic stabilization system is that control of abnormal motion and more physiologic load transmission would relieve pain and prevent adjacent segment degeneration. A remote expectation is that, once normal motion and load transmission is achieved, the damaged disc may repair itself. This is supported by the fact that, many clinical studies suggest that cells of the intervertebral disc respond favorably to reduced but not eliminated mechanical loading through deposition of extracellular matrix proteins into the disc space (27–29). For example, in initial clinical trials with one such system (Wallis®, Abbott Spine; Austin, Texas, U.S.A.) it was observed that the degenerated disc became hydrated over time (26). The pertinent biomechanical questions in dynamic stabilization at present are:

1. How much control of motion is desirable?
2. How much load should be shared by the system to unload the damaged disc?
3. What are the long-term implant failure implications?

The advantages of using dynamic stabilization systems over fusion and arthroplasty techniques are:

1. Ability to be performed posteriorly: familiarity of surgeons with the posterior approach is advantageous for accuracy purposes;
2. Tissue sparing;
3. Load sharing: this is an advantage over the total disc replacement and prosthetic disc replacement, which cannot be used for patients with significant posterior pathology;
4. Can be used adjunct to other non fusion technologies: dynamic stabilization/motion preservation technologies can be utilized with total disc replacements and disc nucleus replacements.

The present day indications for the use of dynamic stabilization systems are for, younger patients with multi-segment disc degeneration, stabilization of decompression surgeries, and adjacent to fusion to avoid adjacent level degeneration (26). However, they cannot be used as stand alones in cases where the disc is completely degenerated.

There are two types of dynamic stabilizations systems, which are currently available:

- Interspinous based systems
- Pedicle screw based systems

Interspinous Ligament Devices

Wires and tension bands have been used for many years in orthopedic surgery. Posterior spinal ligament complex stability is known to be re-established by the use of sublaminar wires and cables. From this concept, interspinous ligament devices have emerged. These devices bind the two adjacent spinous processes using only a ligament, without any metal anchorage. These devices may be used as a stand alone or along with fusion to stabilize adjacent segments. Several investigators have found that these devices are effective as a stand alone for recurrent disc herniation cases (30–34). Suzuki et al. (33) conducted a biomechanical study with the porcine vertebral model to assess the stability offered by Leed-Keio ligament in degenerative lumbar spondylolisthesis. Five porcine motion segments (L4–L5) were tested in the intact, destabilized, and Leeds-Keio-instrumented conditions. Specimens were loaded in flexion and extension, and construct stiffness was measured during the initial loading cycle and at 250 cycle intervals for 1500 cycles. They found that the system was effective in initially stabilizing an unstable degenerative lumbar spondylolisthesis model; it further maintained its stabilizing effect during cyclic loading. The surgery required for interspinous ligament devices is very simple, however they do not unload the disc in extension at all, hence the evolution of interspinous spacer devices (25).

Interspinous Distraction Devices

The interspinous distraction devices are floating devices, which are not rigidly connected to the vertebrae. The interspinous spacers are designed to off load the posterior disc and the facet joint, by distracting the spinous processes (25). Their usage is meant to be for the treatment of early stage intervertebral disc degeneration, or to increase the foraminal space in patients with stenosis (26). There are several interspinous-based distraction devices, with the basic structure being a spacer placed in between the spinous processes and then a set of bands to tie the device to the processes.

Lindsey et al. conducted an in vitro biomechanical test on seven lumbar spines to quantify changes in kinematics following the implantation of the X-stop® (St. Francis Medical Technologies, Inc., Alameda, California, U.S.A.) (Fig. 3A). The spines were tested in flexion/extension, axial rotation, and lateral bending. Images were taken during each test to determine the kinematics of each motion segment. They found that the flexion–extension range of motion was significantly reduced at the instrumented level, while the axial rotation and lateral bending ranges of motion were not affected at the instrumented level. The range of motion at the adjacent segments was not significantly affected by the implant (35).

Fuchs et al. (36) conducted an in vitro biomechanical testing with the X-stop® spacer in conjunction with graded factectomy procedure and found that in bilateral total factectomy the implant significantly decreased the range of motion in flexion and extension; had no effect on axial rotation; significantly increased the ROM for lateral bending.

Swanson et al. (37) conducted a biomechanical investigation using eight cadaver lumbar specimens (L2–L5). The specimens were loaded in flexion, neutral, and extension. A pressure transducer was used to measure the intradiscal pressure and annular stresses during each of the three positions at each of the three disc levels. An appropriately sized interspinous implant (X-stop®) was placed at L3–L4, and the pressure measurements were repeated. The implant did not significantly change the intradiscal pressures at the adjacent levels, and significantly unloaded the intervertebral disc at the instrumented level in the neutral and extended positions (37).

Wiseman et al. (38) measured the facet loading parameters of lumbar cadaver spines during extension; before and after the placement of the X-stop® interspinous spacer in seven cadaver lumbar spines. The specimens were loaded to 15 Nm of extension and 700 N compressions with and without X-stop® placed between the L3–L4 spinous processes. Pressure-sensitive film was placed in the facet joints of the implanted and adjacent levels. After loading, the film was digitally analyzed for peak pressure, average pressure, contact area, and force. These values were compared between the intact and implanted specimens at the adjacent and implanted levels using a paired t-test. They found that the implant significantly reduced the mean peak pressure, average pressure, contact area, and force at the implanted level; no significant change was seen at the adjacent levels. They concluded that stabilization with interspinous implant may not cause adjacent level facet pain or accelerated facet joint degeneration. Furthermore, pain induced from pressure originating in the facets and/or posterior annulus of the lumbar spine may be relieved by surgery with X-stop® (38).

Minns et al. measured the intradiscal pressure and sagittal plane stiffness in compression at four angles of flexion with loads up to 700 N in a cadaveric study using the DIAM™ (Medtronic Sofamar Danek, Memphis, Tennessee, U.S.A.) interspinous system (Fig. 2B). They concluded that the DIAM™ system stabilized the spinal segment with a reduction in intradiscal pressure (39).

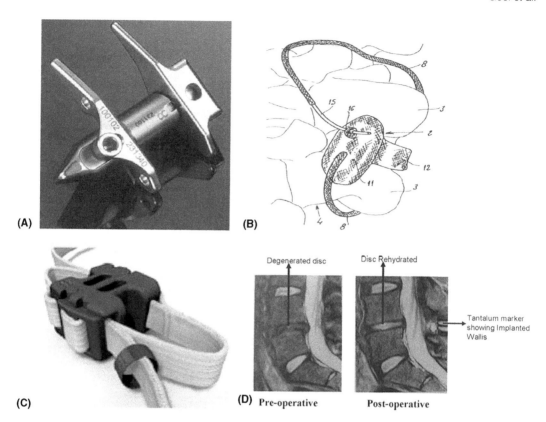

(A) (B)

(C) (D) Pre-operative Post-operative

Degenerated disc Disc Rehydrated

Tantalum marker
showing Implanted
Wallis

FIGURE 3 (**A**) The X-stop® spacer is made of high strength titanium alloy, and consists of two parts. The first part being the main body which has an oval spacer and tissue expander, and the second part is the universal wing. *Source*: Adapted from Ref. 49. (**B**) The device for intervertebral-assisted motion system consists of a polymeric interspinous spacer, with extended wings to act as a posterior shock-absorbing device. It consists of a flexible spacer and dual independent ligaments, which attach the spacer to the spinous process above and below the spinous process. The flexible spacer is made with an inert medical-grade silicone core material, and the ligament is made from the Graf/ Senegas ligament. *Source*: Adapted from Ref. 48. (**C**) The Wallis® interspinous spacer system. The first generation device was a titanium spacer stabilized within the interspinous space by two ligaments attached to the spinous processes of the adjacent segments. The limitations of the first generation implant were, ligament loosening and spinous process fracture due to the titanium spacer. The second generation spacer was made of Polyetheretherketone (PEEK) composite with two attached polyester ligaments. The elastic stiffness of PEEK lies between that of the cortical bone and the cancellous; thus reduces the stress that might be caused at the bone implant interface. *Source*: Adapted from Ref. 48. (**D**) Preoperative and postoperative MRIs distinctly showing a change in the hydration of the level treated with Wallis®. *Source*: From Ref. 26.

Mariottini et al. (40) have used DIAM for 43 patients suffering from back pain and sciatica and have found that in 97% of the cases had satisfying results. Test information from Abbott Laboratories, has shown that the Wallis® system (Figs. 3C and D) increased the segment stiffness, and reduced the segment displacement (26). The international clinical study for patient follow-up with MRI, after implantation with Wallis® showed a distinct change in the hydration of the level treated with the Wallis® system. The study claimed that the increase in hydration was observed in almost 50% of the patients (26). The limitations of the first generation implant were, ligament loosening and spinous process fracture due to the titanium spacer.

Pedicle Screw Based Systems

Some flexible stabilization systems have relied upon fixation to the pedicle of the vertebrae. Such systems consist of pedicle screws threaded into adjacent segments and a member spanning between the heads of the pedicle screws to limit the movements of the spinal segment (Figs. 4A–D).

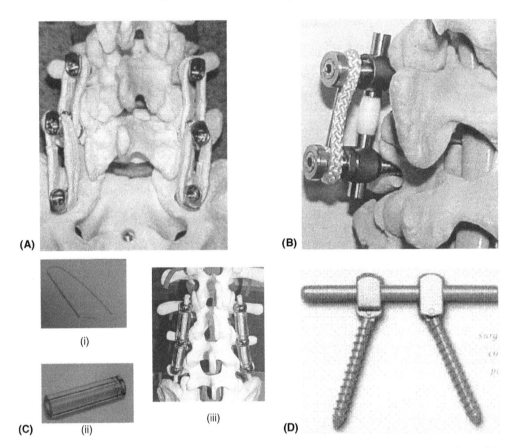

FIGURE 4 (**A**) Graf ligament system. It consists of a nonelastic band as a ligament to connect the pedicle screws across the segment to be stabilized to lock the segment in full lordosis. *Source*: Adapted from Ref. 48. (**B**) Fulcrum assisted soft stabilization (FASS) system. In this system, a fulcrum is placed between the pedicle screws in front of the ligament. The fulcrum distracts the posterior annulus. When the elastic ligament is placed posterior to the fulcrum, to compress the pedicle screw heads, the fulcrum transforms this posterior compression force into an anterior distraction force, which distracts the anterior annulus. The lordosis is not dependent on the patient's ability but is created by the tension in the ligament. *Source*: Adapted from Ref. 48. (**C**) Dynesys system (*dynamic neutralization system*). Dynesys system comprises of three components, (i) pedicle screws, (ii) polyethylene-terephthalate ligaments, and (iii) polycarbonate urethane spacers. *Source*: Adapted from Ref. 48. (**D**) Cosmic system has a hinge between the screw head and threaded portion which helps in load sharing and reduces mechanical stress. *Source*: Adapted from Ref. 47.

Markwalder and Wenger conducted a clinical study with an average follow-up of 7.4 years for 39 patients implanted with Graf ligament (Fig. 4A). The indications for the use of the Graf ligament in this study were young patients with mild or no facet joint degeneration, and minor disc degeneration. 66.6% of the patients participating in the study reported complete disappearance of back pain and 92.5% patients reported a complete disappearance of leg pain. They concluded that soft stabilization of lumbar motion segments yielded favorable long term results only in a highly selected patient population (41).

BrechbuÈhler et al. (42) conducted a clinical and radiological study of surgical outcomes of the Graf system and stated that it had good surgical outcomes in degenerative disc disease with decompression of the lumbar segment. They observed that, regional as well as global lumbar lordosis was maintained. Although statistically not significant, an increase of intervertebral distance was observed in adjacent segments in flexion of the lumbar spine. They concluded that these phenomena might represent pressurization of instrumented as well as adjacent discs after the insertion of ligament prostheses. Graf ligamentoplasty procedure also produced a significant increase in lateral canal stenosis especially in the presence of degenerative change in the facet joints or in the ligamentum flavum, causing early clinical failure of the Graf ligament (43).

The fulcrum assisted soft stabilization system (FASS system) was developed to address the disadvantages of the Graf ligament (Fig. 4B). Experimental studies have shown that the implant unloads the disc, but the flexibility of the segment was lost as greater unloading of the disc occurred by the adjustment of the tension in the ligament and the fulcrum (43).

The present indications for use of Dynesys® (Zimmer Inc.; Warsaw, Indiana, U.S.A.) system shown in Figure 4C are: (*i*) central spinal stenosis, (*ii*) spondylolisthesis, (*iii*) primary discopathy, (*iv*) hyper mobile, functional instability, and (*v*) mono or multisegmental stenosis. The contraindications for the usage of Dynesys are osteoporosis, degenerative, and rotational scoliosis. Dynesys also cannot be used when the spinal disc is completely degenerated. In the Dynesys system the spacers are bilaterally placed between the pedicle screw heads to withstand compressive loads. The ligaments are run through the hollow core of the spacers. A tensile preload of about 300 N is used to stabilize the construct. The plastic cylinder between the screw heads limits the degree of lordosis that can be created. As the ligament is not elastic, flexion compresses the disc, and the axis of flexion is the posterior ligament, which is well posterior to the normal axis of flexion. Active extension will open up the anterior annulus without compression of the posterior annulus. Theoretically, lordosis can be achieved by the action of the spinal extensor muscles and in extension; the cylinder will take increasing load. Thus, the principle of the system is its ability to create load sharing and restoration of disc height, not necessarily motion preservation because the system is rigid.

Freudinger et al. (44) tested the Dynesys system on four cadaveric spine specimens on a lumbar spine simulator, which allowed the simultaneous application of bending moments, compressive and shear loads. They concluded that the Dynesys reduces flexion and extension angles significantly.

Wilson et al. (45) investigated 10 cadaveric lumbar spine specimens, subjected to pure moments of ± 7.5 Nm (axial rotation, flexion, and extension) to compare range of motion and facet loads of intact specimens with those of injured specimens stabilized with Dynesys. The facet loads were measured using thin film electro-resistive pressure sensors. They found that the facet loads decreased in axial rotation after implantation of Dynesys, extension facet load values showed no significant difference compared to the intact case. They however found that the facet loads were significantly higher in flexion with the Dynesys due to device compression. Dynesys system reduced spinal motion from intact and decreased peak facet loading.

Grob et al. (46) did a surgical and patient oriented outcome study in 50 cases after an average of two years with the Dynesys system. Their primary indication for the implantation of Dynesys was degenerative disc and stenosis with associated instability. The surgeries were done at multilevels. They found that both back pain and leg pain on an average were moderately high two years after instrumentation with the Dynesys.

The Cosmic (Ulrich, Ulm, Germany) system (47) is a pedicle screw based dynamic instrumentation system. Equipped with a hinge between the screw head and threaded portion Cosmic is a load sharing system reducing mechanical stress on the implants (Fig. 4D). Thus, protection against implant failure and loosening is achieved. The hinged screw allows only for axial load, due to this, it is important to have a largely intact anterior column for implantation of this system. While Dynesys stabilizes by neutralizing motion, Cosmic corrects the sagittal plane and maintains motion in flexion/extension.

Vishnubhotla and associates (48) have done finite element based studies on various dynamic stabilization systems. A validated 3D nonlinear finite element model of the intact L3–S1 lumbar spine was used to evaluate the biomechanics of various dynamic stabilization systems in comparison with rigid screw rod system that is used in conventional fusion. The intact model was modified at L4–L5 to simulate stabilization with, rigid screw-rod system, rigid screw flexible rod system, Dynesys system, Cosmic system, and Wallis system. These devices were also simulated in decompression surgery to evaluate the stability. The load control and hybrid protocols were used to evaluate these devices. Various biomechanically relevant parameters like range of motion, facet loading, disc stresses, implant stresses, instantaneous axis of rotation and load sharing were evaluated. Results show that the flexible rod systems do not vary much in terms of stiffness and load sharing capabilities from the rigid screw rod system. Dynesys, Cosmic, and Wallis® systems are more flexible than rigid

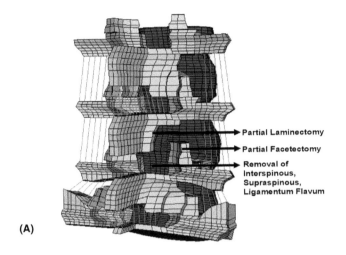

(A)

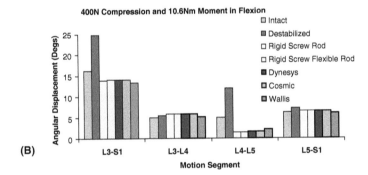

(B)

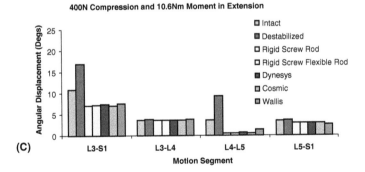

(C)

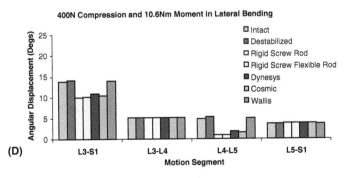

(D)

FIGURE 5 (**A**) Simulation of the decompression surgery at L4–L5 in the L3–S1 lumbar spine finite element model. Relative motions (degrees) at all the levels of the lumbar spine in response to 400 N compression and 10.6 Nm in (**B**) flexion for intact, (**C**) extension for intact, (**D**) lateral bending for intact, and (**E**) axial rotation for intact destabilized spine and stabilization with the instrumentation models. Total facet loads (N) in response to 400 N compression and 10.6 Nm moment in (**F**) extension for intact, (**G**) lateral bending for intact, and (**H**) axial rotation for intact, destabilized spine and stabilization with the instrumentation models. *Source*: Adapted from Ref. 48. (*E–H on next page.*)

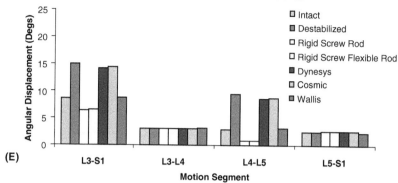

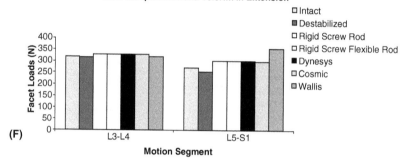

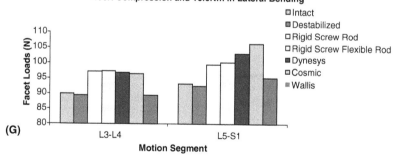

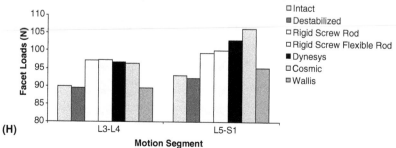

FIGURE 5 *Continued.*

systems but not flexible enough to say that they preserve motion (Figs. 5A–H). However, they have the ability to allow for loading through the intervertebral disc. All the flexible stabilization systems were capable of stabilizing the decompression surgery in flexion and extension and lateral bending, and not that effective in axial rotation.

REFERENCES

1. Goel VK, Panjabi MM. Introduction. In: Vijay K Goel, Manohar M Panjabi, eds. Roundtables in Spine Surgery, Spine Biomechanics: Evaluation of Motion Preservation Devices and Relevant terminology. Vol. 1. Issue 1. St. Louis: Quality Medical Publishing, 2005.
2. Turner JA, Ersek M, Herron L, et al. Patient outcomes after lumbar spinal fusions. JAMA 1992; 268(7):907–911.
3. Park P, Garton HJ, Gala VC, Hoff JT, McGillicuddy JE. Adjacent segment disease after lumbar or lumbosacral fusion: Review of the Literature. Spine Vol. 29, 1938–1944, Sept 1, 2004.
4. Buttner-Janz K. The development of the Artificial Disc Charite SB. Dallas: Hudley and Associates, 1992.
5. Ahrens J. In vitro evaluation of the LINK SB Charité intervertebral prosthesis: stability biomechanical testing project. Final report. Plano, Texas: Institute for Spine & Biomedical Research, 1997.
6. Waldemar Link & Co. GmbH, LINK SB Charite Intervertebral Prosthesis, Product Brochure. Germany: Hamburg, 1989.
7. Gilbertson LG, et al. Biomechanical evaluation of a new lumbar disc implant: in vitro-simulations of disc surgery, implantation, and post-op mobilization. Proceedings of the International Society for the Study of the Lumbar Spine, Melbourne, Australia, 1996.
8. Cunningham BW, Kotani Y, McNulty PS, Cappuccino A, McAfee PC. The effect of spinal destabilization and instrumentation on lumbar intradiscal pressure: an in vitro biomechanical analysis. Spine 1997; 22(22):2655–2663.
9. Cunningham BW, Gordon JD, Dmitriev AE, Hu N, McAfee PC. Biomechanical evaluation of total disc replacement arthroplasty: an in vitro human cadaveric model. Spine 2003; 28(20):S110–S117.
10. Cinotti G, David T, Postacchini F. Results of disc prosthesis after a minimum follow-up period of 2 years. Spine 1996; 21(8):995–1000.
11. Dooris AP, Goel VK, Grosland NM, Gilbertson LG, Wilder DG. Load-sharing between anterior and posterior elements in a lumbar motion segment implanted with an artificial disc. Spine 2001; 26(6):E122–E129.
12. Panjabi MM, Goel VK. Adjacent-level effects: design of a new test protocol and finite element model simulations of disc replacement. In: Goel VK, Panjabi MM, eds. Roundtables in spine surgery; Spine Biomechanics: Evaluation of Motion Preservation Devices and Relevant Terminology. Vol. 1. Issue 1. St. Louis, MO: Quality Medical Publishing, 2005:45–58.
13. Panjabi MM. Biomechanical evaluation of spinal fixation devices: Part1. A conceptual frame work. Spine 1988; 13:1129–1134.
14. Goel VK, Kim YE, Lim T-H, et al. An analytical investigation of the mechanics of spinal instrumentation. Spine 1988; 13:1003–1011.
15. Goel VK, Grauer J, Patel TCh, et al. Effects of charite artificial disc on the implanted and adjacent spinal segments mechanics using a hybrid testing protocol. Spine 2005; 30(24):2755–2764.
16. Dmitriev AE, Cunningham BW, Hu N, Sell G, Vigna F, McAfee PC. Adjacent level intradiscal pressure and segmental kinematics following a cervical total disc arthroplasty: an in vitro human cadaveric model. Spine 2005; 30(10):1165–1172.
17. Faizan A, Goel VK, Bergeron B. The anterior longitudinal ligament is essential to restore disc biomechanics following artificial disc replacement. 52nd annual meeting, Orthopedic Research Society, Chicago, IL, March 19–22, 2006.
18. Goffin J, Van Calenbergh F, van Loon J, et al. Intermediate follow-up after treatment of degenerative disc disease with the Bryan Cervical Disc Prosthesis: Single-level and bi-level. Spine 2003; 28(24):2673–2678.
19. Delamarter RB, Fribourg DM, Kanim LE, Bae H. ProDisc artificial total lumbar disc replacement: introduction and early results from the United States clinical trial. Spine 2003; 28(20):S167–S175.
20. Hallab NJ, Cunningham BW, Jacobs JJ. Spinal implant debris-induced osteolysis. Spine 2003; 28(20):S125–S138.
21. Dooris AP. Experimental and theoretical investigations into the effects of artificial disc implantation on the lumbar spine. Ph.D. Dissertation, University of Iowa, Iowa City, IA, 2001.
22. Lee CK, Goel VK. Artificial disc prosthesis: design concept and criteria. Spine 2004; 4:209S–218S.
23. Zhu QA, Larson CR, Sjovold SG, et al. Biomechanical evaluation of the total facet arthroplasty system: An in vitro human cadaveric model. 51st annual meeting, Orthopedic Research Society, Washington, DC, February 2005.
24. Shaw MN. A biomechanical evaluation of lumbar facet replacement systems. Masters Thesis, University of Toledo, OH.

25. Sengupta DK. Dynamic stabilization devices in the treatment of low back pain. Orthop Clin North Am 2004; 35(1):43–56.
26. Viscogliosi AG, Viscogliosi JJ, Viscogliosi MR. Beyond Total Disc, the Future of Spine Surgery. New York: Viscogliosi Bros., 2004.
27. Ishihara H, McNally DS, Urban JP, Hall AC. Effects of hydrostatic pressure on matrix synthesis in different regions of the intervertebral disk. J Appl Physiol 1996; 80(3):839–846.
28. Handa T, Ishihara H, Ohshima H, Osada R, Tsuji H, Obata K. Effects of hydrostatic pressure on matrix synthesis and matrix metalloproteinase production in the human lumbar intervertebral disc. Spine 1997; 22(10):1085–1091.
29. Hutton WC, Elmer WA, Bryce LM, Kozlowska EE, Boden SD, Kozlowski M. Do the intervertebral disc cells respond to different levels of hydrostatic pressure? Clin Biomech (Bristol, Avon) 2001; 16(9):728–734.
30. Caserta S, La Maida GA, Misaggi B, et al. Elastic stabilization alone or combined with rigid fusion in spinal surgery: a biomechanical study and clinical experience based on 82 cases. Eur Spine J 2002; 11(Suppl 2):S192–S197.
31. Mochida J, Toh E, Suzuki K, Chiba M, Arima T. An innovative method using the Leeds-Keio artificial ligament in the unstable spine. Orthopedics 1997; 20(1):17–23.
32. Marcacci M, Zaffagnini S, Visani A, Iacono F, Neri MP, Petitto A. Arthroscopic reconstruction of the anterior cruciate ligament with Leeds-Keio ligament in non-professional athletes. Results after a minimum 5 years' follow-up. Knee Surg Sports Traumatol Arthrosc 1996; 4(1):9–13.
33. Suzuki K, Mochida J, Chiba M, Kikugawa H. Posterior stabilization of degenerative lumbar spondy-lolisthesis with a Leeds-Keio artificial ligament. A biomechanical analysis in a porcine vertebral model. Spine 1999; 24(1):26–31.
34. Garner MD, Wolfe SJ, Kuslich SD. Development and preclinical testing of a new tension-band device for the spine: the Loop system. Eur Spine J 2002; 11(Suppl 2):S186–S191.
35. Lindsey DP, Swanson KE, Fuchs P, Hsu KY, Zucherman JF, Yerby SA. The effects of an interspinous implant on the kinematics of the instrumented and adjacent levels in the lumbar spine. Spine 2003; 28(19):2192–2197.
36. Fuchs PD, Lindsey DP, Hsu KY, Zucherman JF, Yerby SA. The use of an interspinous implant in con-junction with a graded facetectomy procedure. Spine 2005; 30(11):1266–1272; discussion 1273–1274.
37. Swanson KE, Lindsey DP, Hsu KY, Zucherman JF, Yerby SA. The effects of an interspinous implant on intervertebral disc pressures. Spine 2003; 28(1):26–32.
38. Wiseman CM, Lindsey DP, Fredrick AD, Yerby SA. The effect of an interspinous process implant on facet loading during extension. Spine 2005; 30(8):903–907.
39. Minns RJ, Walsh WK. Preliminary design and experimental studies of a novel soft implant for correct-ing sagittal plane instability in the lumbar spine. Spine 1997; 22(16):1819–1825; discussion 1826–1827.
40. Mariottini A, Pieri S, Giachi S, et al. Preliminary results of a soft novel lumbar intervertebral prothesis (DIAM) in the degenerative spinal pathology. Acta Neurochir Suppl 2005; 92:129–131.
41. Markwalder TM, Wenger M. Dynamic stabilization of lumbar motion segments by use of Graf's liga-ments: results with an average follow-up of 7.4 years in 39 highly selected, consecutive patients. Acta Neurochir (Wien) 2003; 145(3):209–214; discussion 214.
42. BrechbuÉhler D, Markwalder ThMm, Braun M. Surgical Results after soft system stabilization of the lumbar spine in degenerative disc disease: Long term results. Acta Neurochir (Wien) 1998; 140: 521–525.
43. Mulholland RC, Sengupta DK. Rationale, principles, and experimental evaluation of the concept of soft stabilization. Eur Spine J 2002; 11(Suppl 2):S198–S205.
44. Freudinger S, Dubois G, Lorrain M. Dynamic neutralization of the lumbar spine confirmed on a new spine simulator in vitro. Arch Orthopedic Trauma Surgery 1999; 119:127–132.
45. Wilson DC, Niosi C, Zhu Q, et al. How does loading in the facet joint a change with implantation of a dynamic posterior stabilization system? Conference abstract, ISSLS, Porto, Portugal, 2004.
46. Grob D, Benini A, Junge A, Mannion AF. Clinical experience with the Dynesys semi-rigid fixation system for the lumbar spine: surgical and patient-oriented outcome in 50 cases after an average of 2 years. Spine 2005; 30(3):324–331.
47. http://www.ulrich-ulm.de/eng/wirbelsaeule/cosmic-intro.html
48. Vishnubhotla S. A biomechanical evaluation of dynamic stabilization systems. Masters Thesis. Uni-versity of Toledo, OH.
49. http://www.spine-dr.com/site/surgery/surgery_xstop_ipd.html
50. http://www.spine-health.com/research/trials/wallis/wallis.html

26 | The Ideal Artificial Lumbar Intervertebral Disc

Isador H. Lieberman and Edward Benzel
The Cleveland Clinic Foundation, Cleveland, Ohio, U.S.A.

E. Raymond S. Ross
Hope Hospital, Eccles Old Salford, U.K.

INTRODUCTION

The spine is comprised of multiple segments, each one defined by White and Panjabi as a "functional spinal unit" (FSU). The FSU consists of a three-joint complex including the disc (endplate, annulus fibrosis, and nucleus pulposus) and the dorsal facet joints. More recently, it has been redefined to include the passive and active constraints that are provided by the attached ligaments and muscles. The FSU performs as a continuous, semi-constrained joint, where complex three-dimensional movements take place. These movements, which occur through six degrees of freedom, include axial compression/distraction, anterior, posterior and lateral bending, translation, and rotation. These movements are constrained by the need to protect neurological elements and yet maintain the head balanced over the pelvis to facilitate interaction with the surrounding environment.

The FSUs are typically subject to ongoing degenerative changes. These degenerative changes represent a continuum of mechanical deterioration, secondary to multiple etiologies (aging, trauma, metabolic, and so on.) which may or may not be symptomatic (mechanical pain, inflammatory pain, radicular pain, stenotic symptoms). As the FSU degenerates, the normal biomechanical parameters are altered, and compensatory mechanisms (loss of lumbar lordosis, hip and knee flexion posture) are recruited to achieve the goals of spinal balance and motion.

The current clinical surgical "gold standard" strategy for treating symptomatic degeneration of the FSU is to stabilize the degenerated segment by fusing the affected spinal level. The goal of fusion is to restore the native anatomic relationships including disc height and spinal curvature, while relieving the patient's painful symptoms. Surgical strategies have evolved from dorsal, dorsolateral, ventral, instrumented, and un-instrumented fusions to the contemporary techniques involving inter-body cages and synthetic as well as biologic bone substitutes. Despite this evolution, the results of fusion are less than perfect, with fusion rates ranging from 60% to 90% and clinical outcome improvement rates from 60% to 70% (1). Spinal fusion also carries with it the longer-term problem of increasing the strain at the adjacent levels, potentially contributing to premature degenerative changes (2).

To date, none of the increasingly complex implants and instruments has resulted in an improvement on the outcomes of fusion. With this in mind, much like the evolution to arthroplasty from fusion of a peripheral joint, a philosophy of spine arthroplasty instead of spinal fusion is now evolving.

In the development of a spinal arthroplasty system, one must consider five principle issues; (*i*) an understanding of how the spine reacts to loading in the normal and degenerative state, (*ii*) the device's ability to replicate FSU mechanical properties including motion, (*iii*) the clinical effectiveness of the arthroplasty device, (*iv*) the device's ability to prevent adjacent level premature deterioration, and (*v*) the revisability of the implant in the event of infection, dislodgement or device failure.

SPINAL BIOMECHANICS IN THE NORMAL AND DEGENERATED SPINE

Lee has compiled a critical literature review on spinal biomechanics for the lumbar spine, describing the significance of the individual spinal elements and their impact on maintaining a healthy, functioning spine (3). After analyzing what Lee has compiled, it is clear that providing motion is not the primary function of the native disc, but that passive resistance to the forces during motion is the more important factor to be considered when designing a strategy for the long-term restoration of the FSU.

Likewise Ito et al. (4) verified the notion of passive resistance by describing the non-linear relationship between compressive load and disc stiffness. They reported low stiffness at lower loads (800 N/mm at 1000 N) and proportionately higher stiffness at higher loads (2000 N/mm at 4000 N). This differential allows for less resistance to motion at the lower loads of daily activities and more resistance to motion at the higher loads. This phenomenon presumably works to maintain spinal alignment and to protect the neurological structures throughout the full range of motion.

Kimura et al. (5) illustrated and quantified the effect of loading on the lumbar spine in eight volunteers. They described the functional response of the lumbar spine and the ability of the spine to adapt to normal loading. Their key finding was that, when loaded, the spine first responds by increasing the native lordotic or kyphotic curvature, and then subsequently responds by altering disc height. These changes in disc height, and the differential stiffness described by Ito, are reflections of the viscoelastic and biomechanical nature of the nucleus, annulus and endplate complex.

Patwardhan during his development of the "Follower Load" biomechanical model defined the mechanism by which the spinal system attempts to maintain and reduce the localized shear stress on each intervertebral disc at or near zero during body movements (6). The shear stress, if left unchecked, presumably can cause intra-discal disruption and injury, thus possibly contributing to degeneration and mechanical dysfunction. Clinically, any disruption of an index FSU either ventrally or dorsally, by injury, aging or even surgery, may exaggerate the degeneration observed at the adjacent levels, as a result of the spinal system attempting to compensate for a compromised index FSU.

Kirkaldy-Willis schematically depicted the pathophysiology of degeneration of the lumbar spine as a degenerative cascade (Fig. 1) (7,8). He described the three phases of degeneration as dysfunction, instability, and ultimately restabilization. Early degenerative events, such as disc herniation, lead to decreased stiffness of the spine. The natural response of the body is to resist abnormal stresses and strains with physiologic responses such as osteophyte formation. Osteophytes are a manifestation of the body's attempt to reduce the shear stress towards zero and to restore the load bearing capacity of the FSU. The fact that the restoration of stability and load bearing may lead to other clinical pathologies (such as nerve compression and loss of motion) emphasizes the critical importance of stability and load bearing even at the expense of neurologic compromise and loss of flexibility.

With the aforementioned in mind, any surgical intervention, and especially disc arthroplasty, must take the biomechanical responses, the inherent disc function and the degenerative cascade into account. Following Kirkaldy-Willis's algorithm, the body's natural response to degenerative changes is to work toward stabilization, reducing motion through increased stiffness and osteophyte formation. It therefore is imperative to match the proposed treatment to the stage of degeneration. If intervention on the degenerated disc utilizes a replacement prosthesis that introduces unnatural and unconstrained motion, it may reverse the process back toward the abnormally decreased stiffness phase.

FIRST GENERATION ARTIFICIAL DISCS

First generation disc arthroplasty design has evolved from the total joint replacement experience in hips and knees. The designs mimic the ball and socket design used in artificial hips and knees.

Although the first generation devices may offer some benefit over fusion in which they reportedly preserve motion in the spinal segment (9), they do not function like the natural disc.

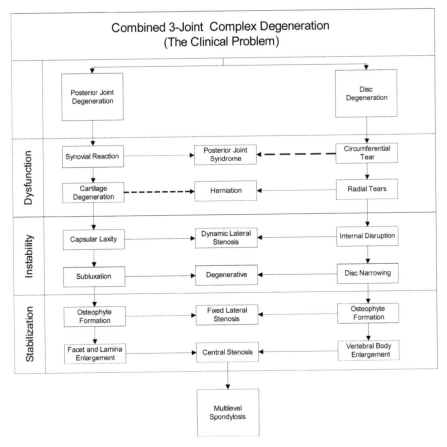

FIGURE 1   Kirkaldy-Willis degenerative cascade: the pathophysiology of degenerative disease of the lumbar spine.

These devices force a fixed axis of rotation on the spine and do not allow for true coupled motion (10). The natural disc provides for three-dimensional motion: flexion and extension, lateral bending, rotation and compression. It is also viscoelastic, where the stiffness varies with the loading rate and magnitude (4). The first generation discs restore only two-dimensional motion, providing no axial compression, and they have no viscoelastic properties. Therefore, while they may prove successful in replacing a painful, degenerated disc with some motion, they cannot replicate the native function of the natural disc. These shortcomings are more than just theoretical limitations and likely will lead to problems and disappointing long-term results.

Lemaire reported on the first, long-term European experience with mechanical disc replacement (11). He described his experience with the Charité® (DePuy Spine, Raynham, Massachusetts, U.S.A.) as the "best disc replacement compromise." He observed that the Charité® provided mobility but fell short of full restoration of the native function of the lumbar FSU. Furthermore, even though mobility and short-term results were favorable, he opined that the long-term clinical implications appeared to be suboptimal. The factors that impeded the Charité® from achieving long-term clinical success were facet arthritis, osteoporosis, structural deformities, and secondary facet pain. Based on these results, one could conclude that motion and/or unconstrained motion alone may be insufficient in restoring normal native motion and FSU function and/or long-term pain relief. Lemaire's observations have been confirmed more recently by a variety of clinical investigators (12,13), suggesting that long-term implantation of the Charité® places the facet joints under abnormal and excessive loading, thus creating an environment for facet degeneration and reoccurrence of localized pain. Introducing unconstrained motion by using an articulating bearing surface certainly seems insufficient to restore normal native motion and function, and appears likely to eventually cause further degenerative problems and pain.

Blumenthal et al. (14) reported the results of the Food and Drug Administration device trial comparing the Charité® disc replacement to fusion using threaded stand alone interbody cages. This was a randomized control trial of 304 patients designed as a non-inferiority study. The follow-up was two years and they reported generic and disease specific outcome measures as well as radiographic fusion rates and implant motion. Their results revealed very similar complication rates and clinical outcome of 42.4% improvement in the fusion group and 48.5% improvement in the disc replacement group. The fusion rate in the fusion group was reported as 91.9%. These fusion results from the control group are consistent with previously reported fusion study results. These results however seem to fall short of proving a significant advantage of disc replacement over fusion. Blumenthal et al. also reported shorter hospital stays and faster time to recovery compared to fusion.

Van-Ooij et al. (15) collected and analyzed a series of failed first generation disc replacements in 27 patients with 11 to 127 month follow-up. Seven of 27 patients developed adjacent level deterioration and 11 of 27 developed facet degeneration. In 18 patients the failure was due to implant subsidence, and in two the failure was due to implant migration. They had primarily revised all patients and reported less than ideal improvement in the patients' symptoms after the revision.

One of the authors [Raymond Ross (RR)] has considerable experience with the Charité® lumbar disc. Abstract presentations at International Society for Study of the Lumbar Spine (ISSLS) and Euro-spine (2004, Porto Portugal) reported indifferent clinical outcomes after an average follow up of ten years. Furthermore, the motion which was occurring in the vast majority of these implants was disappointing, being an average of only four degrees. The reason for this is not as might be predicted; i.e., that the segments are fusing. It is more likely due to deformation of the plastic insert with binding of the movable parts. Kaplan-Maier survival curves were created from the data and survivorship of as little as 55% at ten years was found. Were this data describing hip or knee replacements, they would no longer be used clinically. Adjacent level degeneration still occurred, although it is difficult to say whether this is part of the degenerative cascade, failure to reduce the strain on the adjacent segment, or the effect of reducing motion with time. Further work is in progress (Ross, Oxborrow, Harris, and Patwardhan) to confirm whether or not the differences in quality of motion between the intact spine and the spine with a Charité® disc implanted have some bearing on overall functional results. The prosthesis is described as a "bipolar device with translation of the spacer on flexion and extension." This does occur, but equally there are cases in which only the upper plate moves without translation. Cases have been observed of plastic core trapping by the metal plates, with movement only occurring at the last moment, producing a jerk to the movement.

RR also had experience with a viscoelastic® disc (AcroFlex Disc, DePuy Spine, a Johnson & Johnson Company, Raynham, Massachusetts, U.S.A.). Design faults led to this being halted at the clinical trial stage. However, four surviving patients have been reviewed at five years with no degradation of the rubber. The clinical outcomes showed quite startling falls in Oswestry disability scores from greater than 50% in two cases to zero and the other two with post operative scores of 4% and 10%, respectively. Though a very small series, these results suggest that the viscoelastic properties are of considerable importance in improving the clinical outcome.

After a comprehensive review of the published literature, the available evidence does not support the contention that first generation disc replacements provide normal clinical motion or minimize the stresses on adjacent levels to prevent adjacent level segmental deterioration.

DEFINITION OF THE IDEAL ARTIFICIAL LUMBAR INTERVERTEBRAL DISC

The intervertebral disc is part of a complex system, and its function must be understood in that context. In particular, the importance of all of the components of the FSU on spinal function must be appreciated and respected. The natural disc does not function independently.

As such, any prosthetic replacement should offer more than one dimension of function, and should not act in isolation from the native biomechanics of the spine.

Lemaire suggested that the ideal substitute for the lumbar disc "... should meet the following criteria: geometry, motion, deformability, inherent stiffness, and acoustics" (10). The hallmark of a next-generation design is that it should replicate native function, embracing the four key biomechanical concepts: complex motion, viscoelasticity, load bearing capacity, and passive resistance to loads.

The load bearing capability of the spine is also a function of anatomy and alignment. Kimura illustrated and quantified the effect of loading on the lumbar spine, describing the functional response of the spine and its ability to adapt to normal loading (5). The key finding was that the spinal system responds to loading by first increasing the native lordotic or kyphotic curvature and then subsequently by altering disc height. This highlights the fact that the spinal response to motion is a system-wide response and not just local to the segments. A prosthetic disc replacement should attempt to restore the natural curvature of the FSU. Further, the ability of the disc to compress axially is fundamental to the load response and load-sharing function, so an artificial disc replacement must move in this dimension to fully act as a shock absorber.

The concept of the next-generation design requires full replication of function. A biomechanical basis for an ideal prosthetic disc suggests that it must function in concert with the entire FSU, including the adjacent vertebral bodies, the surrounding ligaments, the facets and the muscles. Additionally, it should replicate the viscoelasticity of the natural disc, responding with increasing stiffness at higher loads and higher rates of load application. It must compress axially, allowing changes in disc height required to respond to loads appropriately and naturally. It should also restore and maintain the proper angle of the spinal curve. Lastly, it should provide passive resistance to forces during motion.

In order to meet the aforementioned requirements, the implant must provide for short-term fixation and long-term fixation. The short-term fixation is needed to allow for initial motion and preservation of biomechanics until the long-term fixation is achieved. The long-term fixation, preferably by osteointegration, is required to maintain the motion and biomechanics and adapt to potential changes over time in bone and endplate architecture.

The fixation of the disc replacement to the bony endplates is also critical for the transmission of forces from one level to the next without creating artificial pathways of least resistance. These artificial pathways would have the propensity to become sites of wear between either the components of the disc replacement or the disc replacement and the vertebral body endplates.

DESIGN OF THE IDEAL ARTIFICIAL LUMBAR INTERVERTEBRAL DISC
Material and Design Optimization

To satisfy the previously described requirements, the material chosen for the core of an artificial disc should possess the viscoelastic characteristics of a natural human disc so that it will be capable of obtaining the geometry, motion, deformability, and inherent stiffness properties of the native disc. As such, an ideal candidate for the designation of next-generation technology is an elastomer-based artificial disc. At low loading rates, the elastomer material should be relatively flexible, and at accelerated loading rates, it should stiffen. This feature is useful for reducing the shock transmitted to the spine during normal day-to-day activities, while allowing the treated segment to function in a manner that is consistent with the rest of the spine.

Fixation of the elastomeric core to the bony end plates may be achieved by metal or composite end plates. The bone-interface surface of the end plates must have an appropriate surface to promote osteointegration and long-term fixation. Fixation of the end plates to the elastomeric core is necessary to provide passive resistance to the forces applied to the spine.

Biomechanical Characterization

An artificial disc should be thoroughly biomechanically characterized to demonstrate its strength and durability. The device should have strength which complements that of the natural disc and/or surrounding anatomy in compression, rotation, shear, flexion, and extension. Since axial compression is the primary load bearing mode in an artificial disc, compressive strength should be of the utmost importance.

Durability evaluations include fatigue testing in compression, rotation, flexion/extension, and lateral bending to determine the endurance limits, failure modes, and potential for wear debris generation. Additionally, coupled motion fatigue testing may be used to predict more physiologically realistic loading scenarios and resulting failure modes. Device creep and resilience are also important properties to characterize in order to predict long term performance.

Device stiffness and range of motion should also be characterized and compared with that of a healthy natural disc. Stiffness and range of motion may be characterized statically and dynamically in compression, rotation, and flexion/extension.

The propensity for subsidence of the device into the vertebral bodies or expulsion of the device from the disc space should be evaluated. Testing in polyurethane foam simulated vertebral bodies eliminates the variability associated with bone specimens.

For multiple-component bonded devices, extensive bond strength and durability testing should be conducted. Evaluations of the bond should be a part of the testing described previously, or alternatively as separate investigations, non-physiologic tests designed to focus the stress on the bond.

Development of Surgical Technique and Instrumentation

In addition to the physiologic and biomechanical requirements, the surgical requirements of the clinician must be met. The device size should be optimized to meet the morphometric restrictions of the lumbar spine, and the device designed and constructed to withstand the challenging environment of the lumbar intradiscal space for decades. The implantation system and surgical technique should accommodate precision and accuracy. The system should provide both a spatial reference and accurate placement of device without adding too much complexity to the implantation method. Ideally, the system could be implanted from either a transperitoneal or retroperitoneal approach within a similar operative time as anterior inter-body fusion procedures. The system should also be optimized to keep the incision small and the number of steps low.

CONCLUSIONS AND FINAL THOUGHTS

While technology based upon artificial hip and knee replacement has helped to "move thinking" regarding the management of spinal degenerative disorders, the clinical strategies that were derived in this environment do not meet many of the criteria of the ideal disc replacement outlined herein. The next generation of disc replacements must more closely replicate the biomechanical properties of the normal human disc. Elastomeric materials, by virtue of their viscoelastic properties, appear to most closely approximate the native properties of the human disc. Discs using these materials must also conform to toxicology and chronicity standards. Internal bonding and suitable mechanical testing of all implant components and characteristics, including failure modes, must be tested. Prevention of displacement in the short and long term is paramount to design. Combining suitable surgical instrumentation designed to achieve accuracy and replicability of placement regarding orientation and position of the prosthesis using known surgical approaches should be part of the design process. Catastrophic failure prevention and contingency management plans should be in place, in the event of disc failure must be preconceived and viable.

REFERENCES

1. Fritzell P, Hagg O, Wessberg P, et al. Lumbar fusion versus nonsurgical treatment for chronic low back pain: a multicenter randomized controlled trial from the Swedish Lumbar Spine Study Group. Spine 2001; 26:2521–2532.

2. Eck JC, Humphreys SC, Hodges SD. Adjacent-segment degeneration after lumbar fusion: a review of clinical, biomechanical and radiologic studies. Am J Orthop 1999; 28(6):336–340.
3. Lee R. Kinematics of the Lumbar Spine. On-line article: http://www.rs.polyu.edu.hk/RLee/Spine/LumbarKin/
4. Ito M, Tadano S, Kaneda K. A biomechanical definition of spinal segmental instability taking personal and disc level differences into account. Spine 1993; 18(15):2295–2304.
5. Kimura S, Steinbach GC, Watenpaugh DE, et al. Lumbar spine disc height and curvature responses to an axial load generated by a compression device compatible with magnetic resonance imaging. Spine 2001; 26(23):2596–2600.
6. Patwardhan AG, Havey RM, Meade KP, Lee B, Dunlap B. A follower load increases the load-carrying capacity of the lumbar spine in compression. Spine 1999; 24(10):1003.
7. Kirkaldy-Willis WH, Bernard T. The three phases and three joints. In: Managing Low Back Pain. 4th ed. Philadelphia, PA: Churchill Livingstone, 1999:249–262.
8. Yong-Hing K, Kirkaldy-Willis WH. The pathophysiology of degenerative disease of the lumbar spine. Orthop Clinics North Am 1983; 14(3):491–504.
9. Cunningham BW. Basic scientific considerations in total disc arthroplasty. Spine 2004; 4:219S–230S.
10. O'Leary P, Nicolakis M, Lorenz M, et al. Response of Charite total disc replacement under physiologic loads: prosthesis component motion patterns. Spine J 2005; 5:590–599.
11. Lemaire JP, Skali W, Lavaste F, et al. Intervertebral disc prosthesis, results and prospects for the year 2000. Clin Orthop Related Res 1997; 337:64–76.
12. Pimenta L, Phillips F, Diaz R. The fate of the facet joints after lumbar total disc arthroplasty: A clinical and MRI study. North American Spine Society 20th Annual Meeting. Philadelphia, 2005.
13. Griffith SL, Shekelov AP, Buttner-Janz K, LeMaire JP, Zeegers WS. A multi-center retrospective study of the clinical results of the LINK SB Charite Intervertebral Disc Prosthesis: the Initial European Experience. Spine 1994; 19(16):1842–1849.
14. Blumenthal S, McAfee PC, Guyer RD, et al. A prospective, randomized, multicenter food and drug administration investigational device exemptions study of lumbar total disc replacement with the Charite™ Artificial Disc versus Lumbar Fusion. Spine 2005; 30(14):1565–1575.
15. Van Ooij A, Oner FC, Verbout AJ. Complications of artificial disc replacement. J Spinal Disord Tech 2003; 16(4):369–383.

27 | Artificial Discs and Their Clinical Track Records

Rick B. Delamarter and Ben B. Pradhan
Spine Research Foundation, The Spine Institute, Santa Monica, California, U.S.A.

INTRODUCTION
Lumbar Spine

The goal of restoring normal painless motion to a joint is not a new concept in orthopedics. Total joint arthroplasty for the hip and knee has been shown to provide excellent pain relief while maintaining motion in scores of clinical studies. In light of the historically wide range of results of fusion for low back pain, and the risk of adjacent segment disease, this concept of motion preservation has been applied to degenerative disc disease of the lumbar spine in four recent large-scale United States Food and Drug Administration (USFDA) clinical trials comparing total disc replacement to spinal fusion. The FDA approved the SB Charité III™ (DePuy Spine, Raynham, Massachusetts, U.S.A.) prosthesis for single level use in November of 2004 (1). The ProDisc-L™ (Synthes Spine, Paoli, Pennsylvania, U.S.A.) trials have also completed enrollment, and a two-year follow-up results are being evaluated prior to FDA approval (estimated early 2006) for single and two-level use. Enrollment for the Maverick™ disc (Medtronic, Memphis, Tennessee, U.S.A.) U.S. clinical trials began in the spring of 2003, and the FlexiCore™ disc (Stryker Spine, Allendale, New Jersey, U.S.A.) U.S. clinical trials are going on as well.

Cervical Spine

As the surgical standard of care to date for intractable neck and arm pain due to cervical degenerative disc disease or disc herniation, anterior cervical discectomy and fusion (ACDF) has been very effective. Delamarter et al. (2–4) at our own center has shown that in the appropriately selected patient, symptoms are relieved reliably and early after surgery. However, the long-term effects of motion-eliminating surgery in the spine, especially at multiple levels, have come under scrutiny recently. Several studies have documented the degeneration of adjacent segments after cervical fusion surgery. Hilibrand et al. (5) reported a 2.9% per year rate of symptomatic degeneration of cervical segments adjacent to a fusion, with a reoperation rate of 66%. Goffin et al. (6) reported a 36% rate of clinical deterioration at eight years, with a re-operation rate of 6%. Katsuura et al. (7) reported a 50% rate of adjacent segment degeneration at 10 years. The apparently accelerated incidence of degenerative changes in discs adjacent to fused levels has led to the hypothesis that elimination of segmental motion leads to abnormal loading and motion of the remaining segment(s).

Anterior lumbar or cervical discectomy, along with the removal of osteophytes, are necessary in order to remove the discogenic source of pain as well as anterior neural compression. It is well accepted that the anterior spinal column must be reconstructed after discectomy. Discectomy alone can lead to loss of intervertebral and foraminal height, kyphotic deformity, and increased pain. Traditionally segmental reconstruction has been done with structural allograft, autologous bone, or various interbody devices. Anterior plating (cervical spine) or posterior instrumentation (lumbar spine) may be added to immobilize the reconstructed segment even further and encourage fusion. Various interbody fusion devices have been developed recently, all designed to impart disc space distraction and stability while fusion takes effect.

However, just as in the case of other major joints in the body, spinal reconstruction does not necessarily have to be immobile. With the increased attention being focused on adjacent segment disease, mobile anterior spinal reconstruction techniques have been developed, beginning with lumbar artificial disc replacement.

DESIGN RATIONALE

The ideal spinal segmental reconstruction technique will preserve as many of the physiologic properties of the intervertebral disc as possible. These include maintaining intervertebral viscoelasticity with as near-normal range of motion as possible. Intervertebral height needs to be maintained, as this will affect foraminal height as well. Furthermore, segmental lordosis is important to maintain spinal alignment. Ideally, the prosthesis design and placement technique should be simple to reduce operative time and morbidity, and to allow early recovery and return to function. Finally, it must be shown in a well-designed clinical trial that the prosthesis is at least as effective as the current standard of care, with the added potential benefit of reducing adjacent segment deterioration.

In summary, when designing or choosing a prosthetic disc implant, desirable device characteristics include the following:

- Biocompatibility of material
- Durability
- Ease of implantation
- Stability (from migration)
- Reproduction of normal mobility
- Reproduction of normal disc height
- Physiologic load sharing with posterior and adjacent structures
- Ease of revision or salvage
- Image friendliness (easy to visualize in radiographic modalities)
- Cost effectiveness

CLINICAL EXPERIENCE—LUMBAR ARTHROPLASTY

There are four lumbar total disc replacements that are actively being implanted in the U.S. today. As mentioned above, the Charité disc has been approved by the FDA for single-level use, and the ProDisc-L disc is expected to receive approval soon for one and two-level use. The Maverick and FlexiCore discs are further behind in this process. Published reports on the clinical outcomes after lumbar disc arthroplasty have been listed in Table 1. The individual prostheses are discussed in detail below, with results in graphical form from selected studies shown in Figures 1–3.

SB Charité III™

Kurt Schellnack and Karin Buttner-Janz created the first generation of the SB Charité disc in 1982 at the Charité hospital of Berlin, Germany (8,9). The first human implantation was performed in 1984. The second generation was developed in 1985. The first two generations failed in clinical use due to material failure and implant migration. The currently used third version was created and manufactured by Waldemar-Link after the company acquired the product rights in 1987 (Fig. 4). This latest version is comprised of three separate pieces: two cobalt chrome endplates and one ultra high molecular weight polyethylene insert. The insert has a biconvex surface which is not attached to either endplates. There is a metal wire around the circumference of the insert to aid in radiographic imaging. The endplates are anchored to the vertebrae by several teeth and textured bony in-growth surfaces. The prostheses used in the U.S. trials did not have the rough bony in-growth surfaces on their endplates. The prosthesis is a nonconstrained device that attempts to mimic normal disc biomechanics by permitting both rotation and translation (in contrast with the ProDisc-L). Biomechanical testing has revealed that the variable instantaneous axis of rotation of the prosthesis is consistent with

TABLE 1 Published Lumbar Disc Replacement Outcome Studies

Study	N	Mean follow-up (yrs)	Results (good/excellent)
SB Charité III™ disc			
Buttner-Janz et al., 1988 (63)	62	1.25	83%
David,1993 (64)	22	1	68%
Griffith et al., 1994 (65)	93	1	65% had less back pain, 41–48% had less leg pain
Cinotti et al., 1996 (16)	46	3.2	63%
David, 1996 (66)	135	3	77%
Shelokov, 1997	67	6	66%
Lemaire et al., 1997 (13)	105	4.25	79%
Zeegers et al., 1999 (15)	50	2	70%
David, 2000 (67)	85	5	68%
Lemaire, 2001	55	10	64%
David, 2002 (68)	142	5	79%
Hochschuler et al., 2002 (69)	56	0.1–1	50% improvement in VAS, 40% improvement in ODI
McAfee et al., 2003 (70)	41	1–3	57% improvement in VAS, 50% improvement in ODI
Guyer et al., 2004 (71)	100	1–3	58% improvement in VAS, 54% improvement in ODI
Lemaire et al., 2005 (14)	100	10–13.4	90%
Blumenthal et al., 2005 (1)	205	2	41% improvement in VAS, 49% improvement in ODI
ProDisc-L™			
Marnay, 2001 (18)	64	7–11	93%
Mayer and Wiechert, 2002 (72)	34	0.5	83%
Marnay, 2002 (73)	53/200	1.4/2	94%
Bertagnoli and Kumar 2002 (24)	108	Up to 2	91%
Delamarter et al., 2003 (23)	35	0.5	41% improvement in VAS, 52% improvement in ODI
Zigler et al., 2003 (74)	28	0.5	30% improvement in VAS, 48% improvement in ODI
Tropiano et al., 2003 (19)	53	1.4	94%
Zigler, 2004 (75)	55	0.5–1	55% improvement in VAS, 67% improvement in ODI
Tropiano et al., 2005 (20)	55	7–11	75%
Bertagnoli et al., 2005 (21)	104	2	61% improvement in VAS, 45% improvement in ODI
Delamarter et al., 2005 (in press)	171	2	43% improvement in VAS, 52% improvement in ODI
Maverick™ disc			
Mathews et al., 2004 (28)	7	1.5	36 point improvement in ODI
Le Huec et al., 2005 (29)	64	1–3	58% improvement in VAS, 47% improvement in ODI

Abbreviations: N, number of patients; ODI, Oswestry disability index; VAS, visual analog score.

the physiologic characterization by Panjabi (10,11). The biconvex shape of the insert allows greater and a more physiologic range of motion, but the nonconstrained kinematics potentially places a greater load on the facet joints.

Since 1987, well over 10,000 SB Charité III discs have been implanted worldwide (12). The United States Food and Drug Administration–Investigational Device Exemption (USFDA–IDE) trial enrollment phase is over for the one-level operation. The control group for the U.S. trials was one-level stand-alone anterior lumbar interbody fusion with Bagby and Kuslich (BAK) cages and autologous bone. As the older of the two most frequently implanted prostheses (the other being ProDisc-L), the SB Charité disc also has the most published results. A comprehensive list of these studies is listed in Table 1. In general, satisfactory outcomes have ranged from 63% to 85% with follow-up period ranging from 12 months to 10 years. Lemaire et al. (13) have reported some of the longest clinical follow-up, with a 79% rate of excellent results and an 87% rate of return to work after more than four years. More recently, the same lead

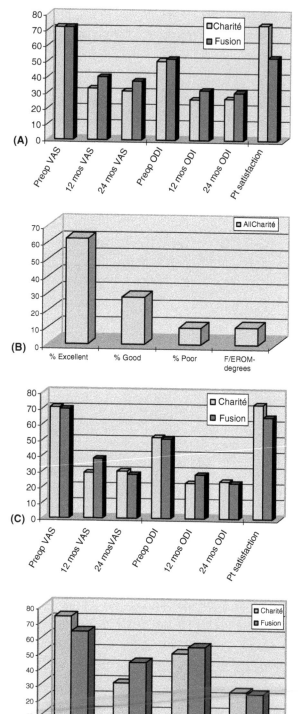

FIGURE 1 Charité III clinical outcomes (**A**) at up to two years; (**B**) at up to 13 years; (**C**) at up to two years; (**D**) at up to three years. *Abbreviations*: F/E ROM, flexion-extension range of motion in degrees; ODI, Oswestry disability index; VAS, visual analog scale. *Source*: From Refs. 1, 14, 70, 71.

author reported on a larger cohort of 100 patients with a follow-up of 10 to 13.4 years, and standardized outcome instruments revealed 90% good to excellent results (14). Lemaire et al. also measured maintenance of segmental mobility at 4.25 years: 15° of flexion-extension at L4–L5 and 9° of flexion-extension at L5–S1. This motion was still preserved at approximately 10°

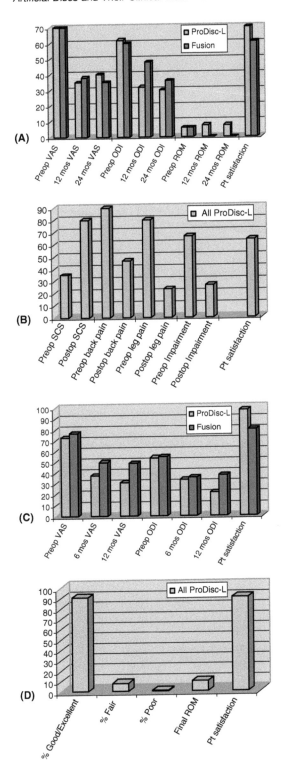

FIGURE 2 ProDisc-L[TM] clinical outcomes (**A**) at up to two years; (**B**) at up to 11 years; (**C**) at up to one year; (**D**) at up to two years. *Abbreviations*: ODI, Oswestry disability index; ROM, flexion-extension range of motion in degrees; SCS, Stauffer-Coventry scores; VAS, visual analog scale. *Source*: From Refs. 20, 24, 75, 79.

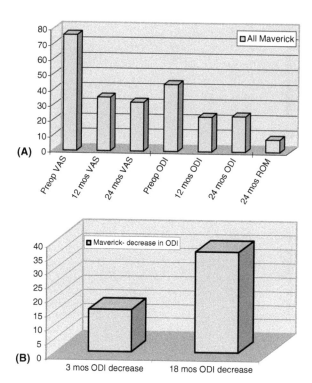

(A)

(B)

FIGURE 3 Maverick™ clinical outcomes (**A**) at up to three years; (**B**) at up to 1.5 years. *Abbreviations*: ODI, Oswestry disability index; ROM, flexion-extension range of motion in degrees; VAS, visual analog scale. *Source*: From Refs. 28, 29.

after 10 to 13 years. Zeegers et al. and Cinotti et al. (15,16) corroborated these results. Cinotti et al. also found that the motion was greatest at segments where the prosthesis covered 80% or greater of the vertebral endplate. Greater motion was also associated with the prosthesis positioned posterior to center of the disc space, implying a kinematically optimal location exists for this disc. Range of motion has been seen to be better for patients who became active as soon as one week after surgery versus those who wore corsets for three months (17).

Recently several studies have been published pertaining to the U.S. FDA clinical trials follow-up experience. These have also been listed in Table 1 and Figure 1. In general, after two to three years Charité disc replacement, the reduction in pain and disability achieved early on seems to have been well maintained, with both being reduced by half or more.

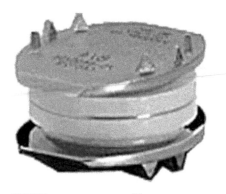
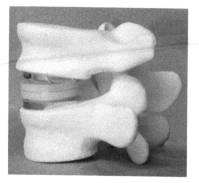

FIGURE 4 The SB Charité™ III lumbar artificial disc.

These results are comparable to the fusion controls in the same studies, but with the added achievement of motion preservation at the operative spinal segment.

ProDisc-L™

Thierry Marnay created the first ProDisc I prosthetic disc in 1989 at Montpellier, France. The first human implantation was in 1990. After implanting to 93 patients, in almost 70 cases, Marnay stopped to evaluate the long-term outcomes of his implant. Finally, he published his results in 2001 after 8 to 10 years follow-up (18). All implants remained intact without any migration or subsidence. Range of motion of the spinal segments was maintained. There was significant reduction in back and leg pain and almost 93% of the patients were satisfied and would have the surgery again. The promising results from his experience paved the way for the pivotal clinical trials recently completed here in the United States.

The first generation ProDisc I had titanium endplates and a double keel. In 1999, it was changed to cobalt chrome endplates with a single keel (ProDisc II, Fig. 5). The single serrated keel over each endplate, two small lateral pegs, along with the plasma-sprayed in-growth surface give the implant immediate stability. The insert is made of ultra high molecular weight polyethylene, which snap-locks to the bottom endplate, and thus has only one articulating convex side. The device is semi-constrained, allowing it to "load-share" with collateral structures such as the facet joints, ligaments, tendons and muscles, especially in shear. This places more load at the device-bone interface, but protects the facet joints. Axial rotation is unconstrained, and the axis of rotation of the cephalad endplate is angled posteriorly in the neutral position due to the intradiscal lordosis of the prosthesis, consistent with the physiologic axis of rotation (11).

Since its inception in 1990, there have been over 14,000 lumbar disc replacement procedures with the ProDisc-L device worldwide, with over 1000 implanted in the United States. There already exists a body of literature on the outcomes of these procedures. These are listed in Table 1 and Figure 2. In general, results have been favorable, with outcomes regularly in the 90% good to excellent results, and with significant decreases in pain and disability scores. In the longest prospective follow-up studies, Marnay and Tropiano et al. (18–20) have reported well to excellent results at a rate of 93% and 75% to 94%, respectively. Pain and disability standardized scores routinely are decreased by about half. As one of the busiest centers participating in the U.S. clinical trials (171 patients with ProDisc-L implanted, excluding approximately 20 patients with 3-level disc replacements), we have noted significantly greater earlier gains with ProDisc-L disc replacement versus fusion, but this significance is lost by about six months. Thereafter, for two to three years, the trend remains—both groups are significantly better off than the earlier surgery. We have not observed any device-related

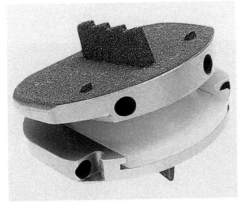
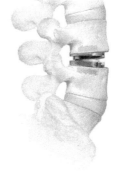

FIGURE 5 The ProDisc-L™ lumbar artificial disc.

complications, and no device has had to be revised or ex-planted. Note that the fusion controls in the ProDisc-L trials were 360° circumferential fusion with autologous iliac crest bone graft, and may explain the early clinical superiority of ProDisc-L over fusion. This was felt by the pertinent study committees to be the standard of care since the ProDisc-L was being studied for multi-level procedures, and by itself points out a significant advantage of multi-level disc replacement versus fusion. Bertagnoli et al. in a large and recent prospective study found similar clinical improvements in 108 patients with the ProDisc-L implants at two years, and his group also did not observe any device-related complications (21). Patient satisfaction rated 96% at two years.

Functionally speaking, in the experience at our institute, the disc replacement patients had significantly greater segmental range of motion (approximately 10° at L4–L5, and 6° at L5–S1) compared to the controlled fusion group (essentially no motion) at up to 24 months (22,23). Bertagnoli and Kumar (24) reported an average range of motion of 10° at L3–L4, L4–L5, and 9° at L5–S1 at one year after ProDisc placement. Tropiano et al. (19) reported a 10° range of motion at L4–L5 and 8° range of motion L5–S1 after a mean of 1.4 years of follow-up. Huang et al. (25) reported that at a mean of 8.7 years, the ProDisc prostheses had a mean measurable motion of 4° at L3–L4, 4.5° at L4–L5, and 3.2° at L5–S1 without any radiographic evidence of loosening or osteolysis. Equally important, only 9 of 34 (26%) junction levels above the prostheses demonstrated transitional degeneration at a mean of 8.7 years, none of them requiring surgery. In a comparable follow-up period, Cauchoix and David (26) reported transitional changes in 79% of patients 10 years after fusion surgery. For a follow-up ranging from two to 15 years, Gillet (27) reported transitional degeneration in 32% after 1-level fusion, but severe enough for 11% to need further surgery.

Maverick™

The Maverick disc was modeled after the ProDisc-L with a keel and employs a metal-on-metal ball-and-socket configuration without a polyethylene component (Fig. 6) (28). The two-piece cobalt–chromium endplates interface directly and attached to the vertebral bodies via keels that are larger than those of the ProDisc-L. The end-result is a semi-constrained artificial disc with a fixed center of rotation. The multi-center U.S. clinical trials began in the spring of 2003, with controls being anterior lumbar interbody fusion with lordotic and tapered (LT) cages (Medtronic, Memphis, Tennessee, U.S.A.) and InFuse (rhBMP-2). As a more recent entry into the field of spinal arthroplasty, there are relatively fewer indexed published articles about the Maverick disc. In a recently published prospective analysis, Le Huec et al. reported on two-year clinical outcomes (Table 1, Fig. 3) with a 58% reduction in back pain and a 47% reduction in disability (29). They also demonstrated maintenance of flexion-extension at the treated level, which averaged over 8°.

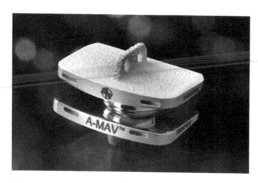 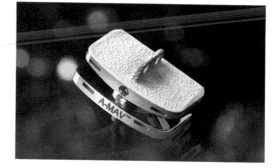

FIGURE 6 The Maverick™ lumbar artificial disc.

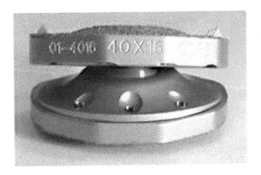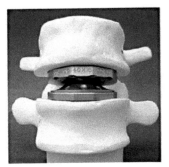

FIGURE 7 The FlexiCore™ lumbar artificial disc.

FlexiCore™

The FlexiCore disc is another metal-on-metal device in which the endplates are linked by a ball-and-socket joint that is captured into the construct (Fig. 7). The endplates are porous-coated with plasma-sprayed titanium, have pegs to anchor into the vertebral bodies, and are dome-shaped to fit into the concavities of the disc space. This produces a fully constrained device with a fixed center of rotation. The multi-center U.S. trial is underway, and the disc is being compared to 360° fusions with femoral ring allograft anteriorly and instrumented fusion with iliac crest autograft posteriorly. Errico has written about the device, but no published results from the clinical trial are available as of yet (30).

CLINICAL EXPERIENCE—CERVICAL ARTHROPLASTY

There have been limited published reports on the clinical results of cervical artificial disc replacement. There are three artificial cervical discs with the most clinical experience, and which have also completed U.S. clinical trials and are currently being evaluated for their two-year results before FDA approval: the ProDisc-C device (Synthes Spine, Paoli, Pennsylvania, U.S.A.), the Bryan™ device (Medtronic, Memphis, Tennessee, U.S.A.), and the Prestige™ device (Medtronic, Memphis, Tennessee, U.S.A.). Newer cervical artificial discs that have been designed are the Porous Coated Motion™ (PCM) disc (Cervitech, Roundhill, New Jersey, U.S.A.), and the CerviCore™ disc (Stryker, Rutherford, New Jersey, U.S.A.). Published reports on the clinical outcomes after cervical arthroplasty are listed in Table 1. Note that all the reports are favorable in terms of standardized outcomes instruments, with flexion-extension range of motion preserved in all studies. The individual discs are discussed below.

ProDisc-C™

The ProDisc-C prosthesis (Fig. 8) shares many of the physical characteristics of the ProDisc-L lumbar prosthesis. The device is essentially a ball-and-socket joint: the endplates are constructed of a cobalt-chrome alloy, and the articulating convex insert is made of ultra high molecular weight polyethylene (UHMWPE). Both are proven materials with an extensive track record in hip and knee arthroplasty. Both upper and lower endplates have slotted keels, and titanium plasma spray coating. These design characteristics allow for immediate fixation onto the vertebral endplates, as well as long-term fixation via bony ingrowth.

The first ProDisc-C implantation was performed in December 2002. Since then, over 3000 prostheses have been implanted worldwide. Multi-level disc replacements have also been performed. In the original European studies, there have been no device failures or need for revision surgeries. The first implantation in the United States was performed at our center in August 2003. Since then, over 300 implantations have been performed in 15 centers across the country as part of the U.S. IDE study.

We reported the early outcomes after ProDisc-C implantation, with significant reductions in visual analog pain and Oswestry disability scores (23). The study enrollment phase is

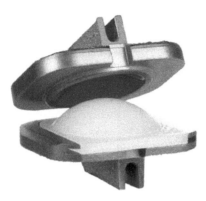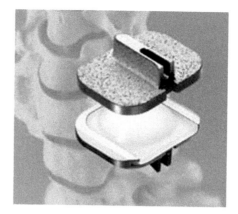

FIGURE 8 The ProDisc-C™ cervical artificial disc.

complete, with the FDA now analyzing the data for two years of follow-up. More recent results from our center are listed in Table 2 and shown in Figure 9. Under FDA-controlled compassionate allowance, approximately 20 patients have received 2 to 3-level disc replacements with ProDisc-C with good clinical results, comparable to the clinical trial for 1-level arthroplasty. No device-related complications have been observed in single or multi-level cervical arthroplasty with ProDisc-C. The average flexion-extension after disc replacement was seen maintained at 12° at approximately two years. Bertagnoli et al. (31,32) also reported clinical results after implantation of the ProDisc-C device, with significant reductions (approximately 40%) in visual analog scale (VAS) and neck disability index (NDI) scores, with motion

TABLE 2 Published Cervical Disc Replacement Outcome Studies

Study	N	Mean follow-up (yrs)	Results (good/excellent)
Bryan™ *cervical disc*			
Goffin et al., 2002 (33)	30	1	90%, maintained motion in 88%
Goffin et al., 2003 (36)	100	1–2	70–80%, ROM 8–9 deg
Duggal et al., 2004 (37)	26	1.25	NDI sig improved, SF-36 trend to improvement, ROM 7.8 deg
Tian et al., 2005 (76)	29	0.31	56% improvement in JOA, ROM 9.4 deg
ProDisc-C™			
Delamarter and Pradhan, 2004 (77)	15	0.5	84% improvement in VAS, 75% improvement in ODI, motion maintained
Bertagnoli et al., 2005 (32)	27	1	40% improvement in VAS, 35% improvement in NDI, motion maintained
Bertagnoli et al., 2005 (31)	16	1	Significant improvement in pain and disability, ROM 4–12 deg
Delamarter et al., 2005 (in press)	24	1.5–2	50% improvement in VAS, 64% improvement in ODI, ROM 12 deg
Prestige™ *disc*			
Wigfield et al., 2002 (38)	14	2	45% improvements in VAS, 31% improvement in NDI
Robertson et al., 2002 (78)	27	2	Maintained motion
Robertson and Metcalf, 2004 (39)	14	4	Improvement in NDI and SF-36, maintained motion
Porchet and Metcalf, 2004 (40)	27	2	Improvements in VAS, NDI, and SF-36, ROM 5.9 deg
PCM disc			
Pimenta et al., 2004 (41)	52	1	97%, 67% improvement in NDI, 76% improvement in VAS
CerviCore™ *disc*			
		No published human studies yet	

Abbreviations: JOA, Japanese Orthopaedic Association outcome scale; N, number of patients; NDI, neck disability index; ODI, Oswestry disability index; ROM, flexion/extension range of motion; deg, degrees; SF-36, short form 36 item health survey; VAS, visual analog score.

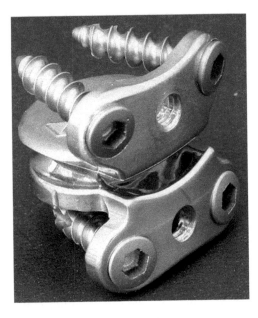

FIGURE 9   CerviCore™ cervical artificial disc.

maintained at the treated level at 1-year follow-up. Their studies also revealed no device-related complications, with maintenance of range of motion at treated levels (mean of 10.2°).

Bryan™ Disc

The Bryan disc consists of a low-friction polyurethane nucleus surrounded by a polyurethane sheath, which is then contained between two titanium alloy shells (Fig. 10). The dual articulating metal-on-polymer possesses elasticity and some compressibility, allowing for unconstrained motion and translation through a relatively normal range of motion. The prosthesis is axially symmetric, allowing for similar range of motion in the sagittal and coronal planes.

As of mid-2005, more than 4000 Bryan discs had been implanted worldwide. Goffin et al. (33) reported a 90% rate of good to excellent results at one to two years after cervical disc arthroplasty with the Bryan prosthesis. No device-related complications were described, or any subsidence or explantation. Device migration was seen in one patient, and suspected in the other, and these were attributed to incomplete milling of the endplates. The endplate milling required for this device has also been implicated in postoperative cervical kyphosis

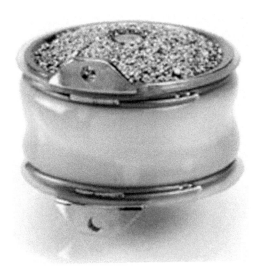

FIGURE 10   The Bryan™ cervical artificial disc.

and heterotopic ossification (34,35). A longer follow-up study by Goffin et al. (36) again resulted in a 90% rate of satisfactory clinical results, with sagittal motion preserved in almost 90% of the patients. Duggal et al. (37) studied the results of Bryan cervical disc replacement in patients with soft versus hard disc herniations, and with myelopathy versus radiculopathy. They found no significant difference in clinical outcome or complication rate in either case.

Prestige™ Disc

This disc was formerly known as the Bristol disc, and before some design change was also known as the Cummins or Frenchay disc. In its current form, the Prestige disc is a two-piece metal-on-metal ball-and-socket joint. The upper endplate includes a hemisphere on its articulating end, and the bottom endplate has a receiving ellipsoid saucer (Fig. 11). Moreover, the endplates have extensions that bend out anteriorly over the respective vertebral bodies, through which fixation screws can be placed.

A pilot study revealed significant improvements in all aspects of patient function and quality of life at two years (38). They reported a 46% improvement in pain and a 31% improvement in disability two years after implantation of the Prestige cervical artificial disc. Mean range of motion was preserved at 6.5°. There were no device-related complications. One device was removed and converted to a fusion due to persistent symptoms, which did not change even after successful fusion. Robertson and Metcalf (39) followed the pilot study patients out to four years, and affirmed maintenance of the good clinical outcomes. Porchet and Metcalf (40) published a multicenter, prospective, randomized controlled study comparing the Prestige disc with fusion at two years out. Both treatment groups achieved significant improvements in VAS, NDI, and short form 36 item health survey (SF-36), with no significant difference between treatments. However, motion was maintained at two years in the Prestige patients with a mean range of motion of 5.9°.

Porous Coated Motion™ Disc

The PCM disc consists of cobalt-chromium endplates with a polyethylene liner fixed to the caudal endplate (Fig. 12). The bearing surface radius is large, allowing minor translation. The endplates are porous coated at the outer surfaces. The only peer reviewed published study is by Pimenta et al. (41). They noted significant improvements in pain and disability in a year of follow-up in 52 patients. Ninety-seven percent of patients achieved good to excellent results. Complications reported were a single case of partial anterior translation of the device, and one case of mild heterotopic ossification.

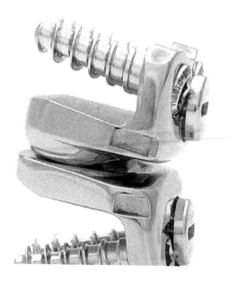

FIGURE 11   The Prestige™ cervical artificial disc.

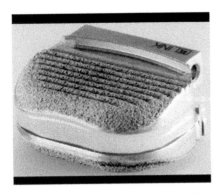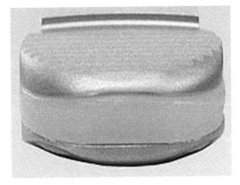

FIGURE 12 The Porous Coated Motion™ cervical artificial disc.

Cervicore™ Disc

The CerviCore (SpineCore, Inc., Summit, New Jersey, U.S.A.) disc is a cobalt-chrome metal-on-metal device with a saddle-shaped articulation, aiming to better mimic physiologic coupled motions (Fig. 13). After placement of the device, bone screws are inserted into the vertebral bodies through the anterior flanges. To date there are no published reports of clinical results from the implantation of this device.

DISCUSSION

Lumbar spine fusion is a commonly performed procedure for various conditions of the spine. In the absence of true instability however, the role of fusion in management of low back pain remains controversial. Fusion in effect achieves removal of the painful disc (if interbody fusion), maintenance or improvement of the intervertebral height, and cessation of abnormal motion—providing pain relief by eliminating function of all intervertebral structures which may generate pain. The continuous search for alternative surgical treatments has led to the development of a number of motion-preserving ideas for reconstruction of the spinal column, both anterior and posterior (42). All of these techniques attempt to maintain physiologic range of motion at the level of pathologic segment, avoiding the "hypomobility" of a fused segment and the "hypermobility" of a segment adjacent to the fusion. Anterior motion-preserving ideas range from biologic regeneration of disc material or mechanical

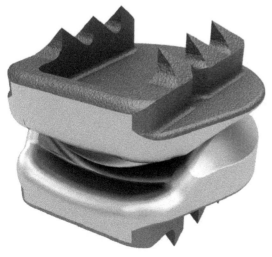

FIGURE 13 CerviCore™ (SpineCore, Inc., Summit, New Jersey, U.S.A.).

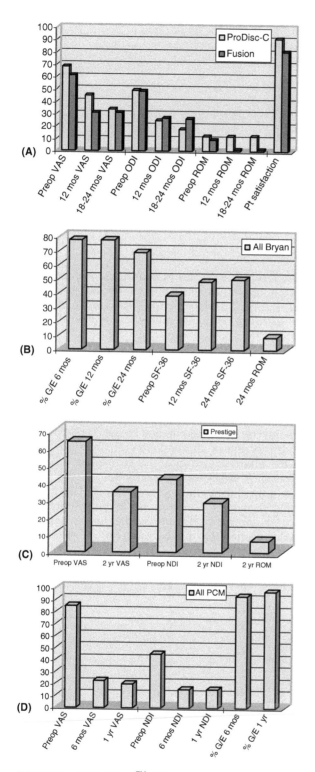

FIGURE 14 (**A**) ProDisc-C™ clinical outcomes at up to two years (**B**) Bryan™ clinical outcomes at up to two years; (**C**) Prestige™ clinical outcomes at up to two years; (**D**) PCM clinical outcomes at one year. *Abbreviations*: G/E, Good to excellent results; NDI, neck disability index; ODI, Oswestry disability index; PCM, porous coated motion; ROM, flexion-extension range of motion in degrees; SF-36, short form 36 item health survey; VAS, visual analog scale. *Source*: From Refs. 36, 38, 41, 79.

replacement of the nucleus pulposus, to total disc replacement. Posterior motion-preserving techniques include ligament reconstructions, interspinous shock absorbers, and dynamic neutralization, and are discussed in other parts of this textbook.

Even though fusion has been the only available end-stage treatment of the degenerative lumbar segment, the clinical outcomes of this procedure are quite variable, leading to continued controversy about its indications (43–50). There are well-regarded studies that have proven fusion to be successful for intractably painful motion segments compared to continued conservative care (51,52). Historically, fusion for low back pain has yielded clinical success in the 60–70% range, which pales in comparison to the 90–95% success range of the most successful surgery in spine–decompression for neurogenic claudication (10,17,53). An important point made in the literature is that radiographic and clinical outcomes do not necessarily correlate. In patients undergoing anterior lumbar interbody fusion (ALIF) with cages, Ray reported a good to excellent result rate of 65%, although 96% had radiographic fusion (54). For a similar group of patients Kuslich et al. (55) reported a 95% radiographic fusion rate, but only 63% of patients were gainfully employed at four years. Boden et al. (56) described a 93% fusion rate and a 72% patient satisfaction rate when using bone morphogenetic protein in cages for ALIF. These were all anterior-only fusions. The literature has shown that posterior spinal fusions are generally more morbid, mostly related to the greater muscle dissection and retraction involved, and thus potentially even less satisfactory to patients, at least in the short term (44,45,49,57,58). In an attempt to prevent graft resorption, collapse, and pseudarthrosis, surgeons have used combined anterior-posterior surgery. Again however, clinical success has not matched radiographic success. Kozak et al. (46) found acceptable clinical results in 80% of their anterior-posterior fusions. Slosar et al. (59) also found an 81% clinical success rate with a 99% fusion rate. Thus even with superlative fusion rates using newer instrumentation, techniques, and combined approaches, reliable clinical success remains elusive.

New treatments for degenerative disc disease must show superiority over the natural history of the disease, or at least equivalency to the current standard of care with the potential of additional benefit (such as prevention of adjacent spinal segment degeneration in the case of artificial discs). Smith et al. (60) followed 25 patients with low back pain and positive discograms who declined surgical intervention. After five years, 68% showed clinical improvement, and 24% had more severe back pain and disability. Fritzell et al. (51), in a landmark series of patients with fusion for chronic low back pain, showed that 60% to 68% rated themselves "better" or "much better" at two years after surgery, and 12% to 16% were "worse." On average, back pain decreased from six to four, and leg pain from four to three on the VAS. The study showed that lumbar fusion can improve back pain, but a controlled comparison to nonoperated patients was not performed. Although fusion surgery has been shown to lead to improvement in symptoms, many patients unfortunately still have significant persistent pain after fusion.

The initial European study on ProDisc-L showed promising results (18,20). A retrospective review of the original ProDisc-L (ProDisc-I) with 7 to 11-year follow-up on 61 patients was conducted. One third of patients had two-level ProDisc-L implantations. There were no cases of subsidence or migration, and no implants had to be removed or revised. Overall, 93% of the patients reported that they were satisfied or entirely satisfied with the procedure. The average VAS for back pain went from 8.5 preoperatively to three postoperatively, and VAS for leg pain from seven preops to two postops.

The European experience with the second generation of ProDisc-L (ProDisc-II) yielded similarly excellent results. In one center in Germany, a total of 134 discs were replaced in 108 patients with three-month to two-year follow-up (24). The study is ongoing, with prospective data collection of clinical exam, VAS, Oswestry disability index (ODI), and SF-36 scores. The preliminary data revealed 91% excellent and good results, 8% fair, and 1% poor results. The authors note that fair and poor clinical outcomes were found primarily in patients with more severe, multilevel degenerative disease including facet arthritis. There were no cases of implant migration or subsidence.

The excellent results obtained with the ProDisc-L device and the lack of any catastrophic failure in Europe paved the way for the FDA pivotal clinical trials currently underway in the United States (23,61). Patients have reported higher satisfaction rates with disc replacement than fusion. The reasons may be multi-factorial. The earlier recovery after disc replacement, patients' preconceived bias against fusion surgery, the promise of a newer technology, rigid patient selection criteria, and so on may have all contributed to the more optimistic outlook in disc replacement patients.

Although with the follow-up available no comment is made yet about adjacent segment degeneration, the potential benefit of disc replacement is indicated by the flexibility or motion at the treated intervertebral level. The logic being that a mobile treated level is less likely to transfer undue stresses to the adjacent segment. At the L4–L5 level, the sagittal motion data suggests that the disc replacement not only preserves motion, but can also increase or restore motion, for the follow-up period of this study. At L5–S1 level an increase in sagittal motion in the disc replacement patients was also observed compared to the fusion patients. At the untreated L3–L4 levels, no significant changes in motion or height were detected at any interval up to two years—however, this may very well change with long-term follow-up.

Theoretically, motion preservation will have a protective effect against future degeneration at adjacent levels. In the future it will be important to evaluate not only whether there is motion, but also to qualify the motion that occurs across the spinal segment, since this may play a role in facet displacement and loading. Various prosthetic designs will have different motion parameters, with different directional constraints. While most disc replacements may be able maintain motion, the local effect on collateral structures such as the facets may a paramount factor. Only long-term follow-up will reveal whether significant benefit is observed at the level adjacent to a disc replacement, and/or whether facet arthrosis will be prevented or even exacerbated depending on the prosthesis design. With the follow-up available, carefully conducted clinical trials have indicated that the lumbar and cervical disc replacements are a viable alternative to motion-sacrificing spinal fusion surgery. The semi-constrained, porous-coated ProDisc-L has withstood the test of 2-level disc replacement at up to four years in clinical trials. Under a "compassionate use" arm of the study, with special consideration from the FDA, some patients have also successfully undergone 3-level lumbar and 3-level cervical disc replacements using the semi-constrained ProDisc-L and ProDisc-C prostheses, with good early success, which will be the subject of a future report (62). Other issues that may exist with disc arthroplasty such as infection, wear particles, subsidence, implant failure, and longevity have not been a factor at this intermediate stage of the study.

CONCLUSIONS

The interim results from published studied in the literature demonstrate decreased postoperative morbidity and improved function after artificial disc replacement. Patients who received disc replacement as opposed to fusion achieved a significant improvement in pain, to less than half of its preoperative intensity, in as early as six weeks after surgery. This reduction in pain has been maintained through at least two years of observation. Functional status in particular was improved in the early postoperative period for the disc replacement patients compared to fusion patients. Patient satisfaction was significantly higher with disc replacement versus fusion. The artificial disc has been shown to preserve motion at the surgical level over at least the first two years after implantation. Longer observation is needed to assess the important potential benefit of protection against adjacent segment degeneration by artificial disc replacement. Long-term results from the U.S. FDA pivotal clinical trials for the lumbar and cervical prostheses (currently having completed enrollment at selected sites across the country) will provide valuable information comparing this new technology to the current mainstay surgical treatment of degenerative disc disease—spinal fusion.

CASE STUDIES
Case 1

A 45-year-old female presented with intractable low back pain of at least five years duration. She works as a park ranger in an Alaskan national park, and her symptoms were significantly hindering her work. Her pain radiated to bilateral buttocks but no further. She had failed the

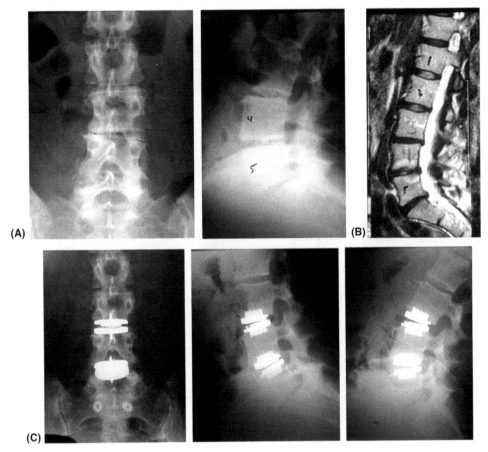

FIGURE 15 Case 1 preoperative radiographs (**A**), magnetic resonance imaging (**B**), and postoperative anteroposterior and flexion extension radiographs (**C**). Note the dynamic correction of local scoliotic deformity at L3–L5 due to asymmetric disc collapse.

gamut of nonoperative treatment, including physical therapy with multiple modalities, epidural steroid injections, facet blocks, and radio frequency ablation of her facet joint nerves. She was on Celebrex and multiple hydrocodone pills a day for pain control. Her radiographs and magnetic resonance imaging (MRI) revealed degenerated discs at L3–L4 and L4–L5 (Figs. 15A,B). Discograms were concordantly positive at L3–L4 and L4–L5. She had markedly asymmetric collapse of the disc spaces at the two affected levels, resulting in local scoliotic deformity. She successfully underwent a two-level artificial disc replacement with the ProDisc-L prosthesis (Fig. 15C). By six months postoperatively she related outstanding pain relief, and continues to do well 24 months out. She was back to work as a park ranger, was swimming, and was off all narcotic pain medications.

Case 2

A 37-year-old female presented with an approximately twenty-year history of low back pain that had been progressively deteriorating over the last several years. She denied any radiation of her pain. She was a multi-sport athlete in high school, and that is when her troubles began. She had tried exhaustive nonoperative measures for her back. She had seen chiropractors, physical therapists, taken multiple nonsteroid anti-inflammatory pills and strong narcotic pain pills, received acupuncture—all to no avail. The pain was keeping her from even her normal activities of daily living at this point. Plain radiographs revealed mild degenerative changes with anterior spurring at L3–L4 and L4–L5, but severe degenerative

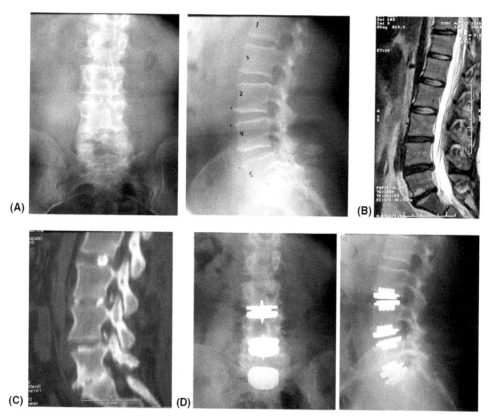

FIGURE 16 Case 2 preoperative radiographs (**A**), magnetic resonance imaging (**B**), CT discogram (**C**), and postoperative anteroposterior and lateral radiographs (**D**).

changes at L5–S1 with collapse of disc space (Fig. 16A). The MRI revealed desiccated discs at L3–L4, L4–L5, and L5–S1 (Fig. 16B). Discogram computed tomography (CT) revealed internal disc disruption as well as positive concordant pain at all three levels (Fig. 16C). A single or two-level fusion would not have addressed all her sources of pain and would have left a compromised disc to bear supraphysiologic loads adjacent to the lever arm of the fusion construct. Her young age also made a three-level fusion a poor surgical choice due to the risk of adjacent segment disease and her desire of leading an active lifestyle. Therefore a special request was made to the FDA to gain permission for the compassionate use of a three-level artificial disc replacement surgery with the ProDisc-L device. This was approved and the patient successfully underwent surgery (Fig. 16D). She is approximately 12 months after surgery and doing very well. She is on an independent walking program and has weaned herself off of all narcotics.

Case 3

Figure 17A shows a lateral radiograph of a 36-year-old female with almost a year long history of worsening axial neck pain, and left-sided radicular arm pain, numbness and tingling. Her diagnosis was a degenerative and herniated disc at C5–C6. Her MRI is shown in Figures 16B and C. She had failed nonoperative treatments including physical therapy and epidural steroid injections. She voluntarily enrolled into the ProDisc-C artificial cervical disc replacement clinical trial at our center, and was randomized to the prosthetic disc (versus anterior cervical discectomy and fusion). Her two-year postoperative radiographs, including flexion-extension are shown in Figures 17D–F. She is almost completely symptom-free and is not taking any medications for her neck or arm.

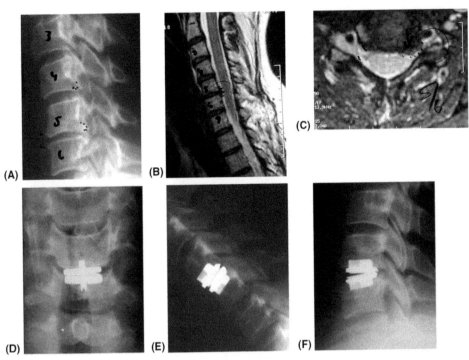

FIGURE 17 Case 3 preoperative radiograph (**A**), magnetic resonance imaging (**B,C**), and postoperative flexion-extension radiographs (**D–F**).

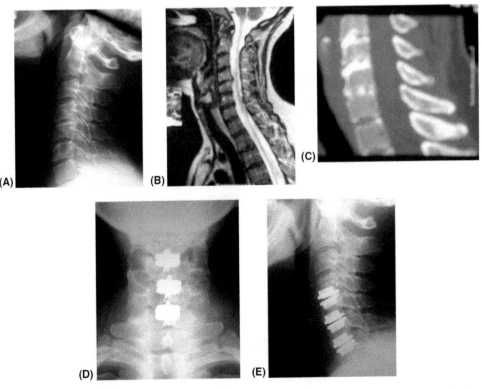

FIGURE 18 Case 4 preoperative radiograph (**A**), magnetic resonance imaging (**B**), Discogram-CT (**C**), and postoperative radiographs (**D,E**).

Case 4

Figure 18A shows a lateral radiograph of a 42-year-old female with a multi-year history of neck pain, occipital headaches, and bilateral upper arm pain, numbness and tingling. Extensive non-operative treatments including physical therapy and epidural steroid injections had not helped definitively. An MRI (Fig. 18B) revealed early degenerative changes with disc herniations, mostly at C4–C5 and C6–C7. A discogram-CT (Fig. 18C) revealed positive concordant pain at three levels C4–C7. She had a very active lifestyle, both professionally and recreationally, and was partially blind in one eye. Having good medical knowledge, she was positively against getting a 3-level discectomy and fusion, for fear of early degeneration of her adjacent segments, and for fear of losing the neck mobility that was especially important to her because of her vision problems. A special request was made to the FDA for compassionate allowance for a 3-level disc replacement for her. Based on the surgeon's experience, and our prior results, this was approved. The one-year postoperative radiographs are shown in Figures 18D and E. She is completely satisfied with her surgery, with an approximately 80% reduction in her Visual Analog Scale and Oswestry Disability Index at one year.

REFERENCES

1. Blumenthal S, McAfee PC, Guyer RD, et al. A prospective, randomized, multicenter Food and Drug Administration investigational device exemptions study of lumbar total disc replacement with the CHARITE artificial disc versus lumbar fusion: Part I. Evaluation of clinical outcomes. Spine 2005; 30(14):1565–1575.
2. Wang JC, McDonough PW, Endow K, Kanim LE, Delamarter RB. The effect of cervical plating on single-level anterior cervical discectomy and fusion. J Spinal Disord 1999; 12(6):467–471.
3. Wang JC, McDonough PW, Endow KK, Delamarter RB. Increased fusion rates with cervical plating for two-level anterior cervical discectomy and fusion. Spine 2000; 25(1):41–45.
4. Wang JC, McDonough PW, Kanim LE, Endow KK, Delamarter RB. Increased fusion rates with cervical plating for three-level anterior cervical discectomy and fusion. Spine 2001; 26(6):643–646; discussion 6–7.
5. Hilibrand AS, Carlson GD, Palumbo MA, Jones PK, Bohlman HH. Radiculopathy and myelopathy at segments adjacent to the site of a previous anterior cervical arthrodesis. J Bone Joint Surg Am 1999; 81(4):519–528.
6. Goffin J, Geusens E, Vantomme N, et al. Long-term follow-up after interbody fusion of the cervical spine. J Spinal Disord Tech 2004; 17:79–85.
7. Katsuura A, Hukuda S, Saruhashi Y, et al. Kyphotic malalignment after anterior cervical fusion is one of the factors promoting the degenerative process in adjacent intervertebral levels. Eur Spine J 2001; 10:320–324.
8. Buttner-Janz K. The development of the artificial disc: SB Charité. Dallas: Hundley and Associates, 1992.
9. Buttner-Janz K, Schellnack K, Zippel H. Biomechanics of the SB Charité lumbar intervertebral disc endoprosthesis. Int Orthop 1989; 13(3):173–176.
10. McAfee PC, Fedder IL, Saiedy S, Shucosky EM, Cunningham BW. Experimental design of total disk replacement-experience with a prospective randomized study of the SB Charité. Spine 2003; 28(20):S153–S162.
11. White AA, Panjabi MM. Clinical biomechanics of the spine. 2nd ed. JB Lippincott Co, 1990:112–115.
12. Guyer RD, Blumenthal SL, Hochschuler SH, Ohnmeiss DD. SB Charité III prospective randomized U.S. trial. Total disc replacement precourse. 18th Annual Meeting of the North American Spine Society. San Diego, CA, 2003.
13. Lemaire JP, Skalli W, Lavaste F, et al. Intervertebral disc prosthesis. Results and prospects for the year 2000. Clin Orthop 1997; 337:64–76.
14. Lemaire JP, Carrier H, Ali el-HS, Skalli W, Lavaste F. Clinical and radiological outcomes with the Charité artificial disc: A 10-year minimum follow-up. J Spinal Disord Tech 2005; 18:353–359.
15. Zeegers WS, Bohnen LM, Laaper M, Verhaegen MJ. Artificial disc replacement with the modular type SB Charité III: 2-year results in 50 prospectively studied patients. Eur Spine J 1999; 8(3):210–217.
16. Cinotti G, David T, Postacchini F. Results of disc prosthesis after a minimum follow-up period of 2 years. Spine 1996; 21(8):995–1000.
17. Guyer RD, Ohnmeiss DD. Intervertebral disc prostheses. Spine 2003; 28(15):S15–S23.
18. Marnay T. Lumbar disc arthroplasty: 8–10 year results using titanium plates with a polyethylene inlay component. American Academy of Orthopaedic Surgeons Annual Meeting. San Francisco, CA, 2001.

19. Tropiano P, Huang RC, Girardi FP, Marnay T. Lumbar disc replacement: preliminary results with ProDisc II after a minimum follow-up period of 1 year. J Spinal Disord Tech 2003; 16(4):362–368.

20. Tropiano P, Huang RC, Girardi FP, Cammisa FP Jr, Marnay T. Lumbar total disc replacement. Seven to eleven-year follow-up. J Bone Joint Surg Am 2005; 87A(3):490–496.

21. Bertagnoli R, Yue JJ, Shah RV, et al. The treatment of disabling single-level lumbar discogenic low back pain with total disc arthroplasty utilizing the ProDisc prosthesis: a prospective study with 2-year minimum follow-up. Spine 2005; 30(19):2230–2236.

22. Bae H, Kanim L, Delamarter R. ProDisc artificial lumbar disc replacement: introduction and results from the USA clinical trial. International Society for Study of the Lumbar Spine, Annual Meeting. Porto, Portugal, 2004.

23. Delamarter RB, Fribourg DM, Kanim LE, Bae H. ProDisc artificial total lumbar disc replacement: introduction and early results from the United States clinical trial. Spine 2003; 28(20):S167–S175.

24. Bertagnoli R, Kumar S. Indications for full prosthetic disc arthroplasty: a correlation of clinical outcome against a variety of indications. Eur Spine J 2002; 11(suppl 2):S131–S136.

25. Huang RC, Girardi FP, Cammisa FP Jr, Tropiano P, Marnay T. Long-term flexion-extension range of motion of the ProDisc total disc replacement. J Spinal Disord Tech 2003; 16(5):435–440.

26. Cauchoix J, David T. Arthrodeses lombaires: resultats apres plus de 10 ans. Rev Chir Orthop 1985; 71:263–268.

27. Gillet P. The fate of the adjacent motion segments after lumbar fusion. J Spinal Disord 2003; 16:338–345.

28. Mathews HH, Lehuec JC, Friesem T, Zdeblick T, Eisermann L. Design rationale and biomechanics of Maverick Total Disc arthroplasty with early clinical results. Spine 2004; 4(suppl 6):S261–S275.

29. Le Huec JC, Mathews H, Basso Y, et al. Clinical results of Maverick lumbar total disc replacement: two-year prospective follow-up. Orthop Clin North Am 2005; 36(3):315–322.

30. Errico TJ. Lumbar disc arthroplasty. Clin Orthop 2005; 435:106–117.

31. Bertagnoli R, Yue JJ, Pfeiffer F, et al. Early results after ProDisc-C cervical disc replacement. J Neurosurg Spine 2005; 2(4):403–410.

32. Bertagnoli R, Duggal N, Pickett GE, et al. Cervical total disc replacement: Part 2. Clinical results. Orthop Clin North Am 2005; 36:355–362.

33. Goffin J, Casey A, Kehr P, et al. Preliminary clinical experience with the Bryan Cervical Disc Prosthesis. Neurosurgery 2002; 51(3):840–845.

34. Johnson JP, Lauryssen C, Cambron HO, et al. Sagittal alignment and the Bryan cervical artificial disc. Neurosurg Focus 2004; 17(6):E14.

35. Leung C, Casey AT, Goffin J, et al. Clinical significance of heterotopic ossification in cervical disc replacement: a prospective multicenter clinical trial. Neurosurgery 2005; 57(4):759–763.

36. Goffin J, Van Calenbergh F, van Loon J, et al. Intermediate follow-up after treatment of degenerative disc disease with the Bryan Cervical Disc Prosthesis: single-level and bi-level. Spine 2003; 28:2673–2678.

37. Duggal N, Pickett GE, Mitsis DK, Keller JL. Early clinical and biomechanical results following cervical arthroplasty. Neurosurg Focus 2004; 17(3):E9.

38. Wigfield CC, Gill SS, Nelson RJ, Metcalf NH, Robertson JT. The new Frenchay artificial cervical joint: results from a two-year pilot study. Spine 2002; 27(22):2446–2452.

39. Robertson JT, Metcalf NH. Long-term outcome after implantation of the Prestige I disc in an end-stage indication: 4-year results from a pilot study. Neurosurg Focus 2004; 17(3):E10.

40. Porchet F, Metcalf NH. Clinical outcomes with the Prestige II cervical disc: preliminary results from a prospective randomized clinical trial. Neurosurg Focus 2004; 17(3):E6.

41. Pimenta L, McAfee PC, Cappuccino A, Bellera FP, Link HD. Clinical experience with the new artificial cervical PCM (Cervitech) disc. Spine J 2004; 4(suppl 6):S315–S321.

42. Mayer HM, Korge A. Non-fusion technology in degenerative lumbar spinal disorders: facts, questions, challenges. Eur Spine J 2002; 11(suppl 2):S85–S91.

43. de Kleuver M, Oner FC, Jacobs WC. Total disc replacement for chronic low back pain: background and a systematic review of the literature. Eur Spine J 2003; 12(2):108–116.

44. 44. Greenough CG, Taylor LJ, Fraser RD. Anterior lumbar fusion: results, assessment techniques and prognostic factors. Eur Spine J 1994; 3:225–230.

45. Greenough CG, Peterson MD, Hadlow S, Fraser RD. Instrumented posterolateral lumbar fusion. Spine 1998; 23:479–486.

46. Kozak JA, Heilman AE, O'Brien JP. Anterior lumbar fusion options. Technique and graft materials. Clin Orthop 1994; 300:45–51.

47. Mayer HM. Microsurgical anterior approaches for anterior interbody fusion of the lumbar spine. In: Young PH, ed. Essentials of Spinal Microsurgery. Philadelphia: Lippincott-Raven, 1998:633–649.

48. Nachemson A. Instrumented fusion of the lumbar spine for degenerative disorders: a critical look. In: Nachemson A, ed. Philadelphia: Lippincott Raven, 1996.

49. Nachemson A, Zdeblick TA, O'Brien JP. Lumbar disc disease with discogenic pain. What surgical treatment is most effective? Spine 1996; 21(15):1835–1838.

50. Szpalski M. The mysteries of segmental instability. Bull Hosp Joint Dis 1996; 55:147–148.

51. Fritzell P, Hagg O, Wessberg P, et al. 2001 Volvo Award Winner in Clinical Studies. Lumbar fusion versus nonsurgical treatment for chronic low back pain: a multicenter randomized controlled trial from the Swedish Lumbar Spine Study Group. Spine 2001; 26:2521–2534.

52. Krismer M. Fusion of the lumbar spine. A consideration of the indications. J Bone Joint Surg Br 2002; 84:783–794.

53. Yukawa Y, Lenke LG, Tenhula J, et al. A comprehensive study of patients with surgically treated lumbar spinal stenosis with neurogenic claudication. J Bone Joint Surg Am 2002; 84A:1954–1959.

54. 54. Ray CD. Threaded titanium cages for lumbar interbody fusions. Spine 1997; 22(6):667–679; discussion 79–80.

55. Kuslich SD, Danielson G, Dowdle JD, et al. Four-year follow-up results of lumbar spine arthrodesis using the Bagby and Kuslich lumbar fusion cage. Spine 2000; 25(20):2656–2662.

56. Boden SD, Zdeblick TA, Sandhu HS, Heim SE. The use of rhBMP-2 in interbody fusion cages. Definitive evidence of osteoinduction in humans: a preliminary report. Spine 2000; 25(3):376–381.

57. Pradhan BB, Nassar JA, Delamarter RB, Wang JC. Single-level lumbar spine fusion: a comparison of anterior and posterior approaches. J Spinal Disord 2002; 15:355–361.

58. Scaduto AA, Gamradt SC, Yu WD, Huang J, Delamarter RB, Wang JC. Perioperative complications of threaded cylindrical lumbar interbody fusion devices: anterior versus posterior approach. J Spinal Disord Tech 2003; 16(6):502–507.

59. Slosar PJ, Reynolds JB, Goldthwaite N. Combined anterior and posterior lateral lumbar fusions. Ninth Annual Meeting of the North American Spine Society. Minneapolis, MN, 1994.

60. Smith SE, Darden BV, Rhyne AL, et al. Outcome of unoperated discogram-positive low back pain. Spine 1995; 20:1997–2000.

61. Zigler JE. Clinical results with ProDisc: European experience and U.S. investigation device exemption study. Spine 2003; 28(20):S163–S166.

62. Pradhan BB, Bae HW, Kropf MA, Kanim LE, Delamarter RB. Sagittal and Coronal Alignment after Multi-level Lumbar Artificial Disc Replacement with ProDisc-L. Spinal Arthroplasty Society. New York, NY, 2005.

63. Buttner-Janz K, Schellnack K, Zippel H, et al. Erfahrungen und ergebnisse mit der lumbalen zwischenwirbelendoprothese SB Charité. Z Klin Med 1988; 43:1785–1789.

64. David T. Lumbar disc prosthesis. Surgical technique, indications, and clinical results in 22 patients with a minimum 12 months follow-up. Eur Spine J 1993; 1:254–259.

65. Griffith SL, Shelokov AP, Buttner-Janz K, LeMaire JP, Zeegers WS. A multicenter retrospective study of the clinical results of the LINK SB Charité intervertebral prosthesis. The initial European experience. Spine 1994; 19(16):1842–1849.

66. David TJ. Lumbosacral disc prosthesis. In: Margulies JY, ed. Lumbosacral and spinopelvic fixation. Philadelphia: Lippincott-Raven, 1996:881–887.

67. David TJ. Lumbar disc prosthesis: five years follow-up study on 96 patients. The 15th Annual Meeting of the North American Spine Society, 2000.

68. David T. Lumbar disc prosthesis: five years follow-up study on 147 patients with 163 SB Charité prosthesis. Eur Spine J 2002; 11(suppl 1):S18.

69. Hochschuler SH, Ohnmeiss DD, Guyer RD, Blumenthal SL. Artificial disc: preliminary results of a prospective study in the United States. Eur Spine J 2002; 11(suppl 2):S106–S110.

70. McAfee PC, Fedder IL, Saiedy S, Shucosky EM, Cunningham BW. SB Charité disc replacement: report of 60 prospective randomized cases in a US center. J Spinal Disord Tech 2003; 16(4):424–433.

71. Guyer RD, McAfee PC, Hochschuler SH, Blumenthal SL, Fedder IL, Ohnmeiss DD, Cunningham BW. Prospective randomized study of the Charité artificial disc: data from two investigational centers. Spine J 2004; 4(suppl 6):S252–S259.

72. Mayer HM, Wiechert K. Microsurgical anterior approaches to the lumbar spine for interbody fusion and total disc replacement. Neurosurgery 2002; 51(suppl 5):159–165.

73. Marnay T. Lumbar disc replacement. Spine J 2002; 2:94S.

74. Zigler JE, Burd TA, Vialle EN, Sachs BL, Rashbaum RF, Ohnmeiss DD. Lumbar spine arthroplasty: early results using the ProDisc II: a prospective randomized trial of arthroplasty versus fusion. J Spinal Disord Tech 2003; 16(4):352–361.

75. Zigler JE. Lumbar spine arthroplasty using the ProDisc II. Spine J 2004; 4(suppl 6):260S–267S.

76. Tian W, Liu B, Li Q, Hu L, Li ZY, Yuan Q, Sun YZ. Early clinical outcomes of cervical artificial disc replacement. Zhonghua Yi Xue Za Zhi 2005; 85(1):37–40.

77. Delamarter RB, Pradhan BB. Indications for cervical spine prostheses, early experiences with ProDisc-C in the USA. Spine Art 2004; 1:7–9.

78. Robertson J, Porchet F, Brotchi J, et al. A multicenter trial of an artificial cervical joint for primary disc disease. Society for Spinal Arthroplasty. Montpellier, France, 2002.

79. Delamarter RB, Bae HW, Pradhan BB. Clinical results after lumbar total disc replacement: an interim report from the United States clinical trial for the ProDisc-II prosthesis. Orthop Clin North Am 2005; 36:301–313.

28 | Dynesys® Spinal Instrumentation System

William C. Welch, Peter C. Gerszten, and Boyle C. Cheng
Department of Neurological Surgery, UPMC Health System, University of Pittsburgh School of Medicine, Pittsburgh, Pennsylvania, U.S.A.

James Maxwell
Scottsdale Spine Care, Scottsdale, Arizona, U.S.A.

INTRODUCTION

The Dynesys® Spinal Instrumentation System (Zimmer Spine, Minneapolis, Minnesota, U.S.A.) is a unique, FDA-approved lumbar spinal instrumentation system that has been implanted in over 15,000 patients in Europe and the United States (1). This system is FDA-approved under the 510(k) process as an adjunct to lumbar fusion in skeletally-mature individuals to supplement bilateral-lateral onlay autograft bone. Dynesys® has recently completed an FDA investigational device exemption (IDE) trial comparing the system without bone grafting to a standard 1 or 2-level lumbar fusion with pedicle screw supplementation and onlay autograft bone. The purpose of this Chapter is to review this spinal system, its potential indications, available biomechanical data and our clinical experience with the system.

INSTRUMENTATION

The Dynesys® system is straightforward and simple. The components include a number of fixed-head pedicle screws available in a large number of configurations. The screws are made of titanium and are designed to promote bone on-growth. The screws have a fairly aggressive self-tapping thread pattern which is designed to strongly engage the cancellous bone of the pedicle and vertebral body. The screws are designed to be oriented in a very lateral-to-medial direction and are placed deeply in the bone. Ultimately, the design is to have the screw heads placed deeply against the bone comprising the transverse process and lateral facet joint (Fig. 1).

The next component of the system is tubular spacers made of polycarbonate urethane (Fig. 2). The spacers are delivered in a fixed length and are trimmed to the appropriate distance to be inserted between the pedicle screw heads. The spacer length is determined with a measuring tool that is inserted into the pedicle screw head cable openings. This measuring tool has a built-in tensionometer so that the surgeon may, in a limited fashion, determine the in vivo rigidity of the functional spinal unit (FSU). The length of the spacers is custom-tailored for each pedicle screw head-pedicle screw head length in the operative field using a specialized cutter (Fig. 3). They are secured to the pedicle screw heads with the third and final component of the system-tensioning cables.

The tensioning cables are made of braided polyethylene terephthalate (PET). These are inserted through one pedicle screw, through the spacer and into the next pedicle screw. The cables have three "zones." The first zone is called the introduction zone. This area is smaller in diameter than the working and functional zones. The introduction zone is quite stiff enabling it to be pushed and pulled during the course of surgery. The working zone is wider in diameter than the introduction zone and the functional zone is the area of the tensioning cable that is ultimately secured to the pedicle screws and remains in the patient.

The surgical tools used to implant the Dynesys® system are equally straightforward and simple. These tools are designed to maximize the bone contact between the pedicle screws and the pedicles/vertebral bodies. As such, the system does not include curved pedicle probes or bone taps. The bone preparation tools include an awl to perforate cortical bone and a small, straight, tapered pedicle probe only (Fig. 4).

There are a number of tools designed to manipulate the tensioning cord and spacers. These instruments include a spacer cutter and spacer holder. A specialized cord manipulator

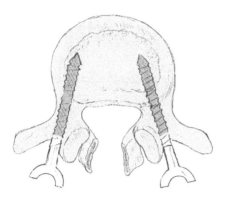

FIGURE 1 Drawing demonstrating direction of pedicle screws and recession of screw heads into facet-transverse process recess.

(essentially a modified Kerrison punch) can be used to place the cord through the screws and spacer. This manipulator is designed to reduce abrasion on the cord during cord placement.

Another tool used prior to tightening of the cables against the pedicle screws and spacers is the tensioner. This hand-held device grasps the cord at one end while pushing it against the pedicle screw head at the other end. This device created the final tension on the cord-spacer-pedicle screw unit as the securing screws are tightened against the cord. A right angle extender is available for this final tightening phase. This device allows the cord to be tensioned outside of the wound and is useful in cases where the exposure is limited.

BIOMECHANICAL ASSESSMENT

The Dynesys® dynamic neutralization system is a posterior pedicle screw based system designed to transmit load from one vertebral body to the connected vertebral body via a two component dynamic rod (2). The unique capabilities of this system stem from the attributes of the rod design and the materials used. Additionally, the surgical technique required by this system potentially contributes to the increased stability of an FSU.

The dynamic rod provides optimal resistance of tensile loading through the use of a PET cord. Moments generated from pure flexion bending or from other bending, for example, from secondary coupled motion or lateral bending, load one or both PET cords in tension. This should be considered "stretching" of the PET cord component. Conversely, in extension bending, the PET cord is offloaded, and the polycarbone urethane (PCU) spacer becomes compressively loaded or "shortened" (Fig. 5). Likewise, this may occur on the opposite side of the tensile loaded PET cord during lateral bending or arise from other coupled motions. This concept allows the components to be appropriately tailored for specific loading profiles. The multi-polymer configuration may be advantageous with appropriate tailoring of these components by providing different types of resistance for different types of bending.

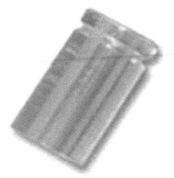

FIGURE 2 Cut polycarbonate urethane (PCU) spacer.

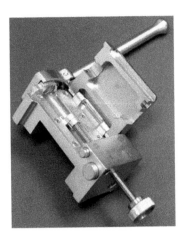

FIGURE 3   Polycarbonate urethane (PCU) spacer cutting device.

Should one compare the Dynesys® system to rigid or semi-rigid pedicle screw-based systems with stiff metal rod constructs, a clearly different load response occurs? Posterior pedicle screws with metal rods provide a stiff construct in all modes of loading. This is attributed to the homogenous isotropic properties of a metal rod. In other words, rigid constructs have the same materials properties in all directions. Regardless of flexion extension or even lateral bending, the structure of a metal rod will provide the same response. The end result is the transfer of loads through the construct to adjacent spinal levels.

Traditional posterior pedicle screw fixation with such metal rods has limited motion, because of this rigid fixation between vertebral bodies. The screw rod interface with metal screws and rods have been shown to be both strong and stiff. The design intent of Dynesys® was to provide the same type of instant fixation and stabilization to a FSU in patients required posterior stabilization with one major design difference, that is, to minimize the load transferred to adjacent levels.

By limiting intersegmental motion, pedicle screw based systems are designed and have been shown clinically to promote fusion. At first glance, this concept may be diametrically opposed to the concept of dynamic neutralization. However, as clinical results from both European history and the preliminary results from the US FDA IDE trial demonstrate, there is evidence that supports successful clinical outcomes with the use of posterior systems that are less rigid and do not use anterior column support.

As this system has been shown to increase stiffness when compared to a normal FSU, this can be attributed to the materials selected and also the surgical technique. The ability to have the base of the screw as close to the anatomy not only provides a lower profile for the system when implanted in the patient, it also serves as a buttress effect. The stability of the construct is more stable when the system mass outside the pedicle is brought closer to the bony surface.

An important caveat with the Dynesys® system is that when it is initially implanted the construct is very rigid (3). Comparison studies of Dynesys® to semi-rigid pedicle screw

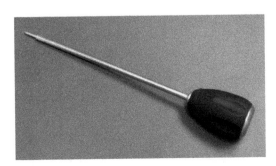

FIGURE 4   Awl used to create a small cortical opening in the dorsal lateral bone prior to pedicle probe insertion.

Flexion   Extension

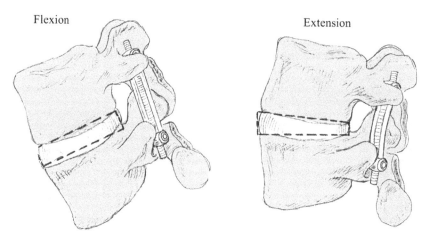

FIGURE 5 Drawing of the Dynesys® construct in flexion and extension causing tension on the PET cord with unloading of the PET spacer and loading of the spacer, respectively.

systems showed that both provided equal stability. This allowed the Dynesys® system to gain FDA fusion adjunct approval. However, following implantation, the Dynesys® system becomes less rigid. This is due to a combination of the system warming-up to the in vivo environment, mechanical "settling in" of the PCU spacers and PET tensioning cord, and mechanical properties of the spacers and tensioning bands. Ultimately, the system equilibrates after approximately 500,000 loading cycles (approximately 6 to 12 months in clinical use).

CLINICAL INDICATIONS

As with any device, clinical indications are critical to the outcomes expected and desired. In general, once a patient has been identified with the appropriate clinical indications, important criteria for success include appropriate surgical site preparation, appropriate implant sizing, and appropriate technique.

As noted earlier in the chapter, the current FDA-approved indication for the Dynesys® system is as an adjunct to fusion when used in skeletally matured individuals in combination with autograft bone in the lateral gutters. Essentially, this is the same indication as most pedicle screw fusion systems.

The indication most surgeons are interested in is the potential for this system to be utilized as a stand-alone device without the intent of fusion. This indication was evaluated in a large (approximately 400 patients) pivotal trial as part of the US IDE trial. Enrollment criteria included skeletally matured patients with a stenosing lesion (either central canal stenosis or lateral recess/neuroforaminal stenosis) at one or two levels. The patients had to have more leg symptoms than lower back symptoms. Patients with no greater than Grade I spondylolisthesis could be randomized.

The usual exclusionary criteria applied to this instrumentation study including the presence of infection, degenerative scoliosis, and prior attempt at fusion at the surgically indicated level, gross obesity, osteoporosis, immunosuppressive therapy, instrumentation component allergies, trauma, and others. Another exclusionary criterion is the exclusion of patients with primarily lower back pain or neurological symptoms of unclear etiology.

The control group is one or two level fusion using a semi-rigid pedicle screw-based fixation system. The test group is Dynesys instrumentation at one or two levels without autograft supplementation. This prospective, randomized trial was performed at a 2:1 Dynesys®:posterior spinal fusion randomization schema.

Safety will be determined by neurological maintenance or improvement, and freedom from further surgical intervention for the system. Efficacy will be determined by the rate of pain relief and functional improvement. Enrollment has been completed for over one year as of this writing and results should be available soon.

Globally, over 17,000 Dynesys® implants have been performed. The global indications are more liberal than the US IDE trial indications and include primary degenerative disc disease, disc rupture, revision surgery, adjacent segment degeneration, revision discectomy and others.

SURGICAL TECHNIQUE

The Dynesys® system was designed for a far lateral approach which provides two important elements to the overall FSU. First, it allows a triangulation approach between the pedicle screws and existing bony anatomy. Specifically, this can be thought of as a triangular structural truss. The screws makeup two sides of the truss while the lamina completes the structural triangle. The structural trusses between vertebrae are then connected via the dynamic rid. This technique promotes high pull out strength and other biomechanical advantages.

The Dynesys construct is FDA-approved as a fusion adjunct and, as such, may be combined with an anterior column support structure. The anterior column device may be placed through an anterior or posterior approach as is the standard practice of the surgeon. Generally speaking, placement of an anterior column device, if so desired by the surgeon, is performed prior to Dynesys placement or augmentation.

The current Dynesys design calls for the placement of pedicle screws in a slightly modified fashion and then the connection of the PET cord and PCU spacers to the screw heads. The pedicle screws are placed from a very lateral position and aimed medially so that the screw tips come close to converging in the anterior vertebral body. This provides for both wide triangulation and allows the screw heads to be placed deeply into the lateral facet-transverse process recess. The screw placement technique is also slightly different from other screw placement techniques in that there is no bony tapping required for the screw placement. An awl is used to create the initial small hole in the cortical bone after which a pedicle probe is passed to the appropriate depth. The screws are then placed using the tract created by the pedicle probe as a guide. In this way, the bone-screw interface is maximized.

After the screws are placed, the distance between the screw heads is measured with a measuring device (Fig. 6). The surgeon may then choose to cut a PCU spacer that is the measured distance, or he may select a longer or shorter length spacer to off-load the facets or provide compression across an anterior column support device. The PET cord is inserted through a screw head and tightened to the head with a crimping screw. The PCU spacer is passed over the cord and the free end of the cord is inserted into the subsequent screw head. A fixed tension is placed against the screw head and spacer and the cord in secured to the screw head using a tensioning device (Fig. 7), effectively creating a tension band against a spacer.

Once this is completed, the surgeon may proceed to the opposite side of the construct and then work in a cephalad direction on any other FSU levels to be fused. After the construct is secured, the excess cord is trimmed with a scapel (Fig. 8). Lateral fusion can be performed with the placement of bone over the transverse processes or lamina (if present).

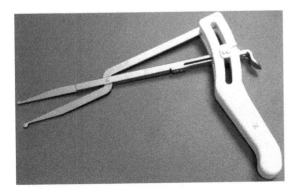

FIGURE 6 Device used to measure interpedicular screw head distance.

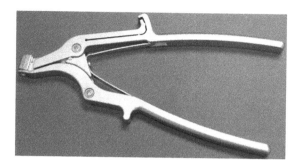

FIGURE 7   Cord tensioner.

CLINICAL OUTCOMES

The results of the U.S. IDE are not yet available. There have been a limited number of published results based on the European experience with this device. A recent, prospective, independent clinical observational trial of 26 patients treated for symptomatic lumbar stenosis with up to grade I spondylolisthesis by Schnake and colleagues was published (4). This study had a minimum follow-up of 24 months and the mean age of the patients was 71 years. The treated patients showed a statistically significant improvement in walking distances and a statistically significant reduction in pain. The overall progression of spohdylolisthesis was 2% and implant failure was seen in four patients (three cases of screw loosening and one screw breakage). Interestingly, implant failure was not associated with poor clinical outcomes and adjacent segment instability developed on one patient.

Another clinical study included a retrospective review of 83 patients who underwent Dynesys® placement between 1994 and 2000 (5). This study examined the indications, safety and efficacy following the application of the Dynesys® system in the European market. The average of the patient was 58 years and the primary indications were spinal stenosis and degenerative disc disease. Most constructs were performed at one or two levels, generally at the L3-4-5 levels. Improvements were noted in the Oswesty Disability Index, Visual Analog Scale (VAS) Pain Scales, functional and economic improvements. Usual instrumentation complications occurred, including misplaced screws and dural tears. Screw loosening requiring instrumentation revision occurred in one patient and radiographic evidence of screw loosening was evident in seven patients. The overall screw loosening rate was 3.6% (10/280 screws).

Not all studies have demonstrated statistically significant clinical improvements. Grob and colleagues performed a retrospective analysis of 50 patients who underwent instrumentation with Dynesys® in the past 40 months (6). Follow-up was performed by mailed questionnaire. The 31 patients had 2 year follow-up. The primary indicating for surgery was degenerative disc disease and one-third of patients had prior spinal surgery. The 11 of the 31 patients underwent decompression during the procedure. At follow-up, approximately two-thirds of the patients improved regarding their back and leg pain. Only 40% of patients improved in their ability to perform physical activities. Half of the patients felt that the

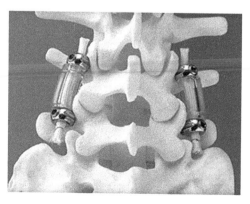

FIGURE 8   Pictorial representation of a single-level construct with cord ends trimmed.

surgery improved their overall quality of life. Six of the 31 patients were to undergo or did undergo further spinal surgeries in the follow-up period. The authors felt that dynamic stabilization did not result in better outcomes than did arthrodesis.

CONCLUSIONS

The Dynesys® system is straightforward in its surgical application. Few new surgical skills are required to technically master the procedure. Rarely the system is robust and instrumentation failure occurs. Overall patient outcomes, based on the limited surgical reports available for review, appear to be generally positive.

The greatest question to be addressed involves patient selection for the procedure. The US IDE trial should yield further light on the direct comparison of Dynesys® to fusion in a specific patient population. The efficacy of the broader role of Dynesys® will be defined as further clinical and radiographic data becomes available.

REFERENCES

1. Dubois B, de Germay B, Schaerer NS, et al. Dynamic neutralization: a new concept for restabilization of the spine. In: Szalski M, Gunzburg R, Pope MH, eds. Lumbar Segmental Instability. Philadelphia, PA: Lippincott Williams and Wilkins, 1999:233–240.
2. Niosi CA, Zhu QA, Wilson DC, Keynan O, Wilson DR, Oxland TR. Biomechanical characterization of the three-dimensional kinematic behavior of the Dynesys dynamic stabilization system: an in vitro study. Eur Spine J 2005; 15:913–922.
3. Schmoelz W, Huber JF, Nydegger T, Claes L, Wilke HJ. Dynamic stabilization of the lumbar spine and its effects on adjacent segments. J Spinal Dis 2003; 16:418–423.
4. Schnake KJ, Schaeren S, Jeanneret B. Dynamic stabilization in addition to decompression for lumbar spinal stenosis with degenerative spondylolisthesis. Spine 2006; 31:442–449.
5. Stoll TM, Dubois G, Schwarzenbach O. The dynamic neutralization system for the spine: a multi-center study of a novel non-fusion system. Eur Spine J 2002; 11:S170–S178.
6. Grob D, Benini A, Junge A, Mannion AF. Clinical experience with the Dynesys semirigid fixation system for the lumbar spine: surgical and patient-oriented outcome in 50 cases after an average of 2 years. Spine 2005; 30:324–331.

29 | Clinical Application of Computer Image Guidance Systems

Michael O. Kelleher, Linda McEvoy, and Ciaran Bolger
Department of Neurosurgery, Beaumont Hospital, Dublin, Ireland

INTRODUCTION

Over the last 10 years there has been a dramatic increase in the number of patients undergoing instrumented spinal fusion. Of these, pedicle screw fixation has become standard. The consequences of mis-directing screws are well documented and have lead to increased interest for more accurate placement methods. The use of image guidance can increase the safety and reliability of lumbar pedicle screw placement. It is especially useful where normal anatomical landmarks have been lost.

Navigation, including noncomputer based technology can allow the surgeon to overcome the problems associated with cannulating small thoracic pedicles. Instrumentation of the dorsal spine is moving away from hazardous hook and claw constructs towards image guided pedicle screw placement. Variability of the pedicle trajectory in the dorsal spine coupled with the relative obscurity of the area to fluoroscopic imaging makes this a difficult pursuit without guidance.

In the cervical spine image guidance has specific benefits. Roy-Camille has described the complex morphology of the cervical lateral mass (1,2). The proximity of the vertebral artery, exiting spinal nerve root and spinal cord considerably reduce the margin of error during cervical screw placement. This is particularly significant for the accurate placement of transarticular screws. With poor visibility of the complex anatomy for the accurate placement of the screw through the center of the cervical vertebral 2 (C2) pars interarticularis, computer generated image guidance is essential. The planning and accurate placement of transarticular C1/C2 screws inserted percutaneously using a minimally invasive exposure to avoid potential damage to either the vertebral artery or the C2 nerve root.

EFFICACY OF SPINAL IMAGE GUIDANCE IN THE LUMBAR SPINE

Since first introduced by Roy Camille in the late 1950s pedicle screw fixation has become one of the most widely used techniques for stabilization of the spine (1,2). The incidence of misplaced pedicle screws using conventional techniques (surgeon's feel, anatomic landmarks and fluoroscopy) ranges from 10% to 55% (3). The consequences of misdirecting screws are well documented and have led to increased interest for more accurate placement methods (4–6).

Due to poor visibility of the actual pedicle during screw placement, surgeons have utilized numerous different aids in the past to try and decrease the frequency of wayward screws and optimize screw placement. Such techniques employed include, mechanical probing, fluoroscopy, electrophysiological monitoring, impedance measurement, postoperative computer tomography (CT) (7–16). Although all of these tools offer varying degrees of help to surgeons, they all have limitations.

With advances in computer technology, image-guidance in the spine has become an interactive means of using a surgical pointer or tool at the time of surgery and visualizes a corresponding virtual tool on images on a computer workstation in the operating theatre. It offers the surgeon many benefits for the safe and accurate placement of spinal instrumentation (17,18). In spinal surgery, there have been two main applications of image-guidance: (*i*) the visualization of trajectories in order to optimize placement of instrumentation, in particular

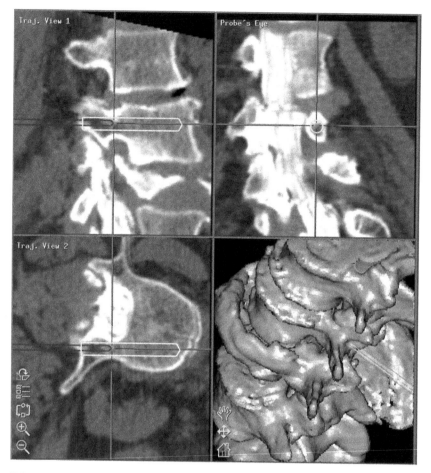

FIGURE 1 Image-guidance allows for preoperative planning and visualization of trajectory for optimal placement of pedicle screw.

of screws (Fig. 1) (15,18–22); (*ii*) orientation with regard to difficult tumors involving the spine (23–26).

In recent years, there have been numerous publications on the accuracy and the utility of image-guidance in the spine. Cadaver studies have compared traditional fluoroscopy with image-guidance based on preoperatively acquired CT and registered at single levels or multiple levels (3,15,19,27–29). Similar clinical studies have used postoperative CT to assess optimal placement of screws with and without image-guidance (30,31). Virtual fluoroscopy techniques have been assessed in a similar manner (18,32,33). By and large, all of these reports have found some advantage of image-guidance (in the form of more consistent screw placement with less cortical violation), especially when the target size is technically challenging (thoracic pedicles) or the anatomy is distorted (spinal deformities and tumors).

Computer-aided stereotactic navigation provides a three-dimensional (3D) guide for pedicle screw placement (18,34). Image guidance can facilitate preoperative planning, allow for measurement of all dimensions of the pedicle and help determine the optimal trajectory for screw placement. For routine lumbar and sacral pedicle screw placement, image-guidance using preoperative CT or intraoperatively acquired fluoroscopy can replace standard fluoroscopy (34,35).

However, computer image-guidance is not suitable for all spinal conditions. In spondylolosthesis, a stress fracture of the pars interarticularis causes detachment of the stabilizing elements posterior to the motion segment causing a biomechanical misbalance resulting in

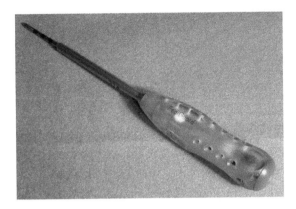

FIGURE 2   Impedance measuring device for navigation through the pedicle.

sheering and eventual displacement of the vertebral body. Because there is no stale anatomy in which to attach a reference frame, image guidance cannot yield accurate navigation.

NONIMAGE BASED NAVIGATION: IMPEDANCE-SENSITIVE DRILLING TOOLS

Alternative technologies to image-based guidance are available. To improve reliability of pedicle screw placement, a new free-hand instrument has been developed to provide the surgeon with feedback in the event of a pedicle violation by discriminating changes of tissue impedance at the tip of a drilling instrument (Fig. 2) (36,37). It consists of an awl instrument with a hollow handle that houses an in-built electronic printed circuit board. Bipolar electrodes situated at the tip of the instrument measure electrical impedance of the tissue as the tip is advanced through the pedicle. The device is integrated in the drilling tool, and the technology allows real-time detection of perforation through two independent parameters, impedance variation and evoked muscular contractions. An initial animal study confirmed the safety and accuracy of this impedance measurement device (37). For clinical validation, a multi-center trial was undertaken (36). Fifty-two percent of the breaches were detected by the impedance device and not by the surgeon. Based on these results and our experience combining image-guidance with the impedance measurement device, we feel that this combination is most reliable in optimizing placement of spinal instrumentation.

IMAGE GUIDANCE PLACEMENT OF THORACIC INSTRUMENTATION

Thoracic pedicle screw instrumentation is gaining in popularity because of its higher stiffness and strength compared with instrumentation using hooks (38,39). The small size of pedicles in the thoracic spine often makes screw insertion difficult and potentially hazardous. Christodoulou et al. (40) found the narrowest external transverse pedicle diameter to be at the T5 level with a mean of 5.09 mm (range: 4.10–6.88 mm) with a mean internal diameter of 3.90 mm (range: 3.10–4.82 mm). The thoracic pedicle is different from that of the lumbar spine because its mediolateral diameter is significantly less than its superoinferior diameter and it has less medial inclination (41).

In scoliosis surgery, pedicle screws have been shown to provide a better correction of the frontal, sagittal, and rotational deformity with a shorter fusion length and less loss of correction and have a higher pullout strength (42,43). Parent et al. (43) found that pedicle width is significantly diminished on the concavity of scoliotic curves and they advocated caution with the use of pedicle screws in the thoracic spine especially on the concave side of the curve.

The use of thoracic pedicle screws remains controversial because of the potential risks of major neurological and vascular complications. Complication rates as high as 25% have been reported with their use (5). However, the neurological risks associated with the use of thoracic pedicle screws have been reported to be fewer than those with hook instrumentation (42). Suk et al. reported a series of 462 patients who underwent thoracic pedicle screw insertion out of which there were screw-related neurological complications in four patients (0.8%), 11

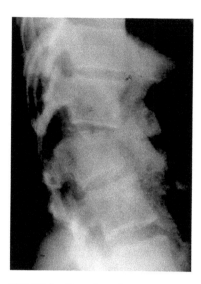
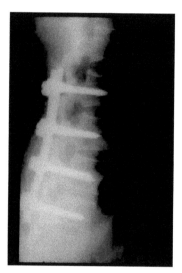

FIGURE 3 Thoracic pedicle screw construct.

intraoperative pedicle fractures, 35 screw loosenings, nine postoperative infections, and one pneumothorax (44).

As spinal fusion has progressed from the hook and claw method to rigid pedicle screw fixation (Fig. 3), there is more need for precise navigation through the pedicle to avoid neurological damage. Advantages over conventional laminar and pedicle hook fixation include not violating the canal and a sounder mechanical construct (45). The analysis of hook positions revealed dislocated pedicle hooks in 16.7% (38).

The major problem encountered in attempting to apply image-guidance systems to the spine is that of maintaining accurate registration coordinates because of problems involving the relative articulation between vertebral bodies (15,17). In the thoracic spine registration is facilitated by the fact that there is relatively little intersegmental movement due to the stabilizing effect of the ribs. There is good body of literature to support the superior results of image-guidance for pedicle screw placement in the thoracic spine (22,34,46).

Spinal fusion rates are significantly greater with pedicle screws but difficulty in assessing correct pedicle screw position by conventional fluoroscopy is well recognized (7). The use of intraoperative fluoroscopy for placement of pedicle screws has resulted in prolonged fluoro time and radiation exposure to the surgical personnel and patient (47). The highly variable pedicle anatomy in the thoracic spine coupled with the proximity of vital neurological, vascular and pulmonary structures makes the application of pedicle screws less inviting (48,49). These factors combined with the variability of the pedicle trajectory and the relative obscurity of the area to fluoroscopic imaging make thoracic pedicle screw insertion a difficult pursuit without guidance. Clinical and cadaveric studies have shown that 15% to 50% of thoracic screws violate the pedicular cortex, when placed by landmarks, fluoroscopic techniques, or both (38,48,50).

Because of the smaller size and more complex three-dimensional morphology of the thoracic pedicle, transpedicular screw placement can be an extremely challenging procedure (51). Medial misplacement of screws is the most feared complication of thoracic pedicle screws. Vacarro et al. (52) reported a medial penetration rate of 23% with nonimage guided pedicle screw placement in the thoracic spine. The accurate identification of pedicle anatomy is a key in avoiding complications. To this end there has been increasing usage of computer image guidance to guide optimal placement of thoracic pedicle screws (46,53,54). We feel that there is often an advantage of using a preoperatively acquired volumetric CT for thoracic instrumentation not only because of the registration advantages just discussed, but also because lateral fluoroscopic images by themselves or acquired for an image-guidance system can be of limited quality.

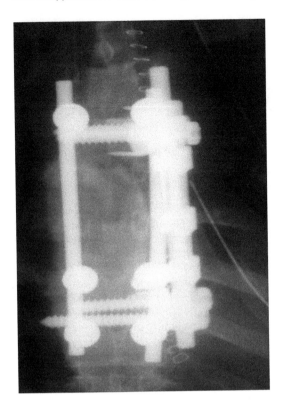

FIGURE 4 Circumferential fusion.

CIRCUMFERENTIAL FUSION

Circumferential fusion has the advantage of producing the strongest construct that restores the functional biomechanical anatomy closest (55,56). It is less invasive in that it results in fewer segments requiring fusion (Fig. 4). However, it has the disadvantage of requiring both an anterior and posterior approach with the instrumentation being placed into the same vertebral body from both approaches. Using image-guidance this may be achieved by an initial approach from the anterior aspect using standard surgical procedure, graft, and instrumentation. Prior to completing the posterior stage of the fusion, the patient undergoes an image-guided protocol scan. Single block registration is achieved and the image-guidance is used to guide the insertion of the posterior instrumentation around the anterior construct for the optimal construct.

CERVICAL SPINE

The morphology of the cervical lateral mass has been described by Roy-Camille et al. (2) and Ebraheim et al. (57). The vertebral artery, nerve root and superior articular process lie in extreme proximity to one another. The vertebral artery lies anterior and in immediate contact with the nerve root, and its ganglia flattens with the pillar of the lateral mass. The close approximation of all these structures to the bony screw trajectory places them at risk during screw placement. C7 is distinguished from the levels above by having a larger spinal nerve and thinner lateral mass (57). Ebraheim et al. (58) has shown that the foramen transversarium lies in line with the midpoint of the lateral mass. As a result, a laterally directed screw will likely miss the vertebral artery (59). Xu et al. (60) suggested that the potential risk of nerve root violation is higher with the Magrel and Anderson techniques than the An method.

Even though the anatomical landmarks for lateral mass screws are fairly reliable, image-guidance using a 3D CT model can occasionally help avoid variants of transverse foramen location, thus avoiding injury to the vertebral artery. In cases of normal or increased cervical motility, care must be taken to register each vertebral level separately, or accuracy can suffer

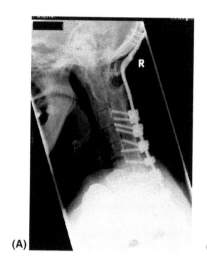

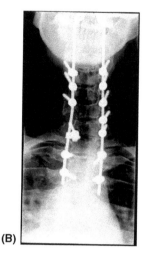

FIGURE 5 Occipital–thoracic lateral mass fusion: (**A**) Lateral view, (**B**) anterior-posterior view.

greatly. When cervical motility is restricted by a halo vest or some preexisting fusion it may be reasonable to perform a single registration for multiple levels either by point matching or by surface matching.

Lateral mass screw fixation techniques have become increasingly popular over the last 10 years (59,61,62). Extensive work has been done both clinically and in the laboratory on lateral mass fixation (59,63–67). The various trajectories have been assessed in terms of their likelihood to cause neurovascular injury. Injury to the spinal nerves associated with insertion of lateral mass screws is the main complication of this procedure (58). The incidence of nerve root injury varies from 1.5% to 6% (59,61,62). Image-guidance is used more frequently for pedicle screw placement at the cervico-thoracic level, since pedicles and lateral masses here are narrower, making optimal placement of screws more challenging (Fig. 5).

Image-guidance is used less commonly in anterior cervical approaches in part because the anterior vertebral bodies make an easier target than pedicles, but also there are less recognizable landmarks that can be used as fiducials for registration. The presence of anterior osteophytes can serve as better landmarks for registration as has been reported (Fig. 6) (19). Anterior image-guidance is useful for optimizing the extent of the decompression (i.e., with a lateral osteophyte) while avoiding damage to the vertebral arteries.

Some authors suggest that fluoroscopic image-guidance is particularly useful in approaches to the odontoid for placement of odontoid screws (68–70). In our experience the usefulness in odontoid peg fixation is limited by the risk of distal displacement of the odontoid fragment

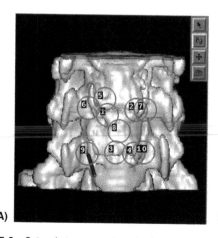

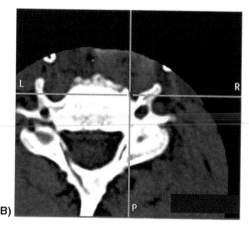

FIGURE 6 Osteophytes can act as landmarks to aid anterior cervical registration: (**A**) 3D model; (**B**) computed tomography scan.

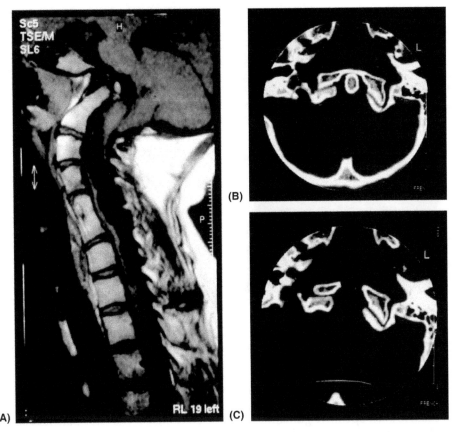

FIGURE 7   Basiliar invagination with pre- and postoperative transoral resection of the odontoid peg: (**A**) Lateral view; (**B**) pre op; (**C**) post op.

when the screw is being placed. This is not apparent with image-guidance and can only be detected with real time screening. 3D image-guidance is also extremely useful for anterior craniocervical surgery (70–72). In our experience the best results are achieved using CT scan based navigation, registered to the cranium rather than the spine (Fig. 7). Fluoroscopic navigation has also been proposed for this approach. However, we feel that there is poor visualization of the anatomy on anterior–posterior (AP) radiography that severely limits its usefulness.

ATLANTOAXIAL FIXATION FOR C1/C2 TRANSARTICULAR SCREW PLACEMENT

Nowhere in the spine is accuracy more crucial and image-guidance more helpful than in the placement of C1/2 transarticular screws. The normal nonpathological anatomy is very complex with many vital structures traversing in close proximity to the bony structures. The close proximity of the spinal cord, exiting spinal nerve roots and above all the tortuous and often variable course of the vertebral artery make C1/C2 anatomy complex and dangerous. A large proportion of patients who develop instability at this level have Rheumatoid Arthritis, which destroys the normal anatomical landmarks, thereby making C1/C2 screw placement in these patients even more hazardous.

Magerl and Seemann first introduced trans-articular screw fixation to treat atlantoaxial subluxation (C1/C2) in 1987 (73). Atlantoaxial instability has the potential to cause neural injury, vascular compromise and cervical pain if left untreated. Transarticular screw fixation provides good pain relief and has superior biomechanical stability than many other techniques of C1/C2 fixation (74). It allows fixation across the plane of movement and prevents basilar invagination. The hazards of screw placement include vascular injury especially for

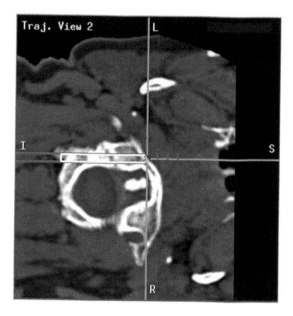

FIGURE 8 Virtual screw trajectory for C1/C2 trans-articular screws.

the vertebral artery within C2, neural damage, haemorrhage from venous plexuses and the potential for poor screw purchase in the presence of metabolic bone disease with subsequent loosening (75).

Image-guidance allows the complex, and often times, variable anatomy of rheumatoid patient to be better appreciated at the time of screw insertion. Up until the advent of computer generated image-guidance, bi-planer fluoroscopic imaging was the pinnacle of what was on offer when it came to intra-operative guidance at the C1/C2 complex. The information obtained by bi-planer fluoroscopy was limited because it offered 2D information on a 3D problem. Image-guidance offers the surgeon more anatomical confidence by producing 3D information, which updates trajectory information in all three planes in real time (Fig. 8).

Technique of C1/C2 Screw Placement

The light emitting diodes (LED) reference arc is attached to the spinous process of C2. Registration is then achieved by a combination of point matching and surface mapping on the posterior arch of C2. Registration is to C2 in isolation.

Using the image-guidance pointer the skin surface projection of the preoperative plan is matched to the patient's skin, lower in the cervical spine. A stab incision is made at this point on

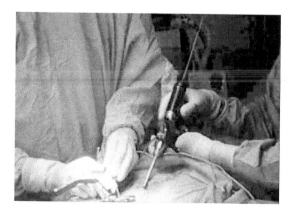

FIGURE 9 Percutaneous image guidance insertion of K-wire.

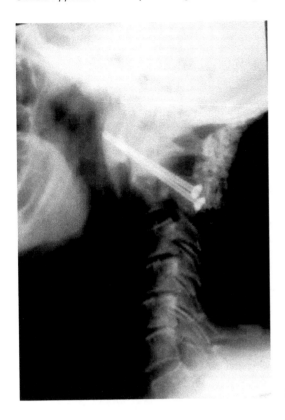

FIGURE 10 C1/2 screws.

both sides. An image-guided drill-guard is introduced through the stab incision to the posterior arch of C2, in the line of the preoperative plan, as identified by referring to the computer screen.

A K-wire is then passed through the drill-guide and then into C2 by continuous reference to the image-guidance system to insure close approximation to the preoperative plan. The relationship of the K-wire and its passage through the C1/C2 joint and on into C1 is evaluated by lateral fluoroscopy (Fig. 9).

Once the K-wire is inserted, a cannled drill and tapping instrument may be passed along the same trajectory, although this is not necessary if using self-tapping screws.

The optimal screw length is identified either from the image-guidance system or direct measurement from the K-wire, and an appropriate cannled screw is inserted over the K-wire. The wire is then removed with C1/2 screw in place.

Previous studies have suggested that failure to fully reduce C1 on C2 screw precludes C1/C2 transarticular screw insertion (76), however in our experience this is not the case. The difficulty with non-image-guidance techniques is that the anatomical landmark is the C1 tubercle. Thus in cases that are not reduced the trajectory into C1 is lowered (Fig. 10). This places the vertebral artery at risk when passing the screw through C2, as the trajectory aligns the screw in close proximity to the vertebral artery in its groove inferior to the C2 pars. With image-guidance the trajectory is guided by the C2 anatomy, the relative position of C1 being irrelevant, thus an optimal trajectory through C2 may be chosen irrespective of the C1 tubercle.

REFERENCES

1. Roy-Camille R, Gaillant G, Bertreaux D. Early management of spinal injuries. In: McKibben B, ed. Recent Advances in Orthopaedics. Edinburgh: Churchill-Livingstone, 1979:57–87.
2. Nohara Y, Taneichi H, Ueyama K, et al. Nationwide survey on complications of spine surgery in Japan. J Orthop Sci 2004; 9(5):424–433.

3. Sagi H, Manos R, Ordway NR, Connolly PJ. Electromagnetic field-based image-guided surgery part one: Results of a cadaveric study evaluating lumbar pedicle screw placement. Spine 2003; 28(17):2013–2018.
4. Davane SH, Myers DL. Complications of lumbar spine fusion with transpedicular instrumentation. Spine 1992; 17:362–367.
5. Esses SI, Sachs BL, Dreyzin V. Complications associated with technique of pedicle screw fixation. Spine 1993; 18:2231–2239.
6. Laine T. Accuracy of pedicle screw insertion with and without computer assistance: a randomized controlled clinical study in 100 consecutaive patients. Eur Spine J 2005; 9(3):235–240.
7. Amiot L, Lang K, Zippel H. Comparison accuracy between conventional and computer-assisted pedicle screw installation. J Bone Joint Surg (Br) 1998; 80:240.
8. Beatty RM, McGuire P, Moroney JM. Continuous intraoperative electromyographic recording during spinal surgery. J Neurosurg 1995; 82:401–405.
9. Gundanna M, Eskenazi M, Bendo J, Spivak J, Moskovich R. Somatosensory evoked potential monitoring of lumbar pedicle screw placement for in situ posterior spinal fusion. Spine J 2003; 3(5):370–376.
10. Herdmann J, Deletis V, Edmonds HL, Morota N. Spinal cord and nerve root monitoring in spine surgery and related procedures. Spine 1996; 21(7):870–877.
11. Laine T, Lund T, Ylikoski M, Lohikoski J, Schlenzka D. Accuracy of pedicle screw insertion with and without computer assistance: a randomised controlled clinical study in 100 consecutive patients. Eur Spine J 2000; 9(3):235–240.
12. Lubicky J, Spadaro J, Yuan H, Fredrickson B, Henderson N. Variability of somatosensory cortical evoked potential monitoring during spinal surgery. Spine 1989; 14(8):790–798.
13. Rampersaud YR, Pik JH, Salonen D, Farooq S. Clinical accuracy of fluoroscopic computer-assisted pedicle screw fixation: a CT analysis. Spine 2005; 30(7):E183–E190.
14. Shi YB, Binette M, Martin WH, Pearson JM, Hart RA. Electrical stimulation for intraoperative evaluation of thoracic pedicle screw placement. Spine 2003; 28(6):595–601.
15. Bolger C, Wigfield C. Image-guided surgery: applications to the cervical and thoracic spine and a review of the first 120 procedures. J Neurosurg 2000; 92:175–180.
16. Darden BV, Wood KE, Hatley MK, Owen JH, Kostuik J. Evaluation of pedicle screw insertion monitored by intraoperative evoked electromyography. J Spinal Disord 1996; 9(1):8–16.
17. Foley K, Smith M. Image-guided spine surgery. Neurosurgical Clinics North Am 1996; 7:171–186.
18. Foley KT, Simon DA, Rampersaud YR. Virtual fluoroscopy: computer-assisted fluoroscopic navigation. Spine 2001; 26(4):347–351.
19. Bolger C, Wigfield C. Frameless stereotaxy and anterior cervical surgery. Comput Aided Surg 1999; 4:322–327.
20. Kalfas IH. Image-guided spinal navigation. Clin Neurosurg 2000; 46:70–88.
21. Kalfas IH, Kormos DW, Murphy MA, et al. Application of frameless stereotaxy to pedicle screw fixation of the spine. J Neurosurg 1995; 83(4):641–647.
22. Youkilis AS, Quint DJ, McGillicuddy JE, Papadopoulos SM. Stereotactic navigation for placement of pedicle screws in the thoracic spine. Neurosurgery 2001; 48(4):771–778.
23. Arand M, Hartwig E, Kinzl L, Gebhard F. Spinal navigation in tumor surgery of the thoracic spine: first clinical results. Clin Orthop Relat Res 2002; (399):211–218.
24. Hufner T, Kfuri M Jr, Galanski M, et al. New indications for computer-assisted surgery: tumor resection in the pelvis. Clin Orthop Relat Res 2004; (426):219–225.
25. Shoda N, Nakajima S, Seichi A, et al. Computer-assisted anterior spinal surgery for a case of recurrent giant cell tumor. J Orthop Sci 2002; 7(3):392–396.
26. Moore T, McLain RF. Image-guided surgery in resection of benign cervicothoracic spinal tumors: a report of two cases. Spine J 2005; 5(1):109–114.
27. Austin MS, Vaccaro AR, Brislin B, Nachwalter R, Hilibrand AS, Albert TJ. Image-guided spine surgery: a cadaver study comparing conventional open laminoforaminotomy and two image-guided techniques for pedicle screw placement in posterolateral fusion and nonfusion models. Spine 2002; 27(22):2503–2508.
28. Benzel EC, Rupp FW, McCormack BM, Baldwin NG, Anson JA, Adams MS. A comparison of fluoroscopy and computed tomography-derived volumetric multiple exposure transmission holography for the guidance of lumbar pedicle screw insertion. Neurosurgery 1995; 37(4):711–716.
29. Choi WW, Green BA, Levi AD. Computer-assisted fluoroscopic targeting system for pedicle screw insertion. Neurosurgery 2000; 47(4):872–878.
30. Carl AL, Khanuja HS, Gatto CA, et al. In vivo pedicle screw placement: image-guided virtual vision. J Spinal Disord 2000; 13(3):225–229.
31. Youkilis AS, Quint DJ, McGillicuddy JE, Papadopoulos SM. Stereotactic navigation for placement of pedicle screws in the thoracic spine. Neurosurgery 2001; 48(4):771–778.

32. Ludwig SC, Kramer DL, Balderston RA, Vaccaro AR, Foley KF, Albert TJ. Placement of pedicle screws in the human cadaveric cervical spine: comparative accuracy of three techniques. Spine 2000; 25(13):1655–1667.
33. Rampersaud YR, Simon DA, Foley KT. Accuracy requirements for image-guided spinal pedicle screw placement. Spine 2001; 26(4):352–359.
34. Holly LT, Foley KT. Intraoperative spinal navigation. Spine 2003; 28(Suppl 15):S54–S61.
35. Resnick DK. Prospective comparison of virtual fluoroscopy to fluoroscopy and plain radiographs for placement of lumbar pedicle screws. J Spinal Disord Tech 2003; 16(3):254–260.
36. Bolger C, McEvoy L, Bourlion M, et al. A new device to detect iatrogenic initial vertebtal cortex perforation: First clinical results [abstr]. Eur Spine J 2003; 12.
37. Bolger C, Carozzo C, Roger T, et al. A preliminary study of reliability of impedance measurement to detect iatrogenic initial pedicle perforation (in the porcine model). Eur Spine J 2006; 15:316–320.
38. Liljenqvist UR, Halm HF, Link TM. Pedicle screw instrumentation of the thoracic spine in idiopathic scoliosis. Spine 1997; 22(19):2239–2245.
39. Zindrick MR, Wiltse LL, Widell EH, et al. A biomechanical study of intrapeduncular screw fixation in the lumbosacral spine. Clin Orthop Relat Res 1986; (203):99–112.
40. Christodoulou AG, Apostolou T, Ploumis A, Terzidis I, Hantzokos I, Pournaras J. Pedicle dimensions of the thoracic and lumbar vertebrae in the Greek population. Clin Anat 2005; 18(6):404–408.
41. Ebraheim NA, Jabaly G, Xu R, Yeasting RA. Anatomic relations of the thoracic pedicle to the adjacent neural structures. Spine 1997; 22(14):1553–1556.
42. Suk SI, Lee CK, Min HJ, Cho KH, Oh JH. Comparison of Cotrel-Dubousset pedicle screws and hooks in the treatment of idiopathic scoliosis. Int Orthop 1994; 18(6):341–346.
43. Parent S, Labelle H, Skalli W, de GJ. Thoracic pedicle morphometry in vertebrae from scoliotic spines. Spine 2004; 29(3):239–248.
44. Suk SI, Kim WJ, Lee SM, Kim JH, Chung ER. Thoracic pedicle screw fixation in spinal deformities: are they really safe? Spine 2001; 26(18):2049–2057.
45. Suk SI, Lee CK, Kim WJ, Chung YJ, Park YB. Segmental pedicle screw fixation in the treatment of thoracic idiopathic scoliosis. Spine 1995; 20(12):1399–1405.
46. Assaker R, Reyns N, Vinchon M, Demondion X, Louis E. Transpedicular screw placement: image-guided versus lateral-view fluoroscopy: in vitro simulation. Spine 2001; 26(19):2160–2164.
47. Rampersaud YR, Foley KT, Shen AC, et al. Radiation exposure to the spine surgeon during flurosco-pically assissted pedicle insertion. Spine 2000; 25(20):2637–2645.
48. Xu R, Ebraheim NA, Ou Y, Yeasting RA. Anatomic considerations of pedicle screw placement in the thoracic spine. Roy-Camille technique versus open-lamina technique. Spine 1998; 23(9):1065–1068.
49. Rampersaud YR, Simon DA, Foley KT. Accuracy requirements for image-guided spinal pedicle screw placement. Spine 2001; 26(4):352–359.
50. Youkilis AS, Quint DJ, McGillicuddy JE, Papadopoulos SM. Stereotactic navigation for placement of pedicle screws in the thoracic spine. Neurosurgery 2001; 48(4):771–778.
51. Youkilis AS, Quint DJ, McGillicuddy JE, Papadopoulos SM. Stereotactic navigation for placement of pedicle screws in the thoracic spine. Neurosurgery 2001; 48(4):771–778.
52. Vaccaro AR, Rizzolo SJ, Balderston RA, et al. Placement of pedicle screws in the thoracic spine. Part II: An anatomical and radiographic assessment. J Bone Joint Surg Am 1995; 77(8):1200–1206.
53. Youkilis AS, Quint DJ, McGillicuddy JE, Papadopoulos SM. Stereotactic navigation for placement of pedicle screws in the thoracic spine. Neurosurgery 2001; 48(4):771–778.
54. Amiot LP, Lang K, Putzier M, Zippel H, Labelle H. Comparative results between conventional and computer-assisted pedicle screw installation in the thoracic, lumbar, and sacral spine. Spine 2000; 25(5):606–614.
55. Christensen FB, Hansen ES, Eiskjaer SP, et al. Circumferential lumbar spinal fusion with Brantigan cage versus posterolateral fusion with titanium Cotrel-Dubousset instrumentation: a prospective, randomized clinical study of 146 patients. Spine 2002; 27(23):2674–2683.
56. Rathonyi GC, Oxland TR, Gerich U, Grassmann S, Nolte LP. The role of supplemental translaminar screws in anterior lumbar interbody fixation: a biomechanical study. Eur Spine J 1998; 7(5):400–407.
57. Ebraheim NA. Posterior lateral mass screw fixation: Anatomic and radiographic considerations. Ortho J 1999; 12:66–72.
58. Ebraheim NA, Xu R, Stanescu S, Yeasting RA. Anatomic relationship of the cervical nerves to the lateral masses. Am J Orthop 1999; 28(1):39–42.
59. Sekhon LH. Posterior cervical lateral mass screw fixation: analysis of 1026 consecutive screws in 143 patients. J Spinal Disord Tech 2005; 18(4):297–303.
60. Xu R, Haman SP, Ebraheim NA, Yeasting RA. The anatomic relation of lateral mass screws to the spinal nerves. A comparison of the Magerl, Anderson, and an techniques. Spine 1999; 24(19):2057–2061.
61. Deen HG, Birch BD, Wharen RE, Reimer R. Lateral mass screw-rod fixation of the cervical spine: a prospective clinical series with 1-year follow-up. Spine J 2003; 3(6):489–495.

62. Houten JK, Cooper PR. Laminectomy and posterior cervical plating for multilevel cervical spondylotic myelopathy and ossification of the posterior longitudinal ligament: effects on cervical alignment, spinal cord compression, and neurological outcome. Neurosurgery 2003; 52(5):1081–1087.

63. Ebraheim NA, Xu R, Stanescu S, Yeasting RA. Anatomic relationship of the cervical nerves to the lateral masses. Am J Orthop 1999; 28(1):39–42.

64. Ebraheim NA, Klausner T, Xu R, Yeasting RA. Safe lateral-mass screw lengths in the Roy-Camille and Magerl techniques. An anatomic study. Spine 1998; 23(16):1739–42.

65. Ebraheim NA, Xu R, Challgren E, Yeasting RA. Quantitative anatomy of the cervical facet and the posterior projection of its inferior facet. J Spinal Disord 1997; 10(4):308–316.

66. Ebraheim NA, Xu R, Challgren E. Radiologic evaluation of the relation of the screw tip to the nerve root in the intervertebral foramen. J Spinal Disord 1997; 10(3):234–239.

67. Ebraheim NA, Xu R, Knight T, Yeasting RA. Morphometric evaluation of lower cervical pedicle and its projection. Spine 1997; 22(1):1–6.

68. Pollack IF, Welch W, Jacobs GB, Janecka IP. Frameless stereotactic guidance. An intraoperative adjunct in the transoral approach for ventral cervicomedullary junction decompression. Spine 1995; 20(2):216–220.

69. Welch WC, Subach BR, Pollack IF, Jacobs GB. Frameless stereotactic guidance for surgery of the upper cervical spine. Neurosurgery 1997; 40(5):958–963.

70. Borm W, Konig RW, Albrecht A, Richter HP, Kast E. Percutaneous transarticular atlantoaxial screw fixation using a cannulated screw system and image-guidance. Minim Invasive Neurosurg 2004; 47(2):111–114.

71. Veres R, Bago A, Fedorcsak I. Early experiences with image-guided transoral surgery for the pathologies of the upper cervical spine. Spine 2001; 26(12):1385–1388.

72. Vougioukas VI, Hubbe U, Schipper J, Spetzger U. Navigated transoral approach to the cranial base and the craniocervical junction: technical note. Neurosurgery 2003; 52(1):247–250.

73. Magerl F, Seemann PS. Stable posterior fusion of the atlas and axis by transarticular screw fixation. In: Kehr P, Weidner A, ets. Cervical Spine 1. Vienna: Springer-Verlag, 1987:322–327.

74. Reilly TM, Sasso RC, Hall PV. Atlantoaxial stabilization: clinical comparison of posterior cervical wiring technique with transarticular screw fixation. J Spinal Disord Tech 2003; 16(3):248–253.

75. Liang ML, Huang MC, Yen YS, et al. Posterior transarticular screw fixation for chronic atlanto-axial stability. J Clin Neurosci 2004; 11(4):368–372.

76. Madawi AA, Casey AT, Solanki GA, Tuite G, Veres R, Crockard HA. Radiological and anatomical evaluation of the atlantoaxial transarticular screw fixation technique. J Neurosurg 1997; 86(6): 961–968.

30 | Image-Guided Angled Rongeur for Posterior Lumbar Discectomy

Masahiko Kanamori
Department of Orthopaedic Surgery, University of Toyama, Toyama, Japan

Kazuo Ohmori
Department of Orthopaedic Surgery, Nippon-Kokan Hospital, Kanagawa, Japan

INTRODUCTION

Computer image-guiding systems, such as those introduced for pedicle screw insertion in spinal surgery can provide accurate three-dimensional surgical information intraoperatively (1–10). Recently, we developed a real-time image-guided angled rongeur for posterior discectomy in patients with lumbar disc herniation. Here, we discuss the efficacy of such an image-guided angled rongeur for posterior discectomy in these patients.

SPINAL NAVIGATION SYSTEM AND NEW DEVICE

We used a commercially available computer-assisted surgery navigation system (Stealth-Station®; Medtronic Sofamor Danek, Memphis, Tennessee, U.S.A.) to monitor the three-dimensional positioning of the surgical field. This system consists of a computer workstation, a reference frame, a standard probe, and an electro-optical camera connected to the computer workstation, which serves as a position sensor. We have originally developed a new image-guided angled rongeur, which indicates the position of the tip of the angled rongeur intra-operatively (Fig. 1). The basic data used for navigation are the pre-operative computer axial tomography imaging data (slice thickness, 1 mm) of the lumbar spine between the proximal and distal levels involving the disc herniation. The data is transferred and recorded on the system computer, and reconstructed into three-dimensional images on a TV monitor. Infrared light-emitting diodes (LEDs) are attached to the reference frame, the probe, and the angled rongeur (Fig. 1). The ultra red-beam from the probe and angled rongeur is tracked by the electro-optical camera, and the position of the tip of the angled rongeur can be identified in real-time in the surgical field.

OPERATIVE PROCEDURES AND RESULTS

We employed this image-guided angled rongeur in 20 posterior discectomies (17 discectomies for central herniation and three for subradicular herniation). All the patients had a single level disc herniation; the level of disc herniation was L2-3 in one case, L4-5 in five, and L5-S in 14.

After the posterior bony elements of the lumbar spine were exposed bilaterally, the reference frame was fixed to the spinous process proximal to the level of the disc herniation. Matched-pair point and surface registration of the vertebra was carried out completely using a standard probe. The image-guided angled rongeur was calibrated by placing the tip of the angled rongeur on the top of the reference frame, and then unilateral or bilateral laminotomy was performed. The nerve root was retracted medially and the intervertebral disc level was explored. The intervertebral disc just beneath the nerve root was removed using a straight rongeur following resection of the posterior longitudinal ligament. The tip of the angled rongeur was monitored in coronal, saggital, and transverse images, using the image-guided angled rongeur, and discectomy was performed in order to remove central herniation with or without ossification and the posterior annulus ventral to the dura mater.

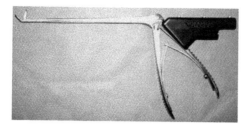

FIGURE 1 Image-guided angled rongeur. Three infrared light-emitting diodes are attached to the angled rongeur.

After discectomy, we confirmed whether or not the discectomy was carried out completely using a standard probe.

In all cases, we could successfully perform registration; the registration error ranged from 0.4 to 0.9 mm with an average of 0.77 mm, and the time necessary for registration ranged from four to nine minutes with an average of 6.5 minutes. All operations were performed successfully and safely. The image-guided angled rongeur provided three-dimensional topographical comprehension during posterior discectomy because the position of the tip of the angled rongeur within the disc space was superimposed in real-time as the crossing point of the two lines on coronal, sagittal, and transverse images (Figs. 2 and 3). Therefore, the positional relationship between the tip of the angled rongeur and the herniated mass could be understood clearly. In most of the cases, approximately one-third of the posterior area of the intervertebral disc was removed using this rongeur. In particular, in cases with central disc herniation, this image-guided angled rongeur was very useful for performing posterior discectomy. In a case of LA-5 central disc herniation accompanied with massive posterior ossification, we could

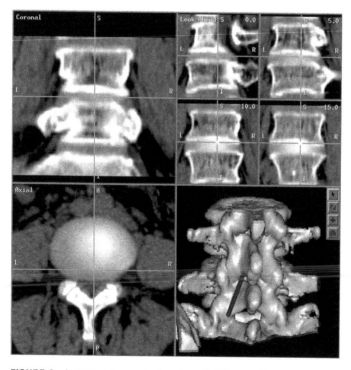

FIGURE 2 Intraoperative navigation view of a 56-year-old male with LA-5 central herniation with segmental stenosis. The crossing point of the two lines indicates the tip of the angled rongeur on navigation view. The tip of the angled rongeur is located just beneath the central disc herniation judging from coronal, sagittal, and transverse images.

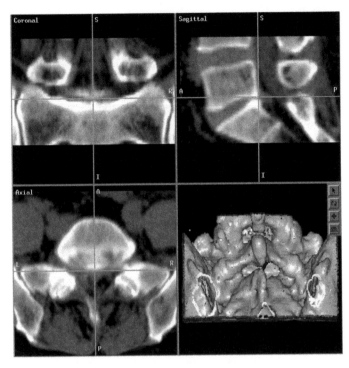

FIGURE 3 Intraoperative navigation view of a 65-year-old male with L5-S central herniation associated with spinal stenosis. Coronal, sagittal, and transverse views indicate that the tip of the angled rongeur is positioned at the top of the posterior edge.

carry out posterior discectomy and resection of the ossification by employing an osteotome and this image-guided angled rongeur.

DISCUSSION

Computer image-guiding systems in spinal surgery were introduced for the insertion of pedicle screw, and the accuracy of pedicle screw insertion has been confirmed in several laboratory and clinical studies (1–8,10). However, it has been considered that the lack of surgical device and computer software limited the application another spinal procedures without instrumentation. A cadaveric study by Klein et al. (11) indicated the efficacy of using a computer-assisted Kerrison punch in performing an anterior cervical foraminotomy. We have also reported that three cases in which vertebral collapse of the thoraco–lumbar spine compressing the spinal cord were successfully treated with image-guided anterior corpectomy (9).

Posterior discectomy following partial laminotomy of the lumbar spine, which was first described by Love (12), has been one of the standard procedures for the surgical treatment of lumbar disc herniation. This procedure is reported to have a good surgical outcome (13,14). However, several reports have documented vascular injuries encountered in posterior discectomy (15–17). Szolar et al. (17) described that intraoperative complications of the great vessels in lumbar disc surgery are relatively frequently caused by the rongeur. Although such a problem is rare, it could be lethal. In this series, we observed the discectomy area to be the posterior one-third area in most cases. We could perform discectomy very safely. This discectomy area seemed to be sufficient for the typical procedure for disc herniation. But for posterior interbody fusion, a wider area of discectomy is necessary. In such cases, the present image-guided rongeur should be a more useful tool.

Furthermore, this rongeur has a great advantage for discectomy procedures for central disc herniation. Knop-Jergas et al. (18) pointed out an unsatisfactory outcome for most patients with a lumbar central disc herniation undergoing posterior discectomy. We suspect that the unsatisfactory outcome in the central herniation patients was due to the inadequate removal of the disc herniation. Indeed, the lumbar central disc herniation cannot be identified under direct vision during posterior discectomy, so it is difficult to identify the position of the tip of the angled rongeur during discectomy and to remove the disc herniation completely. We confirmed the position of the tip of the angled rongeur by real-time monitoring during discectomy. This equipment proved to be very useful to safely perform effective discectomy. However, the time necessary for registration ranged from four to nine minutes with an average of 6.5 minutes, and the average of the operation time was 98 minutes (range: 70–135). Therefore, operation time seemed to become longer due to the registration.

Through our experience using the new image-guided angled rongeur, we are convinced that this rongeur enables the surgeon to navigate the discectomy. In case of the central disc herniation, particularly, this device would aid the surgeon for the safe discectomy.

CONCLUSION

We developed a real-time image-guided angled rongeur for posterior discectomy in patients with lumbar disc herniation. The StealthStation was used to monitor the three-dimensional positioning of the tip of the angled rongeur. The data used for navigation was the preoperative computer axial tomography imaging data of the lumbar spine of each patient. Using this rongeur, we carried out posterior discectomy in 20 patients with lumbar disc herniation. All operations were performed successfully and safely. The position of the tip of the angled rongeur in the disc space was superimposed in real-time on coronal, sagittal, and transverse images, so that the positional relationship between the tip of the angled rongeur and herniated mass could be clearly understood. In particular, in cases with central disc herniation, this rongeur enabled the surgeon to completely remove the disc herniation. This new image-guided angled rongeur provides three-dimensional topographical comprehension and is thus very useful for performing posterior discectomy steadily and safely.

REFERENCES

1. Foley KT, Smith MM. Image-guided spine surgery. Neurosurg Clin N Am 1996; 7:171–186.
2. Girardi FP, Cammisa FP, Sandhu HS, et al. The placement of lumbar pedicle screws using computerised stereotactic guidance. J Bone J Surg 1999; 81-8:825–829.
3. Glossop ND, Hu RW, Randle JA. Computer-aided pedicle screw placement using frameless stereotaxis. Spine 1996; 21:2026–2034.
4. Kalfas IH, Kormos DW, Murphy MA, et al. Application of frameless stereotaxy to pedicle screw fixation of the spine. J Neurosurg 1995; 83:641–647.
5. Kamimura M, Ebara S, Itoh H, et al. Cervical pedicle screw insertion: assessment of safely and accuracy with computer-assisted image guidance. J Spinal Disord 2000; 13:218–224.
6. Kamimura M, Ebara S, Itoh H, et al. Accurate pedicle screw insertion under the control of a computer assisted image guiding system: laboratory test and clinical study. J Orthop Sci 1999; 4:197–206.
7. Kim KD, Johnson JP, Masciopinto JE, et al. Universal calibration of surgical instruments for spinal stereotaxy. Neurosurgery 1999; 44:173–178.
8. Laine T, Schlonzka D, Makitalo K, et al. Improved accuracy of pedicle screw insertion with computer-assisted surgery. A prospective clinical trial of 30 patients. Spine 1997; 22:1254–1258.
9. Ohmori K, Kawaguchi Y, Kanamori M, et al. Image-guided anterior thoracolumbar corpectomy. A report of three cases. Spine 2001; 26:1197–1201.
10. Welch WC, Subach BR, Pollack IF, et al. Frameless stereotactic guidance for surgery of the upper cervical spine. Neurosurgery 1997; 40:958–963.
11. Klein GR, Ludwig SC, Vaccaro AR, et al. The efficacy of using an image-guided Kerrison punch in performing an anterior cervical foraminotomy. Spine 1999; 24:1358–1362.
12. Love JG. Protruded intervertebral disks. JAMA 1939; 113:2029–2035.

13. Abramovitz JN, Neff SR. Lumbar disk surgery: results of the prospective lumbar diskectomy study of the joint section on disorders of the spine and peripheral nerves of the American Association of Neurological Surgeons and the Congress of Neurological Surgeons. Neurosurgery 1991; 29:301–308.

14. Stambough JL. Lumbar disk herniation: an analysis of 175 surgically treated cases. J Spinal Disord 1997; 10:488–492.

15. Brewster DC, May ARL, Darling RC, et al. Variable manifestations of vascular injury during lumbar disk surgery. Arch Surg 1979; 114:1026–1030.

16. DeSaussure RL. Vascular injury coincident to disk surgery. J Neurosurg 1959; 16:222–228.

17. Szolar DH, Preidler KW, Steiner H, et al. Vascular complications in lumbar disk surgery: report of four cases. Neuroradiology 1996; 38:521–525.

18. Knop-Jergas RM, Zucherman JF, Hsu KY, et al. Anatomic position of a herniated nucleus pulposus predicts the outcome of lumbar discectomy. J Spinal Disord 1996; 9:246–250.

31 | Radioscopic Methods for Introduction of Pedicular Screws: Is a Navigator Necessary?

Matías Alfonso, Carlos Villas, and Jose Luis Beguiristain
Department of Orthopaedics, University Clinic of Navarra, Pamplona, Spain

INTRODUCTION
Evolution of Internal Fixation in the Spine

Before Harrington's instrumentation, pseudoarthrosis in surgical treatment of scoliosis was approximately 40% (1). Harrington introduced rods and hooks, and pseudoarthrosis was reduced to 15% (2). Similar results were observed in fractures. Before this treatment bed-rest or plaster was necessary. With Harrington's instrumentation, deformities were much reduced, patients gained earlier, mobilization, and patient care cost was reduced. But the problem of "flat-back" in the lumbar spine appeared with this instrumentation due to distraction.

Luque (3) introduced a new adaptation of rods fixed to the spine by sublaminar wires, which improved the rate of fixation reducing pseudoarthrosis to 5% and allowing correction of curves in several planes. Nowadays this instrumentation is used in neuromuscular scoliosis mainly due to high probability of neural damage.

The next generation of instrumentation attempted to solve the problems of Harrington and Luque instrumentation. Cotrel and Dubousset (4) added multiple sublaminar hooks improving three-dimensional correction and rigidity of instrumentation.

But that instrumentation depended on the presence of posterior structures such as lamina. King (5) in 1944 and Boucher (6) in 1959 introduced transarticular screws with little success due to complications.

The modern age of pedicular screws begins in France in the 1970s. Raymond Roy-Camille was the first to insert screws in the vertebra across the pedicle (7). From 1963 Roy-Camille, under Judet supervision, used plates and pedicular screws successfully, and published his results in 1970 (8). Pedicular screws run along pedicle parallels to the sagittal plane and joined by osteosynthesis plates. This technique was first used for fractures (9) and later was extended to pseudoarthrosis, tumors, espondilolisthesis and surgery of the degenerative spine (10). In 1976, Louis and Maresca (11,12) modify the implant and the method of introduction of Roy-Camille to improve lumbosacral fixation. In 1986, Louis (13) published his results in 455 patients: the fusion percentage was 97.4% in posterolateral fusion, and 100% in 360° fusion. Raymond Roy-Camille and René Louis can be considered the fathers of modern fixation with pedicular screws.

In our country, Spain, in the 1970s Cabot (14) described "crab" plates fixed to the spinous process, and later modified for pedicular screws. In 1980 Beguiristain (15) introduced the Louis technique and instrumentation for spinal diseases.

In the 1980s, Frizt Magerl (16) introduced the concept of rigid fixation giving bases for short instrumentations in toracolumbar fractures. This concept allowed the design of the AO internal spinal fixator by Dick (17).

In 1976 in the United States, Paul Harrington published a report on the use of pedicular screws to reduce and stabilize high-grade listhesis (18). At same time Steffee used standard Association for Osteosynthesis (AO) plates with screws in degenerative listhesis (19). Fixed holes in AO plates made introduction of screws at multiple levels difficult and resulted in the creation of variable screw plates by Steffee (VSP).

Screws were introduced in Cotrel-Dubousset (4) instrumentations improving versatility. Today the spine surgeon can select from a huge number of instrumentations (rigid or semi-rigid), which offer more or less ease of use that facilitates spinal rigidity while the bone graft is healing.

The use of pedicular screws has increased internationally even though limited in the United States due to restrictions imposed by the Food and Drug Administration (FDA).

Complications of Pedicular Screws in the Lumbar Spine

In the lumbar spine there are 2 mm of peridural space adjacent to the pedicle (10), and 2 mm more of subaracnoidal space (20), with 4 mm of space before root damage occurs if the screw is located inside the canal. The lumbar roots take up the top third of the foramen, so the most dangerous places for pedicle breakage are the inferior and internal cortical. If a screw breaks the pedicle on the lateral side, the danger is less, but there may be damage of the superior root similar to an extraforaminal hernia. If the screw crosses, anterior vertebral cortical, major vessels can be punctured. Vascular complications are extremely rare (21) due to anterior vertebral ligament (22) but potentially fatal (23,24). If a screw breaks the vertebral endplate by entering the disc space in a nonfused disc, it may accelerate disc degeneration.

General complications associated with pedicular instrumentation range from 25% (21) to 46% (25) with extreme values of as much as 75% (26) in reinterventions. In a study by the American Back Society (21) of 617 interventions and 3949 screws, the average value of complications was 24%.

Neurological complications in wide series (4,7,21,27–31) range from 0.5% to 3% of all patients reaching 17% (25) depending on the type of pathology [lysthesis (32)] and surgeon experience. Infectious complications range from 0.4% (7) to 11% (27). Implant failure has been described as a complication and can be up to 29% (33).

Vertebral Dimensions Related to the Introduction of Pedicle Screws

An early paper by Saillant in 1976 (34) entitled "Étude anatomique des pédicules vertébraux. Application chirurgicale," which presented a rationalization for screw introduction. He proposes going straight on from the pedicle entrance.

The first studies were carried out using human fresh vertebrae (34–37) and skeletons belonging to osteological collections at Cleveland Museum of Natural History (38,39) or University of New York in Buffalo (40), performing a direct measuring with calipers. New image techniques such as computed tomography (CT) have lately been used in patients (35,37,40–45) with similar results, although thin CT cuts are advisable (1 or 2 mm).

Most studies consider pedicular width and pedicular angle in order to set a course for the screw and its maximum width. Pedicular width is measured considering the external part of pedicle. With CT it is possible to measure the internal part of pedicle [endostal width (35,42)], which permits a more accurate prediction of screw width.

We performed a study to find the pedicular angle and dimensions in Spanish people (46) in lumbar spine from L3 to S1 comparing the right and left sides and gender. Our results conclude that the pedicle can accept screws 5.5 mm wide or wider from L3 to S1, bearing in mind that pedicle width could be 5 mm in L3 or upper levels. Gender has no influence on pedicular width nor does the side affect the result, but bear in mind that there could be a difference of up to 5 mm in L5 or 9 mm in S1. Results of endostal width makes us think that generally it is possible to use screws 5.5 mm wide from L4 to S1, given that in L4 and higher there are pedicles 4 mm wide, and 5 mm wide in L5, and it is not recommended to use screws wider than the endostal width due to the high risk of pedicular fracture. Endostal width is about 80% of the external part of pedicle. Pedicular angles are on average around 28° in S1, 20° in L5, and 10° in L3 and L4. There are no significant differences between two sexes in pedicular angle. There are significant differences in L5 between the right and left sides, but they are not clinically relevant.

The squared shape of L4 (Fig. 1) and above, the rounded shape of about 50% of L5 vertebrae (Fig. 2), the pyramidal shape of another 50% of L5 (Fig. 3), the "rectangular" shape of S1 (Fig. 4) and the "odd" shape of S1 (Fig. 5) determine the right route for the pedicular screw in addition to the pedicular width and pedicular angle.

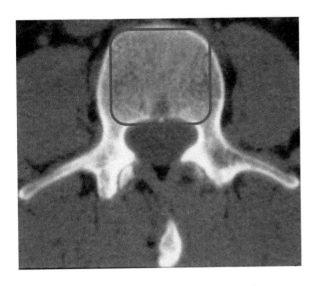

FIGURE 1   Vertebra L4 with squared shape.

So we recommend in L4 and above, screws 45 mm long if we medially incline the screw less than 10°, and 50 mm long if we incline more than 10°. In L5 we can use screws 40 mm long if we incline the screw less than 20°, and 45 mm long if we incline more than 20°. In S1 we can use screws 40 mm long if we incline the screw less than 30°, and 45 mm long if we incline more than 30°.

Insertion Methods for Pedicular Screws

The usual methods for introduction of pedicular screws are the following.

Anatomical Methods

These methods are based on a good knowledge of vertebral anatomy and require a careful learning curve because the sensitivity of the surgeon is important while the screw is penetrating cancellous bone in the pedicle, as is the feeling of resistance of the anterior vertebral cortex and inclining of the screw in the sagittal and axial planes.

Many authors have contributed key points. Ebraheim et al. (47) concluded that the reference point of the pedicle in posterior structures was 3.9 mm above the line passing half-way along the transverse apophysis. In L2 it was 2.8 mm, in L3 1.4 mm, in L4 0.5 mm above and in L5 it was 1.5 mm below the line.

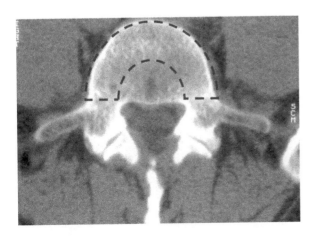

FIGURE 2   Rounded shape in a L5 vertebra.

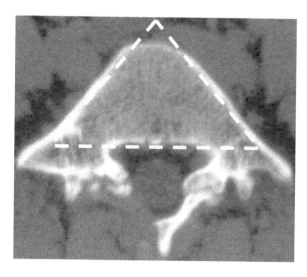

FIGURE 3 Pyramidal shape in a L5 vertebra.

Roy-Camille et al. (10) proposed the entry point as the crossing of two lines: a vertical line passing down the articular facet and a horizontal line passing halfway along the transverse apophysis. In the sagittal plane screws were directed perpendicular to the floor in L4, inclining 10° in L5 and 45° in S1, due to lordosis.

Louis (13) located the entry point in a similar place to Roy-Camille and recommended moving forward without to incline the screw in the lumbar spine.

Magerl (48) and Weinstein et al. (49) chose the entry point lateral to the facet joint being forced to incline the screw inwards.

X-Ray–Assisted Methods

Steinmann et al. (50) and Magerl (48) proposed to incline the C-arm in the pedicular axis to assess the screw position inside pedicle during introduction.

Krag et al. (51) and Whitecloud et al. (52) proposed a modified lateral view (10° oblique view) to assess screws going beyond the anterior vertebral cortex in the lumbar spine. Whitecloud et al. (52) introduced screws in lateral view from the Roy-Camille entry point to the anterior cortex. When the screw reached radiologically to the anterior cortex, there was a 90% probability that it broke through anterior cortex. In S1, Steinmann et al. (53) proposed a modified pelvic view to assess the position and length of screws in the sacrum.

Meter et al. (54) suggest a method to evaluate the position of screws near vertebral plates. They concluded that a screw is in the correct position if, in anteroposterior (AP) or lateral view,

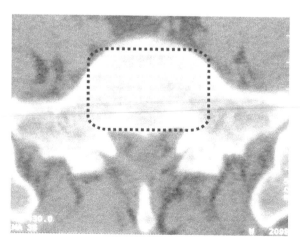

FIGURE 4 Rectangular shape in S1 vertebra.

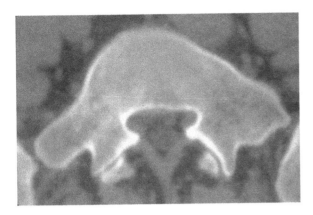

FIGURE 5 Odd shape in S1 vertebra.

it is 3 mm or more away from the vertebral plate due to plate concavity. Horton et al. (55) proved the concurrence of the radiological image of the pedicle. In L5 medial cortex was more reliable than the lateral.

Results using conventional methods are good. CT cortical perforations range from 10% (56) to 67% (57), bearing in mind that anterior cortical perforations and "questionable" positions are measured. Medial pedicular cortical perforations range from 2.6% (58) to 32% (59), reaching more than 4 mm intrusion in the canal in 6.6% (60) of all screws.

Computer-Assisted Methods

These methods are based on computer systems that compare information obtained from the patient by CT with virtual data intraoperative entitled intraoperative navigation. Most common navigators are optoelectronics. The main parts of the system are: (*i*) instruments for screw introduction equipped with light emitting diode (LED); (*ii*) a dynamic reference base fixed to the spine, also equipped with LED, which gives the position of the spine; (*iii*) an infrared camera that can read LED that gives references from instruments and the position of the spine to the computer; (*iv*) a computer that displays information in a monitor.

A CT is necessary before surgery for making reconstructions in 2D and 3D to plan the path of the screws. During the procedure we match points in the patients (e.g., spinous process) with the same points in the CT image to calibrate the system. The system is more reliable when more matched points are done.

Results with computed assisted surgery (CAS) are very good. Assessed by CT, cortical perforations range from 1.8% (61) to 19% (62), in many cases without including anterior cortical perforations [62% (57) if this is considered]. Medial pedicular cortical perforation ranges from 0% (61,63) to 3.7% (64), reaching more than 4 mm in the canal in 1.2% (64) of all screws.

On average, miscalculation between the intraoperative CT virtual image and reality are 1.5 mm and 4° (65–67).

Other Methods

There are many pedicle finders described in Ref. 68. Their success depends on the surgeons, which makes any success calculation subjective.

Recently virtual fluoroscopy has appeared; it is intraoperative navigation that combines fluoroscopic images with computer-assisted surgery. In this case CT images are not necessary and they are replaced by several fluoroscopic images. Its reliability depends on the number of matched points as in CAS, which increases patient radiation. The results of virtual fluoroscopy with multiple points of reference are similar to CAS.

METHODS

As many as 208 pedicular screws were introduced in the lumbosacral spine by three surgeons with different experience in 44 consecutive patients (17 men and 27 women). The average patient age was 42 years. Ten patients had been operated on previously. Arthrodesis was indicated for treatment of chronic lumbar pain or instability, mainly due to lumbar disc disease, lumbar disc disease associated with herniated nucleus pulposus, and listhesis.

Screws were introduced by three surgeons:

1. A senior surgeon with 20 years experience in the introduction of pedicular screws.
2. A fourth-year resident with some experience in spinal surgery and with the learning curve in the introduction of pedicular screws fulfilled.
3. A second-year resident without experience in spinal surgery.

The assignment of patients was randomized. Our own instrumentation at the Clinica Universitaria de Navarra (CUN) (University Clinic of Navarra) was used, composed of titanium (Ti 6 Al 4 V) with pedicular screws and ringed rods (15). Screws were 5.5 mm wide and their length ranged from 30 to 50 mm.

The method for introduction of screws is as follows:

Step 1: Perfect anteroposterior (AP) view. The pedicles are equidistant from the spinous process and both vertebral plates are seen as a line, not as an ellipse (Fig. 6). An incorrect view is when pedicles are not equidistant from spinous process (Fig. 7) or when vertebral plates are seen like an ellipse, not as a line (Fig. 8).

Step 2: Prepointing the pedicle entrance. With a K-wire we mark the superior and external quarter of the pedicle, very often on top of the superior articular process of the lower vertebra (Fig. 9). With a 3.2 mm manual drill we advance into the pedicle without going beyond the medial or inferior cortex (Fig. 10). If the drill goes beyond the medial or inferior pedicular edge we will go on to the next step.

Step 3: Perfect lateral view. In this view vertebral plates are seen as a line, not as an ellipse (Fig. 11). If the drill goes beyond the medial border in the AP view and it is still in the pedicle, the tip of the screw is inside the canal. On the other hand, if the tip of the screw has gone beyond the pedicle, the screw is in the vertebral body.

Step 4: Introducing the screw. Now we introduce the screw in the path created by the drill. Immediately afterwards, we perform a radiological control with AP and lateral view to confirm the position (Fig. 12). If we have doubts about the external position of the screw we will go to next step.

Step 5: Oblique view and Steinmann view. In the lumbar spine an oblique view helps us see if the tip of screw has penetrated the lateral cortex of the pedicle or vertebral body (Figs. 13 and 14). This view is performed beginning from perfect AP view and inclining C-arm on a lateral plane from 10° to 20°.

The Steinmann view (53) is obtained inclining the C-arm cranially until the X-ray beam passes perpendicular to the vertebral plate of S1 and allows assessment of the position of screws in S1 as in a CT-scan view, mainly an anterior break (Fig. 15).

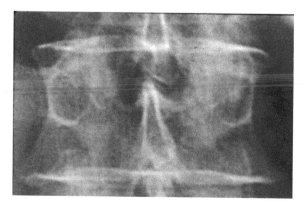

FIGURE 6 Perfect anteroposterior view.

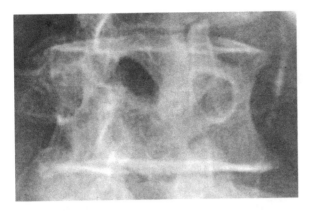

FIGURE 7 Incorrect view. Pedicles are not equidistant from spinous process.

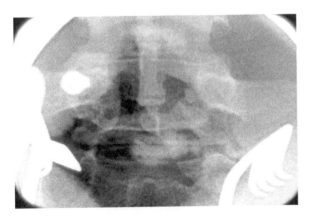

FIGURE 8 Incorrect view. Vertebral plates are seen like an ellipse, not as a line.

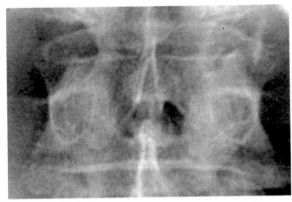

FIGURE 9 Choosing the entry point of S1 pedicle.

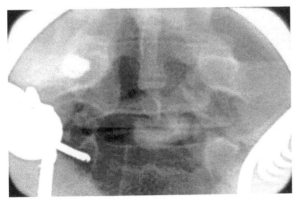

FIGURE 10 Drilling the path of screw in S1 pedicle.

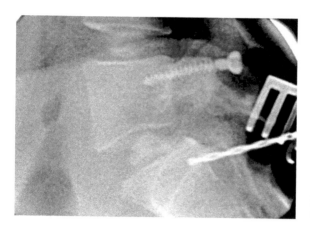

FIGURE 11 Lateral view. The drill is inside vertebral body. In L5 the screw is correct.

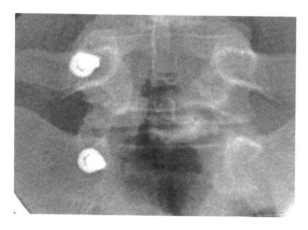

FIGURE 12 Verifying screw position in antero-posterior view. Screws are correct.

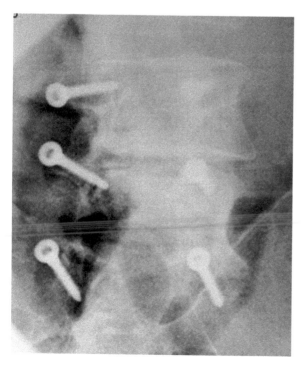

FIGURE 13 Oblique view. Screws are in the correct position.

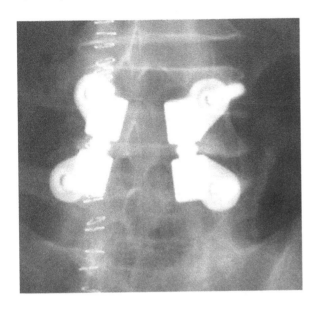

FIGURE 14   Oblique view. L4 screw is out.

After surgery we assess the position of screws with X-rays and with CT scans. In X-rays we perform AP and lateral views classifying them as medial, lateral, superior, inferior or too long (Fig. 16).

CT scans were performed with cuts that passed through the pedicles, 2 mm wide. In CT scans mistakes (Fig. 17) are classified as:

- *Anterior*: Screw is too long and breaks anterior cortex.
- *Medial*: Screw breaks medial cortex of pedicle.
- *Lateral*: Screw breaks lateral cortex of pedicle.

Radiation exposure time is registered in each surgical procedure. Two C-arms have been used: SIREMOBIL 2000®, from Siemens, with double screen which saves images on the monitor, and SIREMOBIL 4K®, from Siemens, with a single screen and unable to save images.

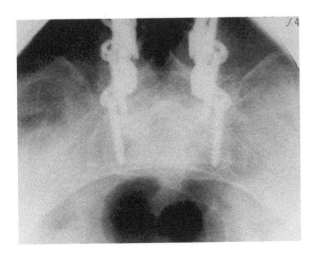

FIGURE 15   Steinmann view.

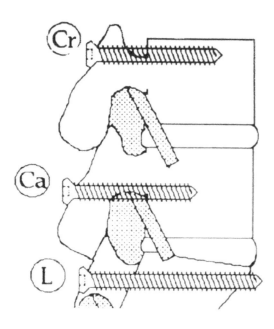

FIGURE 16 Mistakes in lateral view: cranial (Cr), caudal (Ca), and too long (L).

RESULTS

We assess 208 pedicular screws distributed as follows:

- *Senior surgeon*: 147 screws (52 in S1, 56 in L5, 26 in L4, 9 in L3, and 4 in L2).
- *Fourth-year resident*: 32 screws (13 in S1, 15 in L5, 4 in L4).
- *Second-year resident*: 29 screws (7 in S1, 13 in L5, 8 in L4, and 1 in L3).

In 30 patients (142 screws) we used a C-arm which saved images, and in 14 patients (66 screws) the other C-arm. Radiation exposure time was on average 204 seconds (3.4 minutes) per procedure. Using the image-saving C-arm, time was on average 156 seconds per procedure (32 seconds per screw) and using C-arm unable to save images time was on average 306 seconds per procedure (64 seconds by screw). Senior surgeon spent on average 40 seconds per screw, fourth-year resident 48 seconds per screw and second-year resident 51 seconds per screw.

Some cortical breakage (Table 1) was seen in 15 screws (7.2% of all screws): five medial (Figs. 18 to 20), five lateral (Figs. 21 to 23), four anterior cortical breakage (Fig. 24) and one cranial (Fig. 16).

Senior surgeon had 6.8% of screws with cortical breakage, fourth-year resident 9.4% and second-year resident 6.9% (Table 2).

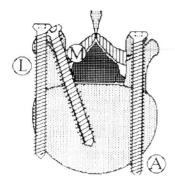

FIGURE 17 Mistakes in computed tomography scans: lateral (L), medial (M), anterior (A).

TABLE 1 Cortical Breakage Distribution by Level

	Medial	Lateral	Anterior	Cranial	Caudal	% Cortical breakage by level
L2 (*n* = 4)	—	1 < 2 mm	—	—	—	25.0
L3 (*n* = 10)	1 < 2 mm	1 < 2 mm	—	—	—	20.0
L4 (*n* = 38)	1 < 2 mm	1...2–4 mm	—	—	—	5.2
L5 (*n* = 84)	1 < 2 mm	2 < 2 mm	1 < 2 mm	1...2–4 mm	—	5.9
S1 (*n* = 72)	2 < 2 mm	—	3 < 2 mm	—	—	6.9
% cortical breakage (*n* = 208)	2.40	2.40	1.92	0.48	0.00	

No significant difference of cortical breakage results of the three surgeons was noted (chi-squared test: $P = 0.876$).

No significant difference was noted comparing cortical breakage results by vertebral level (chi-squared test: $P = 0.199$). L2 and L3 vertebrae were taken in conjunction due to similar shape and low number of vertebrae at each level.

Significant difference was noted between radiation exposure time of the image-saving C-arm and the other C-arm (Mann Whitney U test: $P < 0.001$).

DISCUSSION

Anatomical methods depend on the anatomical knowledge and the experience of the surgeon and have a long training curve. With radiological methods the surgeon is helped by fluoroscopy and can know at any given moment where the screw is in two dimensions and, depending on the radiological views that we use, in three dimensions, with the disadvantage of higher radiation levels for both surgeon and patient. With CAS the image we see is not real. This is a virtual image and there are screws completely outside the pedicle with this technique (69). Radiation levels for the surgeon are very low, but for patient they are very high, due to the extra CT scan for preoperative study.

The high number of screws that appeared out of pedicles in X-rays and the breakage of vertebral cortices in CT scans encouraged us to perform this study. We supposed that by following several fixed steps during the introduction of screws we could avoid most errors (cortical breakage). Our purpose was to have no cortical breakages and to have a method reliable so that even inexperienced surgeons could replicate the results of an experienced surgeon.

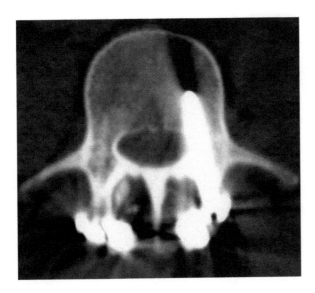

FIGURE 18 L3 left; medial screw.

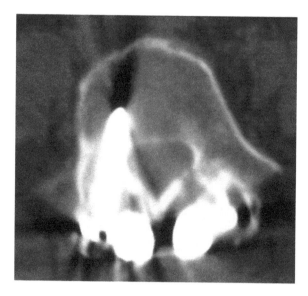

FIGURE 19 L5 right; medial screw.

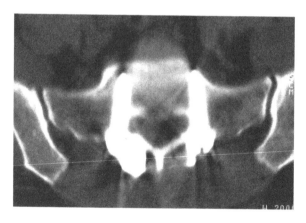

FIGURE 20 S1 right; medial screw.

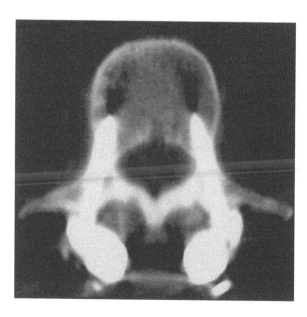

FIGURE 21 L2 right; lateral screw.

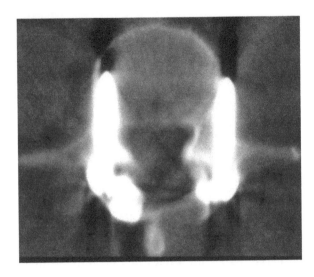

FIGURE 22   L4 left; lateral screw.

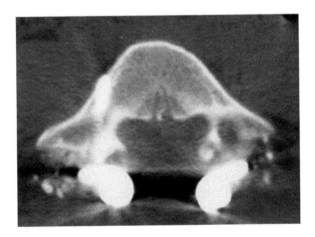

FIGURE 23   L5 right; lateral screw.

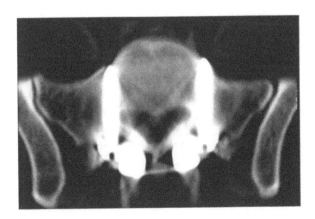

FIGURE 24   S1 left; anterior screw.

TABLE 2 Cortical Breakage Distribution by Surgeon and Level

	Senior surgeon ($n = 147$)	4th Year resident ($n = 32$)	2nd Year resident ($n = 29$)
L2	1 lateral < 2 mm		
L3	1 lateral < 2 mm		
	1 medial < 2 mm		
L4	1 medial < 2 mm	1 lateral 2–4 mm	
L5	2 lateral < 2 mm		1 medial < 2 mm
	1 cranial 2–4 mm		1 anterior < 2 mm
S1	1 medial < 2 mm	1 medial < 2 mm	
	2 anterior < 2 mm	1 anterior < 2 mm	
% cortical breakage	6.8	9.4	6.9

In studies that used CT scans to assess the screw position introduced with radioscopic methods including anterior cortical rupture, most had between 20% and 45% of cortical breakage (58,60,70–76) and neurological complications ranged from 0.5% and 3% of patients (4,11,13,21,27–31) and 0.2% and 0.9% of screws (28). This means that only the few screws that break the vertebral cortex damage the nerve tissues. In screws that go through more than 4 mm into the canal, 33% cause neurological complications (20). A screw that goes through the lateral cortex of the pedicle could cause a root lesion as an extraforaminal hernia (58). What seems indisputable is that a screw inside the pedicle and vertebral body without cortical breakage cannot cause root damage.

The results of cortical rupture were very similar among three surgeons (no significant difference) with under 10% of cortical ruptures in all case. Therefore, we consider the method to be reliable and effective.

With regard to radiation exposure time in all cases it was lower than 60 seconds per screw, which seems an average time in literature (77).

Cortical perforations assessed by CT using fluoroscopic methods range from 10% (56) to 67% (57). Our ruptures (7.2%) are lower than the best published result (56). Medial pedicular cortical perforations range from 2.6% (58) to 32% (59), but in our series it was 2.4%. No screw entered more than 4 mm into the canal.

On the other hand, using CAS the cortical perforations ranged from 1.8% (61) to 19% (62), in many cases without considering anterior cortical perforations [62% (57) if we consider this]. Ours was 7.2%, which is an intermediate value. Medial pedicular cortical perforations ranged from 0% (61,63) to 3.7% (64) in our series it was 2.4% (Table 3).

The possibility of errors using CAS is a given and risky if we trust in CAS, as what you can see in the screen may not be the same in reality. Miscalculation between intraoperative CT virtual image and reality can reach 4.5 mm (78). Accounts have been published of screws completely out of pedicle in the thoracic spine (79) using CAS.

The disadvantages of properative CT-based image guidance according to Holly and Foley (80) are: preoperative CT scan performed using a specific protocol; significant learning curve to select anatomic landmarks and matching them to the image anatomy; in cases of spinal instability (e.g., trauma, listhesis) it is mandatory to make matching in every vertebrae increasing surgical time.

CAS is very useful when vertebral morphology is altered as in a previous fusion mass (81). The time spent in the introduction of a screw with CAS is around 9.5 minutes and with fluoroscopic methods around 5.2 minutes (67).

TABLE 3 Comparison of Medial Cortical Ruptures Between Computer-Assisted Surgery and Our Results

	Total medial	<2 mm	2–4 mm	4–6 mm	>6 mm
Schwarzenbach (79)	3.3%	3.3%	—	—	—
Laine (63)	0%	—	—	—	—
Girardi (61)	0%	—	—	—	—
Merloz (64)	3.7%	2.5%	—	1.2%	—
Alfonso	2.4%	2.4%	—	—	—

Our results are quite similar to that obtained by CAS with the advantage of cost and similar reliability in degenerative spine with a short learning curve. On the other hand, in CAS radiation exposure time is non-existent for the surgeon but not for the patient who receives the extra CT scan. Exposure to radiation can be reduced by using plumbed globes (reducing hand exposure by 40%) and plumbed apron (reducing body exposure by 90%) (50).

RECOMMENDATIONS FOR INTRODUCTION OF PEDICULAR SCREWS IN LUMBAR SPINE

- In L3 and L4 pedicular screws can be introduced with 0° to 10° of medial inclination, 45 mm of length and width of 5.5 mm.
- In L5 pedicular screws can be introduced 45 mm long with 20° of medial inclination and 5.5 mm wide. If the shape is pyramidal we recommend screws 40 mm long if we do not want to cross the anterior cortex.
- In S1 pedicular screws can be introduced 45 mm long with 30° of medial lean and 5.5 mm wide or more. If we cannot incline, the screw length must be 40 mm if we do not want to cross the anterior cortex.

CONCLUSIONS

This inexpensive and easy surgical method that we propose makes for a low incidence of error only comparable to computer-assisted surgery results with low radiation dose.

REFERENCES

1. Shands A. End result study of the treatment of idiopathic scoliosis: Report of the Research Committee of the American Orthopaedic Association. J Bone Joint Surg 1941; 23(A):963–977.
2. Dickson J, Erwin W, Rossi D. Harrington instrumentation and arthrodesis for idiopatic scoliosis: A twenty-one year follow-up. J Bone Joint Surg 1990; 72(A):678–683.
3. Luque ER. Surgical inmovilization of the spine in elderly patients. Clin Orthop 1978; 133:273–274.
4. Cotrel Y, Dubousset J, Guillauman M. New universel instrumentation in spinal surgery. Clin Orthop 1988; 227:10–23.
5. King D. Internal fixation for lumbosacral fusion. J Bone J Surg 1948; 30(A):560–565.
6. Boucher HH. A method of spinal fusion. J Bone J Surg 1959; 41(B):248–259.
7. Louis R. Fusion of the lumbar and sacral spine by internal fixation with screw plates. Clin Orthop 1986; 203:18–33.
8. Roy-Camille R. Ostéosynthése du rachis dorsal, lombaire et lombosacré par plaque métalliques visées dans pédicules vertébraux et les apophyses articulaires. Presse Méd 1970; 78:1447–1448.
9. Roy-Camille R, Saillant G, Berteaux D, Salgado V. Osteosynthesis of thoracolumbar spine fractures with metal plates screwed through the vertebral pedicles. Reconstr Surg Traumatol 1976; 15:2–6.
10. Roy-Camille R, Saillant G, Mazel C. Internal fixation of the lumbar spine with pedicle screw plating. Clin Orthop 1986; 203:7–17.
11. Louis R, Maresca C. Stabilisation chirurgicale avec réduction des spondylolyses et des spondylolysthésis. Int Orthop 1977; 1:215–225.
12. Louis R, Maresca C. Les arthrodèse stables de la lombo-sacrée. Rev Chir Orthop 1976; 62(Suppl 2):70.
13. Louis R. Fusion of the lumbar and sacral spine by internal fixation with screw plates. Clin Orthop 1986; 203:18–33.
14. Cabot JR, Roca J, Fernandez-Fairen M, Diaz J. Cirugía del dolor lumbosacro. Ponencia oficial del XI congreso de Hispano-Portugues de Cirugía Ortopédica y Traumatología (Valladolid 1977). Editorial Garsi. Madrid, 1977:225–265.
15. Beguiristain JL, Villas C, Preite R, Martinez R, Barrios RH. Lumbosacral arthrodesis using pedicular screws and ringed rods. Eur Spine J 1997; 6:233–238.
16. Magerl F. External fixation of the lower thoracic and the lumbar spine. In: Uhthoff H, ed. Current concepts of external fixation of fractures. Berlin: Springer, 1982:353–366.
17. Dick W. The "fixateur interne" as a versatile implant for spine surgery. Spine 1987; 12:882–900.
18. Harrington PR, Dickson JH. Spinal instrumentation in the treatment of severe progressive spondylolisthesis. Clin Orthop 1976; 117:157–163.
19. Steffee AD, Biscup RS, Sitkowski DJ. Segmental spine plates with pedicle screw fixation: A new internal fixation device for disorders of the lumbar and thoracic spine. Clin Orthop 1986; 203:45–53.
20. Gertzbein SD, Robbins SE. Accuracy of pedicular screw placement in vivo. Spine 1990; 15:11–14.

21. Esses SI, Sachs BL, Dreyzin V. Complications associated with the technique of pedicle screw fixation. A selected survey of ABS members. Spine 1993; 18:2231–2239.

22. Asprinio D, Curcin A. Retroperitoneal structures at risk with lumbar pedicle screws: an anatomic and radiographic assessment. Orthop Trans 1995–1996; 19:617.

23. Heini P, Schöll E, Wyler D, Eggli S. Fatal cardiac tamponade associated with posterior spinal instrumentation. Spine 1998; 23:2226–2230.

24. Jendrisak M. Spontaneous abdominal aortic rupture from erosion by a lumbar spine fixation device: A case report. Surgery 1986; 18:2327–2331.

25. Whitecloud TS, Butler JC, Cohen JL, Candelora P. Complications with the VSP system. Spine 1989; 14:472–476.

26. Pihlajamäki H, Myllynen P, Böstman O. Complications of transpedicular lumbosacral fixation for non-traumatic disorders. J Bone Joint Surg 1997; 79(B):183–189.

27. Faraj A, Webb J. Early complications of spinal pedicle screw. Eur Spine J 1997; 6:324–326.

28. Lonstein JE, Denis F, Perra JH, Pinto MR, Smith MD, Winter R. Complications associated with pedicle screws. J Bone J Surg 1999; 81(A):1519–1528.

29. Ohlin A, Karlson M, Düppe H, Hasserius R, Redlund-Johnell Y. Complications after transpedicular stabilization of spine. A survivorship analysis of 163 cases. Spine 1994; 19:2774–2779.

30. Yahiro MA. Review of the "Historical cohort study of pedicular fixation of thoracic, lumbar and sacral spinal fusions" report. Spine 1994; 19(Suppl):S2297–S2299.

31. Yuan HA, Garfin SR, Dickman CA, Mardjetko SM. A historical cohort study of pedicle screw fixation in thoracic, lumbar and sacral spinal fusions. Spine 1994; 19(Suppl):S2279–S2299.

32. Steffee AD, Sitkowski DJ. Reduction and stabilization of grade IV spodylolisthesis. Clin Orthop 1988; 227:82–89.

33. Hsu J, Zuckerman JF, White AH, Wynne G. Internal fixation with pedicle screws. In: White AH, Rothman RH, Roy CD, eds. Lumbar Spine Surgery. St Louis: CV Mosby, 1987: 322–338.

34. Saillant G. Étude anatomique des pédicules vertébraux. Application chirurgicale. Rev Chir Orthop 1976; 62:151–160.

35. Misenhimer G, Peek R, Wiltse L, Rothman S, Widell E. Anatomic analysis of pedicle cortical and cancellous diameter as related to screw size. Spine 1989; 14:367–372.

36. Panjabi MM, Goel V, Oxland T, et al. Human lumbar vertebrae: cuantitative three-dimensional anatomy. Spine 1992; 17:299–306.

37. Zindrick MR, Wilste LL, Doornik A, et al. Analysis of the morphometric characteristics of the thoracic and lumbar pedicles. Spine 1987; 12:160–166.

38. Berry J, Moran J, Berg W, Stefee A. A morphometric study of human lumbar and selected thoracic vertebrae. Spine 1987; 12:362–367.

39. Scoles P, Linton A, Latimer B, Levy M, Digiovanni B. Vertebral body and posterior element morphology: the normal spine in middle life. Spine 1988; 13:1082–1086.

40. Olsewski J, Simmons E, Kallen F, Mendel F, Severin C, Berens D. Morphometry of lumbar spine: Anatomical perspectives related to transpedicular fixation. J Bone Joint Surg 1990; 72(A):541–549.

41. Bernard T, Seibert C. Pedicle diámeter determined by Computed Tomography. Its relevance to pedicle screw fixation in the lumbar spine. Spine 1992; 17(Suppl):S160–S163.

42. Cheung K, Ruan D, Chan F, Fang D. Computed tomographic osteometry of asian lumbar pedicles. Spine 1994; 19:1495–1498.

43. Krag M, Beynnon B, Pope M, Frymoyer J, Haugh L, Weaver D. An Internal fixator for Posterior Application to Short Segments of the Thoracic, Lumbar or Lumbosacral Spine. Design and Testing. Clin Orthop 1986; 203:75–98.

44. Krag M, Weaver D, Beynnon B, Haugh L. Morphometry of the thoracic and lumbar spine related to transpedicular screw placement for surgical spinal fixation. Spine 1988; 13:27–32.

45. Van Schaik J, Verbiest H, Van Schaik F. Morphometry of lower lumbar vertebrae as seen on CT scans: Newly Recognised Characteristics. Am J Roetgenol 1985; 145:327–335.

46. Alfonso M, Villas C, Beguiristain JL, Zubieta JL. Morfometría Vertebral en Población Española. Revista de Ortopedia y Traumatología 2002; 2:158–164.

47. Ebraheim NA, Rollins J, Xu R, Yeasting R. Projection of the lumbar pedicle and its morphometric analysis. Spine 1996; 21:1296–1300.

48. Magerl FP. Stabilization of the lower thoracic and lumbar spine with External Spinal Skeletal Fixation. Clin Orthop 1984; 189:125–141.

49. Weinstein JN, Spratt KF, Sprengler D, Brick C, Reid S. Spinal pedicle fixation: reliability and validity of roetgenogram-based assesment and surgical factors of successful screw placement. Spine 1988; 13:1012–1018.

50. Steinmann JC, Herkowitz HN, El-Kommos H, Wesolowski DP. Spinal pedicle fixation. Confirmation of an image-based technique for screw placement. Spine 1993; 18:1856–1861.

51. Krag MH, Van Hal ME, Beynnon BD. Placement of transpedicular screws close to anterior vertebral cortex: description of methods. Spine 1989; 14:879–883.

52. Whitecloud TS, Skalley T, Morgan E, Cook S. Roetgenografic measurement of pedicle screw penetration. Clin Orthop 1989; 245:57–68.
53. Steinmann JC, Mirkovic S, Abitbol JJ, Massie J, Subbaiah P, Garfin SR. Radiographic assessment of sacral screw placement. J Spinal Disord 1990; 3:232–237.
54. Meter JJ, Polly DW, Miller DW, Popovic NA, Ondra SL. A method for radiographic evaluation of pedicle screw violation of the vertebral endplate. Spine 1996; 21:1587–1592.
55. Horton W, Rodriguez J, Hutton WC. Radiographic control of pedicle screw insertion. Orthop Trans 1993; 17:129.
56. Sim E. Location of transpedicular screws for fixation of the lower thoracic and lumbar spine. Acta Orthop Scand 1993; 64:28–32.
57. Berlemann U, Heini P, Müller U, Stoupis C, Schwarzenbach O. Reliability of pedicle screw assessment utilizing plain radiographs versus CT reconstructions. Eur Spine J 1997; 6:406–411.
58. Beguiristain JL, Berjano P, Alfonso M, Zubieta JL, Villas C. Valoración por Tomografía Axial Computadorizada de la posición de tornillos pediculares en raquis lumbosacro. Rev Ortop Traum 2001; 45:106–113.
59. Schulze CJ, Munzinger E, Weber U. Clinical relevance of accuracy of pedicle screw placement. A computed tomographic-supported analysis. Spine 1998; 23:2215–2220.
60. Gertzbein SD, Robbins SE. Accuracy of pedicular screw placement in vivo. Spine 1990; 15:11–14.
61. Girardi FP, Cammisa FP, Sandhu HS, Alvarez L. The placement of lumbar pedicle screws using computerised stereotactic guidance. J Bone J Surg 1999; 81(B):825–829.
62. Arand M, Hartwig E, Hebold D, Kinzl L, Gebhard F. Precision analysis of navigation-assisted implanted thoracic and lumbar pedicle screws. A prospective clinical study. Unfallchirurg 2001; 104:1076–1081.
63. Laine T, Schlenzka D, Makitalo K, Tallroth K, Nolte L-P, Visarius H. Improved accuracy of pedicle screw insertion with Computer-Assisted Surgery. Spine 1997; 22:1254–1258.
64. Merloz P, Tonetti J, Pittet L, Coulomb M, Lavallee S, Sautot P. Pedicle screw placement using image guided techniques. Clin Orthop 1998; 354:39–48.
65. Carl AL, Khanuja HS, Sachs BL, et al. In vitro simulation. Early results of stereotaxy for pedicle screw placement. Spine 1997; 22:1160–1164.
66. Glossop ND, Hu RW, Randle JA. Computer-Aided pedicle screw placement using frameless stereotaxis. Spine 1996; 21:2026–2034.
67. Schlenzka D, Laine T, Lund T. Computer-assisted spine surgery. Eur Spine J 2000; 9(Suppl 1):S57–S64.
68. Sendino M, Cimarra I, Galeote A, Muñoz J, Deglane R. Introducción de los tornillos pediculares mediante el uso de una cánula de biopsia ósea. Rev Ortop Traumatol 1994; 40:285–288.
69. Mirza S, Wigginsn G, Kuntz C, et al. Accuracy of thoracic vertebral body screw placement using standard fluoroscopy, fluoroscopic image guidance, and computer tomographic image guidance: a cadaver study. Spine 2003; 28:402–413.
70. Castro WH, Halm H, Jerosch J, Malmams J, Steinbeck J, Blasius S. Accuracy of pedicle screw placement in lumbar vertebrae. Spine 1996; 21:1320–1324.
71. Haaker RG, Eickhoff U, Schopphoff E, Steffen R, Jergas M, Krämer J. Verification of the position of pedicle screws in lumbar spinal fusion. Eur Spine J 1997; 6:125–128.
72. Halm HF, Liljenqvist UR, Link TM, Jerosch J, Winkelmann W. Computerized tomography monitoring of the position of pedicle screws in scoliosis surgery. Z Orthop Ihre Grenzgeb 1996; 134:492–497.
73. Laine T, Makitalo K, Schlenzka D, Tallroth K, Poussa M, Alho A. Accuracy of pedicle screw insertion: a prospective CT study in 30 low back patients. Eur Spine J 1997; 6:402–405.
74. Liljenqvist UR, Halm HF, Link TM. Pedicle screw instrumentation of the thoracic spine in idiopatic scoliosis. Spine 1997; 22:2239–2245.
75. Schulze CJ, Munzinger E, Weber U. Clinical relevance of accuracy of pedicle screw placement. A computed tomographic-supported analysis. Spine 1998; 23:2215–2220.
76. Sjöstrom L, Jacobnson O, Karström G, Pech P, Rauschning G. CT analysis of pedicles and screws tracts after implant removal in thoracolumbar fractures. J Spinal Disord 1993; 6:225–231.
77. Slomczykowski M, Roberto M, Schneeberger P, Ozdoba C, Vock P. Radiation dose for pedicle screw insertion. Fluoroscopic method versus computer-assisted surgery. Spine 1999; 24:975–983.
78. Amiot LP, Labelle H, DeGuise JA, Sati M, Brodeuur P, Rivard CH. Computer-assisted pedicle screw fixation. A feasibility study. Spine 1995; 20:1208–1212.
79. Schwarzenbach O, Berlemann U, Jost B, et al. Accuracy of Computer-Assisted pedicle screw placement. Spine 1997; 22:452–458.
80. Holly LT, Foley KT. Intraoperative spinal navigation. Spine 2003; 28(Suppl):S54–S61.
81. Austin M, Vaccaro A, Brislin B, Nachwalter R, Hilibrand A, Albert T. Image-guided spine surgery: A cadáver study comparing conventional open laminoforminotomy and two image-guided techniques for pedicle screw placement in posterolateral fusion and non fusion models. Spine 2002; 27:2503–2508.

32 | Bone Graft Materials Used to Augment Spinal Arthrodesis

Debdut Biswas and Jonathan N. Grauer
Department of Orthopaedics and Rehabilitation, Yale University, New Haven, Connecticut, U.S.A.

Andrew P. White
Department of Orthopaedic and Neurological Surgery, Thomas Jefferson University Hospital, Philadelphia, Pennsylvania, U.S.A.

INTRODUCTION

Spinal fusion may be performed for the treatment of degenerative disc disease, instability, or deformity. This commonly performed procedure aims to eliminate motion between adjacent vertebrae by achieving segmental union. While instrumentation and postoperative bracing are often used to limit spinal motion after fusion surgery, bony union is necessary to achieve long-term stability. There have been significant advances in understanding this process over recent years, but many important details remain incompletely understood (1).

A bone graft material may have one of a number of features. Osteoconductive materials provide a structural scaffold onto which bone can be formed. Osteoinductive materials induce local precursor cells down a bone-forming lineage. Osteopromotive materials lead to proliferation of bone forming cells. Osteogenic materials contain precursor or bone forming cells.

Autograft is bone transplanted form one site to another in the same individual. Although many sites may be used, the iliac crest has been the most common for spinal applications since the 1940s when Abbott first described iliac harvest techniques (2). Autograft possesses all of the bone graft properties listed above is considered the "gold standard" bone graft material.

Although autograft is considered the material most likely to promote fusion, pseudarthrosis rates still range from 5% to 35% (3). There are also well-described morbidities associated with the harvest of autograft (4). These include chronic donor site pain (5,6), infection (7), fracture, herniation (8), and injury to surrounding structures (9,10). Additional operative time is also required, and donor bone may be limited in quantity because of poor bone quality or previous graft harvest.

The limitations and morbidity of autograft have motivated the desire for bone graft alternatives and supplements. This Chapter will review the evaluation of bone graft materials and then discuss a number autograft alternatives or supplements. Allograft options, including structural and morcelized allograft as well as demineralized bone matrix (DBM) will be discussed. The application of platelet gels, bone marrow aspirates, as well as systems of biologic activation, such as electrical stimulation and ultrasound will be reviewed. The recombinant human bone morphogenic proteins (rhBMPs) will be reviewed in a separate Chapter.

FUSION BIOLOGY

Bone graft is incorporated into a developing fusion mass according to a defined series of biologic events. These include hemorrhage, inflammation, vascular invasion, and remodeling (11). Surgical preparation of the fusion bed sets the stage for these events; decortication exposes marrow elements. Mesenchymal stem cells are then recruited to differentiate into chondroblasts and osteoblasts, as directed by local osteoinductive factors. These factors include the bone morphogenetic proteins (BMPs) and other mitogens such as platelet-derived growth factors, interleukins, fibroblast growth factors, insulin-like growth factors, granulocyte colony–stimulating factors, and granulocyte-macrophage colony–stimulating factors. Concurrently, capillary buds invade the graft to provide a local blood supply. Angiogenic factors, such as vascular endothelial-derived growth factor, are also released (12). The osteopromotive influence of these factors delivers a population of cells ready to form new bone.

EVALUATION OF GRAFT MATERIALS

There are varieties of diverse clinical scenarios for which bone graft may be considered. Host risk factors such as smoking and diabetes, as well as factors specific to the local biological and mechanical milieu may all affect fusion success. For example, the anterior interbody environment which heals under compression differs significantly from the posterior environment which heals under tension. In general, a bone graft material should be validated for each specific site for which application is being considered. This is often initiated at the preclinical level and then brought to the clinical setting only when encouraging results are found.

If a material is used to substitute autograft it is considered a bone graft alternative. If it increases the effect of autograft it is considered a bone graft supplement. Similarly, if it is used to augments the coverage or volume of autograft it is considered an extender.

While many bone graft materials contain a single component such as most allograft products, there are products that are composed of more than one agent. For example, rhBMP products are a combination of an osteoinductive protein and a carrier, which is often a collagen based material. When a product has more than one component, each must be specifically considered from both a scientific and regulatory perspective.

Importantly, not all bone graft materials are evaluated with the same level of scrutiny by the U.S. Food and Drug Administration. One categorical difference is that some products are evaluated as implant devices and others are evaluated as minimally manipulated human tissues. The highly publicized development of the rhBMPs for use in spinal surgery can be used as an example. Randomized, prospective clinical studies regarding their use have been reported in the literature (13,14). Only with this high level of scientific data have such products been brought to market. Other products, however, such as DBM and other allograft based formulations, is classified as minimally manipulated human tissues and is not subject to the same regulation as implant devices.

The primary measure used to assess the potency of a bone graft material is fusion success. This outcome measure, however, is often difficult to determine with certainty. The accuracy of plain radiographs has long been noted to be relatively poor at assessing fusion success (15). Clinical findings, such as loss of correction and back pain, are also unreliable (16). Although some investigators have stated their preference for the use of CT scans in the evaluation of fusion, there are no definitive studies documenting its accuracy in comparison to radiographs (17). Clearly, more studies on noninvasive methods to assess spinal fusion are warranted.

The uncertainty of assessing fusion success is complicated by the fact that there is a poor correlation between clinical success and fusion success (18). This discrepancy has been attributed to poor predictability of outcome and inconsistent indications for fusion. Nonetheless, since the goal of bone graft augmentation is typically to achieve biologic union, success is characteristically measured by this outcome.

There is a broad range of bone graft products available for use in spinal arthrodesis. Each material possesses distinct cellular, biochemical, and structural properties that determine its specific clinical indications. As the mechanisms underlying the biology of spinal fusion continue to be elucidated, it is likely that bone graft substitutes will become more refined (11). Regardless, it is the responsibility of the surgeon to evaluate the literature related to their patient's clinical scenario to determine if and when particular bone graft agents might be appropriately indicated.

ALLOGRAFT

Allogeneic bone graft, or allograft, is bone harvested from one individual and transplanted to another. This has traditionally been the most commonly used bone graft material, especially in the United States. Depending on the method of preparation, the characteristics and properties of allograft may vary.

Structural and Morcelized Allograft

Structural and morcelized allografts are osteoconductive. Although there may be some osteoinductive potential, most of this is eradicated in the preparation process. These products do not contain live cells and, as such, are not osteogenic. The remodeling of both cortical and cancellous allograft occurs more slowly than the remodeling of autograft, and there is typically a phase of greater resorption of allograft as compared to autograft (19).

The risk of disease transmission is a potential concern. There have been two documented cases of human immunodeficiency virus (HIV) transmission from allograft bone, both of which involved unprocessed grafts (20). Rigorous donor screening and careful tissue processing has lowered the calculated risk of disease transmission to less than one per million (21). There has, in fact, never been a documented transmission of HIV using current bone graft preparation techniques. Structural allografts are generally fresh-frozen or freeze-dried (lyophilized) in order to decrease their antigenicity and permit storage for extended periods of time (22). Because fresh grafts carry the greatest risk of disease transmission and are the most immunogenic, they are not routinely used. Fresh-frozen allografts may be kept for up to one year at $-20°C$ with no change in structural characteristics and are considerably less immunogenic than fresh grafts while still preserving some BMPs. Lyophilized allografts are dehydrated and vacuum packed, which allows for storage at room temperature and reduces immunogenicity even more than freezing. This preparation, however, destroys most of the BMP in the allograft and is also associated with a decrease in certain mechanical properties (23–25).

Structural allografts may be used for weight bearing reconstructions throughout the spine. These grafts can be cut in the operating room or premilled. Previous studies evaluating patients undergoing single-level fusions of the anterior cervical spine with either allograft or autograft have demonstrated similar fusion rates (26–28). Variation in fusion rates is more significant as the number of levels being addressed increases (29,30). In the lumbar spine, excellent fusion outcomes have been reported with the use of femoral ring allografts (31,32). In cases involving revision anterior lumbar fusions, one study found that the results obtained with tricortical allograft may be comparable to those obtained with autogenous bone graft taken from the iliac crest (33).

Morcelized allograft may be cortical or cancellous. Cortical allograft offers greater structural features than cancellous allograft but is associated with slower incorporation than cancellous grafts (12). In the posterior spine, allograft consistently performs less well than autograft. In two prospective clinical trials comparing autograft with various allograft preparations, patients treated with autograft achieved solid posterolateral fusion more frequently than those receiving allograft (34,35). One clinical counterexample, however, is pediatric scoliosis fusion where the hospitable fusion environment has been associated with comparable fusion rates using autograft or allograft (36).

Collectively, studies suggest that cortical allografts may be acceptable alternatives to autogenous bone graft in certain clinical situations requiring a structural support, such as certain anterior cervical or lumbar applications. Many surgeons also find cancellous allograft to be an acceptable alternative to autograft in the adolescent patient undergoing scoliosis fusion.

Demineralized Bone Matrix

DBM is a form of allograft from which the mineralized component is eluted. The remaining growth factors, collagen, and noncollagen proteins are then prepared for implantation. A partial list of products on the market includes: Grafton® (Osteotech, Eatontown, New Jersey, U.S.A.), Dynagraft® (GenSci Orthobiologics, Irvine, California, U.S.A.), Osteofil® (Regeneration Technologies, Alachua, Florida, U.S.A.), Allomatrix® (Wright Medical Technologies, Arlington, Tennessee, U.S.A.), and DBX® (Musculoskeletal Transplant Foundation, Edison, New Jersey, U.S.A.). The preparation of these products is generally proprietary and not fully disclosed. Carriers are typically collagen or glycerol based.

The ability of demineralized rabbit bone to induce new bone formation when implanted in rabbit muscle pouches was first described by Marshall Urist almost 50 years ago (37). The active osteoinductive agents were subsequently isolated by Urist and others, and ultimately named the BMPs. It is these and other bone growth factors in DBM that are believed to stimulate bone formation. Although the concentration of these factors in DBM is orders of magnitude less than the supraphysiologic amounts provided with rhBMP products (38), the physiologic mixture of cytokines is postulated to be advantageous for bone formation.

DBM products demonstrate an enormous degree of variability in their osteoinductive potentials. A recent study assessed the osteoinductive ability of eight different commercially available DBMs in an athymic rat model of spinal fusion (39), with fusion rates varying from 20% to 80%. Osteofil Paste had the highest radiographic scores at four weeks, whereas Grafton Putty had the best radiographic scores at eight weeks. The spines implanted with Allomatrix had the lowest radiographic scores at both four and eight weeks. With regard to fusions assessed by manual palpation, Osteofil Paste was the most effective at four weeks, whereas Grafton Flex and Grafton Putty had the highest rate of fusion at eight weeks. The lowest rates of fusion were seen in the Allomatrix and Grafton Crunch groups. Another athymic rat study compared the efficacy of Grafton Putty, DBX Putty and AlloMatrix Injectable Putty (40). Fusion rates varied from 0% to 100%, depending on the DBM used. At eight weeks, the investigators reported that the all spines in the Grafton group were fused, half of the spines in the DBX group were fused, and none of the Allomatrix had fused. These preclinical studies show statistically significant variation between different DBMs. Clearly, it is important for the clinician to understand the needs of each individual case as well as the relative strengths and weaknesses of all of the products so that the most appropriate DBM is selected.

Significant variability between different formulations of the same DBM has been reported. Martin and colleagues compared fusion outcomes using multiple formulations of Grafton DBM in a rabbit model. They observed that the putty and flexible sheet forms enhanced spinal fusion to a greater extent than the gel formulation and hypothesized that this effect was related to the improved handling characteristics of these fiber-based preparations (41). Subsequently, a posterolateral rhesus monkey model was used to compare the osteoinductive ability of Grafton Flex and Grafton Matrix. In four animals, autograft (4 g per side) was implanted with a piece of human Grafton Flex demineralized bone matrix. In the other four animals, rhesus Grafton Matrix demineralized bone matrix, was implanted with autograft (4 g) on one side of the spine, and Matrix with half the amount of autograft (2 g) was implanted on the opposite side. The Grafton Matrix formulation performed better than the human Flex, with evidence of larger fusion masses. Evidence of osteoinduction was seen in all four monkeys that received Matrix, which improved the fusion success of autograft (42).

While variability in the fusion performance of similar DBM products may be anticipated by many surgeons, variability between different lots of the same product is unexpected. A recent evaluation of the BMP-2 and BMP-7 content in nine formulations of DBM showed a high degree of BMP inconsistency in different samples of the same DBM product. In fact, there was a higher degree of BMP variability found among samples of the same product than there was among the nine different DBM products altogether (43). In general, the amount of BMP measured was quite low. For example, to achieve the standard commercially available BMP-2 dose of 6 mg, 100 kg of the Grafton Putty evaluated would be required.

Variation between samples of DBM from the same tissue bank has also been reported (44–46). A more recent study also noted significant variability in the osteoinductive abilities in different lots of DBMs from the same tissue bank (47). Using an in vitro assay that correlates alkaline phosphatase (ALP) activity in a pluripotent myoblast cell line to osteoinductivity, the investigators reported that the capacity of DBM to induce ALP varied from bank to bank and from batch to batch within the same bank. Additionally bone forming potential was tested in vivo by implanting DBM intra-muscularly in nude rats. The investigators reported significant variations in bone formation in the explants between DBMs from different banks as well as lots within the same bank.

Studies have suggested that the variability between DBM samples from the same bank could be attributed to inherent differences in the quality of the material. Schwartz examined whether donor age or gender contributed to the variability seen with these preparations. The investigators implanted twenty-seven different batches of DBM from one bank intramuscularly and bilaterally in nude mice. The authors noted that DBM from older donors was less likely to have strong bone-inducing activity. By contrast, no difference in ability to induce new bone was noticed between male or female donors (48). A study by Zhang reported similar results (45,46). The studies suggest that commercial bone banks need to verify the ability of DBM to induce new bone formation and should reconsider the advisability of using bone from older donors.

There are several reports evaluating the safety of glycerol-based DBM products (49,50). In the athymic rat, renal toxicity was noted when very supra-physiologic doses of glycerol-based products were used, at eight times the maximum volume used in humans. In humans, however, there have been no reported cases of glycerol toxicity related to the implantation of DBM products, despite more than 10 years of their use (11).

With regard to the osteoinductivity of DBM, human outcome data is sparse. One retrospective study retrospectively reviewed an age-, gender-, and procedure-matched group of patients who had undergone instrumented posterolateral lumbar spinal fusion with autograft and Grafton gel. There was no difference in radiographic fusion outcome at 3, 6, 12, and 24 months after surgery. The fusion rates in the autograft-with-Grafton group and the autograft-only group were 60% and 56%, however; these rates are lower than those reported in other studies of instrumented posterior fusion (51).

More recently, the effectiveness of Grafton DBM gel and iliac crest autograft in posterolateral spine fusion was evaluated. All patients underwent posterolateral spine fusion with pedicle screw fixation. Iliac crest autograft was implanted on one side of the spine and a Grafton DBM/autograft composite was implanted on the contra-lateral side. Fusion was found in 42 cases (52%) of the Grafton DBM sides and in 44 cases (54%) of the autograft sides. Despite the similar results on each side, the authors concluded that Grafton DBM might offer a means of extending a smaller quantity of autograft than is normally required (52). Overall, the literature suggests that DBM may have limited efficacy as a substitute but may be considered as a potential bone graft extender in combination with other graft materials in certain indications (11).

BONE MARROW ASPIRATES

Osteogenic bone graft materials contain undifferentiated mesenchymal stem cells (MSCs) that retain the ability to proceed down various cell lineages. They also harbor osteoprogenitor cells that are prepared to proceed down bone forming lineages. These cells are present in autograft. The potential to harvest these cells by aspiration in an attempt to circumvent the morbidity associated with bone graft has been appreciated since Goujon in 1869 (12).

The vast majority of cells obtained from needle aspiration are hematopoetic cells which are not of direct benefit from a bone grafting perspective. Osteoprogenitor cells, on the other hand, constitute approximately one out of 20,000 to 30,000 cells in such aspirates (53). It is these relatively rare cells that facilitate bone formation and thus are the goal of aspiration. However, the concentration of osteoprogenitor cells decreases with aspiration volumes over two milliliters, as the volume of returned venous blood increases. This has lead to the recommendation of limiting aspirations from each site to two milliliters. It is recommended to aspirate from additional sites to obtain greater volume, as opposed to drawing larger volumes from a single site.

The number of precursor cells also varies with patient age and gender (53,54). A 57 patient cohort was recruited for bone marrow assay prior to elective orthopedic procedures. Two-milliliter samples of bone marrow were from the anterolateral iliac crest. Aspirates obtained from female subjects demonstrated a significant age-related decline in the number of cell colonies expressing alkaline phosphatase (an early marker for osteoblastic differentiation), while no decline was found in men (55–57). It is hypothesized that these differences may be associated with the pathophysiology of age-related bone loss and post-menopausal osteoporosis (54).

Typically, marrow aspirates are combined with osteoconductive carriers to provide a framework for cell delivery. Synthetic materials, as well as collagen, allograft, and DBM are materials used for this purpose. Long bone fracture and non-union models have been used to investigate the potential role of bone marrow aspirates (58–61). These data provide a foundation upon which animal spinal fusion studies are conducted to evaluate the potential role of bone marrow aspirates (62–66).

The New Zealand white rabbit posterolateral fusion model is commonly used to evaluate potential bone graft formulations for the spine. Curylo et al. (67) studied a bone paucity model (one iliac crest) implanted with either blood or bone marrow aspirate. Fusion rates of 25% and

61%, respectively, were observed suggesting that bone marrow aspirate may be more effective than blood alone as a bone graft extender. A similar rabbit study found a 100% fusion rate with bone marrow aspirate harvested from the iliac crest with a calcium phosphate ceramic carrier (64).

The efficacy of bone marrow aspirate with Healos®, Orquest Inc., Mountainview, California, U.S.A., a Type I collagen sponge with hydroxyapatite coating has also been evaluated in the New Zealand white rabbit posterolateral spinal fusion model. Autologous iliac crest bone graft lead to fusion in 75% of the rabbits, Healos alone in 20% of the rabbits, and bone marrow aspirate harvested from both tibias and both femurs with Healos in 100% of the rabbits (68). In contrast to these findings, Boden found 0/12 fusions with Healos and iliac crest bone marrow in the same model (69). These conflicting results may be related to the site of marrow harvest and relative number of osteoprecursor cells in these two studies, but more work is needed to clarify this discrepancy.

With generally encouraging results in the preclinical arena and in long bone clinical trials, clinical evaluations of bone marrow aspirates have been performed. Kitchel has reported similar fusion rates between a Healos/bone marrow aspirate and autograft in instrumented posterolateral lumbar fusion (70). Welch et al. (71) reported similar results in an evaluation of Healos/bone marrow aspirate or autograft in an anterior lumbar interbody fusion model.

A posterior instrumented scoliosis fusion model has been used to evaluate autograft, allograft, and a composite of bone marrow aspirate and DBM (72). Failure rates, defined as pseudarthrosis or loss of correction, were 12.5% with autograft, 28% with allograft, and 11.1% with marrow + DBM. As no significant morbidity was associated with the marrow aspirate, fusion rates equivalent to with traditional iliac crest autograft, marrow aspirate and DBM seemed to offer an encouraging potential option in this population where fusion is less challenging to achieve than in other situations.

In the cervical spine, a prospective, nonrandomized trial with a minimum two-year follow-up evaluated bone marrow aspirate combined with hydroxyapatite in a titanium alloy cage. A 24% increase in the hydroxyapatite mass was seen two years after surgery. At this point, 92% of the patients experienced relief of their symptoms and none required reoperation. Despite the lack of a control group, significant clinical improvement was seen without the morbidity associated with autograft harvest (73).

In light of the fact that the MSCs seem to provide encouraging results (although studies are still limited), efforts have additionally been made concentrate these cells. One means of achieving this goal is the centrifugation of cells. Using this technique, better response than marrow aspirate alone was observed in a rabbit long bone defect model (74). Additional potential techniques include cell culture amplified (65) or selective retention of desired cell. Further studies on all of these techniques, however, are needed.

PLATELET GELS

Platelets are known to express cytokines such as transforming growth factor beta (TGF-beta), platelet-derived growth factor (PDGF), and insulin-like growth factor (IGF). In their normal role, platelets degranulate at their site of action releasing these products which can act in chemo-attractant and osteopromotive fashions. Platelet gels can be prepared to concentrate and potentially exploit the multiple growth factors that have mitogenic and chemotactic effects on MSCs and osteoblasts.

Although there are a number of commercial schemes to generate platelet gels, the general principles are similar. Patient blood is drawn off and spun. The buffy coat, which includes the platelets, is isolated and activated with products such as thrombin to stimulate the degranulation process. Once combined with a selected carrier, these products are implanted at a bone-grafting site (11). Like DBM, platelet gels are classified as minimally manipulated tissues and are therefore not closely regulated or subjected to rigorous safety and efficacy testing before making it to market.

In animal studies, PDGF has been shown to enhance bone formation. For example, this has been shown in subcutaneous punch studies. Howes et al. (75) reported that a PDGF supplement enhanced the osteoconductive activity of a subcutaneous DBM implant in a rat model. Other studies, however, have found that cytokines such as PDGF and TGF-β may actually interfere with the process of bone healing. In vitro data have raised the possibility that the cytokines in platelet concentrates can inhibit the activity of bone morphogenetic proteins at certain concentrations. Marden et al. (76) reported that the application of PDGF to osteogenin, a bone inductive protein, inhibited bony repair in a rat craniotomy defect model. Harris also reported that TGF-β inhibited the formation of bone nodules in a culture of fetal rat osteoblasts and impaired the expression of genes associated with bone formation (77).

There have been several clinical studies evaluating platelet gels. Autologous growth factor (AGF) concentrate, a form of platelet gel trademarked by Interpore Cross International, has been the subject of many of these studies. Other AGF products are also marketed, such as Symphony™ (DePuy Spine, Raynham, Massachusetts).

Lowery performed a retrospective review of 39 patients undergoing anterior or posterior lumbar fusion who received AGF concentrate with coralline hydroxyapatite. After an average follow-up of 13 months, no pseudarthroses were noted clinically or on plain radiographs. The authors concluded that AGF offered theoretical advantages that needed to be examined in controlled settings (78).

Transformational lumbar interbody fusion with autograft alone has been compared to fusions with a composite of autograft plus AGF (79). Fusion rates of 55% and 36% were observed, respectively. Although there was not a significant clinical difference between groups, the addition of AGF yielded lower fusion rates. The author concluded that the theoretical benefits of AGF platelet gel were not clinically appreciated and cost was not justified based on the results observed.

Another study compared matched cohorts undergoing posterolateral instrumented fusions compared autograft to autograft plus AGF at an average follow-up of three years (80). Fusion rates of 83% and 75% were observed, respectively. Again, this difference was not statistically significant, and the authors did not recommend the use of AGF in spinal fusion.

A retrospective clinical radiographic study compared a group of 27 consecutive patients who underwent a single-level intertransverse lumbar fusion using iliac crest bone graft to a group of 32 patients undergoing similar surgery with autograft used in combination with AGF (81). At two years follow-up, a statistically significant difference in fusion rates of 91% and 62% were noted for the two groups, respectively. This study concluded that there may actually be inhibitory effects seen by the platelet gel product studied.

In general, mixed results have been seen with platelet gel concentrates. Certainly, the biological mechanisms associated with these products and the related clinical results need to be further studied. Some of the neutral or negative data may arise from the fact that concentrations may not be optimized, some platelet factors may be inhibitory to fusion, and/or the carrier may not be optimized. Certainly, all platelet gels may not be the same, but the evidence regarding their efficacy needs to be further elucidated (82).

BIOLOGIC ACTIVATION OF GRAFTS
Electrical Stimulation

For almost five decades, electrical stimulation has been considered in the management of long bone nonunion. Only recently has it been used for spinal fusion. The three major techniques used to deliver electrical stimulation to bones are direct current (DC), pulsing electromagnetic fields (PEMF), and capacitive coupled electrical stimulation. While the DC stimulation is delivered through surgically implanted electrodes, both the PEMF and capacitive coupled devices are externally applied to the skin. Each method has a different mechanism of action. Understanding the scientific data regarding electrical stimulation can help guide the use of these techniques.

DC stimulation involves implanting a cathode in direct contact with the bone graft and decorticated vertebral elements at the time of fusion surgery. DC stimulation has been more thoroughly evaluated for use with spinal surgery than the other modes of electrical stimulation. Statistically significant improvements in fusion rates in patients receiving DC stimulation have been reported (83–86). One advantage of the DC technique is that there is not the possibility of poor compliance. Such an implanted device may increase post surgical risk and cause discomfort, however, and the battery may leak or malfunction. And because the device is internal, malfunction may require revision surgery. The rate of infection or device related complications requiring surgical removal have not been well-described (87).

In the application of PEMF, an external coil generates an electromagnetic field that is intended to induce an electrical current at the fusion site. The effect of pulsed electromagnetic fields for lumbar interbody fusions has been evaluated; fusion rates of 92% and 65% in the experimental and control groups were reported (88). This technique has gained popularity because of its noninvasive nature, but such a device has to be worn eight to 10 hours a day for six to eight months, and as such, its efficacy may be related to long-term patient compliance (87).

Capacitively-coupled electrical stimulation involves a small computer controlled stimulator that delivers alternating current through flexible cables to hydrogel surface electrodes. The leads are placed on either side of the spine at the level of the center of the fusion mass. Patients are instructed to wear the stimulator 24 hours a day until healing has occurred. Goodwin et al. (89) conducted a randomized double-blinded prospective study comparing a capacitively coupled electrical stimulation group with a control group undergoing both interbody and intertransverse lumbar fusion. The authors reported an overall protocol success rate (both clinical and radiographic results rated as successes) of 84.7% for experimental patients and 64.9% for control patients. As with PEMFs, this technique is noninvasive, but it also is dependent on patient compliance (87).

The efficacy of PEMFs and capacitively coupled electrical stimulation are not well verified because of limited study data. These techniques have the advantage of being externally worn, which eliminates the risk of infection and potential removal. The device can only be effective when the patient complies with its use. Notably lower success rates have been reported in patients who did not wear the device for the instructed amount of time (89).

Although some investigations of the ability of electrical stimulation to enhance spinal fusion have shown promising results, they exhibit some limitations. These include poor patient randomization, retrospective design, and in some cases, potential for bias with conflicts of interest. As with other fusion investigations, the lack of an accurate means of assessing the presence of a solid fusion is a confounding factor. Any reported success achieved by the electrical stimulators graded by radiographic criteria must be cautiously interpreted. No direct comparisons of the three electrical stimulation techniques have been made. Future research should provide further insight into the specific mechanisms by which electrical stimulation results in bone growth and thereby lead to further advances in these techniques (87).

Ultrasound

Low-intensity ultrasound has been proposed to accelerate the healing of long bone fractures (17). Accelerated healing with the use of ultrasound in the treatment of tibial shaft fractures has been reported in a prospective, double-blinded study (90). While investigations to evaluate ultrasound in human spinal fusion have not yet been conducted, animal studies have been performed. A study by Glazer (91) reported that rabbits undergoing spinal fusion with ultrasound had a higher rate of fusion as well as increased fusion mass compared to controls. Another study by Aynaci (92) also reported a higher rate of fusion in rabbits using muscle-pediculated bone graft in posterolateral fusion.

CONCLUSIONS

While it is generally accepted that the use of a bone graft or bone graft substitute to augment spinal arthrodesis reduces the risk of pseudarthrosis, it increases cost as well as morbidity in the case of autograft. In evaluating the utility of a particular product, the spinal surgeon must be aware of the data relevant to the arthrodesis application and clinical scenario. Consideration of the biology of healing in different types of spine fusions and the differences between different categories of bone graft substitutes can help surgeons organize the graft selection process.

REFERENCES

1. Boden SD, Schimandle JH. Biology of lumbar spine fusion and bone graft materials. In: International Society for Study of the Lumbar Spine. 2nd ed. The Lumbar Spine, WB Saunders, 1996: 1284–1306.
2. Abbott L. The use of iliac bone in the treatment of ununited fractures. In: Instructional Course Lectures. The American Academy of Orthopedic Surgeons, 1944:13–22.
3. Steinmann JC, Herkowitz HN. Pseudarthrosis of the spine. Clin Orthop Relat Res 1992; (284):80–90.
4. Humphreys SC, Hodges SD, Eck J. Complications of anterior iliac bone graft harvest in anterior cervical fusion. A prospective study of 33 consecutive patients. Loyola Univ Chicago Orthop J 1998; 7:14–16.
5. Fernyhough JC, Schimandle JJ, Weigel MC, et al. Chronic donor site pain complicating bone graft harvesting from the posterior iliac crest for spinal fusion. Spine 1992; 17(12):1474–1480.
6. Summers BN, Eisenstein SM. Donor site pain from the ilium. A complication of lumbar spine fusion. J Bone Joint Surg Br 1989; 71(4):677–680.
7. Arrington ED, Smith WJ, Chambers HG, et al. Complications of iliac crest bone graft harvesting. Clin Orthop Relat Res 1996; (329):300–309.
8. Banwart JC, Asher MA, Hassanein RS. Iliac crest bone graft harvest donor site morbidity. A statistical evaluation. Spine 1995; 20(9):1055–1060.
9. Catinella FP, De Laria GA, De Wald RL. False aneurysm of the superior gluteal artery. A complication of iliac crest bone grafting. Spine 1990; 15(12):1360–1362.
10. Escalas F, DeWald RL. Combined traumatic arteriovenous fistula and ureteral injury: a complication of iliac bone-grafting. J Bone Joint Surg Am 1977; 59(2):270–271.
11. Whang PG, Wang JC. Bone graft substitutes for spinal fusion. Spine J 2003; 3(2):155.
12. Khan SN, Cammisa FP Jr, Sandhu HS, et al. The biology of bone grafting. J Am Acad Orthop Surgeons 2005; 13(1):77.
13. Burkus JK, Sandhu HS, Gornet MF, et al. Use of rhBMP-2 in combination with structural cortical allografts: clinical and radiographic outcomes in anterior lumbar spinal surgery. J Bone Joint Surg Am 2005; 87(6):1205–1212.
14. Vaccaro AR, Patel T, Fischgrund J, et al. A 2-year follow-up pilot study evaluating the safety and efficacy of op-1 putty (rhbmp-7) as an adjunct to iliac crest autograft in posterolateral lumbar fusions. Eur Spine J 2005; 14(7):623–629.
15. Brodsky AE, Kovalsky ES, Khalil MA. Correlation of radiologic assessment of lumbar spine fusions with surgical exploration. Spine 1991; 16(Suppl 6):S261.
16. Dawson EG, Clader TJ, Bassett LW. A comparison of different methods used to diagnose pseudarthrosis following posterior spinal fusion for scoliosis. J Bone Joint Surgery (American volume) 1985; 67(8):1153.
17. Boden SD. Overview of the biology of lumbar spine fusion and principles for selecting a bone graft substitute. Spine 2002; 27(16 Suppl 1):S26.
18. West JL 3rd, Bradford DS, Ogilvie JW. Results of spinal arthrodesis with pedicle screw-plate fixation. J Bone Joint Surg Am 1991; 73(8):1179–1184.
19. Tsuang YH, Yang RS, Chen PQ, et al. Experimental allograft in spinal fusion in dogs. Taiwan Yi Xue Hui Za Zhi 1989; 88(10):989–994.
20. Tomford WW. Transmission of disease through transplantation of musculoskeletal allografts. J Bone Joint Surg Am 1995; 77(11):1742–1754.
21. Asselmeier MA, Caspari RB, Bottenfield S. A review of allograft processing and sterilization techniques and their role in transmission of the human immunodeficiency virus. Am J Sports Med 1993; 21(2):170–175.
22. Stevenson S, Emery SE, Goldberg VM. Factors affecting bone graft incorporation. Clin Orthop Related Res 1996; (324):66.
23. Hamer AJ, Strachan JR, Black MM, et al. Biochemical properties of cortical allograft bone using a new method of bone strength measurement. A comparison of fresh, fresh-frozen and irradiated bone. J Bone Joint Surg (British volume) 1996; 78(3):363.
24. Ehrler DM, Vaccaro AR. The use of allograft bone in lumbar spine surgery. Clin Orthop Relat Res 2000; (371):38.
25. Pelker RR, Friedlaender GE, Markham TC. Biomechanical properties of bone allografts. Clin Orthop Relat Res 1983; (174):54.
26. Cloward RB. The anterior approach for removal of ruptured cervical discs. J Neurosurg 1958; 15:602.
27. Brown MD, Malinin TI, Davis PB. A roentgenographic evaluation of frozen allografts versus autografts in anterior cervical spine fusions. Clin Orthop Relat Res 1976; (119):231–236.

28. Young WF, Rosenwasser RH. An early comparative analysis of the use of fibular allograft versus autologous iliac crest graft for interbody fusion after anterior cervical discectomy. Spine 1993; 18(9):1123–1124.
29. Zdeblick TA, Ducker TB. The use of freeze-dried allograft bone for anterior cervical fusions. Spine 1991; 16(7):726–729.
30. Zhang ZH, Yin H, Yang K, et al. Anterior intervertebral disc excision and bone grafting in cervical spondylotic myelopathy. Spine 1983; 8(1):16–19.
31. Kozak JA, Heilman AE, O'Brien JP. Anterior lumbar fusion options. Technique and graft materials. Clin Orthop Relat Res 1994; (300):45–51.
32. Silcox DH 3rd. Laparoscopic bone dowel fusions of the lumbar spine. Orthop Clin North Am 1998; 29(4):655–663.
33. Buttermann GR, Glazer PA, Hu SS, et al. Revision of failed lumbar fusions. A comparison of anterior autograft and allograft. Spine 1997; 22(23):2748–2755.
34. Jorgenson SS, Lowe TG, France J, et al. A prospective analysis of autograft versus allograft in posterolateral lumbar fusion in the same patient. A minimum of 1-year follow-up in 144 patients. Spine 1994; 19(18):2048–2053.
35. An HS, Simpson JM, Glover JM, et al. Comparison between allograft plus demineralized bone matrix versus autograft in anterior cervical fusion. A prospective multicenter study. Spine 1995; 20(20):2211–2216.
36. Dodd CA, Fergusson CM, Freedman L, et al. Allograft versus autograft bone in scoliosis surgery. J Bone Joint Surg Br 1988; 70(3):431–434.
37. Urist MR. Bone: formation by autoinduction. Science 1965; 150(698):893–899.
38. Finkemeier CG. Bone-grafting and bone-graft substitutes. J Bone Joint Surg Am 2002; 84A(3):454–464.
39. Lee YP, Jo M, Luna M, et al. The efficacy of different commercially available demineralized bone matrix substances in an athymic rat model. J Spinal Disord Tech 2005; 18(5):439.
40. Peterson B, Whang PG, Iglesias R, et al. Osteoinductivity of commercially available demineralized bone matrix. Preparations in a spine fusion model. J Bone Joint Surg (American volume) 2004; 86A(10):2243.
41. Martin GJ Jr, Boden SD, Titus L, et al. New formulations of demineralized bone matrix as a more effective graft alternative in experimental posterolateral lumbar spine arthrodesis. Spine 1999; 24(7):637.
42. Louis-Ugbo J, Murakami H, Kim HS, et al. Evidence of osteoinduction by Grafton demineralized bone matrix in nonhuman primate spinal fusion. Spine 2004; 29(4):360.
43. Kanim LEA, Bae H, Zhao L, et al. Inter and intravariability of BMPs in commercially available demineralized bone matrices. Spine J 2003; 3(5, Suppl 1):81.
44. Schwartz Z, Mellonig JT, De La Fontaine J, et al. Ability of commercial demineralized freeze-dried bone allograft to induce new bone formation. J Periodontol 1996; 67(9):918.
45. Zhang M, Powers RM Jr, Wolfinbarger L Jr. Effect(s) of the demineralization process on the osteoinductivity of demineralized bone matrix. J Periodontol 1997; 68(11):1085–1092.
46. Zhang M, Powers RM Jr, Wolfinbarger L Jr. A quantitative assessment of osteoinductivity of human demineralized bone matrix. J Periodontol 1997; 68(11):1076–1084.
47. Han B, Tang B, Nimni ME. Quantitative and sensitive in vitro assay for osteoinductive activity of demineralized bone matrix. J Orthop Res 2003; 21(4):648.
48. Schwartz Z, Somers A, Mellonig JT, et al. Ability of commercial demineralized freeze-dried bone allograft to induce new bone formation is dependent on donor age but not gender. J Periodontol 1998; 69(4):470–478.
49. Bostrom MPG, Yang X, Kennan M, et al. An unexpected outcome during testing of commercially available demineralized bone graft materials: How safe are the nonallograft components? Spine 2001; 26(13):1425.
50. Wang JC, Kanim LE, Nagakawa IS, et al. Dose-dependent toxicity of a commercially available demineralized bone matrix material. Spine 2001; 26(13):1429.
51. Sassard WR, Eidman DK, Gray PM, et al. Augmenting local bone with Grafton demineralized bone matrix for posterolateral lumbar spine fusion: avoiding second site autologous bone harvest. Orthopedics 2000; 23(10):1059–1064; discussion 1064–1065.
52. Cammisa FP Jr, Lowery G, Garfin SR, et al. Two-year fusion rate equivalency between Grafton DBM gel and autograft in posterolateral spine fusion: a prospective controlled trial employing a side-by-side comparison in the same patient. Spine 2004; 29(6):660–666.
53. Muschler GF, Boehm C, Easley K. Aspiration to obtain osteoblast progenitor cells from human bone marrow: the influence of aspiration volume. J Bone Joint Surg Am 1997; 79(11):1699–1709.
54. Muschler GF, Nitto H, Boehm CA, et al. Age- and gender-related changes in the cellularity of human bone marrow and the prevalence of osteoblastic progenitors. J Orthop Res 2001; 19(1):117–125.
55. Bianco P, Riminucci M, Bonucci E, et al. Bone sialoprotein (BSP) secretion and osteoblast differentiation: relationship to bromodeoxyuridine incorporation, alkaline phosphatase, and matrix deposition. J Histochem Cytochem 1993; 41(2):183–191.

56. Lee K, Deeds JD, Bond AT, et al. In situ localization of PTH/PTHrP receptor mRNA in the bone of fetal and young rats. Bone 1993; 14(3):341–345.
57. Turksen K, Aubin JE. Positive and negative immunoselection for enrichment of two classes of osteo-progenitor cells. J Cell Biol 1991; 114(2):373–384.
58. Strates BS, Stock AJ, Connolly JF. Skeletal repair in the aged: a preliminary study in rabbits. Am J Med Sci 1988; 296(4):266–269.
59. Connolly JF. Common avoidable problems in nonunions. Clin Orthop Relat Res 1985; (194):226–235.
60. Lippiello L, Chavda D, Connolly J. Colony-forming efficiency response of bone marrow stromal cells to acute blood loss. J Orthop Res 1992; 10(1):145–148.
61. Stegemann P, Lorio M, Soriano R, et al. Management protocol for unreamed interlocking tibial nails for open tibial fractures. J Orthop Trauma 1995; 9(2):117–120.
62. Tiedeman JJ, Connolly JF, Strates BS, et al. Treatment of nonunion by percutaneous injection of bone marrow and demineralized bone matrix. An experimental study in dogs. Clin Orthop Relat Res 1991; (268):294–302.
63. Boden SD, Martin GJ Jr, Morone M, et al. The use of coralline hydroxyapatite with bone marrow, auto-genous bone graft, or osteoinductive bone protein extract for posterolateral lumbar spine fusion. Spine 1999; 24(4):320–327.
64. Kai T, Shao-qing G, Geng-ting D. In vivo evaluation of bone marrow stromal-derived osteoblasts-porous calcium phosphate ceramic composites as bone graft substitute for lumbar intervertebral spinal fusion. Spine 2003; 28(15):1653–1658.
65. Cui Q, Ming Xiao Z, Balian G, et al. Comparison of lumbar spine fusion using mixed and cloned marrow cells. Spine 2001; 26(21):2305–2310.
66. Muschler GF, Nitto H, Matsukura Y, et al. Spine fusion using cell matrix composites enriched in bone marrow-derived cells. Clin Orthop Relat Res 2003; (407):102–118.
67. Curylo LJ, Johnstone B, Petersilge CA, et al. Augmentation of spinal arthrodesis with autologous bone marrow in a rabbit posterolateral spine fusion model. Spine 1999; 24(5):434–438; discussion 438–439.
68. Tay BK, Le AX, Heilman M, et al. Use of a collagen-hydroxyapatite matrix in spinal fusion. A rabbit model. Spine 1998; 23(21):2276–2281.
69. Kraiwattanapong C, Boden SD, Louis-Ugbo J, et al. Comparison of Healos/bone marrow to INFUSE(rhBMP-2/ACS) with a collagen-ceramic sponge bulking agent as graft substitutes for lumbar spine fusion. Spine 2005; 30(9):1001–1007; discussion 1007.
70. Kitchel S. Prospective randomized evaluation of healos/bone marrow aspirate versus autologous iliac crest bone graft in posterolateral lumber spine fusion. In: IMAST. Bermuda, 2004.
71. Welch W, Gerszten P, Sherman J, et al. A prospective randomized study of interbody fusion: bone substitute or autograft. Halle, Germany: DePuy, 2002.
72. Price CT, Connolly JF, Carantzas AC, et al. Comparison of bone grafts for posterior spinal fusion in adolescent idiopathic scoliosis. Spine 2003; 28(8):793–798.
73. Papavero L, Zwonitzer R, Burkard I, et al. A composite bone graft substitute for anterior cervical fusion: assessment of osseointegration by quantitative computed tomography. Spine 2002; 27(10):1037–1043.
74. Connolly J, Guse R, Lippiello L, et al. Development of an osteogenic bone-marrow preparation. J Bone Joint Surg Am 1989; 71(5):684–691.
75. Howes R, Bowness JM, Grotendorst GR, et al. Platelet-derived growth factor enhances demineralized bone matrix-induced cartilage and bone formation. Calcified Tissue International 1988; 42(1):34.
76. Marden LJ, Fan RS, Pierce GF, et al. Platelet-derived growth factor inhibits bone regeneration induced by osteogenin, a bone morphogenetic protein, in rat craniotomy defects. J Clin Investigation 1993; 92(6):2897.
77. Harris SE, Bonewald LF, Harris MA, et al. Effects of transforming growth factor beta on bone nodule formation and expression of bone morphogenetic protein 2, osteocalcin, osteopontin, alkaline phosphatase, and type I collagen mRNA in long-term cultures of fetal rat calvarial osteoblasts. J Bone Miner Res 1994; 9(6):855–863.
78. Lowery GL, Kulkarni S, Pennisi AE. Use of autologous growth factors in lumbar spinal fusion. Bone 1999; 25(2, Suppl 1):47S.
79. Castro FP Jr. Role of activated growth factors in lumbar spinal fusions. J Spinal Disord Tech 2004; 17(5):380–384.
80. Carreon LY, Glassman SD, Anekstein Y, et al. Platelet gel (AGF) fails to increase fusion rates in instru-mented posterolateral fusions. Spine 2005; 30(9):E243.
81. Weiner BK, Walker M. Efficacy of autologous growth factors in lumbar intertransverse fusions. Spine 2003; 28(17):1968.
82. Boden SD. Point of view [Editorial]. Spine 2003; 28(17):1971.
83. Kane WJ. Direct current electrical bone growth stimulation for spinal fusion. Spine 1988; 13(3): 363–365.

84. Meril AJ. Direct current stimulation of allograft in anterior and posterior lumbar interbody fusions. Spine 1994; 19(21):2393.

85. Kucharzyk DW. A controlled prospective outcome study of implantable electrical stimulation with spinal instrumentation in a high-risk spinal fusion population. Spine 1999; 24(5):465–468; discussion 469.

86. Rogozinski A, Rogozinski C. Efficacy of implanted bone growth stimulation in instrumented lumbo-sacral spinal fusion. Spine 1996; 21(21):2479–2483.

87. Hodges SD, Eck JC, Humphreys SC. Use of electrical bone stimulation in spinal fusion. J Am Acad Orthop Surgeons 2003; 11(2):81.

88. Mooney V. A randomized double-blind prospective study of the efficacy of pulsed electromagnetic fields for interbody lumbar fusions. Spine 1990; 15(7):708.

89. Goodwin CB, Brighton CT, Guyer RD, et al. A double-blind study of capacitively coupled electrical stimulation as an adjunct to lumbar spinal fusions. Spine 1999; 24(13):1349.

90. Heckman JD, Ryaby JP, McCabe J, et al. Acceleration of tibial fracture-healing by non-invasive, low-intensity pulsed ultrasound. J Bone Joint Surg (American volume) 1994; 76(1):26.

91. Glazer PA, Heilmann MR, Lotz JC, et al. Use of ultrasound in spinal arthrodesis. A rabbit model. Spine 1998; 23(10):1142.

92. Aynaci O, Onder C, Piskin A, et al. The effect of ultrasound on the healing of muscle-pediculated bone graft in spinal fusion. Spine 2002; 27(14):1531.

33 | Current Concepts in Vertebroplasty and Kyphoplasty

Hwan Tak Hee
Department of Orthopaedic Surgery, National University of Singapore, Singapore

INTRODUCTION

With an aging population around the world, osteoporotic and osteolytic vetrebral compression fractures are increasingly common. Peak bone mass is obtained by age 35, after which all individuals lose a small amount each year. Half of all women older than 65 have radiographic evidence of osteoporosis, and 90% are affected by age 75. The most serious consequence of osteoporosis is the occurrence of pathological fracture, In the past, osteoporotic compression fractures were often treated with benign neglect, whereas much attention had been paid to the management of osteoporotic hip fractures. The irony is that the number of osteoporotic compression fractures per year in the United States far exceed the number of osteoporotic hip fractures (1).

Though less common than osteoporotic compression fractures, osteolytic vertebral fractures due to metastasis, multiple myeloma, or aggressive benign tumors (e.g., hemangiomas) can be extremely painful, with a clinical presentation not unlike that of osteoporotic compression fractures.

Complications of osteoporotic or osteolytic fractures include spinal cord compression, urinary retention, and ileus (2). Other complications reported include chronic pain (3) and pulmonary compromise (4). There is a 9% loss of predicted forced vital capacity with each vertebral fracture (4). These patients can suffer considerable physical, functional, and psychosocial impairments manifesting as depression and insomnia (5). One study showed that osteoporotic compression fractures are associated with 30% age-adjusted increase in mortality (6).

Traditional treatment of osteoporotic compression fractures include bed rest, analgesics, brace, and gradual mobilization. Unfortunately, many patients still have intractable pain and are unable to return to their activities of daily living. This is understandable because medical management fails to restore or prevent worsening of spinal alignment, and the immobility status of the patients can further lead to other complications, for example, atelectasis, pneumonia, decubitus ulcers, deep vein thrombosis, pulmonary embolism, urinary tract infection, and worsening osteoporosis. It is known fact that one week of prolonged recumbency will result in 10% loss of bone mass.

In spinal tumors resulting in osteolytic compression fractures, traditional treatment option includes the use of radiotherapy (7). It has been reported that about 50% of patients with spinal metastasis do well with this treatment, particularly with radiosensitive tumors, for example, breast, prostate, and myeloma. However, the spine is still prone to progressive osteolytic collapse.

Surgery has been the traditional treatment of choice in osteoporotic and osteolytic compression fractures if the patient fails non-surgical treatment. Surgical approaches may vary from anterior only decompression and instrumentation, posterior only decompression and instrumentation, and combined anterior–posterior surgery (either staged or same day). Indications for surgical intervention are usually reserved for gross spinal deformity or impending neurological deficit. Caution is exercised when recommending surgery because of the adverse risk–benefit ratio in the elderly/cancer population with poor bone stock and co-morbidities.

Vertebroplasty describes a surgical technique using bone graft, cement, or metal implants to modify or reconstruct damaged or destroyed vertebra. This was traditionally done via open surgery. Percutaneous vertebroplasty was first performed by Galibert and Deramond in 1984. They injected polymethylmethacrylate (PMMA) into a C2 vertebra that had been destroyed by an aggressive hamangioma (8). Dusquenel, subsequently, used this technique to treat compression fractures associated with osteoporosis and malignancy (9). In 1993, the technique of percutaneous vertebroplasty was introduced in the United States by Dion and colleagues, and they reported 85% to 90% significant pain relief for painful osteoporotic compression fractures (10). Percutaneous vertebroplasty has, since, grown in popularity to become the standard of care for painful osteoporotic compression fractures of the spine (11).

VERTEBROPLASTY—PATIENT WORKUP AND SELECTION

Successful results form vertebroplasty require vigorous patient selection. A good history is mandatory, taking particular attention to define whether the compression fractures belong to osteoporotic or osteolytic category. A thorough review of body systems, including checking for night pain, fever, loss of weight, loss of appetite, bladder, or bowel changes should be performed. It is helpful to check if the patient has had medical treatment for osteoporosis before. One should also ask for any previous history of cancer, tuberculosis, and other systemic infection. A history of cancer does not always denote that the vertebral fracture is osteolytic, as one-third of compression fractures in known malignancy are benign.

Good candidates for vertebroplasty describe a focal, intense, deep pain in the midline of the spine. The pain should be mechanical, that is, worse with loading and better with recumbency (12). Vertebroplasty may be considered if the pain is worsening or there is a plateau of functional recovery with significant pain remaining. The type of pain, that is, axial versus radicular pain is also important to note, as those with significantly more radicular pain suggests nerve root compression, which may not benefit from vertebroplasty, It is not uncommon to find patients having referred pain, and this finding is not considered a contraindication to vertebroplasty. Some authors advocate placing a metallic marker at the maximal point of tenderness and correlate this fluoroscopically with the anatomical location of the pain. They found the accuracy to be limited to no better than plus or minus one vertebral level in most cases (13).

The time between fracture occurrence and initial consult should be noted. There is no definite exclusion criteria based on the time of the fracture. However, older fractures (more than three months) are less likely to benefit from vertebroplasty. The exceptions to this rule are the presence of nonunion or recurrent fracture. Nonunion is indicated by abnormal persistent motion on fluoroscopy and the finding of a fluid cleft on MRI which shows up as high signal intensity on T2 weighted scans. Nonunion is not infrequently associated with osteonecrosis (Kümmell's disease), which some authors consider a good indication for vertebroplasty (14). An MRI finding of marrow edema may imply new or recurrent fracture which maybe amenable to vertebroplaty.

Clinical examination should include assessing for spinal deformity and body posture. One may also find associated rib tenderness due to osteoporotic fractures. The pain over the vertebra should increase with flexion, and relieved with extension. Neurological assessment is mandatory since some patients may have "senile burst fractures," which have greater propensity for bony retropulsion leading to neurological deficit.

Good quality imaging is mandatory to allow for proper decision making regarding treatment strategy for these patients. The aims of imaging are several fold, including extent of vertebral collapse, extent of lytic process, degree of involvement of pedicles, posterior cortical wall breach, central and/or foraminal stenosis, and age of fracture. The initial imaging investigation of choice is plain X-rays. It may be helpful to do an erect X-ray of the whole spine to better evaluate the overall spinal balance of the patient. The number of deformities should be noted. Comparison with previous X-rays is useful as they may demonstrate further collapse. Signs suggestive of posterior wall breach include widening of inter-pedicular distance and greater than 50% collapse in height of the vertebra. The level of fractures is important to note, since one study found that fractures occurring above T6 are more likely than not to be neoplastic (15).

Dual energy absorptiometry (DEXA) should be obtained for osteoporotic cases. The data can be used to predict future fracture risks, and can also be used as a baseline for effectiveness of medical treatment of osteoporosis.

Bone scan may help to differentiate the age of the fracture, as a recent fracture will show up as a "hot" spot. However, it does not demonstrate other details, for example, posterior wall integrity, pedicle involvement, presence of paraspinal soft tissue masses which the MRI is able to delineate. For this reason, magnetic resonance imaging (MRI) is now the imaging modality of choice for assessing compression fractures in finer details. Acute fractures will demonstrate edema as decreased T1 and increased T2 or short T1 inversion recovery (STIR) signals (16). MRI is also useful in differentiating between osteoporotic fractures from pathological fractures due to metastasis or infections. Features suggestive of osteolytic fractures as opposed to osteoporotic fractures are heterogeneous bone marrow appearance, absence of fracture clefts, involvement of pedicles, paraspinal soft tissue extension, epidural extension, and multilevel involment.

VERTEBROPLASTY—INDICATIONS AND CONTRAINDICATIONS

Persistent pain after occurrence of compression fracture is an indication for vertebroplasty. The question is how long to wait before offering vertebroplasty to these patients. To the best of my knowledge, there is still no consensus to this question. Some authors will persist with conservative treatment (not applicable to osteolytic fractures) for four to six weeks before performing vertebroplasty (12). In my practice, I am offering vertebroplasty to patients earlier than when I first started performing this procedure. One of the reasons is the significantly good results in terms of pain relief after this procedure. Another is my hypothesis that early aggressive treatment of vertebral compression fractures may prevent progressive kyphosis and its sequelae (17).

Continuing collapse of the fractured vertebra on follow-up, especially with concomitant pain, is also an indication for vertebroplasty. Other fracture patterns that may benefit from vertebroplasty are those occurring at the thoraco-lumbar junction, those greater than 30° kyphosis, and those with presence of vacuum shadow in the vertebra signifying ischemic necrosis. There is currently no role for prophylactic vertebroplasty except at the ends of long posterior spinal instrumentation to prevent "topping-off syndrome."

There are several contraindications to performing vertebroplasty. Presence of neurological deficit is a contraindication, since any cement leakage albeit minor, may lead to catastrophic neurological deficit. Younger patients (younger than 65 years of age) are also not advised to undergo this procedure for two reasons. First, these patients do have the capability for bony healing, and they should not be denied the opportunity for the fracture to unite. Vertebroplasty will prevent the fracture from healing. Secondly, we still do not know the long-term effects of PMMA in the vertebrae. Perhaps, the future lies in the improvement of biomaterials for example, biodegradable and bioabsorbable materials.

Pregnant patients should not undergo vertebroplasty since they are young, and this procedure needs fluoroscopy. Allergy to any of the materials used in vertebroplasty, presence of coagulopathy, active systemic infection, and severe cardiopulmonary compromise to the extent that the patient is unable to lie prone are also contraindications for vertebroplasty.

High velocity injuries leading to burst fractures, chance fractures, or fractures- dislocations are contraindications to vertebroplasty, as they are more appropriately treated with traditional surgery.

Technical reasons, for example, vertebra plana or severe vertebral collapse (>70% reduction in height) (18), posterior cortical wall disruption, and presence of osteoblastic tumor may pose a technical challenge in vertebroplasty. As one gets over the learning curve, these may be listed instead as "extended indications" for vertebroplasty. I have performed vertebroplasty on cases with posterior cortical wall breach and osteoblastic tumor. Others no longer routinely consider vertebra plana as a contraindication (19).

VERTEBROPLASTY—BIOMECHANICS

The most intuitive explanation for the mechanism of pain relief involves simple mechanical stabilization of the fracture. The PMMA stabilizes the vertebral bodies and offloads the facet joints. Another possibility is that analgesia results from local chemical, vascular or thermal effects of PMMA on nerve endings in surrounding soft tissues (20). Supporting this theory is the fact that there is lack of correlation between cement volume and pain relief (21).

Restoration of vertebral stiffness and load-bearing capacity is postulated to eliminate painful micromotion in compression fractures (22). Small amounts of PMMA (14% fill or 3.5 cm^2) can restore the stiffness to the previous level (23). Less cement is required to restore strength; more cement is required to restore stiffness (24). Larger vertebral bodies require more cement for restoration of strength and stiffness, though complete fill is not needed. Similar clinical results are attained for both uni- and bipedicular PMMA fill of the vertebral bodies. Recent studies have focused on new biomaterials, for example, bioresorbable cements. Most are able to restore mechanical integrity of the vertebral body in vitro (25).

One concern about vertebroplasty is the possible increased adjacent fracture risk by placing a hard material in close proximity to osteoporotic bone of the adjacent levels. One study showed that vertebrae adjacent to treated level had an odds ratio of 2.27 for fracture versus 1.44 odds ratio for vertebrae in the vicinity of uncemented fractured vertebra (26). However, if there is correction of spinal deformity by postural reduction during positioning prior to vertebroplasty, the procedure may actually reduce the risk of adjacent level fracture by restoring the spinal column to a more physiological alignment.

This also explains why a modification of vertebroplasty using balloon tamps (kyphoplasty) may reduce the fracture risk at adjacent levels, as inflation of the tamps will restore lost vertebral height of the fractured vertebra.

VERTEBROPLASTY—TECHNIQUE

Vertebroplasty is usually perfomed under local anesthesia and sedation, with close monitoring of the patient's parameters by the anesthesiologist. The preferred sedation used in my institution consists of 3 to 4 mg of midazolam and 50 to 100 mg of fentanyl. Prophylactic antibiotic (1 g of cefazolin) is routinely given, since this procedure involves injecting foreign material (PMMA) into the body. I prefer to use a completely radiolucent table [e.g., Jackson Orthopedic Systems Inc. (OSI) table (OSI, Union City, California, U.S.A.) illustrated in Fig. 1] so that the C-arm has complete access in performing true AP and lateral images of the spine, which is critical to the success of the procedure. Degenerative scoliosis and spinal metastasis with destroyed pedicles may impair proper visualization of the pedicles. Some authors (usually radiologists) prefer to perform vertebroplasty under CT guidance (19). The patient is initially placed prone on the table. Patients who cannot tolerate this position for an hour may not be suitable candidates for vertebroplasty under local anesthesia. Performing vertebroplasty under general

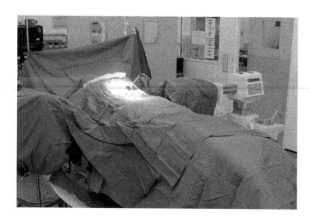

FIGURE 1 Illustration of the radiolucent Jackson OSI table used in vertebroplasty, as well as patient/C-arm positioning. Note the two needle trocars in place for a bipedicular approach to the vertebral body.

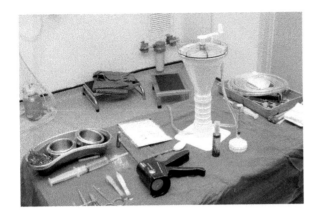

FIGURE 2 Illustration of the set-up of the vertebroplasty system.

anesthesis maybe the next best option, but the major disadvantages are the risk of general anesthesia in these elderly patients and the inability to gather verbal feedback from the patients regarding leg symptoms should there be cement extravasation into the spinal canal.

The operative field is subsequently cleaned and draped in a sterile fashion. Figure 2 illustrates the set-up of the vertebroplasty system. Localization of the pedicles is performed with the aid of the fluoroscopy. Local anesthesia is subsequently given from the skin, subcutaneous layer, and the periosteum of the bone at the bone entry site. A 0.5 cm paramedian incision is made on either side of the spine, for insertion of the 11-gauge trocar-cannula system. The most frequently used route is the transpedicular. This is a familiar route for surgeons used to placement of pedicle screws. It also offers several advantages over the parapedicular route. First of all, the pedicle provides a definite anatomical landmark for needle targeting. Secondly, it is an effective route for vertebroplasty and biopsy of lesions (osteolytic fractures) inside the vertebra. Thirdly, it does not carry the danger of needle damage to adjacent structures, for example, nerve root and lung, as long as one maintains an intrapedicular route throughout.

The parapedicular approach may be useful in the middle to upper thoracic spine, where the pedicles may be small and unable to accommodate the standard 11-gauge trocar-cannula system. This approach allows the needle tip to be angled more toward the center of the vertebra than the transpediclar route. This may allow easier filling of the vertebra with a single needle. The inherent dangers lie in iatrogenic damage to surrounding structures mentioned earlier. It is also harder to tamponade any paraspinous hematoma formed after needle removal from the lateral side of the vertebral body.

Using the transpedicular route, the needle is centered at the 10 o'clock over the left pedicle and 2 o'clock over the right pedicle on the anteroposterior (AP) view with the help of a long needle holder, thus avoiding radiation to the surgeon's hands. One may have to start the entry point slightly more superior, so that the needle is able to traverse the vertebral body without penetrating the fractured and collapsed superior end plate. The needle should also be medialized through the cylinder of the pedicle to reach the middle of the vertebra. Once a footprint is obtained by the needle in the pedicle, and the position is considered ideal on the AP view, advancement of the needle will be done under the guidance of the lateral fluoroscopy (Fig. 3). In osteoporotic bone, penetrating the bony cortex and advancing the needle into the vertebral body is easy. In contrast, the bone in osteoblastic tumor may be hard and dense, except where it is destroyed by tumor. One may consider in this scenario to use a mallet to advance the needle rather than manual manipulation. The tip of the needle should lie beyond the midpoint of the vertebral body on the lateral view. The ideal endpoint is the junction between the anterior and middle thirds of the vertebral body, since this area is relatively devoid of venous plexuses.

I routinely place two needles into the vertebral body, that is, bipedicular approach even though clinical results are reportedly similar with single-versus double-needle approach (27). There are several advantages of the two needle technique. I am more confident of a complete vertebral fill using this technique. The second cannula may act as a "vent" during cement

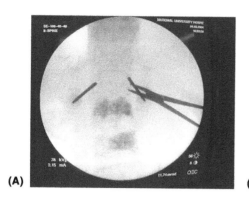 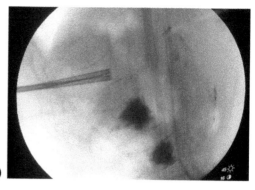

(A) **(B)**

FIGURE 3 (**A**) Illustration of the technique of needle placement of L1 vertebra under the guidance of the C-arm. (**B**) Vertebroplasty had already been performed at the L3 and L2 vertebrae.

injection through the other cannula, reducing the risk of cement extravasation. I can terminate injection through one cannula if there is cement leakage on fluoroscopy, and move on to the other cannula without the worry about not being able to achieve a complete vertebral fill.

Venogram or vertebrogram is used next to identify potential leak sites (particularly into the spinal canal via the epidural venous plexus), which if present, may warrant adjustment of the needle position (Fig. 4). The commonly used agents are omnipaque 300 or isovue 300. Some authors have found no benefits from using venogram/vertebrogram, because the contrast material and the bone cement differ greatly in viscosity (28). Others have found no added benefits in terms of increasing the safety of the procedure with the use of venogam (29). Nevertheless, I still find venography necessary and useful in my practice. If there is no significant extravasation on venography, I am very confident that there will be no cement leakage during cement injection.

Cement is prepared when the position of the needles is ideal and there is no significant extravasation on venography. Cement with adequate opacification (barium or tantalum beads) is used so that injection can be monitored in real time to detect any extravasation. It is shown that barium sulfate in quantities of about 30% by weight mixed with PMMA will provide adequate opacification (30). Certain cement (for example, Simplex P) only contains 10% by weight of barium. Therefore, additional barium should be added to obtain adequate opacification. I will remove about one teaspoon of cement powder (10 mL), and substitute with one teaspoon (6 g) of barium. Current cement manufactured for vertebroplasty, for example, Spineplex® (Stryker, Kalamazoo, Michigan, U.S.A.) and Cranioplastic® (Johnson & Johnson, Raynham, Massachusetts, U.S.A.) contains sufficient barium.

One can slow the polymerization and thus increase the working time by chilling the cement once mixed. Syringes to be used for injection are placed in sterile cold cardioplegic solution.

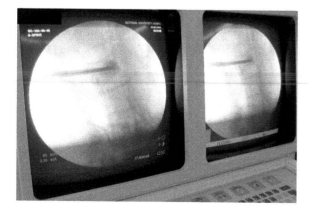

FIGURE 4 Illustration of venography being carried out to confirm that there was no significant leakage of the injected dye (Omnipaque or Isovue).

Using a monomer that has been chilled at near 0°C for 24 hours or more can also slow the polymerization of the cement.

Some authors will routinely add tobramycin to the PMMA before injection. I rely more on prophylactic intravenous antibiotic and maintenance of sterility throughout the procedure. I prefer closed vacuum mixing of the cement as this maintains a sterile environment Open mixing increases the chance of cement contamination and reduces the cement strength by inclusion of air bubbles.

One should inject the cement when it is no longer in a liquid consistency, in order to minimize the risk of extravasation. The cement injection should be monitored real time or small amounts (0.1–0.2 mL) and the result verified before further cement injection takes place. This is done under the guidance of lateral C-arm image. I usually work through one cannula first before moving to the second cannula. This preserves a route for subsequent injection, should a leak be discovered. Moving to the second cannula will complete the vertebral fill without further leak as the original leak will be occluded by the initial cement, which will have hardened. Additional amounts of cement can be delivered by pushing the trocar into the cannula, allowing a further 0.9 mL cement per cannula (1 1-gauge) to be introduced into the vertebra.

The amount of cement required to produce pain relief is still uncertain. One study performed in vitro showed that prefracture stiffness and strength can be restored by 2.5 to 4 mL of cement in the thoracic vertebra, and 6 to 8 mL in the lumbar vertebra (31). This amounts to 50% to 70% fill of the residual volume of the compressed vertebra. Significant strength restoration can be provided with a unipedicular approach if the cement filling crosses the midline of the vertebra (32).

The maximum number of levels to be injected at one setting is also not determined. According to one author, there is no limit as to the number of levels that can be performed, especially if the patient is under general anesthesia (33). However, the current consensus by most experts is that no more than three levels should be attempted at one setting. This minimizes the risk of hemodynamic compromise to the patient from micro-embolization (cement and fat emboli) that may not be apparent from fluoroscopy. The risk of cement leakage is almost twice in osteolytic fractures as compared with osteoporotic compression fractures, and thus I will recommend that this rule be even more stringently applied to spinal metastasis.

After injection of cement is completed, the patient is kept prone until the cement completely hardens, I will rest the patient in bed for the rest of the day, and only start ambulation the following day. This is especially so for the slower setting cement, for example, cranioplastic.

VERTEBROPLASTY—PITFALLS AND COMPLICATIONS

The complications encountered with vertebroplasty can be related to anesthesia, misplacement of instruments, cement extravasation, adjacent level fracture, and infection.

Cement leakage can occur via fracture clefts, improper instrument position, or vertebral venous plexus. This can be overcome by high-quality imaging, adequate barium for opacification, and slow application of PMMA in a viscous state. The cement leakage rate is approximately 6% in osteoporotic compression fractures (26) and 10% in metastasis (34). Cement leakage into adjacent disc space via a pre-existing fracture cleavage plane that extends into the disc space may greatly increase the risk of adjacent level fractures. The rate of asymptomatic leak into the disc space and spinal canal varies from 0% to 65% (10,16,19,26,27,34). The disc normally is the least stiff structure in the spinal column, and helps to dissipate the stress. Leakage of cement into the disc will stiffen-up the disc, and therefore, increases the chance of adjacent level fracture.

The risk of neurological sequelae ranges from 0% to 4% according to various reports (10,16,19,26,27,34) Cement leaking from the vertebra adjacent to a nerve root may produce radicular pain. Analgesics, local steroid, and anesthetic injections should provide adequate relief, provided there are no motor deficits (including bladder and bowel). CT scan on an emergent basis should be arranged if there are significant motor deficits, and is usually associated with large volume leaks resulting in neurological compression.

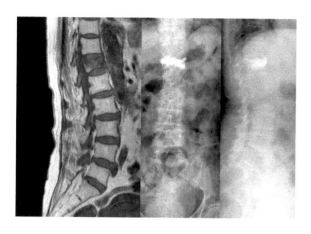

FIGURE 5 Vertebroplasty performed on a patient with T12 osteoporotic compression fracture.

Cement leakage via the venous system has also been associated with pulmonary embolism (10). These are usually not symptomatic, but may rarely produce clinical symptoms accompanying pulmonary infarct. With a right to left shunt, this may result in the development of cerebral infarct (35).

Complication rate is considerably higher in spinal metastasis due to lytic areas involving the vertebral cortex and the propensity for cement leakage into the surrounding tissues (estimated at 10%). Because the introduction of cement involves pushing marrow out of the intertrabecular space, there is concern about fat emboli as well as cement emboli.

CLINICAL RESULTS

There are currently no randomized prospective trials evaluating the efficacy of vertebroplasty. Evans conducted a prospective evaluation of 72 patients pre and postvertebroplasty, and found substantial lasting reduction in pain and improvement in ability to perform activities of daily living (36). Zoarski presented a prospective non-randomized study of the effectiveness of vertebroplasty in relieving pain (37). Utilizing the Musculoskeletal Outcomes Data Evaluation and Management Scale (MODEMS), 22 out of 23 cases improved and remained satisfied during 15 to 28 month follow-up.

In our institution, we have performed vertebroplasty on 54 patients with a minimum of two years follow-up. There were 46 cases of osteoporotic compression fractures (Fig. 5). There were eight cases of spinal metastasis (Fig. 6) leading to osteolytic compression fractures (four breast and four lung). The male to female ratio was 1:4. Thirty-eight patients had single level fractures; 10 had double level fractures; six had triple level fractures. The total number of levels injected were 73. Three levels had to be abandoned because of persistent leakage on

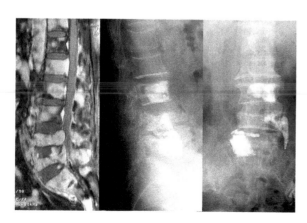

FIGURE 6 Vertebroplasty performed on a case of breast carcinoma with multilevel spinal metastasis and symptomatic pathological fractures from L3 to L5 vertebra. Note the extracorporeal cement leak at L4 vertebra.

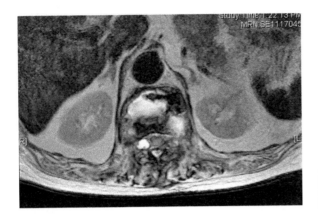

FIGURE 7 Illustration of cement leak in the intervertebral foramen of T12LI on the right, evident only on MRI.

venography, despite adjustment of needle position. Ten injected levels were performed via a unipedicular approach due to persistent dye extravasation through the contralateral pedicle. The length of hospital stay ranged from 1 to 27 days (mean 6 days; median 2 days). At latest follow-up, significant pain relief (defined as decrease of VAS scores of more than 5%) was reported in 52 patients (96%). One patient did not have significant relief because he also had concomitant sacral insufficiency fracture that was not injected with cement, as we did not have experience in sacroplasty (vertebroplasty in sacrum) during the early part of our learning curve. We had one case who developed congestive heart failure after vertebroplasty, and had to be managed in the ICU for 5 days. He had carcinoma of the lung with metastasis to L2 vertebra. He also had poor cardiac function with an ejection fraction of only 26%. We noted three cases of cement extrusion: intradiscal (1), extra-corporeal (1), and neural foramen (1). The extracorporeal leak was due to inadvertent penetration of the anterior border of the L4 vertebra in a case of osteolytic breast metastasis in L3 to L5 vertebrae (Fig. 6). There was one case of cement leak into the intervertebral foramen T12L1 on the right. The leak was not apparent on plain radiographs, and the patient was asymptomatic till four months, later when she presented with sudden weakness of both legs. MRI of the spine was ordered which revealed the above-mentioned finding (Fig. 7). Her weakness spontaneously improved after a week. The cause of the weakness was probably due to hypokalemia which was corrected. Till now, we have not documented any adjacent level fractures in all patients who underwent vertebroplasty. Perhaps, a longer follow-up is needed to assess the incidence of adjacent level fractures.

Favorable results have also been reported using vertebroplasty to manage spinal metastasis. Alvarez reported his experience with vertebroplasty in vertebral tumors (38). In his series, he found excellent results in 66%, decreased pain in 22%, and no change in 12% of his patients. He would not perform vertebroplasty if there is evidence of epidural compression and/or if the posterior wall of the vertebra is not intact on the side of the vertebroplasty. Fourney reported significant pain relief over time in his patients who had painful vertebral body fractures secondary to cancer spread (39). In his series, the absence of cement leakage-related complications probably reflects the use of high-viscosity cement, kyphoplasty in selected cases, and relatively small amounts of cement injected.

A recent study examined predictors of outcome of percutaneous vertebroplasty for osteoporotic vertebral fractures (40). They found better results to be expected in patients with American Society of Anesthesiologists score of 1 and when the vertebral level managed is confirmed by MRI, and the vertebral body height loss is less than 70%.

The future advances in vertebroplasty will probably come from improvements in biomaterials. Although PMMA is widely used in vertebroplasty with good clinical results, they are not ideal. They are not bioabsorbable and biocompatible, and cannot participate in any bony healing. Exothermic reaction of PMMA can cause thermal necrosis to surrounding soft tissues. Any significant cement leakage can have deleterious clinical consequences. Monomer toxicity is also an issue that the physician has to contend with. Newer substitutes are currently being on trial and may offer viable alternatives to PMMA in the future.

Examples are calcium sulfate cement and calcium phosphate cement (CPC). These cements are biocompatible, osteoconductive, euthermic, and are bioabsorbable. One study recently examined vertebral augmentation with calcium sulfate cement in osteoporotic compression fractures (41). They found similar strength and stiffness between the use of calcium sulfate and PMMA. The degree of restoration of strength and stiffness was greater than expected. They concluded that the lower potential stiffness of calcium sulfate may reduce the complications of adjacent level fractures. They may also be suitable agents for the incorporation of growth factors that facilitate bony ingrowth.

Another article evalualed the use of CPC in vertebroplasty (42). They found reliable early relief of pain with his procedure. However, maintenance of pain relief and kyphosis is not encouraging. Union rate was 80%, with the remaining 20% still exhibiting intravertebral clefts. They concluded that CPC alone may not offer sufficient anterior column support.

A recent biomechanical study examined the feasibility of using polypropylene fumarate (PPF) as an injectable bone cement for kyphoplasty. They concluded that addition of barium sulfate for visualization by up to 50% did not adversely affect the compressive strength and stiffness properties of PPF. PPF imparts comparable strength and stiffness to vertebral bodies to PMMA (43).

KYPHOPLASTY

Kyphoplasty is a newer technique, and may be potentially safer than vertebroplasty. It was developed to reduce vertebral body deformity while providing similar pain relief as vertebroplasty. Theoretically, the reduction of kyphosis has several advantages. First of all, the risk of subsequent vertebral fractures maybe reduced, as spinal realignment offered by kyphoplasty may reduce the deformity and the forces on other adjacent vertebrae (44). The second advantage related to the lower extravsation rate during cement delivery, as the cement is delivered at a lower pressure into the void created by the kyphoplasty device. The other advantage may improve the vital lung capacity and gastrointestinal function by reducing the kyphosis associated with compression fractures (45). One maybe tempted to perform kyphoplasty at every level, but spinal balance and curve progression must be taken into consideration when planning for this procedure (44).

There are currently two systems in the market for kyphoplasty, to the best of my knowledge. One uses a balloon-like device (bone tamp) to create a void in the vertebral body before cement delivery (Kyphon, Sunnyvale, California, U.S.A.). The other uses a plastic device which is expandable once placed in the vertebral body (Sky bone expander, Disc-O-Tech, Monroe Township, New Jersey, U.S.A.). Fractures treated within the first three to four weeks offered the best opportunity for height restoration, as they are unlikely to heal to a substantial degree. The exclusion criteria for kyphoplasty are somewhat similar to that of vertebroplasty. There must be sufficient residual height for the kyphoplasty instruments to be inserted into the vertebral body, as the instruments used in kyphoplasty are larger than vertebroplasty. Small pedicles may pose an obstacle to performing kyphoplasty, as the surgeon may need to consider using an alternative route via the parapedicular approach. Most studies showed that kyphoplasty can be safely performed from T7 to L5 (46).

The technical aspects to performing kyphoplasty are similar to vertebroplasty. A 10° en face fluoroscopy view looking straight down at the pedicle has the advantage, in which the surgeon can see the edges of the pedicle and is able to ensure that his working instrument stays within the pedicle. As the learning curve progresses, one may just opt for the standard AP view for needle placement to reduce C-arm movements.

The needle position should also be tailored to the individual fracture patterns. For example, if the fracture is superior, the needle should be positioned inferior to the midline. If the fracture is inferior, the needle is best placed superior to the midline. If the height of the vertebral body is less than 1.5 cm the needle should be aimed at the center or the vertebral body on lateral view. If the height of the body is less than 0.9 mm, then the fracture may not be amenable to kyphoplasty (47). Optimal cement injection should fill the anterior two-thirds of the vertebral body. The patient should remain prone until the cement hardens completely.

The future of kyphoplasty may include the use of this technique in compression fractures in young adults. Furthermore, methods to seal-off the posterior portion of the vertebral body may facilitate augmentation of burst fractures (currently a contraindication) with minimal risk of retropulsion (44). The balloon tamp can also be made biocompatible and resorbable. This will fruther enhance the safety of the procedure by allowing the balloon to be left inside the vertebral body as a barrier to cement extravasation.

SUMMARY

With the increasingly aging population in many countries, symptomatic osteoporotic compression fractures are becoming common and important conditions to manage. Osteolytic compression fractures from spinal metastasis are also becoming more frequent because of the longer life expectancy from improvements in chemotherapy. Percutaneous vertebroplasty with PMMA has been shown to be an effective procedure to treat pain due to these fractures. It is a minimally invasive procedure performed under local anesthesia and sedation. Injection of PMMA provides immediate stability when it hardens, allowing the patient to ambulate without pain. Appropriate patient selection is the key to clinical success. However, this procedure must be treated with respect, and has to be performed by physicians with the necessary training. Otherwise, increased pain, paralysis, and even death may occur. Balloon vertebroplasty or kyphoplasty also reliably reduces pain in these patients, and maybe associated with a lower incidence of complications from cement extravasation, Kyphoplasty is also able to restore partially the sagittal spinal alignment, thereby reducing the possibility of adjacent level fractures, when compared with vertebroplasty. In this Chapter, I will deal with the background issues of osteoporotic and osteolytic vertebral compression fractures, patient selection, surgical technique, complications, and review of current literature on vertebroplasty and kyphoplasty.

CONCLUSION

Osteoporotic and osteolytic vertebral compression fractures pose significant clinical problems including spinal deformity, pain, reduced pulmonary function, reduced mobility, and overall increase in mortality. Traditional forms of treatment may be ineffective in some cases. However, without Level 1 evidence establishing the benefits of vertebroplasty over conservative treatment in osteoporotic compression fractures, the majority of these fractures should initially be managed conservatively. Conducting prospective randomlized studies comparing radiotherapy versus vertebroplasty may be difficult in osteolytic fractures secondary to menstasis, as their lifespan may be limited. Nevertheless, in carefully selected cases, percutaneous vertebroplasty has been shown to be very efficacious in relieving the pain associated with both osteoporotic and osteolytic compression fractures. It is a relatively noninvasive procedure that has gained widespread acceptance as the standard of care for compression fractures unresponsive to traditional forms of treatment. Higher chance of complications is expected for vertebroplasty in spinal metastasis, and part of this drawback arises because of the toxicity and poor handling characteristics of PMMA, rather than the procedure itself. Future advances lie in kyphoplasty, which is a modification of vertebroplasty. It is a higher margin of safety, since it is associaled with a lower cement leakage rate. Other areas of progress may lie in defining the role of prophylactic augmentation and development of synthetic osteoconductive composites to replace PMMA.

REFERENCES

1. Melton LJ. Epidemiology of vertebral fractures in women. Am J Epidemiol 1989; 129:1000–1011.
2. Bostrom MP, Lane JM. Future directions. Augmentation of osteoporotic vertebral bodies. Spine 1997; 15(suppl 24):38–42.
3. Cooper C. Atkinson EJ, O'Fallon WM, Melton LJ. Incidence of clinically diagnosed vertebral fractures: a population-based study in Rochester, Minnesota, 1985–1989. J Bone Miner Res 1992; 7:221–227.

4. Leech JA, Dulberg C, Kellie S, Pattee L, Gay J. Relationship of lung function to severity of osteoporosis in women. Am Rev Respir Dis 1990; 141:68–71.
5. Lyles KW, Gold DT, Shipp KM, Pieper CF, Martinez S, Mulhausen PL. Association of osteoporotic vertebral compression fractures with impaired functional status. Am J Med 1993; 94:595–601.
6. Kado DM, Browner WS, Palermo L. Vertebral fractures and mortality in older women: a prospective study. Study of osteoporotic fractures research group. Arch Intern Med 1999; 159:1215–1220.
7. Sundaresan N, Krol G, Digiacinto G, Hughes J. Metastatic tumors of the spine. In: Sundaresan N, Schmidek HH, Schiller AL, Rosenthal D, eds. Tumors of the Spine; Diagnosis and Clinical Management. London: Saunders, 1990:279–304.
8. Galibert P, Deramond H, Rosat P, Le Gars D. Preliminary note on the treatment of vertebral angioma by percutaneous acrylic vertebroplasty. Neurochirurgie 1987; 33:166–168.
9. Lapras C, Mottolese C, Deruty R, Lapras C Jr, Remond J, Duquesnel J. Percutaneous injection of methyl-methacrylate in osteoporosis and severe vertebral osteolysis (Galibert's technique). J Ann Chir 1989; 43:371–376.
10. Jensen ME, Evans AJ, Mathis JM, Kallmes DF, Cloft HJ, Dion JE. Percutaneous polymethylmethacrylate vertebroplasty in the treatment of osteoporotic vertebral body compression fractures: technical aspects. Am J Neuroradiol 1997; 18:1897–1904.
11. Mathis JM, Barr JD, Belkoff SM. Percutaneous vertebroplasty: a developing standard of care for vertebral compression fractures. Am J Neuroradiol 2001; 22:373–381.
12. Truumees E, Hilibrand A, Vaccaro AR. Percutaneous vertebral augmentation. The Spine J 2004; 4:218–229.
13. Mathis JM. Percutaneous vertebroplasty. In: Mathis JM, ed. Image-guided Spine Interventions. New York: Springer, 2004:245–272.
14. Jensen ME, Dion JE. Percutaneous vertebroplasty in the treatment of osteoporotic compression fractures. Neuroimaging Clin N Am 2000; 10:547–568.
15. Tamayo-Orozco J, Arzac-Palumbo P, Peon-Vidales H, Mota-Bolfeta R, Fuentes F. Vertebral fractures associated with osteoporosis: patient management. Am J Med 1997; 103:44S–48S.
16. Cyteval C, Sarrabere MP, Roux JO. Acute osteoporotic vertebral collapse: open study on percutaneous injection of acrylic surgical cement in 20 patients. Am J Roentgenol 1999; 173:1685–1690.
17. Hee HT. Vertebroplasty—local experience. Minimally invasive spinal surgery workshop, Hong Kong, August 5, 2004.
18. Cotten A, Boutry N, Cortet B. Percutaneous vertebroplasty: state of the art. Radiogaphics 1998; 18:311–320.
19. Barr JD, Barr MS, Lemley TJ, McCann RM. Percutaneous vertebroplasty for pain relief and spinal stabilization. Spine 2000; 25:923–928.
20. Mathis JM, Petri M, Naff N. Percutaneous vertebroplasty treatment of steroid-induced osteoporotic compression fracture. Arthritis Rheum 1998; 41:171–175.
21. Dean JR, Ison KT, Gishen P. The strengthening effect of percutaneous vertebroplasty. Clin Radiol 2000; 55:471–476.
22. Belkoff SM, Mathis JM, Fenton DC, Scribner RM, Reiley ME, Talmadge K. An ex vivo biomechanical evaluation inflatable bone tamp used in the treatment of compression fracture. Spine 2001; 26:151–156.
23. Liebschner MAK, Rosenberg WS, Keaveny TM. Effects of bone cement volume and distribution on vertebral stiffness after vertebroplasty. Spine 2001; 26:1547–1554.
24. Heini PF, Berlemann U, Kaufmann M. Augmentation of mechanical properties in osteoporotic vertebral bodies—a biomechanical investigation of vertebroplasty efficacy with different bone cements. Eur Spine J 2001; 10:164–171.
25. Belkoff SM, Mathis JM, Jasper LE, Deramond H. An ex vivo biomechanical evaluation of a hydroxyapatite cement for use with vertebroplasty. Spine 2001; 26:1542–1546.
26. Grados F, Depriester C, Cayrolle G. Long-term observations of vertebral osteoporotic fractures treated by percutaneous vertebroplasty. Rheumatology (Oxford) 2000; 39:1410–1414.
27. Kim AK, Jensen ME, Dion JE. Unilateral transpedicular percutaneous vertebroplasty: initial experience. Radiology 2002; 222:737–741.
28. Wong W, Mathis JM. Commentary: is intraosseous venography a significant safety measure in performance of vertebroplasty? J Vasc Intervent Radiol 2002; 13:137–138.
29. Gaughen JR, Jensen ME, Schweickert PA. Relevance of antecedent venography in percutaneous vertebroplasty for the treatment of osteoporotic compression fractures. Am J Neuroradiol 2002; 23:594–600.
30. Jasper L, Deramond H, Mathis JM, Belkoff SM. Material properties of various cements for use with vertebroplasty. J Mater Sci Mater Med 2002; 13:1–5.
31. Belkoff SM, Mathis JM, Jasper LE. The biomechanics of vertebroplasty: the effect of cement volume on mechanical behavior. Spine 2001; 26:1537–1541.
32. Tolmeh AG, Mathis JM, Fenton DC, Levine AM, Belkoff SM. Biomechanical efficacy of unipedicular versus bipedicular vertebroplasty for the management of osteoporotic compression fractures. Spine 1999; 24:1772–1776.

33. Martin JB. Cementoplasty. Minimally invasive spinal surgery workshop, Hong Kong, August 5, 2004.
34. Deramond H, Depriester C, Galibert P, Le Gars D. Percutaneous vertebroplasty with polymethyl-methacylate: technique, indications, and results. Radiol Clin North Am 1998; 36:533–546.
35. Scroop R, Eskridge J, Britz GW. Paradoxical cerebral arterial embolization of cement during intraoperative vertebroplasty: case report. Am J Neuroradiol 2002; 23:868–870.
36. Evans AJ, Kip KE, Boutin SM. Evaluation of 72 patients pre and post vertebroplasty: a prospective study. The Spine J 2004; 4(5S):45–46.
37. Zoarski GH, Snow P, Olan WJ. Percutaneous vertebroplasty for osteoporolic compression fracture: quantitative prospective evaluation of long-term outcomes. J Vasc Intervent Radiol 2002; 13:139–148.
38. Alvarez L, Perez-Higueras A, Rossi RE, Calvo E. Vertebroplasty in the treatment of vertebral tumors. Eur Spine J 2001; 10(Suppl l):125.
39. Fourney DR, Schomer DF, Nader R, et al. Percutaneous vertebroplasty and kyphoplasty for painful vertebral body fractures in cancer patients. J Neurosurg Spine 2003; 98:21–30.
40. Álvarez L, Pérez-Higueras A, Granizo JJ, de Miguel I, Quinones D, Rossi RE. Predictors of outcomes of percutaneous vertebroplasly for osteoporotic vertebral fractures. Spine 2005; 30:87–92.
41. Perry A, Kim C, Mahar A, et al. Biomechanical evaluation of vertebral augmentation with calcium sulfate cement in cadaveric osteoporotic vertebral compression fractures. The Spine J 2004; 4(5S):46–47.
42. Ishida T, Hashimoto T, Shigenobu K, Kanayama M, Oha F, Yamane S. Clinical results of vertebroplasty for osteoporotic vertebral collapse with a minimum of 1 year follow up: percutaneous transpedicular injection of calcium phosphate cement under local anesthesia. The Spine J 2004; 4(5S):84.
43. Kim C, Perry A, Mahar A, et al. Biomechanical evaluation of an injectable radiopaque polypropylene fumarate bone cement for kyphoplasty The Spine J 2005; 5(4S):113.
44. Bono CM, Kauffman CP, Garfin SR. Vertebral body augmentation: kyphoplasty. In: Corbin TP, Connolly PJ, Yuan HA, Bao Q, Boden SD, eds. Emerging Spine Surgely Technologies. Evidence and Framework for Evaluating New Technology St Louis: Quality Medical Publishing, 2006:365–376.
45. Wong WH, Olan WJ, Belkoff SM. Balloon kyphoplasty. In: Mathis JM, Deramond H, Belkoff Sm, eds. Percutaneous Vertebroplasty. New York: Springer-Verlag, 2002:109–124.
46. Lieberman IH, Dudeney S. Reinhardt MK. Initial outcome and efficacy of kyphoplasty in the treatment of painful osteoporotic vertebral compression fractures. Spine 2001; 26:1631–1638.
47. Reiley MA. Technique and pitfalls of kyphoplasty. In: Resnick DK, Garfin SR, eds. Vertebroplasly and Kyphoplasty. New York: Thieme, 2005:62–75.

34 Opportunities and Challenges for Bioabsorbable Polymers in Spinal Reconstruction

David D. Hile
Stryker Biotech, Hopkinton, Massachusetts, U.S.A.

Kai-Uwe Lewandrowski
University of Arizona and Center for Advanced Spinal Surgery, Tucson, Arizona, U.S.A.

Debra J. Trantolo
A.G.E., LLC, Princeton, Massachusetts, U.S.A.

INTRODUCTION

The ability to manipulate the chemical and physical properties of bioabsorbable polymers makes them attractive materials for spinal reconstruction. Polymers may be used as manufactured devices (e.g., interbody fusion devices or pedicle screws), for reconstruction of hard tissue (e.g., bone graft substitute), and repair of soft tissue (e.g., disc repair). This Chapter focuses on the manipulation of bioabsorbable polymers specific for the repair and regeneration of the spine. The demands for materials' performance create unique challenges with respect to development of bioabsorbable spinal products. Mechanical properties may be controlled by polymer molecular weight, polymer degradation rates, and/or reinforcement techniques used in a polymer-based repair composite. Biological properties may be adjusted by incorporation of bioactive molecules or surface modification. While degradation and concurrent replacement with native tissue is a significant advantage for bioabsorbable polymers, the degradation process leads to potentially harmful (i.e., acidic) byproducts. The generation of acidic byproducts and mechanisms to control this process is discussed. With the diverse and unique properties of bioabsorbable polymers, the interest in using these materials for spinal reconstruction will continue.

The history of bioabsorbable polymers in clinical use includes devices such as sutures, screws for bone-bone and bone-tendon-bone fixation, and plates for craniofacial and maxillofacial applications. In addition, bioabsorbable polymers have been used as drug delivery vehicles for controlled release of small molecule and large molecule therapeutics. Homopolymer and copolymers of lactide and glycolide [polylactide (PLA), polyglycolide (PGA), poly(lactide-co-glycolide) (PLGA)] possess many desirable chemical, mechanical, and biological characteristics. These polymers making a favorite in the preparation of bioabsorbable devices (1,2). Despite their long history, the tissue response to bioabsorbable implants fabricated from the family of aliphatic polyesters has not been uniformly acceptable. Investigators have reported a late sterile inflammatory foreign body response associated with implant degradation (3,4). This Chapter will review the opportunities and development challenges for bioabsorbable polymers specific to applications in the spine including interbody fusion devices, bone graft substitutes, and drug delivery applications.

PROPERTIES OF BIOABSORBABLE POLYMERS

The terms bioabsorbable, biodegradable, bioerodible, and bioresorbable or resorbable are often used interchangeably in the literature. In the case of the aliphatic polyesters, which include PLA, PGA, and PLGA, the term degradable refers to hydrolysis of the ester linkage to yield a carboxylic acid (RCOOH) and hydroxy acid (ROH). The *bio*-prefix refers to the hydrolysis

TABLE 1 Properties of Materials Under Compression

Material	Strength (MPa)	Modulus (GPa)
poly(D,L-lactide) (56, 57)	60–100	2.4
Human Cancellous Bone (58)	1–10	0.1–0.9
Human Cortical Bone (58)	167–209	15–20
Human Vertebral Bone (59)	1.55–4.6	0.0228–0.0556

in a biological system. In the case of PLGA, in vivo degradation occurs as a result of water impregnation of the polymeric matrix and subsequent reaction between water and the ester linkage rather than an enzymatic reaction. The term bioerodible is linked to polymer erosion. The erosion process occurs as degraded acids become water-soluble and the dissolution of the degraded species causes mass loss from the polymer matrix to the physiological environment. Because degradation necessarily precedes erosion, mass loss of the polymer matrix lacks behind actual bond cleavage. The terms *resorbable* or *bioresorbable* refer to the breakdown of an implant by a biological process, such as the replacement of hydroxyapatite by native bone during the remodeling process. Finally, the term *bioabsorbable* has been used as a general term to encompass both degradation and resorption. The term bioabsorbable is used in this Chapter as a broad definition of polymer degradation, erosion, absorption into the physiological environment, and clearance from the body.

The degradation and erosion properties of bioabsorbable polymers are dictated by multiple factors. Higher molecular weights require additional hydrolysis or chain cleavage of the elongated polymer chains. The erosion rate is decreased due to the prevalence of longer water-insoluble chains and limits water uptake within the bulk implant. Another significant factor is the ratio of glycolide to lactide in PLGA copolymers. Glycolide units degrade at a faster rate than lactides. Glycolide homopolymers may degrade in several weeks, while PLA will degrade in many months to several years. In addition, the degradation rates of PLA are dependent on the chirality of the lactide unit. Polymers of poly(L-lactide) have increased degradation rates due to the polymer's crystalline structure, while racemic poly(D,L-lactide) materials degrade at a faster rate. Semi-crystalline materials prepared from copolymers of poly(L-lactide) and poly(D,L-lactide) [e.g., 70:30 poly(L-lactide-co-D,L-lactide)] are typically used in orthopedic applications. Implants consisting of 70:30 poly(L-lactide-co-D,L-lactide) with molecular weights between 200,000 and 300,000 yield degradation rates significantly beyond the course of bone healing [2–4 years (5)] and mechanical properties (Table 1) between cancellous and cortical bone.

Clearance of Poly(Lactide Co-Glycolide) Polymers

PLGA degradation yields glycolide and lactide subunits that are ultimately cleared from the body (6). Glycolide subunits are not further metabolized and are removed in the urine. Unlike lactide, glycolide has limited solubility in aqueous environments and is not involved in any metabolic pathways in physiological systems. Conversely, lactide is converted to lactic acid then pyruvic acid and ultimately metabolized by the tricarboxylic acid cycle. The relatively slow hydrolysis and erosion process provides ample time for the degraded species to be cleared from the body.

BIOABSORBABLE POLYMERS FOR SPINAL FUSION

Commercially available devices for stabilizing spinal segments to promote fusion include crafted allograft bone, carbon fiber, or metallic devices (7–9). These devices provide structural support and encourage bone union with osteoinductive agents, such as morselized autograft (9) or therapeutics, including the family of bone morphogenetic proteins (10–13). However, of the ~200,000 spinal fusion procedures that are performed each year in the United States, it is estimated that between 10% to 40% of cases result in nonunion or failed fusion dependent upon risk factors (14, 15). Repair materials based upon bioabsorbable polymers, such as PLA or

PLGA, provide the potential to create devices specifically designed for spinal fusion procedures based on the potential of these polymers to respond to material criteria.

Bioabsorbable devices have shown promise in stabilizing spinal segments and supporting new bone formation. Preliminary outcomes suggest that the replacement of metallic implants with bioabsorbables can ameliorate the problems associated with implant loosening, implant migration, and imaging complications (16). The mechanics of bioabsorbable polymers are closer to the native bone than metallics, and, thus, may alleviate complications from stress sharing. Moreover, a potential advantage of a bioresorbable fusion implant is the ability to modify the initial strength of the device. Reducing the stiffness of cages demonstrated improved lumbar interbody fusion rates in goats (17). In this study, fusion increased with decreasing cage stiffness by comparing healing associated with titanium cages to two less rigid poly (L-lactide) (PLLA) cages. In addition, long-term evaluation (36 months) indicated decreased bone formation when titanium cages were used to stabilize the spinal segment compared to PLLA cages (18). The change in the net fusion rates indicated that a stress-shielded environment might have existed within the titanium devices. The ability to control the initial strength of the device and the progressive loss of strength due to polymer degradation may increase the mechanical stress on the fusion site during the healing process, thus enhancing fusion rates and improving surgical outcomes (16).

Bioabsorbable materials provide initial mechanical integrity capable of supporting the defect site and progressive stress sharing during the concomitant stages of polymer degradation and bone healing. This dynamic mechanical environment ultimately permits stress sharing between the device and the fused site at a rate commensurate with new bone formation. Therefore, bioabsorbable polymer devices have a potential advantage in that the temporal mechanical properties can provide an initially rigid structure that progressively shares the load with healing bone.

Clinical Use of Bioabsorbable Implants

Commercial bioabsorbable products have been introduced for spinal applications. A graft containment system consisting of 70:30 poly(L-lactide-co-D,L-lactide) has been cleared for use in the United States by MacroPore, Inc. (San Diego, California, U.S.A.). The MacroPore *OS* Spinal System and MacroPore Hydrosorb™ Spine System are comprised of PLA plates (either porous or nonporous) and associated screws. The devices are intended for maintenance of autograft or allograft position, such as in placement of bone graft to generate vertebral fusion. An interbody fusion device made by MacroPore, Inc. has received approval in Europe (Telamon® Hydrosorb™ Cage).

A two-year clinical study was conducted in 27 patients to evaluate spinal fusion using a 70:30 poly(L-lactide-co-D,L-lactide) interbody spacer (19). Instrumented transforaminal lumbar interbody fusion (TLIF) surgeries were conducted and evaluated at two-year clinical follow-up. The percentage of solid fusions (92.6%, 25/27) was comparable to the field of commercially available interbody devices. Twenty-two patients (82%) had well to excellent outcomes after two years. There was one reported mechanical failure of the bioabsorbable device during insertion. None of the complications following the procedure (3/27) was attributable to the bioabsorbable implant. The study provides clinical support for the continued development of bioabsorbable interbody fusion devices.

COMPLICATIONS WITH BIOABSORBABLE POLYMER IMPLANTS

The use of internal fixation devices consisting of bioabsorbable polymers, such as PGA, PLA, and PLGA, has been linked to late-stage inflammatory responses. Between 0% and 22% of patients treated with bioabsorbable devices consisting of lag screws, interference screws, and plates developed sterile abscess formations at the implant site (3,4,20–22). Bacterial cultures of the drainage routinely tested negative indicating that the biological response was a consequence of the chemical irritation accompanying acidic polymer degradation products (23). The inflammatory response was observed after a relatively long induction period ranging from seven to 20 weeks dependent upon the degradation kinetics of the polymer (3).

Clinical management of these inflammatory responses involved operative drainage at the site. A clinical review of 516 patients receiving PGA screws indicated that 8% developed the inflammatory response (23). A separate review of PLGA screws demonstrated that 11% of patients had inflammatory reactions within three months after surgery (3). Degradation kinetics played a significant role in the manifestion of sterile abscesses, as the inflammatory response occurred more frequently in patients treated with rapidly degrading devices. A comprehensive review of 3200 patients receiving bioabsorbable implants found complications in ~10% of cases ranging from bacterial wound infection (4%), failure of fixation (4%), or sterile abscess formation (2%) (24). Sterile abscesses occurred in patients receiving polyglycolide implants.

In order to lessen the potential for sterile abscess formation, clinicians have adopted the use of implants consisting exclusively of PLA. Lactide homopolymers degrade much more slowly than glycolide homopolymers and copolymers of lactide and glycolide. The degradation of PGA, PLA, and PLGA via hydrolysis produces carboxylic acids, and pH values as low as 2.5 have been measured within degrading systems (25). The slower degradation rates of PLA, especially polymers with molecular weights in excess of 200,000, allow removal of the degraded species by diffusion of the water-soluble carboxylic acid byproduct through the bulk degrading implant. Faster degrading systems produce acids at a rate greater than removal, and these results in the accumulation of acids at the implant site. Although, the exclusive use of PLA has alleviated the potential for sterile abscess formation, information on the clinical outcomes of PLA implants is somewhat limited. This is due, in part, to the fact that commercial bioabsorbable implants consisting of PLA with molecular weights greater than 200,000 have in vivo degradation times in excess of four years (26).

The extended degradation time of PLA implants implies that the bioabsorbable material will outlive its intended use. The clinical use of PLA implants may range between several weeks to fracture fixation to several months for spinal fusion applications. PLA implants have been considered *ghosts* in that these materials have a prolonged presence in vivo. Thus, the body must replace the degrading implant with new tissue long after the repair site has healed.

The presence of polymer degradation byproducts in the spine has not been examined and documented. The degradation behavior of the materials is influenced by the localization of the implant in the body, as well as chemistry and device design (22). Preclinical studies of bioabsorbable implants in the spine have presented mild to moderate inflammatory response related to spinal device degradation (16,18,27). Moderate to severe foreign body reactions (8/8 PLA implants) and implant migration (5/8) during a 12-week feasibility study in sheep have been reported (28). The complications were attributed to polymer degradation and lack of device osteointegration. Because the degradation rate of PLA implants may range from two to four years, there is a long-term potential for tissue reactions to acidic degradation byproducts that may result in chronic complications for bioabsorbable spinal implants.

POLYMER COMPOSITES

The practice of polymer composites may be used to modify the properties of bioabsorbable polymers. Incorporation of particles or fibers may be used to alter degradation rates, buffer the degrading implant, enhance mechanical properties, increase radioopacity, and/or support the eroding implant matrix. Bioabsorbable composites are commercially available including: the family of BioCryl® products (polylactide and tricalcium phosphate composites marketed by DePuy Mitek, Inc., Raynham, Massachusetts, U.S.A.), Biosteon® and Bilok® products (composites of polylactide and hydroxyapatite manufactured by Biocomposites, Ltd., Stafford shire, UK), and the WISORB™ Screw (a composite of polylactide and hydroxyapatite produced by Cambridge Scientific, Inc., Cambridge, Massachusetts, U.S.A. Fig. 1).

Incorporating an osteoconductive buffer into PLA implants mitigates acid generation during degradation and promotes intimate bone healing at the tissue-implant interface. Hydroxyapatite (HA) enables buffering throughout the polymer degradation process because the low water solubility of HA permits a long-term presence. Furthermore, HA is osteoconductive

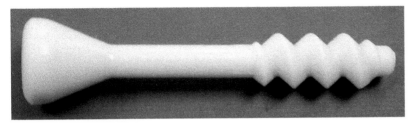

FIGURE 1 The WISORB™ Screw (Cambridge Scientific, Inc., Cambridge, Massachusetts, U.S.A.) prepared by injection molding of polylactide and hydroxyapatite (25% w/w). Hydroxyapatite acts as a long-acting buffer to control the generation of acidic polymer degradation byproducts. In addition, the osteoconductive filler promotes osteointegration of the device. *Source*: Adapted from Ref. 5.

(29–31) and thus is capable of promoting device osteointegration regeneration of bone following implant degradation. Inclusion of HA in PLA constructs has been used to produce osteoconductive materials for the repair of bone defects and fracture fixation (32–35). In addition, HA may be used as a reinforcement agent in the polymer, resulting in improved mechanical properties, osteoconductivity, and radioopacity (33,36). Despite its similarity to rapidly absorbed tricalcium phosphate (TCP), HA is a quasi-permanent material when used to fill defects, with several years required for complete remodeling and replacement by native bone. The solubility of HA, with pKs of approximately 120 (37), is less than that of a degrading polymer. Thus, HA has the potential to serve as a long-acting buffer for neutralizing acid degradation products in situ (5,38).

The effect of HA incorporation within a 70:30 PLLA:PDLA polymer screw was evaluated in vitro. The addition of 25% (w/w) HA neutralized acidic byproducts within a PLA screw without changing the mechanical properties or degradation rates of the device compared to PLA only (5). Neutralization of the resulting carboxylic acids by HA ($Ca(OH)_2 \cdot 3Ca_3(PO_4)_2$) is represented by the following reactions:

$$2RCO_2H + Ca(OH)_2 \cdot 3Ca_3(PO_4)_2 \longrightarrow 2RCO_2^- + Ca^{2+} + 2H_2O + 3Ca_3(PO_4)_2 \quad (1)$$

$$12\,RCO_2H + 3Ca_3(PO_4)_2 \longrightarrow 12\,RCO_2^- + 9Ca^{2+} + 6H_2PO_4 \quad (2)$$

The net reaction may be represented by the following:

Net: $14\,RCO_2H + Ca(OH)_2 \cdot 3Ca_3(PO_4)_2 \longrightarrow 14RCO_2^- + 10\,Ca^{2+} + 2H_2O + 6H_2PO_4$

Incorporation of 25% [weight/weight (w/w)] HA effectively buffered the bioabsorbable screws through 52 weeks of degradation in vitro. The pH of the phosphate buffer incubated with the PLA/HA devices maintained values above 7.3 throughout the course of this study in contrast to PLLA screws where a significant pH decrease from 7.9 to 3.0 was observed between 24 and 52 weeks (Fig. 2). Degradation of bulk PLA generates water-soluble segments

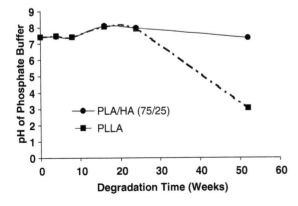

FIGURE 2 Acidic degradation byproducts were monitored by measuring the pH of a phosphate buffer in contact with bioabsorbable screws through 52 weeks of in vitro degradation. The incorporation of 25% (w/w) hydroxyapatite effectively neutralized the phosphate buffer. *Abbreviations*: HA, hydroxyapatite; PLLA, poly (L-lactide); PLA, polylactide; *Source*: Adapted from Ref. 5.

TABLE 2 Percent Change in Screw Dimensions

TIME (WEEKS)	PLA/HA						PLLA					
	0	4	8	16	24	52	0	4	8	16	24	52
%TOTAL LENGTH CHANGE	—	0.18 ± 0.16	0.59 ± 0.13[a]	0.69 ± 0.19	0.58 ± 0.12	2.16 ± 0.63[a]	—	0.24 ± 0.05	0.16 ± 0.07	0.61 ± 0.21	0.46 ± 0.34	0.23 ± 0.12
%THREAD DIAMETER CHANGE	—	1.12 ± 0.14[a]	1.94 ± 0.18[a]	2.02 ± 0.40[a]	4.27 ± 0.95[a]	16.80 ± 2.23[a]	—	0.04 ± 0.09	0.30 ± 0.23	0.41 ± 0.27	0.68 ± 0.38	2.94 ± 0.86

[a]Indicated statistically significant difference compared to PLLA device ($p < 0.05$, unpaired t-test).
Abbreviations: HA, hydroxyapatite; PLA, polylactide; PPLA, poly (L-lactide).

at $\sim$10 monomeric units, suggesting that the yield of carboxylic acids will not approach the theoretical maximum. However, inclusion of the HA buffer increased the degree of swelling as evident in the PLA/HA device by a significant increase change in the diameter of the PLA/HA screw with respect to time versus the PLLA device (Table 2).

In Vivo Testing of Polymer Composites

Incorporation of HA into PLA fracture fixation devices demonstrated greater osteoconductivity in comparison to PLA only devices. In vivo tests revealed improved bone-implant interfaces in PLA/HA composites (32,34,35). Preliminary studies with PLA/HA cancellous lag screws demonstrated benign tissue reactions and promoted osteotomy union in vivo (34,35). In this study, biocompatibility and osteoconductivity of a PLA/HA composite screw in comparison to a PLA only device was evaluated via healing of an osteochondral fragment created in the distal sheep femur in response to fixation with either a PLA or PLA/HA composite screw (34). At follow-up times of 4 and 8 weeks, the specimens were examined with standard radiography, computed tomography, as well as macro- and microhistomorphometry. The intact contralateral femur served as a control. At 8 weeks, nearly all osteotomies had healed and no association between implant type and delayed osteotomy healing was found. The width of the repair tissue at the tissue-implant interface was 250 ± 48 μm representing a clear transition zone of newly formed trabecular bone separating the implant from the surrounding plexiform bone. Composite PLA/HA screws were intimately surrounded by newly formed bone. In contrast, the PLA only implants were noted to have an intervening layer of fibrous tissue (Fig. 3). Histology indicated that integration of the PLA/HA screw was greater at all

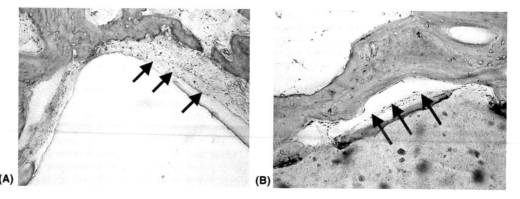

(A)   **(B)**

FIGURE 3 **(A)** Longitudinal section through PLLA screw after eight weeks implantation: Fibroconnective tissue was present along the shaft of the PLLA specimens (*arrows*). **(B)** Longitudinal section through polylactide/hydroxyapatite screw after eight weeks implantation: Evidence of intimate bone contact is visible at the device surface (*arrows*). *Source*: Adapted from Ref. 34.

time points, thereby suggesting at least equal, if not enhanced, bone healing as compared to the PLA-only device.

Bioabsorbable cage composites prepared from PLA and tricalcium phosphate were investigated in a sheep cervical fusion study (28). Fusion was assessed at 12 weeks by radiograph measurement of disc height and biomechanical evaluation of the fusion mass. The PLA and TCP composite demonstrated a significant increase in disc height, stiffness of the fused vertebrae and decreased range of motion compared to a PLA only cage and autologous iliac crest bone. Although fusion outcome measures were superior in the composite cage, evidence of cage cracking was seen in 6 of 8 cages. Similar cracking behavior was observed in PLA/HA composite cages following ex vivo compressive loading of vertebral lumbar segments fixed with the PLA/HA test device (39). In addition, the swelling behavior observed in PLA/HA composites (5) may make the materials susceptible to deformation and cracking. The influences of physiological loading and polymer degradation on the structure of bioabsorbable composites and permissiveness of tissue ingrowth still need to be investigated in additional long-term (e.g., 24 months) preclinical studies.

BIOABSORBABLE BONE GRAFT SUBSTITUTES

Spinal fusion is the most common bone grafting procedure conducted in the United States, comprising some 50% of the estimated half-million bone grafting procedures performed annually (29). It has been estimated that more than 350,000 spinal fusions are performed annually (40). Bone graft substitutes are evaluated based on their ability to provide immediate structural support while encouraging bone ingrowth as fusion progresses. The use of a bioabsorbable and osteoconductive bone graft substitute would allow for immediate mechanical stabilization, while allowing for replacement by new bone growth as the polymer degrades.

An osteoconductive bone graft substitute based on the bioabsorbable polymer, poly(propylene glycal-co-fumaric acid) (PPF) has been investigated as an adjunct for spinal fusion (41). PPF is a subset of the bioabsorbable polyester family, and the degradation and erosion mechanisms of PPF are comparable to PLGA. The bioabsorbable graft substitute is prepared as an injectable paste of PPF and crosslinker, for example, 1-vinyl-2-pyrollidone. PPF, an unsaturated polyester, can be crosslinked in the presence of effervescent and osteoconductive fillers and cured in situ, yielding a porous bone-like scaffold in intimate contact with host tissue (Fig. 4). The use of a bioabsorbable scaffold could, at least, extend the working volume of autograft without compromising its osteoconductive properties and, at best, improve upon the mechanical and bioactivity properties of the graft material as graft consolidation occurs. The fact that the proposed graft substitute sets or cures in a surgical relevant timeframe would also be advantageous in the placement of fusion instrumentation, such as screws, cages, and plates.

Porous bone repair materials provide a structural construct to enable a more rapid ingrowth of bone cells while stabilizing the defect site (42,43). A porous construct with

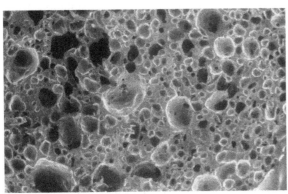

×20

500 μm

FIGURE 4 Scanning electron micrograph of the cured poly(propylene fumarate-co-fumaric acid) scaffold. Pore diameters range between 50 μm and 500 μm, and the average pore size as shown is ~170 μm. The immediate porosity of the cured scaffold enables bone ingrowth. Polymer degradation and erosion permits concurrent replacement with new bone. *Source*: Adapted from Ref. 41.

mechanical properties comparable to native bone will initially provide structural support to the defect site. Thereafter, as the implant degrades, the net result of newly formed bone plus residual implant, the *repair-composite*, is expected to provide continued support to the defect reconstruction, while yielding to the establishment of native bone. A bioabsorbable material for spinal fusion is expected to provide rigid stabilization initially, and enable progressive stress-sharing with the surrounding, healed bone that may prevent osteopenia and/or long-term implant failure.

Bioabsorbable Bone Graft Substitute as a Mechanical Adjunct

The temporal mechanical properties of the PPF scaffold may be advantageous for use in spinal fusion. Mechanical properties of the PPF-based bone graft substitute are comparable to cancellous bone (44). The initial compressive strength of the porous PPF scaffold is ~5 MPa, which approximates that of cancellous bone. Degradation of the polymeric structure yields a decrease in the mechanical properties of the bone graft substitute. Bone ingrowth within the porous scaffold is expected to augment the mechanics of the implant-bone construct during degradation. The loss of compressive strength of the PPF bone graft substitute (50% after three weeks of degradation) is approximately commensurate with the healing rate of cancellous bone (45). The temporal mechanics of the PPF bone graft substitute may be controlled through formulation parameters (such as the starting molecular weight of the PPF polymer, porosity, the degree of crosslinking, and so on) to modify the system for desired mechanical properties and degradation rates.

An ex vivo biomechanical study demonstrated that bioabsorbable cages were capable of supporting lumbar spinal segments in a simulated fusion. Bioabsorbable cages with and without HA osteoconductive buffering were compared to autograft and metallic cages (BAK® Cage, Centerpulse, Minneapolis, Minnesota, U.S.A.) by determining the stiffness and failure load of the L4/5 motion segment of cadaveric human spines (39). The average age of the donors was 50 ± 3 years (donors, 36–55-years old). The L4/5 motion segment was tested by a non-destructive flexibility method using a non-constrained testing apparatus (46). Pure bending moments were applied using a system of cables and pulleys to induce flexion, extension, left and right lateral bending, and left and right axial rotation. Bioabsorbable cages, including a buffered composite of PLA/HA (80/20 w/w), stabilized lumbar spinal segments similar to a clinical standard (BAK cage). In comparison to the unstable L4/5 motion segment, the BAK cage, PLA cage, and PLA/HA cage similarly stabilized the L4/5 motion segment above the level intact motion segment with comparable limitation of ROM in flexion/extension, left and right lateral bending, and to rotation with statistically significant difference ($p < 0.01$, ANOVA). Furthermore, all cages showed a significantly higher flexional/extensional and bending stiffness when compared to the intact motion segment ($p < 0.05$). The HA buffered composite cage and the PLA-only cage yielded comparable range of motion (ROM) and stiffness results when compared to the BAK® Cage, even though the stiffness of the individual devices were different. The respective data was normalized to ROM and stiffness (Fig. 5) of the intact L4/5 motion segment. Augmentation of the bioabsorbable, PLA, cage with the PPF bone graft substitute decreased the ROM and increased the stiffness compared to intact segments and the BAK cage. Thus, coimplantation of the PPF scaffold was able to stiffen the segments in a way that could not be achieved by increasing the mechanical properties of the cage. The PPF scaffold serves as a mechanical adjunct with mechanical properties comparable to local bone.

In Vivo Evaluation of a Bioabsorbable Bone Graft Substitute

The feasibility of using a PPF-based bone repair material as a graft substitute was tested in a posterolateral intertransverse process lumbar spinal fusion model. Intertransverse process fusion in rabbits was evaluated using the osteoconductive and bioabsorbable PPF bone repair scaffold as an alternative or adjunct for autograft (41). Fusion was assessed by bimanual palpation, radiography, computed tomography (CT) imaging, and histomorphometric outcomes (Table 3). Augmentation of the PPF bone graft substitute with morselized autologous

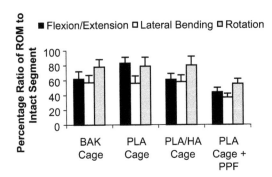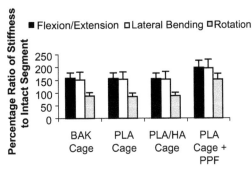

FIGURE 5 Bioabsorbable cages yielded comparable ROM and stiffness results in comparison to currently used clinical standard (BAK cage). Augmentation of a bioabsorbable cage with the PPF bone graft substitute decreased the ratio of ROM to intact segments and increased the stiffness compared to intact. *Abbreviations*: HA, hydroxyapatite; PLA, polylactide; PPF, poly(propylene glycol-co-fumaric acid). *Source*: Adapted from Ref. 39.

bone procured from the iliac crest achieved fusion rates equivalent to if not greater than autograft bone alone. The results suggest that the PPF material might be used in conjunction with autologous bone graft to achieve equivalent fusion rates than the use of autologous bone alone. The mechanical properties of the PPF scaffold may be used to augment the rigidity associated with internal fixation, while promoting bone ingrowth and lumber fusion. These findings have immediate applicability to the further development of a biopolymeric and bioabsorbable bone graft extender for spinal applications with emphasis on the influence of porosity and mechanical strength on the outcome of spinal fusion procedures.

The PPF scaffold supported fusion by serving as a mechanical adjunct and osteoconductive matrix for facilitating bone thrugrowth. The application of the porous bone graft substitute may lesson the need for autologous bone graft or bone morphogenetic proteins (e.g., BMP-2 or BMP-7), which do not provide any mechanical advantage. The PPF repair material may be used as a graft substitute or graft extender by mixing in local bone graft within the injectable material prior to administration at the defect site. Preferably, the use of local autograft as an osteoinductive factor in the PPF material will be collected during the surgery, that is, produced during defect induction for the cage device or harvested locally. Thus, the need for a second surgical procedure to collect autograft from the iliac crest is eliminated.

BIOABSORBABLE POLYMERS FOR CONTROLLED DRUG DELIVERY

Before their application to orthopedics, bioabsorbable polymers developed a long history as vehicles for controlled drug delivery. Drug incorporation within bioabsorbable matrices enables local and sustained release of biologicals. Drug release rates are controlled by drug concentration in the polymer matrix, porosity of the polymer matrix, polymer degradation rate, and drug solubility. The use of bioabsorbable drug delivery systems may prove advantageous for sustained release of osteoinductive bone growth factors in spinal applications. Commercial BMP products approved for spinal fusion applications are applied with collagen-based materials that provide a biocompatible matrix for bone growth (10, 47). Bioabsorbable materials

TABLE 3 Summary of Spinal Fusion Rates by Experimental Group

	Bimanual palpation	Radiographic fusion rate	CT fusion index	Histomorphometric fusion index
Group 1 (Autograft)	40% (2/5)	60% (3/5)	69 ± 9%	72 ± 12%
Group 2 (PPF)	50% (3/6)	50% (3/6)	48 ± 6%	53 ± 12%
Group 3 (Autograft + PPF)	67% (4/6)	67% (4/6)	89 ± 13%	91 ± 17%

Abbreviation: CT, computed tomography.

can provide a longer drug residence time in vivo through extended release and may enable lower effective treatment doses.

Sustained release of proteins from bioabsorbable matrices is achieved through impregnation or encapsulation of the drug through the polymer matrix. Drug release from bioabsorbable carriers occurs via two mechanisms: diffusion and erosion. The *diffusion* mechanism controls the initial drug release as the molecule diffuses through the polymer matrix. *Water impregnation* of the polymer matrix enables diffusion of the drug from the carrier interior to the surface where it is released to the surrounding local environment. As polymer degradation proceeds, erosion of the matrix releases additional drug. The two mechanisms can result in a biomodal release rate dependent upon the diffusivity of the drug and erosion rate of the polymer matrix.

Nonpolymeric devices used in the spine may be modified with bioabsorbable polymers to enable drug delivery. The modification is analogous to drug-coated stents where a polymeric coating is used to enhance the performance of an existing device. A dip-coating method has been tested to coat titanium interbody fusion cages with growth factors such as transforming growth factor (TGF)-β1, insulin-like growth factor (IGF)-1, and BMP-2 (48). The coating method produces a drug-loaded, poly (D,L-lactide) (PDLLA) surface that extends ~10 μm from the surface of titanium implants. The application of PDLLA (with and without BMP-2) promoted increased bone mineral density and fusion mass in a sheep cervical fusion model compared to an uncoated titanium cage (12). Furthermore, incorporation of 150 μg BMP-2 significantly improved the quantity of fusion mass and stiffness of the fused cervical segments. The polymer coating demonstrated greater interbody callus formation compared to BMP-2 delivered in a collagen sponge carrier. Similarly, codelivery of TGF-β1 and IGF-1 enhanced cervical fusion in sheep (49). A dose-dependent response in bone fusion mass and biomechanical properties was achieved up to a loading of 150 μg IGF-I and 30 μg TGF-β1. Higher drug loadings did not produce any significant improvement in fusion outcomes.

An alternative to surface modification is to deliver drugs from polymer microparticles. The microparticles may be used alone or in conjunction with a bioabsorbable scaffold (50) or a resorbable bone graft substitute (51). The purpose of microparticle incorporation is to augment the scaffold or matrix with a biologically active molecule (such as a bone growth factor) and provide a sustained release of bioactive molecules from the matrix (52). The controlled release of bone growth factors from scaffolds is expected to initiate migration of bone progenitor cells from surrounding tissues and ultimately promotes proliferation of bone forming cells. Combinations of growth factors and transplanted cells may be used to enhance bone formation and minimize the effective drug dose (53). Further research is needed to establish effective doses, delivery rates, and treatment combinations for effective bone stimulation in spine applications.

DISC REGENERATION

Repair or replacement of degenerated intervertebral discs may mitigate the need for fusion procedures. Bioabsorbable polymers may prove beneficial as scaffold components in tissue-engineered discs. The repair of degenerated discs represents significant technical challenges due to the complex biomechanics, highly avascular tissue environment, and multiple factors required for a successful product. Biomimetic systems combining appropriate growth factors to stimulate cell growth, soft tissue matrices for cell adhesion and proliferation, and synthetic polymers to support scaffold architecture and mechanical properties have the potential to replace damaged discs. The use of bioabsorbable polymers alone does not appear sufficient; nucleus pulposus cells cultured on PLA scaffolds had less cellular activity and desired morphology than those observed on gelatin scaffolds (54). Composite matrices consisting of PLGA and collagen proved more able to support nucleus pulposus cell growth and resembled native disc tissue after 12 weeks of implantation in athymic mice (55). Composite bioabsorbable scaffolds may prove more robust than soft tissue matrices alone because synthetic polymer materials are more easily scaled to different sizes, provide more mechanical rigidity, and may be used to deliver growth factors to stimulate cell growth.

CONCLUSIONS

Bioabsorbable polymers represent exciting opportunities for materials used for repair, stabilization, and reconstruction of the spine. The ability to manipulate the physicochemical properties of bioabsorbable polymers provides a wide range of materials that can be adapted for specific applications. Polymeric implants have immediate applicability as devices for maintenance of graft placement, pedicle screws, and interbody fusion devices. Polymer degradation enables progressive stress sharing from the implant to healing tissue. In addition, degradation and erosion of the implant mitigates the need for a secondary surgical procedure to remove the device. Furthermore, provided sufficient stimulus, new and functional tissue may replace the eroding polymer matrix. Modification of bioabsorbable devices with fillers can be used to buffer the acidic degradation byproducts, improve mechanical properties, and enhance bioactivity of the matrix. The potential to create new products for spine repair and reconstruction exists through modification of existing devices with bioabsorbable materials, for example, drug-coated implants. Finally, bioabsorbable polymers may become an important component of new treatment paradigms or disease modifying products for replacing or repairing diseased or damaged spine tissue. The range of future bioabsorbable products may include artificial discs, and minimally invasive, injectable treatments for osteoporosis and disc degeneration.

REFERENCES

1. Elisseeff JH, Yamada Y, Langer R. "Biomaterials for tissue engineering." In: Lewandrowski KU, Wise DL, Trantolo DJ, Gresser JD, Yaszemski MJ, Altobelli DE, eds. Tissue Engineering and Biodegradable Equivalents. New York: Marcel Dekker, Inc., 2002:1–24.
2. Verheyen CC, deWijn JR, vanBlitterwijk CA, deGroot K. Evaluation of hydroxylapatite/poly(L-lactide) composites: Mechanical behavior. J Bio Med Mat Res 1992; 26:1277–1296.
3. Bostman OM, Hirvensalo E, Partio E, Tormala P, Rokkanen P. Resorbable rods and screws of polyglycolide in stabilizing malleolar fractures: A clinical study of 600 patients. Unfallchirurg 1992; 95:109–112.
4. Bucholz RW, Henry S, Henley MB. Fixation with bioabsorbable screws for the treatment of fractures of the ankle. J Bone Joint Surg Am 1994; 76:319–324.
5. Hile DD, Doherty SA, Trantolo DJ. Predication of resorption rates for composite polylactide/hydroxylapatite internal fixation devices based on initial degradation profiles. J Biomed Mater Res Part B: Applied Biomaterials 2004; 71B:201–205.
6. Hollinger JO, Battistone GC. Biodegradable bone repair materials: Synthetic polymers and ceramics. Clinical Orthopedics and Related Research 1986; 207:290–305.
7. Brantigan JW, Steffee AD, Geiger JM. A carbon fiber implant to aid interbody lumbar fusion. *Spine* 1991; 16(6/Supplement):s277–s282.
8. Rapoff AJ, Ghanayem AJ, Zdeblick TA. Biomechanical comparison of posterior lumbar interbody fusion cages. Spine 1997; 22(20):2375–2379.
9. Rauzzino MJ, Shaffrey CI, Nockels RP, Wiggins GC, Rock J. Anterior lumbar fusion with titanium threaded and mesh interbody. Neurosurg Focus 1999; 7(6):1–11.
10. Boden SD, Kang J, Sandhu H, Heller JG. Use of recombinant human bone morphogenetic protein-2 to achieve posterolateral lumbar spine fusion in humans: A prospective, randomized clinical pilot trial. Spine 2002; 27:2662–2673.
11. Kandziora F, Schmidmaier G, Bail H, et al. IGF-1 and TGF-β1 application by a poly(D,L-lactide)-coated cage promotes intervertebral bone matrix formation in the sheep cervical spine. Spine 2002; 27(16):1710–1723.
12. Kandziora F, Bail H, Schmidmaier G, et al. Bone morphogenetic protein-2 application by a poly(D,L-lactide)-coated interbody cage: *In vivo* results of a new carrier for growth factors. J Neruosurg (Spine 1) 2002; 97:40–48.
13. Vaccaro AR, Patel T, Fischgrund J, et al. A pilot safety and efficacy study of OP-1 putty (rhBMP-7) as an adjunct to iliac crest autograft in posterolateral lumbar fusions. Eur Spine J, October 2003; 12(5): 495–500.
14. Boden SD. Biology of lumbar spine fusion and use of bone graft substitutes: Present, future, and next generation. Tissue Engineering 2000; 6:383–399.
15. Toth JM, Wang M, Scifert JL, Cornwall GB, Estes BT, Seim HB, Turner AS. Evaluation of 70/30 D,L-PLA for use as a resorbable interbody fusion cage. Orthopedics 2002; 25:s1131–s1140.
16. Vaccaro AR, Madigan L. Spinal applications of bioabsorbable implants. Orthopedics 2002; 25: s1115–s1120.
17. Van Dijk M, Smit TH, Sugihara S, Burger EH, Wuisman PI. The effect of cage stiffness on the rate of lumbar interbody fusion. Spine 2002; 27:682–688.

18. Wuisman, PIJM, van Dijk M, Smit TH. Resorbable cages for spinal fusion: An experimental goat model. Orthopedics 2002; 25(10):s1141–s1148.
19. Coe JD, Vaccaro AR. Deformity surgery. Spine 2005; 30(17 suppl):s76–s83.
20. Matsusue Y, Nakamura T, Suzuki S, Iwasaki R. Biodegradable pin fixation of osteochondral fragments of the knee. Clinical Orthopedics and Related Research 1996; 322:166–173.
21. Partio EK, Bostman O, Hirvensalo R, et al. Self-reinforced absorbable screws in the fixation of displaced ankle fractures: A prospective clinical study of 152 patients. J Orthop Trauma 1992; 6(2):209–215.
22. Claes L, Ignatius A. Development of new, biodegradable implants. Chirurg 2002; 73(10):990–996.
23. Bostman OM. Current concepts review: Absorbable implants for the fixation of fractures. J Bone and Joint Surg 1991; 73A:148–152.
24. Rokkanen PU, Bostman O, Hirvensalo E, et al. Bioabsorbable fixation in orthopaedic surgery and traumatology. Biomaterials 2000; 21:2607–2613.
25. Trantolo DJ, Gresser JD, Wise DL, Lewandrowski KU. Buffered biodegradable internal fixation devices. In: Wise DL, Trantolo DJ, Lewandrowski KU, Gresser JD, Yaszemski MJ, eds. Biomaterials and Bioengineering Handbook. New York: Marcel Dekker, Inc., 2000:603–618.
26. Laitinen O, Pihlajamaki H, Sukura A, Bostman O. Transmission electron microscopic visualization of the degradation and phagocytosis of a poly-L-lactide screw in cancellous bone: A long-term experimental study. J Biomed Mater Res 2002; 61:33–39.
27. Toth JM, Estes BT, Wang M, et al. Evaluation of 70/30 poly (L-lactide-co-D,L-lactide) for use as a resorbable interbody fusion cage. J Neurosurg 2002; 97:423–432.
28. Kandziora F, Pflugmacher R, Scholz M, Eindorf T, Haas NP. Bioabsorbable interbody cages in a sheep cervical spine fusion model. Orthopaedic Research Society Annual Meeting, Paper 287, San Francisco, CA, 2004.
29. Bucholz RW. Nonallograft osteoconductive bone graft substitutes. Clinical Orthopaedics and Related Research. 2002; 395:44–52.
30. Khan SN, Tomin E, Lane JM. Clinical applications of bone graft substitutes. Tissue Engineering Ortho. Surg 2000; 31:389–398.
31. LeGeros RZ, LeGeros JP, Daculsi G, Kijkowska R. Calcium phosphate biomaterials: Preparation, properties, and biodegradation. In: Wise DL, Trantolo DJ, Altobelli DE, Yaszemski M, Gresser JD, Schwartz E, eds. Encyclopedic Handbook of Biomaterials and Bioengineering Part A: Materials. New York: Marcel Dekker, Inc. 1995:1429–1464.
32. Verheyen CC, deWijn JR, vanBlitterwijk CA, deGroot K, Rozing PM. Hydroxylapatite/poly(L-lactide) composites: An animal study on push out strengths and interface histology. J Bio Med Mat Res 1993; 27:433–444.
33. Rizzi SC, Heath DJ, Coombes AGA, Bock N, Textor M, Downes S. Biodegradable polymer/hydroxyapatite composites: Surface analysis and initial attachment of human osteoblasts. J Bio Med MaRes 2001; 55:475–486.
34. Lewandrowski KU, Bondre SP, Shea M, et al. Composite poly(lactide)/hydroxylapatite screw for fixation of osteochondral osteotomies. A morphometric, histological and radiographic study in sheep. J Biomater Sci (Poly Ed) 2002; 13:1241–1258.
35. Lewandrowski KU, Bondre SP, Wise DL, Trantolo DJ. Healing of osteochondral osteotomies after fixation with a hydroxylapatite-buffered poly-lactide screw: A histomorphometric and radiographic study in rabbits. Biomed Mater Eng 2002; 12:259–270.
36. Shikinami Y, Okuno M. Bioresorbable devices made of forged composites of hydroxyapatite (HA) particles and poly-L-lactide(PLLA): Part I. Basic characteristics. Biomaterials 1999; 20:859–877.
37. Aoki H. Science and Medical Applications of Hydroxyapatite. Tokyo: Takayama Press System Center Co. Inc., 1991:1–10.
38. Agrawal CM, Athanasiou KA. Technique to control pH in vicinity of biodegrading PLA-PGA implants. J Biomed Mater Res (Appl Biomater) 1997; 38:105–114.
39. Kandziora F, Pflugmacher R, Kleemann R, et al. Biomechanical analysis of biodegradable interbody fusion cages augmented with poly(propylene glycol-fumaric acid). Spine 2002; 27(15):1644–1651.
40. DiAngelo DJ, Kitchel S, McVay BJ, Scifert JL, Cornwall GB. Bioabsorbable anterior lumbar plate fixation in conjunction with anterior interbody fusion cages. Orthopaedics 2002; 25(10/Supplement): s1157–s1165.
41. Hile DD, Kandziora F, Lewandrowski KU, Doherty SA, Kowaleski MP, Trantolo DJ. A Poly(propylene glycol-co-fumaric acid) based bone graft extender for lumbar spinal fusion: In vivo assessment in a rabbit model. Eur Spine J 2005; in press.
42. Ishaug SL, Crane GM, Miller MJ, Yasko AW, Yaszemski MJ, Mikos AG. Bone formation by three-dimensional stromal osteoblast culture in biodegradable polymer scaffolds. J Biomed Mater Res 1997; 36(1):17–28.
43. Thomson RC, Yaszemski MJ, Powers JM, Mikos AG. Hydroxyapatite fiber reinforced poly(alpha-hydroxy ester) foams for bone regeneration. *Biomaterials* 1998; 19(21):1935–1943.

44. Hile DD, Kirker-Head C, Doherty SA, et al. Mechanical evaluation of a porous bone graft substitute based on poly(propylene glycol-co-fumaric acid). J Biomed Mater Res (Applied Biomaterials) 2003; 66B(1):311–317.
45. Heppenstall RB. Fracture healing. In: Mow VC, Hayes WC, eds. Basic Orthopaedic Biomechanics. New York: Raven Press, 1991:35–64.
46. Kandziora F, Kerschbaumer F, Starker M, Mittlmeier T. Biomechanical assessment of the transoral plate fixation for atlantoaxial instability. Spine 2000; 25:1555–1561.
47. Ripamonti U, Van Den Heever B, Crooks J, et al. Long-term evaluation of bone formation by osteogenic protein 1 in the baboon and relative efficacy of bone-derived bone morphogenetic proteins delivered by irradiated xenogeneic collagenous matrices. J Bone Miner Res 2000; 15(9):1798–1809.
48. Wildemann B, Kandziora F, Krummey G, et al. Local and controlled release of growth factors (combination of IGF-1, TGF-beta I, and BMP-2 alone) from a polylactide coating of titanium implants does not lead to ectopic bone formation in sheep muscle. J Controlled Release 2004; 95:249–256.
49. Kandziora F, Pflugmacher R, Scholz M, et al. Dose-dependent effects of combined IGF-I and TGF-beta1 application in a sheep cervical spine fusion model. Eur Spine J 2003; 12(5):464–473.
50. Hedberg EL, Tang A, Crowther RS, Carney DH, Mikos AG. Controlled release of an osteogenic peptide from injectable biodegradable polymeric composites. J Control Release 2002; 84(3):137–150.
51. Ruhe PQ, Hedberg EL, Padron NT, Spauwen PH, Jansen JA, Mikos AG. rhBMP-2 release from injectable poly(DL-lactic-co-glycolic acid)/calcium-phosphate cement composites. J Bone Joint Surg Am 2003; 85-A Suppl 3:75–81.
52. Malafaya PB, Silva GA, Baran ET, Reis RL. Drug delivery therapies II. Strategies for delivering bone regenerating factors. Current Opinion in Solid State and Materials Science 2002; 6:297–312.
53. Simmons CA, Alsberg E, Hsiong S, Kim WJ, Mooney DJ. Dual growth factor delivery and controlled scaffold degradation enhance in vivo bone formation by transplanted bone marrow stromal cells. Bone 2004; 35(2):562–569.
54. Brown RQ, Mount A, Burg KJ. Evaluation of polymer scaffolds to be used in a composite injectable system for intervertebral disc tissue engineering. J Biomed Mater Res A. 2005; 74(1):32–39.
55. Mizuno H, Roy AK, Vacanti CA, Kojima K, Ueda M, Bonassar LJ. Tissue-engineered composites of anulus fibrosus and nucleus pulposus for intervertebral disc replacement. Spine 2004; 29(12):1290–1297; discussion 1297–1298.
56. Kohn J, Langer R. Bioresorbable and bioerodible materials. In: Ratner BD, Hoffman AS, Schoen FJ, Lemons JE, eds. Biomaterials Science: An introduction to materials in medicine. New York: Academic Press, 1996:64–73.
57. Thomas KA. Biomechanics and biomaterials. In: Brinker MR, Review of Trauma. Philadelphia: WB Saunders, 2001:43–51.
58. An YH. Mechanical properties of bone. In: An YH, Draughn RA, eds. Mechanical Testing of Bone and the Bone-Implant Interface. Boca Raton: CRC Press, 2000:41–63.
59. Panjabi MM, White AA. Physical properties and functional biomechanics of the spine. In: White AA, Panjabi MM, eds. Clinical Biomechanics of the Spine, 2nd ed., Philadelphia: Lippincott-Raven Publishers, 1990.

35 | Biomechanical Properties of a Newly Designed Bioabsorbable Anterior Cervical Plate

Christopher P. Ames and Frank L. Acosta, Jr.
Department of Neurological Surgery, University of California, San Francisco, California, U.S.A.

Robert H. Chamberlain, Adolfo Espinoza Larios, and Neil R. Crawford
Barrow Neurological Institute, Phoenix, Arizona, U.S.A.

INTRODUCTION

A variety of effective surgical options exists for the treatment of patients with symptomatic cervical disc herniation. The anterior approach allows direct visualization of the interspace and decompression of the cervical spinal cord and nerve roots. The anterior approach also allows interbody fusion, if required. This approach has proven to be safe and effective and may be used for treating multiple segment disease. It is associated with minimal morbidity and mortality in large retrospective studies (1).

Biomechanical studies have demonstrated added stability provided by anterior cervical plates compared with bone graft alone (2). The risk-to-benefit ratio of the addition of an anterior plate to a single-level discectomy and fusion is controversial because the fusion rate is high in uninstrumented fusions in this region (3). Recent studies, however, demonstrated an increase in fusion rates in single-level anterior cervical discectomy of 90% to 96% with the addition of anterior cervical plating to the procedure (4–6). There were no clinically significant complications related to the instrumentation in the plated group. These studies also reported a significant decrease in graft-related complications in the instrumented cohort. In multilevel anterior cervical discectomies, the pseudoarthrosis rates are significantly higher in patients treated without plate fixation. In two-level anterior cervical discectomies without plating, pseudoarthrosis rates of 25% to 28% have been reported in large series (5). The addition of plating to a two-level discectomy without autograft has been reported to reduce fusion failure (7).

Anterior cervical screw plates function mechanically as a tension band and a buttress plate. These devices are relatively efficient at resisting cervical extension, axial rotation, and lateral bending. However, they are weakest in resisting neck flexion, particularly if the posterior elements of the cervical spine have been disrupted (i.e., after laminectomy, facet fracture, hyperflexion injuries with ligamentous tears). The extent of fixation depends on patients' bone mineral density. Dense bone provides a strong anchor for the screws, whereas osteoporotic bone holds screws poorly. Cervical screw plates can act to prevent movement of unstable vertebrae, prevent graft extrusion or displacement, and to maintain compression of graft materials.

Currently, most cervical plates are composed of titanium alloys, the most popular of which is Ti-6AI-4V. These plates provide significant rigidity across the fused segment and typically demonstrate low rates of hardware-related complications such as infection, fracture, and screw backout. Nevertheless, titanium produces substantial magnetic resonance imaging (MRI) artifact that may make postoperative imaging difficult to interpret at the instrumented levels. Computed tomography (CT) myelography is often required if imaging is necessary to accurately assess the spinal canal after a titanium plate has been implanted. Also, it has been postulated that the addition of a plate may increase the incidence of next-segment degenerative disease. The etiology of this finding is uncertain, but has been hypothesized to be related to increased dissection of the anterior longitudinal ligament close to the adjacent levels (4). It is possible that the high-rigidity conferred to the fusion segment by the addition of a stiff titanium plate may contribute to the development of next-segment degenerative disease, particularly if the ends of the plate are close to the adjacent levels.

The minimum mechanical characteristics that are necessary for a specific material to function effectively as a plate, to increase fusion rates above bone graft alone, and to prevent complications such as graft dislodgement for the anterior cervical discectomy indication are unknown. Most likely, there is a minimum rigidity that the implant must create and maintain across the segment to allow arthrodesis. A minimal amount of load sharing with the graft must be maintained and a minimal amount of time must pass while the fusion is occurring. These minimal properties of the construct are a function of the mechanical properties of the implant material, the design elements of the implant, the way in which the implant is applied, the preexisting biomechanical properties of the cervical segment, implant-host reaction characteristics, and native and induced host bone biology (Table 1).

Resorbable polylactide polymers have been used for several years in numerous human clinical applications, particularly craniofacial fixation (8,9). The potential advantages of utilizing a fully MRI-compatible, resorbable nonmetallic material for a cervical plate include:

1. Complete radiolucency and lack of MRI artifact from time of implantation.
2. Increased load sharing at immediate and long-term time points as the plate and screws bend as the material slowly resorbs.
3. No permanent encroachment on adjacent segments if subsidence occurs and the plate position shifts because the implant resorbs.
4. The implant is completely transparent so it is easy to visualize the graft position at time of plate insertion.
5. Revision surgery is theoretically much easier as the plate is completely resorbed by 18 months and does not need to be removed if the adjacent segment requires plate fixation.
6. There is no permanent foreign material in the retropharyngeal space.

Vaccaro et al. (10) found that seven of nine (77%) patients treated with allograft interbody fusion followed by application of a HYDROSORB™ (MacroPore Biosurgery, San Diego, California, U.S.A.) resorbable anterior cervical plate had radiographic evidence of fusion at six-month follow up. In a previous study, we examined the stability offered by a mesh of MacroPore™ (Macropore Biosurgery, San Diego, California, U.S.A.) brand 70/30 poly(L-lactide-co-D,L-lactide), or polylactic acid (PLA), placed with two or three screws per vertebra across a single-level discectomy and bone graft (11). The mesh offered a slight improvement in stability over graft alone but did not perform as well as a metallic plate (11–13). Newly designed MacroPore™ anterior cervical fusion plates have since become available. The rationale for utilizing these implants is that they are shaped more like standard metallic anterior cervical fusion plates and may therefore provide stability that is more comparable to a metal plate while still offering the advantages of a bioabsorbable material (Fig. 1). The purpose of the current research is to examine the biomechanical stability offered by the newly designed plate and to compare the stability to that offered by the earlier MacroPore cervical mesh and by a conventional metallic plate.

TABLE 1 Implant Variables Determining Construct Success

Variable	Sample characteristics
Material mechanical properties	Elastic modulus, ductility, compressive strength
Implant design	Dynamism, fixed moment arm, screw size, thread design, screw/plate interface
Method of implant application	Compression, distraction
Native segment biomechanics	Normal (intact stabilizers), three-column injury
Host-implant interaction	Mechanisms of fatigue (fretting, corrosion), osteointegration, resorption
Host bone biology (native or induced)	Osteopenia, bone morphogenic protein

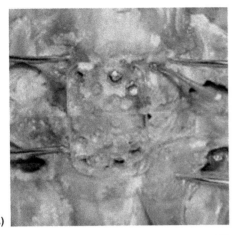 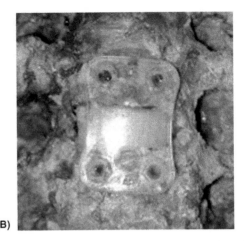

(A)　　　　　　　　　　　　　　　　　　(B)

FIGURE 1　Comparison of (**A**) old-style MacroPore™ mesh previously tested biomechanically, and (**B**) newly designed MacroPore™ anterior cervical fusion plate. The shape of the new plate is more similar to the shape of a standard metallic anterior cervical fusion plate.

MATERIALS AND METHODS
Specimens

Seven human cadaveric specimens were studied (Table 2). In all cases, the level operated was C6 to C7. Specimens were thawed in a bath of 0.9% saline solution at 30°C for preparation and testing. All muscular tissues were dissected with care taken to preserve all ligaments, joint capsules, discs and osseous structures. Household wood screws were inserted in the distal ends of the specimen and the heads of the screws were embedded in polymethylmethacrylate poured in metal testing fixtures. During testing, specimens were wrapped in saline-soaked gauze to prevent dehydration. Each specimen required four freeze-thaw cycles to complete testing such as dissecting and potting, normal testing, surgery, and post-surgical testing. Repeated freezing and thawing has minimal impact on the biomechanical properties of cadaveric specimens (14).

Instrumentation

For discectomies, distraction and endplate preparation were conducted in an identical fashion in every specimen. A scalpel, curette, and pituitary rongeurs were first used to remove disc material at C6 to C7. Then, the distractor from the CORNERSTONE-SR™ (Medtronic Sofamor Danek, Memphis, Tennessee, U.S.A.) set was used to achieve linear distraction of the interspace. The Cornerstone-SR cutter and interspace sizers were used to standardize graft size and thus graft compression forces.

After placing the graft, a one-level resorbable plate was attached (Fig. 1B). In all cases, the rostrocaudal hole spacing was 26 mm. The plate was contoured by hand using standard surgical tools (forceps, curette handle) to match the anterior surface of the spine after dipping in a

TABLE 2　One-Level Specimen Data

ID	Levels	Age (years)	Sex
AM1	C5-T2	59	F
AM2	C4-T1	59	M
AM3	C5-T1	35	F
AM4	C5-T2	53	F
AM5	C5-T2	59	M
AM6	C5-T1	55	M
AM7	C5-T1	64	M

Note: Mean age $\pm$ SD = 55 $\pm$ 9 years.

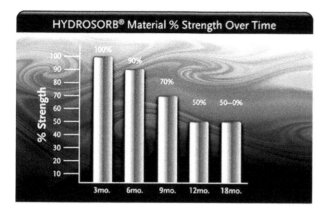

FIGURE 2 Mechanical properties of 70/30 PLA HYDROSORB™ (MacroPore Biosurgery, San Diego, CA, U.S.A.). HYDROSORB retains 100% strength at three months; 90% at six months; 70% at nine months; 50% at 12 months; and 50% to 0% at 18 to 36 months.

hot water bath at 65°C. Two resorbable screws were used in each vertebra of the motion segment to secure the plate. We chose the 70/30 PLA polymer as our plate material due to its ability to retain a significant amount of its initial strength over time (Fig. 2).

Importantly, all procedures in this study and in the previous study in which MacroPore mesh was used were performed by the same surgeon, Christopher P. Ames. Results between the two studies should therefore be directly comparable.

Flexibility Testing

Specimens were nondestructively tested using a standard flexibility testing method (15). Specimens were flexibility tested once in the normal intact condition and a second time after discectomy, graft, and plate. For flexibility testing, nonconstraining, nondestructive pure moment (torque) loading was applied to each specimen through a system of cables and pulleys in conjunction with a standard servohydraulic test system (MTS, Minneapolis, Minnesota, U.S.A.), as described earlier (16). Three cycles of preconditioning (ramp from 0–1.5 Nm) were used. Loads were applied about the appropriate anatomical axes to induce three different types of motion such as flexion-extension, lateral bending, and axial rotation. After allowing the specimen to rest for 60 sec at zero load, specimens were loaded quasistatistically to a maximum of 1.5 Nm in 0.25-Nm increments. Each load was held for 45 seconds. Data were collected at 2 Hz.

Three-dimensional specimen motion in response to the loads was determined using the Optotrak® 3020 system (Northern Digital, Waterloo, Ontario, Canada). This system measures stereophotometrically the three-dimensional displacement of infrared-emitting markers rigidly attached in a noncollinear arrangement to each vertebra. Marker position was related to the x (lateral), y (rostrocaudal), and z (anteroposterior) axes of the specimens by identifying landmarks with a digitizing probe and custom software (17). This software also converted the marker coordinates to angles about each of the anatomical axes using a method that models the vertebrae as stacked cylinders (17,18).

Data Analysis

Three parameters were generated from the quasistatic load-deformation data such as angular range of motion (ROM), lax zone (LZ, zone of ligamentous laxity), and stiff zone (SZ, zone of ligamentous stretching) (Fig. 3). The LZ and SZ are components of the ROM and represent the low-stiffness and high-stiffness portions of the typically biphasic load-deformation curve, respectively (19). The lax zone is similar to Panjabi's (20) neutral zone but is more reproducible and refers to the zone in which there is minimal ligamentous resistance, whereas the neutral zone is the zone in which there is only frictional joint resistance (19). The location at which the LZ crossed to SZ was calculated by extrapolating the load-deformation slope at data points corresponding to 0.75 Nm, 1.00 Nm, 1.25 Nm, and 1.50 Nm to zero load using the method of least squares in Microsoft Excel™ (Microsoft Corp., Redmond, Washington, U.S.A.). Larger values of LZ, SZ, or ROM indicate greater instability.

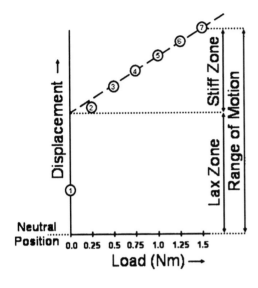

FIGURE 3 Schematic showing the different parameters studied. Each circle represents angular position data recorded quasistatically (after holding steady load for 45 seconds) at the seven different loads applied. The boundary between lax zone (LZ) and stiff zone (SZ) is the displacement where a line through the upper SZ is extrapolated to zero load. LZ and SZ sum to form the range of motion. Shown here is the positive half of a bidirectional motion (e.g., flexion). Each positive curve has a corresponding negative curve (e.g., extension). The neutral position is by definition halfway between the positive LZ/SZ boundary and the negative LZ/SZ boundary.

Flexibility testing data were statistically analyzed using paired 2-tailed Student's t-tests to determine whether significant differences existed in stability between normal and plated specimens. Stability in specimens from the current study during each loading mode was compared to that of the previous study (mesh with two or three screws per vertebra) using nonpaired 2-tailed Student's t-tests. Stability in MacroPore[TM]-plated specimens versus specimens with one-level Atlantis plates from a previous data set (8) was compared using nonpaired 2-tailed Student's t-tests. Student's t-tests were used in all cases rather than analysis of variance to allow direct comparison to the previous study in which only two groups were compared.

RESULTS

After testing, no bone fractures were found in specimens and any screw, rod, or plate showed signs of fracture, loosening, or breakage.

The angular LZ and ROM were statistically significantly smaller than normal after instrumentation with any plate type (Table 3, Fig. 4). The angular SZ was also smaller than normal after plating of any type, although this was not statistically significant in any loading mode. The new MacroPore[TM] plate allowed a significantly smaller non-normalized ROM during extension and SZ during axial rotation, than the MacroPore[TM] mesh (2 screws; Table 3). The new MacroPore plate did not exhibit a significantly different LZ than the previous MacroPore mesh during any loading mode. The new MacroPore plate also allowed a ROM, LZ, and SZ that was closer in magnitude to that of the Atlantis[®] (Medtronic Sofamor Danek, Memphis, Tennessee, U.S.A.) plate than the old MacroPore mesh, and showed almost no significant differences compared to Atlantis. During some loading modes, the new MacroPore plate actually decreased ROM, LZ, and SZ to a value slightly smaller than was allowed by the Atlantis plate (not significant), although the destabilization was more severe in the Atlantis study. However, the SZ was significantly smaller with the Atlantis plate than with the MacroPore plate during flexion (Table 4).

DISCUSSION
Comparison to Normal

It was found that the new MacroPore plate reduced LZ and ROM to significantly within normal during most loading modes. As a rule of thumb, fusion hardware should reduce motion to well within what was observed in the normal case for a good fusion environment. However, the ideal amount of immobilization required to promote fusion is unknown.

TABLE 3   Mean Single-Level Angular Motion in Each Condition Studied in Degrees ± SD

Loading mode and parameter		Normal	MacroPore™ plate	Graft only	MacroPore™ mesh (2 screws)	MacroPore™ mesh (3 screws)	Atlantis® plate
Flexion	LZ	7.64 ± 4.76	1.76 ± 1.96	3.64 ± 3.75	3.97 ± 2.48	4.01 ± 3.34	1.17 ± 1.48
	SZ	2.51 ± 0.81	1.91 ± 1.01	3.03 ± 0.83	2.68 ± 0.66	2.67 ± 0.62	1.00 ± 0.36
	ROM	6.33 ± 2.73	2.75 ± 1.82	4.85 ± 2.41	4.66 ± 1.73	4.67 ± 2.10	1.58 ± 1.08
Extension	LZ	7.64 ± 4.76	1.76 ± 1.96	3.64 ± 3.75	3.97 ± 2.48	4.01 ± 3.34	1.17 ± 1.48
	SZ	1.82 ± 0.88	0.64 ± 0.78	2.20 ± 0.58	1.16 ± 0.44	1.12 ± 0.52	1.27 ± 1.16
	ROM	5.64 ± 2.78	1.53 ± 0.98	4.02 ± 2.18	1.47 ± 1.14	3.12 ± 1.88	1.85 ± 1.87
Lateral bending	LZ	5.90 ± 3.42	2.09 ± 3.07	3.49 ± 3.35	3.47 ± 2.69	4.13 ± 3.88	1.62 ± 1.73
	SZ	1.41 ± 0.30	1.33 ± 0.61	1.69 ± 0.56	1.79 ± 0.62	1.68 ± 0.54	1.38 ± 0.71
	ROM	4.36 ± 1.88	2.38 ± 1.93	3.43 ± 2.05	3.53 ± 1.87	3.75 ± 2.30	2.19 ± 1.45
Axial rotation	LZ	3.80 ± 1.52	1.52 ± 1.59	2.20 ± 2.34	2.41 ± 2.30	2.79 ± 3.34	1.71 ± 1.82
	SZ	1.26 ± 0.37	0.25 ± 0.07	1.62 ± 0.54	1.68 ± 0.55	1.62 ± 0.61	1.55 ± 0.80
	ROM	3.16 ± 0.93	1.07 ± 0.29	2.72 ± 1.59	2.89 ± 1.65	3.02 ± 2.22	2.41 ± 1.69

Abbreviations: LZ, lax zone; ROM, range of motion; SZ, stiff zone.

Comparison to Mesh

During all loading modes, the new MacroPore plate consistently outperformed the older MacroPore mesh. Only a few statistical comparisons were significant, but all mean values of ROM, LZ, and SZ during all loading modes were smaller with the plate attached than with the mesh attached. The validity of comparisons between MacroPore mesh and MacroPore plate is exceptionally good since the same surgeon applied both types of hardware using the same tools for discectomy and grafting. Values of normal ROM, LZ, and SZ between groups are nearly identical in most cases, lending further validity to this comparison.

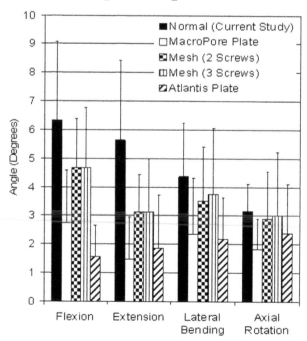

FIGURE 4   Mean angular range of motion (ROM) for specimens in the normal condition, and after discectomy, grafting, and placement of new MacroPore™ plates. For comparison, ROMs of specimens receiving single-level MacroPore™ mesh and single-level Atlantis® plates are included. Error bars show standard deviation.

TABLE 4 P-values for Comparisons of Stiff Zone, Lax Zone, and Range of Motion Among Hardware Conditions

Comparison	Flexion			Extension			Lateral bending			Axial rotation		
	LZ	SZ	ROM	LZ	SZ	ROM	LZ	SZ	ROM	LZ	SZ	ROM
MacroPore™ plate vs. mesh (2 screws)	0.0808	0.1003	0.0577	0.0808	0.1270	*0.0376*	0.3683	0.1751	0.2626	0.4065	*0.0214*	0.1709
MacroPore™ plate vs. mesh (3 screws)	0.1432	0.0994	0.0840	0.1432	0.1775	0.0865	0.2836	0.2575	0.2360	0.3797	*0.0494*	0.2217
MacroPore™ plate vs. Atlantis® plate	0.5351	0.0437	0.1675	0.5351	0.2535	0.6850	0.7313	0.8992	0.8402	0.8420	0.1639	0.4637

Note: Values in *italic* are statistically significant ($p < 0.05$).
Abbreviations: LZ, lax zone; ROM, range of motion; SZ, stiff zone.

Comparison to Previous Metal Plate Data

The comparison to the previous data set of specimens receiving single-level fusion with a metallic (Atlantis) plate showed that the metal plate tended to resist motion only slightly better than the MacroPore plate. In one case (SZ during flexion) did the metal plate allow significantly less motion than the MacroPore plate (Table 4). These findings support the argument that new MacroPore plates are approximately equivalent to metal plates in resisting loading. The difference observed in SZ without differences observed in ROM or LZ implies that the MacroPore plate and/or the bone-screw-plate interface was able to bend more easily than was the metal plate and/or interface between the bone, metal screw, and metal plate.

Limitations

This in vitro research quantifies how the new MacroPore plate performs in resisting particular loads in an immediate postoperative condition without the stabilizing influence of surrounding musculature or (substantial) gravitational compression. These limitations should be kept in mind when considering how our findings apply to patients.

Another limitation of this research is the relatively small number of specimens studied per group, which leads to low statistical power (probability of avoiding type 2 or false-negative error). Typically, a power of 0.8 is desired when making assertions that there was no significant difference between groups. However, in many instances, the power was less than 0.8. Type 2 error is difficult to avoid in this type of research because of the expense and time required to test large numbers of samples. We assumed that differences that were small enough that they would not become apparent with seven specimens were too small to be important clinically.

CONCLUSIONS

Based on our findings, the new MacroPore plates provide better stability than the previous MacroPore mesh and would be preferred clinically. Although our results do not necessarily indicate that, the new MacroPore plate is equivalent to a metal plate in the stability it provides. The new plate provides stability that is certainly closer to what would be expected from a metal plate than was provided by the previous mesh. Although graft containment was not measured, screw design was similar in the new plate and the previous mesh. Therefore, as with the mesh, the surgeon can consider the new MacroPore plate as an excellent alternative if a graft containment device is needed.

SUMMARY

We presented a biomechanical analysis of a newly designed bioabsorbable anterior cervical fusion plate in the treatment of one-level degenerative disc disease of the cervical spine with anterior cervical discectomy and fusion (ACDF) in a human cadaveric model. Cervical spinal stability after placement of the bioabsorbable fusion plate was compared with that after placement of a bioabsorbable mesh, as well as after placement of a more traditional anterior cervical metallic fusion plate.

Seven human cadaveric specimens underwent ACDF at the C6–C7 level with placement of a fibular allograft. A one-level anterior cervical resorbable plate was then placed and secured with bioabsorbable screws. Flexibility testing was performed on both intact and instrumented specimens using a servohydraulic system to create flexion-extension, lateral bending, and axial rotation motions. After data analysis, three parameters were calculated: angular range of motion (ROM), lax zone (LZ), and stiff zone (SZ). Results were compared to a previous study of a resorbable fusion mesh, and to metallic fusion plates. For all parameters studied, the resorbable plate consistently offered more stability than the resorbable mesh. Moreover, the resorbable plate system offered comparable stability to that measured using metallic fusion plates.

CONCLUSIONS

Bioabsorbable plates provide better stability than resorbable mesh. Although, our results do not necessarily indicate that a resorbable plate is equivalent to a metal plate in the stability it provides, certainly, it is more comparable than is the resorbable mesh. Bioabsorbable fusion plates should therefore be considered as alternatives to metal plates when a graft containment device is required.

ACKNOWLEDGMENT

This work was supported by a grant from Macropore Biosurgery. The senior author (CPA) is a paid consultant for MacroPore (MacroPore Biosurgery, San Diego, California) and Medtronic Sofamor Danek (Memphis, Tennessee).

REFERENCES

1. Cauthen JC, Kinard RE, Vogler JB, et al. Outcome analysis of noninstrumented anterior cervical discectomy and interbody fusion in 348 patients. Spine 1998; 23:188–192.
2. Grubb MR, Currier BL, Shih JS, Bonin V, Grabowski JJ, Chao EY. Biomechanical evaluation of anterior cervical spine stabilization. Spine 1998; 23:886–892.
3. Branch CL Jr. Anterior cervical fusion: the case for fusion without plating. Clin Neurosurg 1999; 45:22–24; discussion 21.
4. Kaiser MG, Haid RW Jr, Subach BR, Barnes B, Rodts GE Jr. Anterior cervical plating enhances arthrodesis after discectomy and fusion with cortical allograft. Neurosurgery 2002; 50:229–236; discussion 236–228.
5. Martin GJ Jr, Haid RW Jr, MacMillan M, Rodts GE Jr, Berkman R. Anterior cervical discectomy with freeze-dried fibula allograft: Overview of 317 cases and literature review. Spine 1999; 24:852–858; discussion 858–859.
6. Wang JC, McDonough PW, Endow KK, Delamarter RB. Increased fusion rates with cervical plating for two-level anterior cervical discectomy and fusion. Spine 2000; 25:41–45.
7. Wang JC, McDonough PW, Endow K, Kanim LE, Delamarter RB. The effect of cervical plating on single-level anterior cervical discectomy and fusion. J Spinal Disord 1999; 12:467–471.
8. Cohen SR, Holmes RE. Internal Le Fort III distraction with biodegradable devices. J Craniofac Surg 2001; 12:264–272.
9. Kaptain GJ, Vincent DA, Laws ER Jr. Cranial base reconstruction after transsphenoidal surgery with bioabsorbable implants. Neurosurgery 2001; 48:232–233; discussion 233–234.
10. Vaccaro AR, Venger BH, Kelleher PM, et al. Use of a bioabsorbable anterior cervical plate in the treatment of cervical degenerative and traumatic disc disruption. Orthopedics 2002; 25:s1191–s1199; discussion s1199.
11. Ames CP, Crawford NR, Chamberlain RH, Cornwall GB, Nottmeier E, Sonntag VK. Feasibility of a resorbable anterior cervical graft containment plate. Orthopedics 2002; 25:s1149–1155.
12. Ames CP, Cornwall GB, Crawford NR, Nottmeier E, Chamberlain RH, Sonntag VK. Feasibility of a resorbable anterior cervical graft containment plate. J Neurosurg 2002; 97:440–446.
13. Ames CP, Crawford NR, Chamberlain RH, Deshmukh V, Sadikovic B, Sonntag VK. Biomechanical analysis of a resorbable anterior cervical graft containment plate. Spine 2005; 30(9):1031–1038.
14. Panjabi MM, Krag M, Summers D, Videman T. Biomechanical time-tolerance of fresh cadaveric human spine specimens. J Orthop Res 1985; 3:292–300.
15. Jeanneret B, Magerl F, Ward EH, Ward JC. Posterior stabilization of the cervical spine with hook plates. Spine 1991; 16:s56–s63.
16. Crawford NR, Brantley AGU, Dickman CA, Koeneman EJ. An apparatus for applying pure nonconstraining moments to spine segments in vitro. Spine 1995; 20:2097–2100.
17. Crawford NR, Dickman CA. Construction of local vertebral coordinate systems using a digitizing probe: Technical note. Spine 1997; 22:559–563.
18. Crawford NR, Yamaguchi GT, Dickman CA. A new technique for determining 3-D joint angles: The tilt/twist method. Clinical Biomechanics 1999; 14:153–165.
19. Crawford NR, Peles JD, Dickman CA. The spinal lax zone and neutral zone: Measurement techniques and parameter comparisons. J Spinal Disord 1998; 11:416–429.
20. Panjabi MM. The stabilizing system of the spine: Part II. Neutral zone and instability hypothesis. J Spinal Disord 1992; 5:390–397.

36 | The Role of Electrical Stimulation in Enhancing Fusions with Autograft, Allograft, and Bone Graft Substitutes

Donald W. Kucharzyk and Thomas J. Milroy
The Orthopaedic, Pediatric and Spine Institute, Crown Point, Indiana, U.S.A.

With the expanding knowledge of the lumbar spine and our increasing diagnostic skills and technology, greater pathology of the spine is being identified. These tools have lead the spine surgeon to identify pathologic processes that can be treated surgically. With this ability and the increase in spinal surgery and fusion surgeries being performed, surgeons are still frustrated with the high incidence of potential nonunions. In situ fusion has had good success but was not perfect with its incidence of nonunion (1–3). With the advent of instrumentation and the technologies that go along with this, the incidence of pseudoarthrosis has decreased but it is still a known risk (4–11). Also, greater awareness of underlying metabolic conditions and risk factors has also enhanced our understanding of fusion technology and what contributes to a nonunion. But we still see pseudoarthrosis in spinal fusion surgeries and question whether we can further decrease this incidence (5,7,3,12).

Electrical stimulation has been an area that has shown promise and carries many years of basic science and research. Such means include direct current (DC) stimulation, pulsed electromagnetic field (PEMF), and capacitive coupling with all currently in use and have been shown to be safe and, for specific indications, efficacious in promoting improved fusions over nonstimulated spinal fusions and potentially overcoming many of the risk factors that lead to a pseudoarthrosis. To understand electrical stimulation of the spine, we must look at the basic science and research behind the development of these technologies. Electrical stimulation has its roots in long bone fracture model studies where an electrical current and signal is generated by the applied stresses of a fracture and the body responding by initiating an osteogenic process and leading to bone healing. Fukada and Yasuda (13) presented their work on electrical stimulation in bony injuries and confirmed its positive effect (14–16). From this significant research has been conducted on the role and use of electrical stimulation (17–23). Concluding that if additional electrical current is applied, theses studies have shown an increase in the maximal amount of new bone formation. Kahanovitz in 1984 was the first to examine this effect in the canine spine and showed an accelerated osteogenic response in initial histologic and radiographic studies (24–26). Nerubay in 1986 (27), in their animal studies revealed increased osteoblastic activity and enhanced bone formation and fusion mass in those spine that were stimulated via direct current. Further works by Kahanovitz et al. in 1990 (24–26), showed enhanced fusion success rates and fusion masses in the canine spine and even took it one step further, showing that if the current density was increased five and fifteen fold, there was a significant increase in the quality, quantity, and the rate of formation of the fusion mass. All these studies dealt with DC stimulation and when PEMF studies were undertaken in the canine model, not one study came close to enhancing fusion mass when compared to the nonstimulated canine spine model and when compared to the results with DC stimulation.

Clinical studies have been undertaken to look at the efficacy of DC stimulation, PEMF and capacitive coupling. With reference to DC stimulation, the first study to look at this was that of Dwyer. When in 1974 and 1975, this study revealed an enhanced fusion success rate of 85% when compared to the nonstimulated group in a high-risk pool of patients and it was the first major study to look at the potential and positive effect of DC stimulation (28–30). Kane in 1988 published his hallmark study on implantable DC stimulation and supported the basic science research with his results showing enhanced fusion rates of 91% compared to the control of 81% (31). Furthermore, in a randomized, prospective cohort of patients stimulated, patients had a higher fusion rate 81% compared to the nonstimulated control group 54% and in the open trial, those with DC stimulation had fusion rates of 93% (31). Meril in 1994 (8), studied the effect of DC stimulation on allograft posterior interbody fusions and found a positive effect with a fusion rate of 93%. Tejano in 1996 (32), looked at non-instrumented lumbar fusions treated with DC stimulation and showed enhanced fusion rates to 91.5% with these being the most difficult patients to fuse. Rogozinski in 1996 (3), revealed in instrumented fusion patients an enhanced fusion rate of 96% in those receiving DC stimulation versus 85% in those without stimulation (33). Kucharzyk in 1999 showed again enhanced fusion rates with DC Stimulation to 96% in high risk multiply operated patients, but went one step further. No other study had looked at clinical outcomes and in this study, Kucharzyk reported enhanced clinical success rates of 91% in those receiving DC stimulation versus 79% in the nonstimulated group (6). Grottkau and Lipson (34) studied the effect that DC stimulation had on fusion consolidation revealing greater consolidation earlier in the stimulated group versus the nonstimulated. In addition, Jenis and An (2) have shown that in those patients receiving DC stimulation, the fusion mass was greater in quantity than those not receiving DC stimulation (Fig. 1).

PEMF has been recently studied and when we look at prior clinical studies, these studies have focused on its use in interbody fusions. Simmons in 1985 (35,36) reported a 77% fusion success rate in failed posterior lumbar interbody fusions that were treated with PEMF. In 1989, Lee et al. (7), reported on their use of PEMF in posterior pseudoarthrosis repair and this study revealed only a 67% fusion success rate. Simmons in 1989 (35,36) reported his results on the use of PEMF in posterolateral fusions with the results reported at only 71% fusion success which when compared to DC stimulation was inferior. Mooney in 1990 (37) reported his results of PEMF in either anterior or posterior interbody fusions without posterior fusion revealed a fusion success rate of 92%. Attention was then turned to PEMF's role in posterolateral fusions and Bose in 2001 reported his results in 48 high-risk patients treated with instrumentation, posterolateral fusion and PEMF with this study revealing a fusion rate of 97.9% (38). Silver in 2001 (39) reported his experience with PEMF in patients having undergone a posterior lumbar interbidy fusion (PLIF) and/or a posterolateral fusion with fusion s rates similar to that of Bose at 97.7%. Finally, with the experience of PEMF in lumbar interbody fusions, attention was turned to its role in cervical interbody fusion and its ability to enhance fusion rates. In the randomized prospective controlled clinical trial (2004), 323 cervical high-risk fusion patients were studied with the results revealing in those with stimulation, 84% of the patients achieving fusion in six months compared to 69% in those without stimulation (Fig. 2).

Capacitative coupling (CC) is the third type of technology that has been used to enhance fusion success rates in spinal fusion surgeries. It utilizes an electrical signal that has been derived from in vitro, in vivo, and mathematical modeling studies. Goodwin et al. (40) reported on their work with CC revealing a combined clinical and radiographic success rate of 84.7% in the stimulated versus 64.9% in the nonstimulated groups.

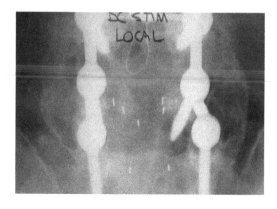

FIGURE 1 Twelve-month follow-up of direct current stimulation with local bone and instrumentation with interbody stabilization device.

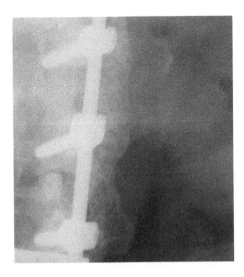

FIGURE 2 Nine-month follow-up of pulsed electromagnetic field with iliac crest bone graft, instrumentation and interbody fusion implant.

All these devices have been studied utilizing autograft harvested from the iliac crest. As we know there are inherent risks in this procedure with reported major and minor complications ranging from drainage to infection to persistant pain and nerve injury. To avoid this, other sources have been identified such as allograft and research with electrical stimulation has been carried out and has shown positive effects although the results have not been as good as autograft except in interbody fusions. But concerns exist about the use of allograft from a safety standpoint and the incidence of nonunion. As a result, bone graft substitutes have recently been used in spinal fusion surgery and these include demineralized bone matrix (DBM) products such as Grafton or Osteofil (Fig. 3), and bone graft extenders such as ProOsteon™, OsteoStim™, or Mastergraft™ (Fig. 4). Reports on their use in the spine have shown promise when combined with local bone or bone marrow aspirate. But can electrical stimulation enhance these bone graft substitutes? The first study to look at the role of DC stimulation and bone graft substitutes was by Bozic and Glazer in Spine 1999 (41). This study looked at the effect of DC stimulation in a rabbit model and found significantly higher fusion rates in those receiving DC stimulation versus those without. This study went even further contributing to our knowledge of DC stimulation and bone-graft extenders. This study showed that with stimulation and a bone-graft substitute, an enhanced fusion mass and a stiffer fusion mass can be achieved compared to the gold-standard autograft (41). Kucharzyk et al. looked at this role in a human model and reported his experience with coralline hydroxyapatite and DC

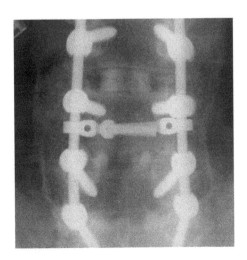

FIGURE 3 Nine-month follow-up of direct current stimulation with DBM Grafton and local bone combined with spinal instrumentation and interbody cortical bone graft.

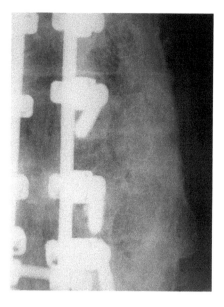

FIGURE 4 Twelve-month follow-up combining direct current stimulation and coralline hydroxyapatite with local bone and spinal instrumentaion.

stimulation showing enhanced fusion rates as high as 92% and 96% in two separate yet unpublished studies and concluded that a positive effect does exist when DC stimulation is used with a bone-graft extender or substitute. Thalgott in Spine 2001 supported his work and concluded that their exists a positive role for a bone-graft substitute or extender such as coralline hydroxyapatite, with fusion rates of 92.5%, in spine fusion surgery and especially the difficult to fuse patient (Fig. 4) (42).

As technology has progressed and new products continue to be developed such as Infuse[TM], research has now allowed us to further investigate on a cellular and genetic level how electrical stimulation works and allows us to compare DC stimulation to the newer technology, that is, BMP. Recently, electrical stimulation has been shown to enhance multiple gene expressions including TGF-Beta, BMP 2, BMP 4, and BMP 7. Capacitative coupling has been shown to increase the production of DNA, PGE 2, and TGF Beta. Fredericks et al. (29) at NASS 2004 reported these positive effects with electrical stimulation namely capacitative coupling and Peterson et al. (43) at the bioelectromagnetic society meeting 2003 showed the similar up regulation of these genes with direct current technology. But when looking at PEMF and compared to these studies, little has been shown on a cellular or genetic level, the positive effects of PEMF on these similar gene expressions. Additionally, these reports reveal the

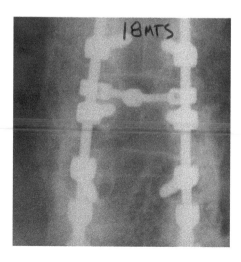

FIGURE 5 Eighteen-month follow-up of a revision spinal fusion for pseudoarthrosis combining Mastergraft with local bone and BMP Infuse[TM] and revision instrumentation.

prolonged enhancement of these elements with DC stimulation as well as the sustained enhancement of these factors for longer periods of time when compared to Infuse™ (BMP 2) or OP-1™ (BMP 7). DC stimulation also has been shown to enhance multiple genes expressions and not only just one as seen with the other products currently on the market. As a result, when one compares DC stimulation against Infuse or OP-1, DC stimulation has greater potential to enhance multiple gene expressions for bone morphogenic proteins as well as prolonged enhancement than those on the market now. Figure 5 and when cost is entered into the discussion, electrical stimulation: via DC, CC, or PEMF are more cost effect with DC stimulation being the only one that has the basic science, research and clinical studies to support its use in enhancing spine fusion surgery. But one final thought exists, and that is, what about combining these two emerging technologies and seeing if with a lower dose of BMP and stimulation either DC, CC, or PEMF, can results be produced that are similar to or exceeding that of autograft. A few cases have been performed in unpublished reports and the results look promising with lower doses of BMP-Infuse and DC stimulation. As research continues, electrical stimulation of complex spine fusion surgery should be included in your thought process and added to your treatment arm for any revision surgery or for patients with significant risk factors.

REFERENCES

1. Dawson EG, Lotysch M, Urist MR. Intertransverse process lumbar arthrodesis with autogenous bone graft. Clin Orthop 1981; 154:90–96.
2. Jenis LG, An HS, Stein R, Young B. Prospective evaluation of electric stimulation in instrumented lumbar fusion. NASS 1997.
3. Rogozinski A, Rogozinski C. Efficacy of implanted bone growth stimulation in instrumented lumbo-sacral spinal fusion. Spine 1996; 21:2393–2398.
4. Kaneda K, Kazaman H, Satoh S, Fujiya M. Followup study of medial facetectomies and posterolateral fusion with instrumentation in unstable degenerative spondylolisthesis. Clin Orthop 1986; 203: 159–167.
5. Kornblatt MD, Casey MP, Jacobs RR. Internal fixation in lumbar spine fusion. Clin Orthop 1996; 203:141–150.
6. Kucharzyk D.A controlled prospective outcome study of implantable electrical stimulation with spinal instrumentation in a high risk spinal fusion population. Spine 1999; 24:465–468.
7. Lorenz M, Zindrick M, Schwaegler P.A comparison of a single level fusion with and without hardware. Spine 1991; 16:S455–S458.
8. Meril AJ. Direct current stimulation of allograft in anterior and posterior lumbar interbody fusions. Spine 1994; 19:2393–2398.
9. Steffee AD, Biscup RS, SItkowski DJ. Segmental spine plates with pedicle screw fixation. Clin Orthop 1986; 203:45–53.
10. Steffee AD, Brantigan JW. The variable screw placement spinal fixation system: Report of a prospective study of 250 patients in FDA clinical trials. Spine 1993; 18:1160–1172.
11. Zdeblick TA. A prospective randomized study of lumbar fusion. Spine 1993; 18:983–991.
12. Stauffer RN, Coventry MB. Posteroloateral lumbar spine fusion: analysis of mayo clinic series. J Bone Joint Surg [Am] 1972; 54:1195–1204.
13. Fukada E, Yasuda I. On the piezoelectric effect of bone. J Physiol Soc Japan 1957; 12:1158.
14. Yasuda I. Electrical callus and callus formation by electret. Clin Orthop 1997; 124:53.
15. Yasuda I. Fundamental aspects of fracture treatment. J Kyoto Med Soc 1953; 4:395.
16. Yasuda I. Dynamic callus and electric callus. J Bone Joint Surg [Am] 1955; 37:1292.
17. Baranowski TJ, Black J. The mechanism of faradic stimulation of osteogenesis. In: Blank M, Findl E, eds. Mechanistic Approaches to Interaction of Electric and Electromagnetic Fields with Living Systems. New'York: Plenum Press, 1987:399.
18. Bassett CAL, Pawluk RJ, Becker R. Effects of electric current on bone in vivo. Nature 1964; 204–652.
19. Black J, Baranowski TJ, Brighton CT. Electrochemical aspects of DC stimulation of osteogenesis. "Bioelectrochem Bioenergy 1984; 12:323.
20. Black J, Brighton CT. Mechanisms of stimulation of osteogenesis by direct current. In: Brighton CT, Black J, Pollock SR, eds. Electrical Properties of Bone and Cartilage: Experimental Effects and Clinical Applications. Grune and Stratton, 1979:215.
21. Brighton CT, Friedenberg ZB, Black J. Electrically induced osteogenesis: Relationship between charge, current density and bone formation. Clin Orthop 1981; 161:122.
22. Friedenberg ZB, Andrews ET, Smolenski B, Perl BW, Brighton CT. Bone reactions to varying amounts of direct current. Surg Gynecol Obstet 1970; 131:894.

23. Friedenberg ZB, Zemsky LM, Pollis RP, Brighton CT. The response of non-traumatized bone to direct current. J Bone Joint Surg [Am] 1974; 56:1023.
24. Kahanovitz N, Arnoczky S. The efficacy of direct current electrical stimulation to enhance canine spinal fusions. Clin Orthop 1990; 251:295–299.
25. Kahanovitz N, Dejardin L, Nemzek J, Arnoczky SP. Effect of varied electrical direct current densities on the healing posterior spinal fusion in dogs. AAOS 1996.
26. Kahanovitz N, Pashos C. The role of implantable direct current stimulation in the critical pathway for lumbar spinal fusion. J Care Management 1996; 2:2.
27. Nerubay J, Marganit B, Bubis J, Tadmor A, Katz NA. Stimulation of bone formation by electrical current on spinal fusion. Spine 1986; 11:167.
28. Dwyer AF. The use of electrical current stimulation in spinal fusion. Orthop Clin North Am 1975; 6:265.
29. Fredericks D, Pertersen E, Bobst J, Simon BJ, Nepola J. Effect of capacitive coupling electrical stimulation on expression of growth factor in a rabbit posterolateral spine fusion model. NASS 2004.
30. Dwyer AF. Direct current stimulation in spinal fusion. Med J Aust 1974; 1:73–75.
31. Kane WJ. Direct current electrical bone growth stimulation for spinal fusion. Spine 1988; 13:363–365.
32. Tejano NA, Puno R, Ignacio JMF. The use of implantable direct current stimulation in multilevel spinal fusion without instrumentation: A prospective clinical and radiographic evaluation with long term follow-up. Spine 1996; 21:1904–1908.
33. Birney TJ. A retrospective review of patient outcomes using internal fixation and implantable direct current stimulation in lumbar spinal fusion. Mid-American Orthopedic Association Hilton Head Island, April 1997.
34. Grottkau B, Lipson SJ. A controlled pilot study to determine the effect of direct current stimulation on fusion mass in lumbar spine fusion patients. NASS 1995.
35. Simmons JW. Treatment of failed posterior lumbar interbody fusion with pulsed electromagnetic fields. Clin Orthop 1985; 183:127–132.
36. Simmons JW, Hayes MA, Christensen DK. The effect of postoperative pulsing electromagnetic fields on lumbar fusion. NASS 1989.
37. Mooney V. A randomized double blind prospective study of the efficacy of pulsed electromagnetic fields for interbody lumbar fusion. Spine 1990; 15:708–712.
38. Bose B. Outcomes after posterolateral lumbar fusion with instrumentation in patients treated with adjunctive pulsed electromagnetic field stimulation. Advances in Therapy 2001; 18(1):12.
39. Silver RA. Application of pulsed electromagnetic fields after lumbar interbody or posterolateral spinal fusion surgery in a heterogeneous patient population. J Neurol Orthop Med Surg 2001; 21:51–62.
40. Goodwin C, Brighton CT, Guyer R, Johnson J, Yuan H. A double blind study of capacitively coupled electrical stimulation as an adjunct to lumbar spinal fusions. Spine 1999; 24:1349.
41. Bozik, Glazer. In vivo evaluation of coralline hydroxyapatite and DC stimulation in lumbar fusion model. Spine 1999; 24(20):2127.
42. Thalgott JS, Giuffre JM, Fritts K, Timlin M, Klezl Z. Instemented posterolateral lumbar fusion using coralline hydroxyapatite with or without dimineralized bone matrix. Spine J 2001; 1(2):131–137.
43. Peterson EB, Friedericks DC, Simon BJ, Nepola J. Effects of direct current electrical stimulation on expression of BMP 2,4,6,7,VEGF and ALK2 receptors in a rabbit posterolateral spine fusion model. Bioelectromagnetics Society Meeting, June 2003.

37 An Analysis of Physical Factors Promoting Bone Healing or Formation with Special Reference to the Spine

Mark R. Foster
Department of Orthopaedic Surgery, University of Pittsburgh School of Medicine, Pittsburgh, Pennsylvania, U.S.A.

INTRODUCTION

Physical factors have been demonstrated to be a naturally occurring component part of the process of osteogenesis or bone formation, regeneration, and repair. Beyond the mechanical forces, generally referred to as a manifestation of Wolff's law (1), where form follows function, electrical currents have been widely studied and recognized in biological organisms and processes, including bone healing and homeostasis. In cases where routine fracture healing has been interrupted and fails to occur, stimulation of the healing process by exogenously introducing electrical currents to simulate the endogenous phenomenon of electric currents in bone healing have been demonstrated effective to assist in supplementing healing, and as an adjunct for causing a bony fusion to occur in the spine. These technologies have been developed and considered particularly promising in the difficult and challenging environment of forming a spinal arthrodesis, which is not absolutely reliable and where failure of healing holds such significant consequences. This Chapter will provide physical intuition regarding the electromagnetic processes being observed and simulated and introduce some additional mechanisms, not previously considered, in an attempt to complete the analysis and as a stimulus to further research and development.

HISTORY/LITERATURE REVIEW

Electrical stimulation of osteogenesis has been available and widely accepted for many years, but not universally utilized. Historically, empirically derived electrical treatments were available in the nineteenth-century (2), including Franklinism, and other devices, such as Leyden jars and electrostatic generators. Wolff's law had been presented as an observation that the structural arrangement of the trabecular architecture of bones was in a morphologic pattern resembling structures designed from engineering calculations to provide maximum strength using minimum material.

Electric currents had been utilized medically, and specifically as an adjunct to healing bones in the 19th century (3,4). Fukada and Yasuda (5) described a phenomenon of bone formation in the vicinity of a cathode, or the negative lead, with a battery pack. Bioelectric potentials were documented (6) to be present at a fracture site and at the growth plate, and these were specifically dependent upon cellular or biological activity. These currents were consistent with an *injury potential* on an organ level, although also observed at the epiphysis as an intermediate signal directing growth and development. Repair at a fracture site may be considered a recapitulation to this initial developmental process; this is consistent with the observation that an externally applied electric current, as a simulation of the observed endogenous current, could stimulate healing in a nonunion, when natural healing had become quiescent (7). Subsequent studies used varying currents at the cathode or area of electronegativity to evaluate an optimum to maximize the response (8). A current of 20 μA was selected from this data for subsequent clinical evaluation, although deleterious effects were noted at the positive electrode and particularly necrosis as the current was increased (9).

Invasive electrical stimulation provides an environment around the cathode favorable to bone healing, of decreased oxygen tension and increased pH (10), and Baranowski confirmed these conditions are achieved by measurement of oxygen tension and pH in the medullary canal with a cathode carrying 20 microamperes of direct current (DC) (11). An alternating current (AC) has also been demonstrated efficacious with conducting electrodes (capacitative coupling) at a long bone nonunion site, as well as over the paravertebral musculature of the spine. Studies have demonstrated that the current flow is within an order of magnitude of the direct current case (12), but the electrode effects (13) are absent. The relatively low water content of cortical bone would be a poor electrical conductor, compared to the nonunion or fusion bed, and thus would preferentially shunt this current through the appropriate area of soft tissue in contact with bone.

Transient electrical potentials were also observed in bone as a result of stress, electronegative in areas of bone under compression and electropositive areas under tension; these results were replicated (14,15) and the biological, cellular, and molecular mechanisms were enthusiastically speculated as a potential explanation (16) for the observations described as Wolff's law. However, the stress-generated potentials persisted in dried tissues, and hence were mechanical and not biological phenomena. Living tissues were not required to generate these potentials, whereas Wolff's law involves the remodeling of bone in response to stress and thus required living, cellular activity. The observed stress generated potentials (SGP) were initially thought to be piezoelectric (17); however, the extra cellular, osseous matrix is not a piezoelectric crystal and does not require the presence of living cells for generation of the electric waveforms. The voltages are a result of charge separation, the amplitude varies with the rate of deformation and the amplitude increases linearly with load (18). Collagen (19) was demonstrated capable of generating potentials, including after demineralization of collagen (20) as ionized fluids flowed past fixed charges and created charge separation, or streaming potentials (SPs), which have been subsequently investigated as the mechanism for the SGP observation. Physiologically, this endogenous signal would be an essential part of bone homeostasis; its absence would be consistent with disuse osteoporosis.

The noninvasive induction (by Faraday's Law) of an electrical potential by a time-varying magnetic field, pulsed electromagnetic field (PEMF) has been utilized, initially at the cadence of gait (14), to simulate these physiologic, homeostatic electrical signals. PEMFs have also been demonstrated effective to initiate bone healing in nonunions, or to promote and accelerate the healing of bone, as well as stimulation of healing in avascular necrosis of bone.

The pulsed electromagnetic signal was not successful in stimulating posterior spine fusion in dogs (21), although anterior interbody fusions were reported to have accelerated healing (22). Dwyer demonstrated that direct current stimulation of osteogenesis was not only effective for long bone fractures, but also stimulated and accelerated lumbar fusions (23), documenting efficacy and recommending a specific technique—a current regulated DC generator with the electrode in the bone-fusion bed. The underlying physical mechanism, which is an electrical current exogenously applied to simulate the observed phenomena or a physical factor effecting bone healing, was confirmed. More recently, a *combined* technique has been presented, where a magnetic field is combined with an electric field as an adjunct to bone healing including spinal fusions. This technology has clinically been presented with results, which are not statistically significant, except in subgroups, but was approved by the Food and Drug Administration (FDA). Further, there is no mechanism presented in parallel with the above techniques and prior technology.

ANALYSIS AND PHYSICAL INTUITION
Direct Current

Friedenberg demonstrated the clinical utility of direct current by placing an electrode in a nonunion of a medial malleolus (24), demonstrating the utility of the phenomena described by Fukada and Yasuda (5) which ushered in the modern era of electrical stimulation. A low voltage from the negative electrode of the battery was in one direction and constant, until exhaustion of the battery and apparently this simulation of the current observed (bioelectric potentials) could be used to reinitiate the osteogenic process where it had not succeeded in healing a fracture. This form of an injury current was shown stimulating growth factors, quiescent in the tissue, and attracting, in a chemotactic sense, and transforming in a morphogenic sense, the residual stem cells to differentiate towards bone.

While, the endochondral ossification for fracture healing may be a recapitulation to the growth process, the electronegative potential was noted also in the growth plate but extinguished with either the end of growth or the healing of a fracture. The response curve for this technique was derived with a fibular osteotomy which is nonweight bearing (25) as it is synostosed with the tibia distally but essentially the results showed acceleration of healing, a result which has been applied to nonunions. Initially electrodes were drilled into the fracture site and a constant current circuit was connected to a battery pack externally with a return pack through a positive skin electrode (Quad Pak™, Zimmer Warsaw Indiana; EBI, Electro Biology Incorporated, Parsippany, New Jersey, U.S.A.; now part of Biomet), which caused superficial skin irritation and had to be moved frequently but was later encapsulated and implanted with a battery pack. Further studies confirmed an electrochemical mechanism at the electrode causing a depression in oxygen tension and a rise in pH consistent with encouraging bone formation and consistent with the observed phenomena.

Alternating Current

Many efforts with conductive electrodes passed a current through the skin (26) to avoid this invasive procedure to stimulate bone. These studies considered various frequencies, pulse durations, pulse intensities and some investigators specifically considered asymmetric pulses, perhaps because the electronegative electrode was the location where bone formed (27). From an engineering standpoint, it is evident that any pulse delivered through the skin would be essentially capacitively coupled through the dielectric of the skin and thus would become electrically neutral, the necessity of being a displacement current, but many such studies proliferated. Other experiments were performed which showed stimulation of bone formation, but unfortunately involved very high electrical fields and were considered unsafe and were not further pursued. Analysis of some of these experiments showed that essentially parallel capacitors allowed the majority of the voltage drop to occur across parts of the apparatus not involving any biological materials, large air gaps with the majority of the voltage drop (28) but when this was recognized, stimulation within the media or at least without large air gaps also developed appropriate stimulation at very safe and reasonable voltages.

From the standpoint of physical intuition, if we consider a simple model of the two ends of an unhealed bone, with an interposed fibrous, failed union or nonunion, we would essentially see the bone as relatively anhydrous and thus a poor conductor. The interposed fibrous tissue would be of much higher water content and thus constitute a shunt or a short circuit through which the voltage would preferentially pass. Using realistic voltages from simulation experiments, and a dielectric constant of 78 for 60 kHz, it was estimated to an order of magnitude that a 20-μA current would flow to that conducting gap of the nonunion. This is consistent with the optimum current flow in the invasive stimulation case but does not have any electrode effects, as it is noninvasive or referred to as capacitive coupling (Spinal Pak™).

Pulsed Electromagnetic Field

In addition to bioelectrical potentials at a fracture site, it was noted from the standpoint of homeostasis, that electrical currents were generated by the application of force to a bone. Thus, long bones were stimulated while walking at the frequency of gait with an electrical current, which resulted from weight bearing. It was well known that nonuse (a lower extremity in a cast after an ankle sprain or fracture resulting in disuse osteoporosis) was not physiologically healthy for a weight bearing bone, as there was neither gravity stress, nor muscle forces across bones to activate and move joints; thus the origin of this electrical signal was sought.

Subsequently, bone healing or fracture stimulation was stimulated by an exogenous electrical current, at the frequency of gait which would be a simulation of weight bearing stresses and intended to reinitiate the healing process (29). Electrical fields shown to reduce disuse osteoporosis had the greatest osteogenetic response at frequencies consistent with those of normal functional activities, suggesting that electricity plays a role in the retention of normal remodeling within bone, as a result of activities of daily living, as is consistent from a standpoint of homeostasis with the fact that electric currents are generated from the application of force to bone either from gravity or a muscle contraction and these are essential to maintain normal bone stock (30).

Initially, it was felt that there was a piezoelectric phenomena which occurred as mechanical stress was applied the bone, and generated electricity, which would be from the displacement of charges from a neutral center but then it was recognized that unlike quartz which is piezoelectric, the analogous crystalline structure in bone, hydroxyapatite, the main mineral constituent of bone, is a symmetric crystal and thus is charge neutral, so it can not be piezoelectric. It was later, found that stress generated potentials (SGP) occurred in collagen, demineralized, without the presence of bone, so this was a material property such that potentials were generated by the application of stress to bones (stress-related potentials) but other materials in the organic phase of bone were responsible for this electrical potential. In fact, it was later recognized that in bone there was a current of charge carriers [streaming potentials (SPs)] which resulted from mechanical stress and which passed fixed charges, primarily electronegative on fixed charges of long chains of proteoglycans, and this interaction was physiologically present within bone.

Electrical signals were created in bone (Faraday's induction law), by the rapid change in a magnetic field under which the bone was in the influence or cut lines of magnetic flux with PEMF, which was at a repetition similar to gait found helpful in the healing of failed bone healing or nonunions. Unfortunately, the large magnetic field required to induce the appropriate level of electric field within the bone required electric power more than a battery pack could provide a person was restrained to have their stimulator device plugged in and hence they became immobile in the clinical application of that device. The advantage of this device was that it was noninvasive; it required x-rays for careful centering of the electromagnetic field over the failed fracture, nonunion site but did not require an operative procedure.

Combined Electric and Magnetic Fields

Finally, combined electric and magnetic fields have been suggested for the reinitiation of healing in a failed fusion or for stimulation as an adjunct to promote bone formation in a spinal fusion. The DC case simulates observed and measured bioelectric potentials, the PEMF case simulates homeostatic maintenance of bone health and density by Faraday induction of electric currents and would cause SPs, which are otherwise a result of stress, and capacitive coupling provides a current on the same order of magnitude as the invasive case, but where the applied potentials are without electrode effects. The combined field has not had a credible, proposed mechanism to allow any physical intuition or suggest a phenomenological basis. As the magnetic susceptibility of biological tissue is about unity, we are all aware that patients enter magnetic resonance imaging (MRI) machines and are subjected to magnetic fields a thousand times greater than the earth's magnetic field without any noted adverse affect or in fact, any effect other than to have their inner organs and tissues imaged without being adversely affected. However, bones are in a magnetic field, which is the earth's magnetic field, and the combined fields do have a field intensity, which is of that order of magnitude, the earth's magnetic field (400 mG). Thus, if we consider in the bone, the flow of ionized charge carriers past fixed carriers, or the stream of potentials, we have a conductive fluid flowing in a magnetic field. This would suggest from the magnetohydrodynamic (MHD) standpoint, conducting fluids in a magnetic field, that a Hall Effect voltage could be produced, as when plasma (which is an ionized gas) may be propelled through a magnetic field and generate electrical power (an MHD generator). Dimensional analysis of a magnetic field similar to the earth's field with charges flowing and colliding with fixed charge carriers would result in essentially a drift velocity or a net rate of speed at which these charge carriers would be displaced and replaced we then calculate a Hall voltage that would result from this current in the magnetic field. The time constant of pressure relaxation is estimated (31) to be from 0.1 milliseconds to 0.1 seconds for a *step* deformation, as bone streaming potentials (SPs) and streaming currents (SCs) are generated in response to mechanical loading and are being considered a signal which cells may read or interpret to transduce into the subsequent cellular action to remodel bone in response (32). Streaming potentials and streaming currents were studied in Haversion canals, laminar tissue of both radial and tangential flow and the relationship was very complex with similar results in these different geometries. Transcortical streaming potentials have been measured and shown to be correlated with the magnitude of strain; the relationship between streaming potentials and strain was similar under differing loading conditions with an in vivo bone preparation (33). The usual electrokinetic responses were studied in fully hydrated bone and the streaming potentials in high ionic strength solutions reveal a flow-dependent streaming potential in the absence of mechanical deformations not previously observed (34). Further, streaming potentials studied in healing, remodeling and intact cortical bone show that there is a modification of the streaming potential magnitude and frequency in response to loading with stages of healing which confirms that they are capable of providing structural feedback information for the repair and remodeling process (35). Modeling of the system has demonstrated the sensitivity of interfacial permeability that is between the canalicular system and matrix microporosity of the collagen-hydroxyapatite bone matrix (36). Deformation-induced hierarchical flow in the structured composite of bone results in drag forces which have been suggested that with the characteristic dimension of Haversian canals the time constant for pressure relaxation through these vascular channels is about 0.1 milliseconds or up to 1 milliseconds (37) consist with transients of streaming potentials at least to an order of magnitude.

The Hall voltage would be essentially the magnetic field times the drift velocity, which could be estimated for a time constant of 0.1 milliseconds over a realistic dimension of one centimeter, or we would have a 10 m/sec net drift velocity in a 0.5 G, 5×10^{-5} Wb/m of magnetic field, which would produce a Hall voltage of $\sim$0.5 mvolts/M or 5 μvolts/cm. Consequently, a two order of magnitude increase in the magnetic field would be required for an effect consistent with calculations with other forms of electrical stimulation, at least to activate voltage gated Ca^{2+} channels. Unfortunately, this was tested with saline flow through bone in a normal and parallel magnetic field of 220 G but was without detectable difference (38); however, a Hall voltage would be at a right angle to the streaming potentials or at least their direction of flow, so that measurement would have missed the result and could potentially represent a mechanism which exists in normal bone healing physiologic situations as bone in the body is in the earth's magnetic field, if effective at levels they propose.

CLINICAL APPLICATIONS WITH SPECIAL REFERENCE TO THE SPINE

Anthony Dwyer showed that a constant direct current was useful in promoting lumbar fusion in early experiments (39,40). An invasive technique used with an electronegative electrode and accomplished the formation of bone. Simulation has been studied and demonstrated in experimental animals as well, demonstrating the statistically significant increase of osteoblastic activity with bone formation near an active bone-growth stimulator (41). Anterior lumbar interbody fusions (42) were treated with PEMF and demonstrated an increased formation in bone fusion with statistical significance. Studies with stimulation posteriorly demonstrated lack of efficacy (43). The SpinalPak[TM] was shown to be effective in the same sense that it treated nonunions (44), the developing fusion mass after posterolateral fusion for the lumbar spine had a statistically significant success rate of 84.7% for active patients versus 64.9% for placebo control. The distribution of field intensity occurring in a human body was mapped out (45) and shown to have appropriate signals consistent with clinical efficacy (46) and the intertransverse process of space was mapped and shown to have appropriate signal and clinical efficacy (47).

Combined fields unfortunately have not had dramatic results and in fact, the clinical study used to support and achieve FDA release failed to show statistical significance for a group of patients, (although the subgroup of females did show statistical significance it was a less than dramatic result).

BASIC SCIENCE STUDIES

When the electrical signals are as a phenomenon demonstrated effective in causing bone to form, questions arise as to mechanism. In particular, what receptor is essentially listening for the signal and through what mechanism is the signal promulgated?

Results with various electrical stimulation protocols have shown positive responses not only of fracture callus cell cultures (48) osteochondral explants (49) in terms of proliferation of cells (50) in culture and differentiation towards bone. However, various growth factors such as IGF-II and increased hydroxylproline (51) have stimulated which is clearly a significant step away from the actual mechanism (52) but is our present state of knowledge. In addition to healing fractures or forming bone, electrical signals may stimulate gene expression and matrix production in articular cartilage (53). Capacitively-coupled fields selectively unregulated gene expression and matrix accumulation of cartilage-specific macromolecules (aggrecan and type II collagen) which may be a non-invasive way to promote cartilage healing or ameliorate the effects of osteoarthritis.

DISCUSSION

Spinal fusion is not the same as fracture healing, because bone was not previously present, or essentially causing heterotopic bone formation. On the other hand, models that have been used for the demonstration of electrical stimulation have usually been acceleration of fracture healing, although the applications have been nonunion or failed fracture healing. Further, bioelectric potentials are a part of healing a fracture or of the growth plate and the intertransverse process heals by endochondral ossification. PEMF coils stimulate with homeostatic signals at the cadence of gait, which should maintain normal bone, but in cases where cartilage has failed to complete the healing towards bone both are demonstrated effective for nonunions or failed healing. Anterior healing has been demonstrated in the favorable interbody space, posterior healing has been markedly less successful. The combined fields as presented and are considered as electrical stimulation in the presence of a magnetic field, which is simulation of the natural condition with the earth's magnetic field. However, combined fields do not have the same intensity for Faraday induction of a voltage as the PEMF, so consequently any results with high intensity pulsed magnetic fields would not apply to the combined magnetic field situation.

CONCLUSIONS

Considering these physical mechanisms should help to understand the circumstances under which bone is formed or fusion is enhanced and supplemented in the spine as a simulation of actual phenomena, and better understanding of the underlying mechanisms should facilitate research. The receptor or the biological mechanisms are not understood, which signals are recognized or transduced. It is certainly unsupported and mere speculation to consider electrical signals to have some special amplitude sequence and the form to act as a specific key, like enzymes, which are recognized conformationally, as proteins shape act as a key in lock, but we may consider the electrical effects as clues and an intermediate step towards understanding the underlying molecular mechanisms.

REFERENCES

1. Wolff J. translated by Maquet PGJ, Furlong R. *Des Gesetz der Transformation der Knochen*. The Law of Bone Remodeling. New York: Springer-Verlag, 1986.
2. Cambridge NA. Electrical apparatus used in medicine before 1990. Proceedings of the Royal Society of Medicine, September 1977; 70:635–671.

3. Hartshorne E. The causes and treatment of pseudarthrosis and especially form of it sometimes called supernumerary joint. Am J Med 1841; 1:21–156.
4. Lente RW. Cases of ununited fracture treated by electricity. NYS J of Medicine, 1850; 5:317–319.
5. Fukada E, Yasuda I. On the piezoelectric effect of bone. J of Phys Soc of Japan, October 1957; 12:1158–1162.
6. Freidenberg ZB, Brighton CT. Bioelectric potentials in bone. JBJS, July 1966; 48A(5):915–923.
7. Freidenberg ZB, Harlow MC, Brighton CT. Healing of non-union of the medial malleolus by means of direct current: A case report. J Trauma, October 1971; 11(10):883–885.
8. Friedenberg ZB, Andrews ET, Smolenski BI, Pearl BW, Brighton CT. Bone reaction to varying amounts of direct current. Surgery, Gynecology & Obstetrics, November 1970; 131:894–899.
9. Friedenberg ZB, Kohanim M. The effect of direct current on bone. Surgery, Gynecology & Obstetrics, July 1968; 127:97–102.
10. Black J, Brighton CT. Mechanisms of stimulation of osteogenesis by direct current. Electrical Properties of Bone and Cartilage 1979; 215–224.
11. Black J, Baranowski TJ. Electrochemical aspect of D.C. stimulation of Osteogenesis. 1984; 173(1–2); 323–327.
12. Carter EL Jr, Vresilovic EJ, Pollack SR, Brighton CT. Field distributions in vertebral bodies of the rate during electrical stimulation: A parametric study. IEEE Transactions on Biomedical Engineering March 1989; 36(3):333–345.
13. Pilla AA. Mechanism of electrochemical phenomena in tissue repair and growth. Bioelectric Chemistry and Bioenergetics 1974; 1:227–245.
14. Bassett CAL, Becker RO. Generation of electric potentials by bone in response to electromagnetic stress. Science 1962; 137:1063–1064.
15. Shamos MH, Levine LS. Physical basis for bioelectric effects in mineralized tissues. Clinical Orthopaedics 1964; 35:177–188.
16. Marino AA, Becker RO. Piezoelectric effect and growth control in bone. Nature, October 31, 1970; 228:473–474.
17. Reinish GB, Nowick, AS. Piezoelective properties of bone as function of moisture content. Nature, February 20, 1995; 253:626–627.
18. Bassett CAL. Biologic significance of piezoelectricity. Calcified Tissue Research 1968; 1:252–272.
19. Anderson JC, Eriksson C. Electrical properties of wet collagen biphysics. Nature, April 13, 1969; 218(5137):166–168.
20. Marino AA, Becker RO, Sodeerholm SC. Origin of the piezoelectric effect in bone. Calcified Tissue Research 1972; 8(3):178–179.
21. Kahanowvitz N, Arnoczky SP, Nemzek J, Shores. The effect of electromagnetic and posterior lumbar spinal fusions in dogs. Spine 1994; 19(6):705–709.
22. Mooney V. A randomized double-blind prospective study on the efficacy of pulsed electromagnetic fields for interbody lumbar fusion. Spine 1990; 15:708–712.
23. Dwyer AF. The use of electrical current stimulation in spine fusion. Orthopaedic Clinics of North America, January 1975; 6(1):265–273.
24. Friedenberg ZB, Harlow MC, Brighton CT. Healing of nonunion of the medial malleolus by direct current: a case report. J Trauma 1971; II(10):873–885.
25. Friedenberg ZB, Roberts PG Jr, Didizian NH, Brighton CT. Stimulation of fracture healing by direct current in the rabbit fibula. JBJS, October 1971; 53-A(7):1400–1408.
26. Piekarski K, Demetriades D, MacKenzie A. Osteogenic stimulation by externally applied DC current. Acta orthop. Scand 1978 49:113–120.
27. Klapper L, Stallard RE. Mechanisms of electrical stimulation of bone formation; electrically mediated growth mechanism in living systems. Ann NY Acad Sci 1974; 238:530–542.
28. Brighton CT, Cronkey JC, Osterman AL. In vitro epiphyseal plate growth in various constant electrical fields. JBJS, October 1976; 58A(7): 971–978.
29. Jorgensen TE. Electrical stimulation of human fracture healing by means of a slow pulsating, asymmetrical direct current. Clinical Orthopaedics and Related Research, May 1977; 124:124–127.
30. McLeod KJ, Rubin CT. The effect of low-frequency electrical fields on osteogenesis. J Bone Joint Surg Am (United States), Jul 1992; 74(6):920–929.
31. Pollack SR, Petrov N, Salzstein RS, Brankov G, Blagoeva G. An anatomical model for streaming potentials in osteons. J Biomech 1984; 17(8):627–636.
32. MacGinite LA, Stanley GD, Bieber WA, Wu DD. Bone streaming potentials and currents depend on anatomical structure and loading orientation. J Biomechanics 1997; 30(11/12):1133–1129.
33. Beck BR, Qin Y-X, McLeod KJ, Otter MW. On the relationship between streaming potential and strain in an in vivo bone preparation. Calcif Tissue Int 2002; 71:335–343.
34. Walsh WR, Guzelsu N. Ion concentration effects on bone streaming potentials and zeta potentials. Biomaterials 1993; 14(5):331–336.
35. Macginitie LA, WU DD, Cochran GVB. Streaming potentials in healing, remodeling, and intact cortical bone. J Bone Miner Res 1993; 8(11):1323–1335.

36. Mak AFT, Huang DT, Zhang JD, Tong P. Deformation-induced hierarchical flows and drag forces in bone canaliculi and matrix microporosity. J Biomech 1997; 30(1):11–18.
37. Johnson MW, Chakkalakal, Harper RA, Katz JL, Rouhana SW. Fluid flow in bone in vitro. J Biomech 1982; 15(11):881–885.
38. El-Messiery MA. Magnetic field interaction with streaming potentials in cancellous bone. Biomaterials 1982; 1(3):168–171.
39. Dwyer AF. The use of electrical current stimulation in spinal fusion. Orthopaedic Clinics of North America, January 1975; 691:265–273.
40. Dwyer A, Wickham GG. Direct current stimulation in spinal fusion. Med J Aust 1974; 1:73–75.
41. Nerubay J, Marganit B, Bubis JJ, Tadmor A, Katznelson A. Stimulation of bone formation by electrical current on spinal fusion. Spine (United States), Mar 1986; 11(2):167–169.
42. Mooney V. A randomized double-blind prospective study of the efficacy of pulsed electromagnetic fields for interbody lumbar fusions. Spine 1986; 15:708–712
43. Zoltan JD. Electrical stimulation of bone: An overview. Seminars in Orthopaedics, December 1986; 1(4):242–252.
44. Brighton CT, Pollack SR. Treatment of a recalcitrant non-union with a capacitively coupled electric field. JBJS, April 1985; 67-A(4):577–585.
45. Carter EL, Pollack SR, Brighton CT. Theoretical determination of the current density distributions in human vertebral bodies during electrical stimulation. IEEE, Transactions on Medical Engineering 1990; 37(6):606–614.
46. Carter E, Vreslovic EJ, Brighton CT. distributions in vertebral bodies of the rat and electrical stimulation: A metric study. EEE Transactions on Biomedical Engineering, March 1989; 36(3):333–345.
47. Goodwin CE, Brighton CT, Guyer RD, Johnson JR, Light KI, Yuan HA. A double-blind study of capacitively coupled electrical stimulation as an adjunct to lumbar spine fusion. Spine, July 1999; 24(13):1349–1356.
48. Yen-Patton GPA, Patton WF, Beer DM, Jacobson BS. Endothelial cell response to pulsed electromagnetic fields: Stimulation of growth rate and angiogenesis in vitro. J Cell Physiol 1988; 134:37–46.
49. Aaron RK, Wang S, Ciombor DMCK. Upregulation of basal TGF[beta]$_1$ levels by EMF coincident with chondrogenesis: Implications of skeletal repair and tissue engineering. J Orthop Res 2002; 20:233–240.
50. Monhan S, et al. Endrochoronology 1990; 126:2534–2542.
51. Woessner JS. Archives of Biochemistry and Biophysics 1961; 93:440.
52. Ryaby J, Fitzsimmons RG, Khin NA, Baylink DJ. The role of insulin-like growth factor II in magnetic field regulation of bone formation. Bioelectrochem Bioenerg 1994; 35:87–91.
53. Wang W, Wang Z, Zhang G, Clark CC, Brighton CT. Up-regulation of chondrocyte matrix genes and products by electric fields. Clinical Orthopaedics & Related Research, October 2004; 427S:S163–S173.

38 | Results of Extended Corpectomy, Stabilization, and Fusion of the Cervical and Cervico-Thoracic Spine

Frank L. Acosta, Jr.
Department of Neurological Surgery, University of California, San Francisco, California, U.S.A.

Carlos J. Ledezma
Department of Neurological Surgery, University of Southern California, Los Angeles, California, U.S.A.

Henry E. Aryan and Christopher P. Ames
Department of Neurological Surgery, University of California, San Francisco, California, U.S.A.

INTRODUCTION

Decompression for multilevel degenerative, traumatic, neoplastic, or infectious disease of the cervical spine can be achieved via several approaches, including laminectomy, laminoplasty, segmental anterior cervical discectomy, and fusion (ACDF), or anterior corpectomy and fusion (ACF) (1–3). Although, laminectomy and laminoplasty are associated with less perioperative morbidity and have been found to be effective for the treatment of multilevel cervical myelopathy (4), the potential for progressive cervical kyphosis and axial neck pain are two significant disadvantages of these procedures (5,6). In addition, neither allows for adequate spinal cord decompression in cases of significant anterior compressive lesions. Segmental ACDF does allow for decompression of the anterior cervical spinal canal. Nevertheless, although single-level ACDF has been shown to be a very efficacious procedure with successful decompression and fusion occurring in up to 94% of patients (7,8), multilevel ACDF has been associated with nonunion rates as high as 53% (9,10). As successful arthrodesis has been correlated with improved clinical outcomes (11–13), multilevel ACDF may lead to unacceptably high rates of recurrent pain and/or neurological symptoms for patients with pathology of multiple levels of the anterior cervical spine.

Advantages of ACF for multilevel cervical decompression include improved visualization allowing for a more extensive decompression, as well as fewer graft-host interfaces requiring fusion (compared to segmental ACDF), theoretically leading to improved rates of arthrodesis. Indeed, ACF with strut grafting has been found to result in higher rates of successful fusion and improved clinical outcomes compared to multilevel ACDF (11). However, extensive ACF involving three or more levels has been associated with increased rates of graft-related complications including graft dislodgment, spinal cord compression, and pseudoarthrosis (14–17). For example, graft failure rates have been found to increase from 6% after two-level ACF to as high as 71% after three-level ACF (18). That the interbody graft is subject to significant compressive forces after multilevel ACF has been confirmed in biomechanical studies (19,20). As such, reconstruction and, ultimately fusion of the cervical spine after extensive corpectomy represents a significant challenge. Although, past studies have evaluated the clinical and radiographic results of multilevel (>1 level) ACF with strut graft (11) and titanium mesh cage (TMC) reconstruction (3), no study has focused specifically on outcomes after extended (≥3 levels) anterior cervical corpectomy and fusion (EACF) using various spinal reconstruction, instrumentation, and fusion techniques.

This retrospective study involves patients with symptomatic degenerative, infectious, or traumatic pathology of the anterior cervical and/or cervicothoracic spine who were surgically treated with EACF, TMC, or strut graft reconstruction, anterior plate, with or without supplemental posterolateral fixation or osteoinductive factors. We also provide a review of the literature on EACF. The purpose was to evaluate and compare the clinical and radiographic efficacy, and complication rates of EACF using various spinal reconstruction techniques.

MATERIALS AND METHODS
Patient Population

All medical, surgical and radiological records were reviewed for patients who underwent EACF at University of California, San Francisco (UCSF) between the years 2000 and 2004.

Fourteen patients (6M:8F, average age 58 years, range 35–78) with extensive pathology of the anterior cervical spine treated with anterior corpectomy and fusion across three or more levels (EACF) at UCSF between 2000 and 2004 were included in this analysis (Table 1). All patients presented with pain and/or myelopathy attributed to pathology of the anterior cervical and/or cervicothoracic spine. Myelopathy was caused by spondylostenosis in four patients, and by osteomyelitis, deformity, and ossified posterior longitudinal ligament (OPLL) in one patient each. Osteomyelitis and deformity caused intractable neck pain in one patient each. Painful myelopathy was caused by spondylostenosis in two patients, and by trauma, deformity, and osteomyelitis in one patient each. The average period between onset of symptoms and surgery was 5.6 months (range 1–28 months).

Diagnostic Evaluation

All patients with myelopathy and/or severe neck pain had diagnostic plain radiographs, computed tomographic (CT) scans with sagittal and coronal reconstructions, and/or magnetic resonance imaging (MRI) demonstrating extensive degenerative, traumatic, or infectious pathology of the anterior cervical and/or cervicothoracic spinal column with or without evidence of mechanical spinal cord compression (Fig. 1).

Operative Technique

Surgical treatment was recommended for patients with severe and/or progressive myelopathy with or without pain and documented evidence of cervical spinal deformity and/or spinal cord compression.

Anterior corpectomy and decompression was performed in all patients, using standard techniques previously described (21). A 14 to 16 mm wide corpectomy trough was created in the vertebral body using a high-speed diamond burr drill. The posterior longitudinal ligament (PLL) was resected in all cases. An interbody fibular strut graft or titanium mesh cage (TMC) with vertebral body autograft was positioned into the corpectomy defect, and the traction subsequently relieved. Traction was provided by halo ring, garner wells tongs or traction on the head provided by anesthesia since caspar posts cannot span defects of three or more levels.

TABLE 1 Summary of Patient Population Treated with Multilevel Cervical Corpectomy

Patient no.	Age (yrs)	Sex	Presentation	Diagnosis	Corpectomy levels (no.)	Follow-up (months)	Outcome at last follow-up
1	52	F	Myelopathy	Spondylostenosis	C3–C6 (4)	47	Resolved
2	68	F	Myelopathy	Osteomyelitis	C4–C6 (3)	47	Resolved
3	35	F	Myelopathy + neck pain	Deformity	C4–C7 (4)	29	Resolved
4	73	F	Myelopathy + neck pain	Spondylostenosis	C4–C6 (3)	25	Resolved
5	63	M	Myelopathy	Spondylostenosis	C4–C6 (3)	25	Resolved
6	60	M	Myelopathy	Spondylostenosis	C4–C6 (3)	23	Resolved
7	59	M	Myelopathy	Deformity	C4–C6 (3)	22	Resolved
8	78	F	Myelopathy	Spondylostenosis	C3–C6 (4)	19	Resolved
9	53	F	Myelopathy + neck pain	Trauma	C4–C6 (3)	18	Resolved
10	50	F	Neck pain	Osteomyelitis	C4–T2 (6)	16	Resolved
11	52	M	Neck pain	Deformity	C4–C6 (3)	14	Improved
12	64	M	Myelopathy + neck pain	Spondylostenosis	C4–C6 (3)	14	Resolved
13	44	F	Myelopathy + neck pain	Osteomyelitis	C3–C6 (4)	13	Resolved
14	56	M	Myelopathy	OPLL	C4–C6 (3)	13	Resolved

Abbreviation: OPLL, ossified posterior longitudinal ligament.

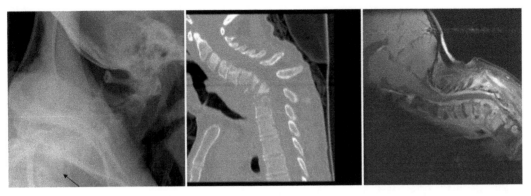

FIGURE 1   *Left*: Lateral plain radiograph in a 50-year-old woman (no. 10) presenting with neck pain. Marked kyphosis related to C3-T2 osteomyelitis is evident. Arrow points to the apex of the kyphosis at the C7-T1 level with significant osseous erosion. *Middle*: Sagittal reformatted CT scan in the same patient showing extensive vertebral body erosion of the anterior cervico-thoracic spine in the same patient. *Right*: Sagittal T1 post gadolinium MR sequence demonstrating an extensive prevertebral and circumferential enhancing epidural abscess and C4-T2 osteomyelitis causing a severe kyphoptic deformity.

TMC and allograft were used in cases for osteomyelitis in which local vertebral body bone was not available because of infection. Recombinant human bone morphogenic protein-2 (rhBMP-2) became available at our institution in 2003 and was thereafter used as an adjunct for anterior cervical spinal reconstruction and fusion after all cases of corpectomy of four or more levels. An anterior cervical titanium plate was used in all cases. Posterolateral screw-rod fixation and fusion after laminectomy was performed in a single-stage manner in eight patients, and in a delayed manner in four patients (Fig. 2).

Follow-Up

All patients underwent a basic neurological examination, an evaluation of neck pain, and an evaluation of neurological deficit at each follow-up visit. Outcome was defined as worsened, unchanged, improved, or resolved. Flexion-extension plain radiographs and/or CT scans were taken in the immediate post-operative period and at follow-up of 3, 6, and 12 months to evaluate for instrumentation positioning and fusion. Fusion was determined based on lack of motion on flexion and extension plain X-rays. CT scans were performed for patients in whom plain radiographs were nondiagnostic for fusion using these criteria. The presence of bridging trabecular bone was considered positive for fusion on CT scans.

RESULTS

The average follow-up period was 23 months (range 13–37 months).

Operative Data

Table 2 summarizes the operative data. Corpectomies were performed across an average of 3.5 levels between C3–T2. Nine patients underwent a three-level corpectomy, four patients underwent a four-level corpectomy, and one patient underwent a six-level corpectomy.

Expandable TMC was used in the majority of cases regardless of the number of levels resected (Fig. 3). Vertebral body autograft was also used in almost all cases except when the vertebra was actively infected, as previously mentioned. Recombinant human bone morphogenic protein-2 (rhBMP-2) was used in all cases involving four or more levels after 2003. rhBMP-2 was also used after a three level corpectomy in one patient (No. 4) with rheumatoid arthritis and severe osteopenia. Anterior plates were used in all cases: dynamic plates were used in 10 patients, and fixed plates in four. Laminectomy with posterolateral screw-rod fixation was performed in all but two patients. Both of these patients underwent three level corpectomy and

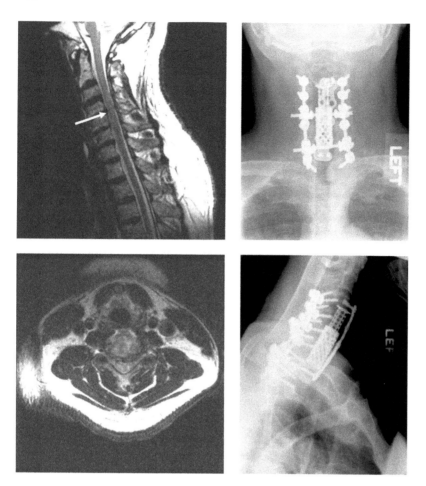

FIGURE 2   *Top left*: Sagittal T2-weighted MRI of the cervical spine in a patient (no. 11) who presented with severe neck pain and early myelopathy demonstrating a straightening of the normal cervical lordosis as well as spondylotic changes extending from C4-C6 causing narrowing of the normal CSF space (*arrow*). *Lower left*: Axial MRI of the same patient at the level of C5-6 demonstrating severe stenosis of the cervical canal with abnormal intramedullary T2 signal. *Top right*: Postoperative AP and lateral. *Lower right*: Plain radiographs after C4-C6 anterior corpectomy with expandable cage and allograft reconstruction. An anterior cervical plate and posterior lateral mass screw-rod fixation from C3-C6 and pedicle screw-rod fixation from C7-T1 were used for supplemental stabilization.

fusion without laminectomy: one for fracture, and another one for osteomyelitis. The length of the posterior fixation was directly correlated to the number of anterior corpectomy levels (Fig. 4).

Twelve patients were immobilized with a Miami-J collar postoperatively for at least six weeks, or until radiographic evidence of fusion. Two patients were immobilized in halo braces for three months postoperatively: one patient after six level corpectomy, and one after four level corpectomy out of concern for noncompliance with a standard rigid cervical collar.

TABLE 2   Techniques for Spinal Reconstruction and Fusion after Extensive Anterior Cervical Corpectomy

Total levels	No. of patients	Expandable TMC (%)	Fibular strut (%)	Autograft (%)	Allograft (%)	rhBMP2[a] (%)	Anterior plate (%)	Posterolateral fixation (%)
3	9	7 (77)	2 (22)	8 (88)	1 (11)	1 (11)	9 (100)	7 (77)
4	4	3 (75)	1 (250	3 (75)	1 (25)	2 (50)	4 (100)	4 (100
6	1	1 (100)	0	0	1 (100)	1 (100)	1 (100)	1 (100)

[a]Available at UCSF after 2003.

Summary of anterior reconstruction and fusion techniques after EACF

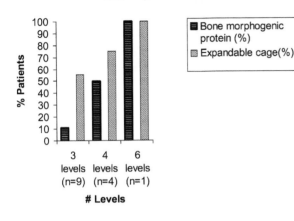

FIGURE 3 Bar graph demonstrating the use of TMC and rhBMP-2 for anterior reconstruction after EACF. *Abbreviations:* TMC, titanium mesh cage; rhBMP-2, recombinant human bone morphogenic protein-2; EACF, extended anterior cervical corpectomy.

Clinical Outcome

Postoperatively, no patient experienced a new neurological deficit. All patients experienced improvement in neurological symptoms when present, and 88% (6/7) experienced complete resolution of pain symptoms. There were no deaths.

Radiographic Outcome

All patients had normal cervical sagittal alignment postoperatively, although a greater degree of correction was possible with the use of TMC compared to fibular strut graft for patients with preoperative kyphosis. No patient experienced loss of sagittal cervical alignment postoperatively. Successful fusion on plain flexion-extension radiographs was achieved in 100% of cases (Figs. 4, 5). Five patients had CT scans documenting fusion when there was a question of motion on plain radiographs. The use of TMC, strut graft, autograft or allograft was not associated with differences in rates of fusion.

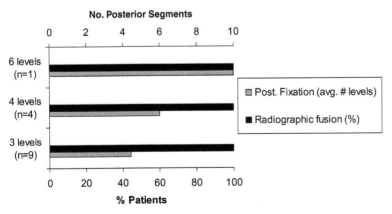

FIGURE 4 Bar graph showing the average number of segments included in posterolateral fixation and the corresponding rates of arthrodesis according to number of corpectomy levels.

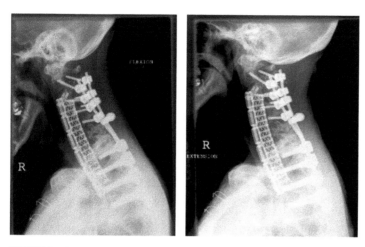

FIGURE 5 Lateral flexion (*right*) and extension (*left*) plain radiographs after six-level cervicothoracic corpectomy and circumferential reconstruction for osteomyelitis (patient no. 10, Fig. 1) after removal of halo brace demonstrating lack of motion of instrumentation as evidence for satisfactory arthrodesis.

Complications

There were no intraoperative or major complications, including injury to the vertebral artery, recurrent laryngeal nerve, and esophagus. Two (14%) of patients experienced postoperative complications. One patient who underwent a four level corpectomy experienced transient dysphagia postoperatively. Displacement of the fibular strut graft occurred in the second patient necessitating reoperation with removal of the strut graft and placement of an expandable TMC (Fig. 6). This patient went on to a satisfactory fusion. None of the TMC grafts became displaced.

DISCUSSION

Since first developed in the 1950s and 1960s by surgeons such as Robinson (22), Cloward (23), and Bailey and Badgley (24), surgical decompression, stabilization, and fusion of the anterior cervical spine has evolved along with advancements in anesthesia and perioperative care, spinal instrumentation, and more recently, novel osteoginductive factors. Currently, ACF is perhaps the most effective procedure for wide spinal cord decompression in patients with severe canal stenosis or pathology of the anterior spine (3). Compared to more conventional surgical techniques for multilevel (>1 level) spinal cord decompression such as segmental ACDF, laminectomy, and laminoplasty, patients treated with ACF have improved rates of arthrodesis, neurological recovery, less axial neck pain, and lower incidences of postoperative loss of sagittal plane alignment (6,11,25,26). The efficacy of EACF, however, is less clear, as fusion rates and clinical outcomes for patients after EACF are often grouped together with patients treated with procedures of single or two level. Moreover, the overall reported experience with EACF is much less than with single- or two-level procedures. Table 3 provides a summary of studies in which >10% of the patient population underwent EACF. When the appropriate data was reported, every attempt was made to determine outcomes and complication rates specifically after EACF.

Stabilization after EACF
Anterior Reconstruction
Anterior column reconstruction after multilevel ACF may be performed using tricortical strut grafts or TMC. Although comparable rates of fusion have been reported with both types of implants (3,11,17,27,28), allo or autograft struts have traditionally been associated with higher rates of subsidence into adjacent vertebral bodies or dislodgement after multilevel

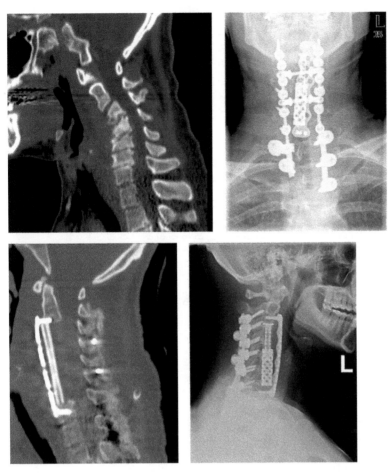

FIGURE 6 *Upper left*: Preoperative sagittal CT reconstruction in a patient with osteomyelitis (no. 13) showing significant prevertebral soft tissue swelling extending from C2 to C6. The endplates of the C3-C6 vertebrae are irregular and sclerotic with collapse of the vertebral bodies and resultant kyphosis. *Lower left*: Postoperative sagittal CT reconstruction after C3-C6 anterior corpectomy with strut graft reconstruction and circumferential fixation. Note the anterior dislodgment of approximately 50% of the superior graft from the corpectomy defect. This patient was subsequently treated with reoperation and removal of the strut graft with placement of an expandable TMC, as demonstrated in the postoperative AP (*upper right*) and lateral (*lower right*) plain radiographs. *Abbreviations:* TMC, titanium mesh cage; AP, anteroposterior.

ACF (1,6,17,29). Sevki et al. (3) reported no occurrences of implant-related complications or failures in 26 patients after multilevel ACF with TMC reconstruction. EACF was performed in nine patients in this series and anterior plating with posterolateral plate fixation was performed in all nine. Vanichkachorn et al. (30), however, found that the rate of strut graft-related complications may be significantly lowered when combined with anterior and posterolateral plate fixation after EACF. Nevertheless, TMC does offer several advantages over strut grafts, including improved biomechanical stability, better correction of sagittal alignment (with pre-contoured lordotic cages), better endplate purchase, variable height and diameter options, and the ability to be packed with auto or allograft bone to provide a larger surface area available for fusion (27,31–33).

Although one found no differences in rates of fusion using either tricortical strut graft or TMC for reconstruction after EACF in our 14 patients, our only incident of implant-related failure occurred from dislodgment of a tricortical strut graft after a four-level corpectomy with both anterior plating and posterolateral screw-rod fixation.

TABLE 3   Summary of the Surgical Techniques and Radiographic and Clinical Outcomes for Reports of Extended Anterior Cervical Corpectomy (EACF)[a]

Author(s), yr, (ref.)	Total no. of cases	No. of cases ≥3 levels (total # levels)	%EACF (out of total # cases)	No. strut/TMC (% total)	% Supplemental anterior fixation	% Posterolateral fixation	% Successful fusion	% Complications (% hardware failure)[b]	Excellent–good outcome[c] (average follow-up)
Hanai et al., 1982 (64)	15	6 (3); 7 (4)	87%	Strut (100%)	0%	0%	NR	21%[d] (7%)[d]	60%[d] (NR)
Boni et al., 1984 (54)	39	9 (3); 20 (4); 9 (5); 1 (6)	100%	Strut (100%)	0%	0%	100%	31% (3%)	92% (6 months–13 yrs)
Bernard et al., 1987 (53)	21	13 (3); 4 (4)	81%	Strut (100%)	0%	0%	100%	5% (5%)	76% (32 months)
Brown et al., 1988 (21)	13	4 (3)	31%	Strut (100%)	100% (ACP)	0%	100%[d]	50%[d] (17%)[d]	100% (15 months)
Tippets et al., 1988 (29)	18	5 (3)	28%	Strut (100%)	100% (ACP)	0%	90%	20% (0%)	(1–15 months)
Kojima et al., 1989 (65)	45	12 (3); 3 (4); 2 (5)	38%	Strut (100%)	0%	0%	100%[d]	24% (9%)	87% (NR)
Zdeblick et al, 1989 (55)	14	6 (3); 2 (4)	57%	Strut (100%)	0%	0%	100%	25%[d] (25%)[d]	100% (NR)
Okada et al., 1991 (52)	37	14 (3); 7 (4)	54%	Strut (100%)	0%	0%	100%	21% (10%)	74% (49 months)
Saunders et al., 1991 (61)	40	22 (3)	55%	Strut (100%)	0%	0%	98%	48% (3%)	57.5 % (NR)
Ebraheim et al., 1995 (66)	25	4 (3); 1 (4)	20%	Strut (100%)	100% (ACP)	0%	100%[d]	33%[d] (17%)[d]	83%[d] (31.2 months)
Macdonald et al., 1997 (16)	36	19 (3); 6 (4)	69%	Strut (100%)	42% (ACP)	0%	97%	56% (8%)	58% (31 months)
Fessler et al., 1998	93	7 (3); 1 (5)	9%	Strut (100%)	29% (ACP)	0%	88%	23% (12%)	86%[d] (39 months)
Saunders et al., 1998 (60)	31	31 (4)	100%	Strut (100%)	0%	0%	90%	26% (10 %)	80%
Vanichkachorn et al., 1998 (10)	11	5 (3); 5 (4)	91%	Strut (100%)	100% (CBP)	100%	90%	9% (9%)	91 % (30.8 months)
Eleraky et al., 1999 (12)	185	28 (3)	15%	Strut (100%)	97% (ACP)	0%	96 %[d]	27% (4%)	87% (36 months)
Majd et al., 1999 (24)	34	5 (3); 7 (4)	35%	TMC (100%)	100% (ACP)	0%	97%	12% (6%)	79 % (32 months)
Riew et al., 1999 (42)	14	12 (3)	86%	Strut (100%)	100% (CBP)	25%[d]	75%[d]	33%[d] (8%)[d]	100%[d] (28 months)[d]
Schultz et al., 2000 (4)	72	30 (3); 2 (4)	44%	Strut (100%)	100% (CBP)	100%	100%[d]	38% (1%)	100%[d] (29 months)
Edwards et al., 2002 (68)	26	11 (3); 2 (4)	50%	Strut (100%)	100% (ACP)	0%	NR	69% (15%)	77% (49 months)
Hilibrand et al., 2002 (47)	59	20 (3); 2 (4)	37%	Strut (100%)	0%	0%	100%[d]	NA (10%)	88% (57 months)
Mayr et al.., 2002 (13)	261	31 (3); 1 (4)	12%	Strut (100%)	100% (ACP)	0%	87 %	36% (5.4%)	99 % (25.7 months)
Dorai et al., 2003 (23)	45	5 (3)	11%	TMC (100%)	100% (ACP)	0%	100%[d]	0%[d] (0%)[d]	NR (12.9 months)[d]
Sasso et al., 2003 (5)	40	7 (3)	18%	Strut (100%)	100% (ACP)[d]	0%	29%[d]	NR (71%)[d]	NR (21 months)[d]
Wang et al., 2003 (41)	249	71 (3); 6 (4); 1 (5)	31%	Strut (100%)	0%	0%	100 %[d]	(10%)[d]	100% (4.7 yrs)
Sevki et al., 2004	26	6 (3); 3 (4)	35%	TMC (100%)	100%[d]	100%[d]	100%	38% (0%)	100% (30 months)
Current study	14	9 (3); 4 (4); 1 (6)	100%	Strut (21%); TMC (79%)	100%	86%	100%	14% (4%)	100% (23 months)

[a]Only including reports in which EACF accounted for >10% of the total study population.
[b]Hardware failure—cage migration, dislodgment, telescoping, instability, plate dislodgment, and screw complications (screw backout or breakage, plate pullout, or pseudoarthrosis).
[c]Excellent—all preoperative symptoms relieved; Good – minimal persistence of preoperative symptoms.
[d]Only patients that underwent ≥3-level corpectomy.
Abbreviations: ACP, anterior cervical plate; CBP, cervical buttress plate; TMC, titanium mesh cage.

Anterior Cervical Plates

The incidence of graft-related complications after multilevel ACF has been found to be as high as 30% (1,6,29,34,35). The addition of anterior cervical plate (ACP) fixation after interbody reconstruction enhances the rigidity and stability of the construct and therefore lowers the risk of graft-related complications and endplate fracture, leading to improved fusion rates even after multisegment decompression (3,14,36–39). DiAngelo et al. (37) and Foley et al. (40) demonstrated that the use of an anterior plate shifts the instantaneous axis of rotation anteriorly, which protects the graft from high stresses that may cause graft collapse. Unicortical locking plate systems are currently favored as they have yielded a lower rate of screw backout, are easier to use, and reduce the risk of spinal injury compared to bicortical plate systems (41,42). Concern that unicortical constrained plates may cause significant graft stress shielding and prevent subsidence-related gap closure after ACF led to the development of multiangle nonconstrained (dynamic) plates (43–45). Dynamic plates have been found to allow for more graft load sharing after ACF (43) and may offer superb biomechanical stability compared to constrained (rigid) plates, particularly in flexion-extension (46). As load sharing by the interbody implant is important to successful fusion, dynamic plates may be particularly useful after EACF. Moreover, in our experience, there is generally a higher degree of graft subsidence after EACF than after one- or two-level procedures, which would not be accommodated by a fixed plate. Constrained plating systems, though, are generally preferred after ACF for trauma with disrupted posterior elements (47).

Other options to prevent graft stress-shielding or subsidence-related failure of the anterior plate include using a cage only (no plate), cervical buttress plates (CBP), or creating flanges in the cage that overlap the adjacent vertebral bodies and are secured with nonconstraining screws (48). Given the high stresses at the inferior end of long plate constructs, CBP (which are fixed usually at the inferior end of the graft) have been advocated as a way to prevent inferior graft dislodgement while allowing for adequate load sharing (30). As the CBP provides less rigid internal fixation than the ACP, however, it is generally accepted that CBP should be used in combination with supplemental posterolateral fixation to avoid graft dislodgment after multilevel ACF (30,49).

Posterolateral Fixation

Isomi et al. (20) evaluated the use of ACP in a single-level and three-level corpectomy model reconstructed with a strut graft without posterolateral fixation. After 1000 cycles of fatigue, instability and a significant increase in motion at the inferior end of the plate was observed in the three-level corpectomy group. Other biomechanical studies have shown that the graft is subject to excessive loading after EACF without posterolateral fixation (19). Vaccaro et al. (14) showed that ~10% of two-level graft and plate constructs and up to 50% of three-level strut graft and plate constructs are at risk for early failure when not supplemented with a posterior segmental stabilization procedure. Sasso et al. (18) reported a 71%-graft failure rate after EACF with strut graft and ACP only. Sevki et al. (3) performed posterolateral fixation with a screw-plate system in nine out of nine patients, who underwent EACF without an occurrence of implant-related complications in this group. It is clear from these and other studies (19,50,51) that supplemental posterolateral fixation after EACF improves biomechanical stability and decreases the rates of graft-related complications, deformity correction loss, and pseudoarthrosis rates. Some studies have shown screw and rod systems (52) to have better biomechanical stability than posterior screw-plate constructs, particular for flexion–extension (53,54). We used posterior lateral mass screw-rod fixation in all of our patients. Tapered rods were used for posterior constructs that spanned the cervicothoracic junction and were connected to pedicle screws from C7-T2.

Osteoinductive Growth Factors

Although osteoinductive agents, such as rhBMP-2, are approved for use in lumbar interbody fusion, there has been no Phase 4 trial to evaluate their efficacy for anterior cervical fusion. In a Phase 1 prospective trial, Baskin et al. (55) showed that rhBMP-2 is safe for use in the cervical spine and experienced a 100% fusion rate. In animal models, rhBMP-2 has been shown to facilitate bony ingrowths after single or multilevel ACDF with interbody cage (56,57).

Beginning in 2003, we used rhBMP-2 as an adjunct to anterior fixation for corpectomies of four or more levels.

Patient Outcomes

Using outcome scales such as Nuric score, the modified Japanese Orthopaedic Association Score (JOA), and others, the reported frequency of overall improvement in clinical status after any ACF ranges from 73% to 100% (29,34,58–60). After EACF in particular, excellent (i.e., resolution of symptoms) or good outcomes (i.e., overall improvement in symptoms) have been reported in 60% to 100% of cases (Table 3). The reported time to the initiation of neurological recovery after surgery, and the duration of this recovery after ACF is extremely variable. Fessler et al. (2) and Majd et al. (27) assert that most neurological recovery occurs within the first six months after surgery. In their series of 26 patients (EACF in 9), Sevki et al. (3) observed neurological recovery from three weeks to 12 months postoperatively. Other studies have found that recovery may be observed up to two years postoperatively (51,61,62). Ebersold et al. (63) noted immediate clinical improvement in 23 (70%) of 33 patients after one- or two-level ACF, with late deterioration in 18%. Interestingly, although age, severity of disease, number of levels decompressed, and preoperative Nurick grade were not predictive of outcome, the duration of symptoms preoperatively was found to be the only factor related to potential postoperative deterioration in this study. This study, however, did not include patients who underwent EACF. After an average follow-up of 30 months, Sevki et al. (3) reported no cases of late neurological deterioration in any of the nine patients treated with EACF.

All patients in our series experienced in improvement or complete resolution of neurological symptoms after an average follow-up of 23 months, and all but one patient had complete resolution of neck pain. We experienced no cases of late neurological deterioration. That there was a relatively short time between onset of symptoms and surgery (mean 5.6 months) in our population may indeed be a factor contributing to our clinical success after EACF.

Fusion Rates

The fusion rate achieved in our series was 100%. In general, fusion rates after EACF have been acceptable, ranging from 75% to 100% (Table 3). Hilibrand et al. (11) reported a 100% union rate for 22 patients who underwent EACF (20 patients three-level, two patients four-level ACF), while Eleraky et al. (47) reported a rate of 96% in 28 patients who underwent three-level ACF. Although, the use of posterolateral fixation has been associated with lower rates of graft-related complications, it has not been correlated with improved rates of arthrodesis.

Complication Rates

Complication rates after EACF range from 0% to 50% (Table 3).

Surgical Complications

Given the complex soft tissue anatomy of the anterior cervical region, the majority of significant surgical complications are secondary to soft tissue retraction and dissection required for adequate surgical exposure. Inadequate release of fascial tissue planes can result in damage to the esophagus, trachea, carotid or vertebral arteries, or the recurrent laryngeal nerve (RLN) and lead to complications such as transient sore throat, dysphagia, hoarseness, dysphonia, RLN paralysis, esophageal perforation, or respiratory insufficiency. In a series of 40 patients undergoing ACF, Saunders et al. (21) reported a perioperative complication rate of 47.5%, the majority of which were due to soft tissue retraction and dissection. Beutler et al. (64) found the overall risk of RLN injury during anterior cervical spine surgery to be 2.7% and that there is no association between the side of the surgical approach and the incidence of RLN symptoms.

Dysphagia, which results from prolonged traction on the esophagus during surgery, seems to exhibit a transient course as it has been reported to have an incidence of 50.2%

at 1 month, and 4.8% incidence at 12 months (65). Spinal cord or nerve root injury is less frequent, but when it occurs generally is a transient C-5 radiculopathy (21).

Soft tissue complications associated with ACF can be minimized by deliberate, extensive dissection, and adequate release of all fascial tissue planes over the cervical spine. Given the risk of dissection and retraction injuries with the anterior cervical approach, the anterior soft tissue structures are carefully protected with the secure positioning of self-retaining retractors. When in place, the retractors should be intermittently released to limit the effect of long-term pressure on the adjacent anatomical structures. This is particularly true during EACF, which requires prolonged periods of extensive soft tissue retraction.

Graft-Related Complications

The mechanism of graft failure is multifactorial (Table 4). Biologic factors include the diagnosis, extent of disease, bone quality, comorbidities, and other host factors. Mechanical factors include the number of surgical levels, fused level (i.e., cervicothoracic involvement), alignment, stability, and the use of internal and external immobilization. Technical factors include long graft length, and stable reconstruction or restoration of alignment.

Long-segment autologous iliac crest bone harvesting has been associated with significant donor site complications and morbidity: postoperative donor-site pain, paresthesias in the distribution of the related peripheral nerves, vascular injury, adjacent bone fracture (pelvic crest), and wound infection (1,34,59). In addition, the natural curvature of the iliac crest may preclude its use in a corpectomy defect spanning a distance of more than two vertebral bodies. Fibular allograft use has several advantages: it avoids harvest-associated complications, facilitates longer bone grafts, and provides a central cavity for the packing of autologous cancellous bone harvested from the corpectomy site to enhance the fusion rate. Nevertheless, despite these advantages, the migration or dislodgement of these long fibular allograft strut grafts may impinge on vital anatomic structures or result in pseudoarthrosis (1,66). Posterior migration can lead to compression of the spinal cord, resulting in paralysis or neural injury. The esophagus can become compressed or perforated by an anteriorly dislodged graft, and tracheal impingement may produce airway obstruction (17). The incidence of graft collapse, telescoping (subsidence >5 mm), extrusion, and pseudoarthrosis increases with each additional level (1,17), even in the presence of internal fixation and stable postoperative immobilization (14,17).

TABLE 4 Summary of Complications after EACF

Surgical complications
  Soft tissue complications
    Recurrent laryngeal nerve injury
    Transient dysphagia
    Transient C5 radiculopathy
    Wound infection
  Airway complications
Graft-related complications
  Donor site
    Graft site pain
    Graft site infection
  Implant site
    Telescoping (subsidence >5 mm)
Plate-related complications
  Screw pullout
  Screw-plate migration
Medical complications
  Deep vein thrombosis
  Pneumonia
  Respiratory distress
  Death

TABLE 5 Factors Contributing to Graft-Related Complications

Biological factors
  Disease process (diagnosis, extensive disease, poor bone quality)
  Comorbidities
  Impaired healing/malnutrition
Graft-related factors
  Graft displacement/fracture
  Telescoping (subsidence >5 mm)
  Nonunion
Hardware-related factors
  Screw pullout/fracture
  Screw-plate migration
  Plate fracture
Technical/mechanical factors
  Long graft length
  Greater number or vertebral bodies removed (i.e., number of surgical levels)
  Graft selection
  Level fused (C7 or cervicothoracic junction involvement)
  Restoration of normal alignment/stability
  Graft preload
  Posterior element load sharing
  Surface area at the graft-host interface
  Use of internal and external immobilization

CONCLUSIONS

Advances in surgical techniques and spinal stabilization methods have expanded the role of corpectomy for the management of complex cervical spine disorders. In this limited retrospective series, we have found that EACF leads to excellent clinical outcomes for patients treated within one year of symptom onset. Reconstruction with precontoured TMC, autograft is ideal. The use of a dynamic ACP facilitates graft load sharing and accommodates postoperative implant subsidence. Supplemental posterolateral screw-rod instrumentation should be used in all cases of EACF and tailored to the length of the anterior interbody implant to decrease graft-related complications. While there is no Class 1 data available, we have used rhBMP-2 as an adjunct to circumferential instrumentation and fusion after corpectomies of four or more levels with good results. Although, multilevel and EACF have traditionally been associated with higher (and, in some reports, unacceptable) rates of graft-related and perioperative complications, modern advancements in spinal instrumentation have made extensive decompression, reconstruction, and bony fusion of the anterior cervical spine an effective treatment, leading to satisfactory clinical and radiographic results, even when performed across three or more levels.

KEY POINTS

- Extended anterior cervical corpectomy and fusion (EACF) is performed across 3 or more levels of the cervical and/or cervico-thoracic spine.
- Reconstruction after EACF is ideally performed using expandable titanium mesh cages with autograft and dynamic anterior cervical plates combined with supplemental posterolateral screw-rod fixation.
- rhBMP-2 can be safely and effectively used to augment anterior fusion after EACF involving four or more levels.
- The length of posterolateral fixation should be based on the number of corpectomy levels.
- With proper reconstruction and fixation techniques, EACF is an effective treatment for symptomatic multilevel degenerative, traumatic, or infectious pathology of the anterior cervical spine, and is not associated with lower fusion rates or higher complication rates compared to more limited corpectomy procedures.

REFERENCES

1. Fernyhough JC, White JI, LaRocca H. Fusion rates in multilevel cervical spondylosis comparing allograft fibula with autograft fibula in 126 patients. Spine 1991;16:s561–s564.
2. Fessler RG, Steck JC, Giovanini MA. Anterior cervical corpectomy for cervical spondylotic myelopathy. Neurosurgery 1998; 43:257–265; discussion 65–67.
3. Sevki K, Mehmet T, Ufuk T, et al. Results of surgical treatment for degenerative cervical myelopathy: anterior cervical corpectomy and stabilization. Spine 2004; 29:2493–2500.
4. Edwards CC, 2nd, Heller JG, Murakami H. Corpectomy versus laminoplasty for multilevel cervical myelopathy: An independent matched-cohort analysis. Spine 2002; 27:1168–1175.
5. Herkowitz HN. A comparison of anterior cervical fusion, cervical laminectomy, and cervical laminoplasty for the surgical management of multiple level spondylotic radiculopathy. Spine 1988; 13:774–780.
6. Yonenobu K, Hosono N, Iwasaki M, et al. Laminoplasty versus subtotal corpectomy. A comparative study of results in multisegmental cervical spondylotic myelopathy. Spine 1992; 17:1281–1284.
7. Emery SE, Bolesta MJ, Banks MA, et al. Robinson anterior cervical fusion comparison of the standard and modified techniques. Spine 1994; 19:660–663.
8. Brodke DS, Zdeblick TA. Modified Smith-Robinson procedure for anterior cervical discectomy and fusion. Spine 1992; 17:s427–s430.
9. Emery SE, Fisher JR, Bohlman HH. Three-level anterior cervical discectomy and fusion: Radiographic and clinical results. Spine 1997; 22:2622–4; discussion 5.
10. Bolesta MJ, Rechtine GR, 2nd, Chrin AM. Three- and four-level anterior cervical discectomy and fusion with plate fixation: A prospective study. Spine 2000; 25:2040–2044; discussion 5–6.
11. Hilibrand AS, Fye MA, Emery SE, et al. Increased rate of arthrodesis with strut grafting after multilevel anterior cervical decompression. Spine 2002; 27:146–151.
12. Emery SE, Bohlman HH, Bolesta MJ, et al. Anterior cervical decompression and arthrodesis for the treatment of cervical spondylotic myelopathy. Two to seventeen-year follow-up. J Bone Joint Surg Am 1998; 80:941–951.
13. Bohlman HH, Emery SE, Goodfellow DB, et al. Robinson anterior cervical discectomy and arthrodesis for cervical radiculopathy. Long-term follow-up of one hundred and twenty-two patients. J Bone Joint Surg Am 1993; 75:1298–1307.
14. Vaccaro AR, Falatyn SP, Scuderi GJ, et al. Early failure of long segment anterior cervical plate fixation. J Spinal Disord 1998; 11:410–415.
15. Swank ML, Lowery GL, Bhat AL, et al. Anterior cervical allograft arthrodesis and instrumentation: Multilevel interbody grafting or strut graft reconstruction. Eur Spine J 1997; 6:138–143.
16. Macdonald RL, Fehlings MG, Tator CH, et al. Multilevel anterior cervical corpectomy and fibular allograft fusion for cervical myelopathy. J Neurosurg 1997; 86:990–997.
17. Wang JC, Hart RA, Emery SE, et al. Graft migration or displacement after multilevel cervical corpectomy and strut grafting. Spine 2003; 28:1016–1021; discussion 21–22.
18. Sasso RC, Ruggiero RA Jr, Reilly TM, et al. Early reconstruction failures after multilevel cervical corpectomy. Spine 2003; 28:140–142.
19. Wang JL, Panjabi MM, Isomi T. The role of bone graft force in stabilizing the multilevel anterior cervical spine plate system. Spine 2000; 25:1649–1654.
20. Isomi T, Panjabi MM, Wang JL, et al. Stabilizing potential of anterior cervical plates in multilevel corpectomies. Spine 1999; 24:2219–2223.
21. Saunders RL, Bernini PM, Shirreffs TG Jr, et al. Central corpectomy for cervical spondylotic myelopathy: A consecutive series with long-term follow-up evaluation. J Neurosurg 1991; 74:163–170.
22. Robinson RA. Fusions of the cervical spine. J Bone Joint Surg Am 1959; 41-A:1–6.
23. Cloward RB. The anterior approach for removal of ruptured cervical disks. J Neurosurg 1958; 15:602–617.
24. Bailey RW, Badgley CE. Stabilization of the cervical spine by anterior fusion. Am J Orthop 1960; 42-A:565–594.
25. Yonenobu K, Fuji T, Ono K, et al. Choice of surgical treatment for multisegmental cervical spondylotic myelopathy. Spine 1985; 10:710–716.
26. Wada E, Suzuki S, Kanazawa A, et al. Subtotal corpectomy versus laminoplasty for multilevel cervical spondylotic myelopathy: A long-term follow-up study over 10 years. Spine 2001; 26:1443–1447; discussion 8.
27. Majd ME, Vadhva M, Holt RT. Anterior cervical reconstruction using titanium cages with anterior plating. Spine 1999; 24:1604–1610.
28. Dorai Z, Morgan H, Coimbra C. Titanium cage reconstruction after cervical corpectomy. J Neurosurg Spine 2003; 99:3–7.
29. Zdeblick TA, Bohlman HH. Cervical kyphosis and myelopathy. Treatment by anterior corpectomy and strut-grafting. J Bone Joint Surg Am 1989; 71:170–182.
30. Vanichkachorn JS, Vaccaro AR, Silveri CP, et al. Anterior junctional plate in the cervical spine. Spine 1998; 23:2462–2467.

31. Hoshijima K, Nightingale RW, Yu JR, et al. Strength and stability of posterior lumbar interbody fusion. Comparison of titanium fiber mesh implant and tricortical bone graft. Spine 1997; 22:1181–1188.
32. Eck KR, Bridwell KH, Ungacta FF, et al. Analysis of titanium mesh cages in adults with minimum two-year follow-up. Spine 2000; 25:2407–2415.
33. Wilke HJ, Kettler A, Claes L. Primary stabilizing effect of interbody fusion devices for the cervical spine: An in vitro comparison between three different cage types and bone cement. Eur Spine J 2000; 9:410–416.
34. Bernard TN Jr, Whitecloud TS, 3rd. Cervical spondylotic myelopathy and myeloradiculopathy: Anterior decompression and stabilization with autogenous fibula strut graft. Clin Orthop Relat Res 1987; 221:149–160.
35. Zdeblick TA, Hughes SS, Riew KD, et al. Failed anterior cervical discectomy and arthrodesis: Analysis and treatment of thirty-five patients. J Bone Joint Surg Am 1997; 79:523–532.
36. Kanayama M, Cunningham BW, Weis JC, et al. The effects of rigid spinal instrumentation and solid bony fusion on spinal kinematics: A posterolateral spinal arthrodesis model. Spine 1998; 23:767–773.
37. DiAngelo DJ, Foley KT, Vossel KA, et al. Anterior cervical plating reverses load transfer through multilevel strut-grafts. Spine 2000; 25:783–795.
38. Epstein NE. The value of anterior cervical plating in preventing vertebral fracture and graft extrusion after multilevel anterior cervical corpectomy with posterior wiring and fusion: indications, results, and complications. J Spinal Disord 2000; 13:9–15.
39. Wang JC, McDonough PW, Kanim LE, et al. Increased fusion rates with cervical plating for three-level anterior cervical discectomy and fusion. Spine 2001; 26:643–646; discussion 6–7.
40. Foley KT, DiAngelo DJ, Rampersaud YR, et al. The in vitro effects of instrumentation on multilevel cervical strut-graft mechanics. Spine 1999; 24:2366–2376.
41. Spivak JM, Chen D, Kummer FJ. The effect of locking fixation screws on the stability of anterior cervical plating. Spine 1999; 24:334–338.
42. Kostuik JP, Connolly PJ, Esses SI, et al. Anterior cervical plate fixation with the titanium hollow screw plate system. Spine 1993; 18:1273–1278.
43. Reidy D, Finkelstein J, Nagpurkar A, et al. Cervical spine loading characteristics in a cadaveric C5 corpectomy model using a static and dynamic plate. J Spinal Disord Tech 2004; 17:117–122.
44. Paramore CG, Dickman CA, Sonntag VK. Radiographic and clinical follow-up review of Caspar plates in 49 patients. J Neurosurg 1996; 84:957–961.
45. Brodke DS, Gollogly S, Alexander Mohr R, et al. Dynamic cervical plates: Biomechanical evaluation of load sharing and stiffness. Spine 2001; 26:1324–1329.
46. Dvorak MF, Pitzen T, Zhu Q, et al. Anterior cervical plate fixation: a biomechanical study to evaluate the effects of plate design, endplate preparation, and bone mineral density. Spine 2005; 30:294–301.
47. Eleraky MA, Llanos C, Sonntag VK. Cervical corpectomy: Report of 185 cases and review of the literature. J Neurosurg Spine 1999; 90:35–41.
48. Bilsky MH, Boakye M, Collignon F, et al. Operative management of metastatic and malignant primary subaxial cervical tumors. J Neurosurg Spine 2005; 2:256–264.
49. Riew KD, Sethi NS, Devney J, et al. Complications of buttress plate stabilization of cervical corpectomy. Spine 1999; 24:2404–2410.
50. Singh K, Vaccaro AR, Kim J, et al. Biomechanical comparison of cervical spine reconstructive techniques after a multilevel corpectomy of the cervical spine. Spine 2003; 28:2352–2358; discussion 8.
51. Kirkpatrick JS, Levy JA, Carillo J, et al. Reconstruction after multilevel corpectomy in the cervical spine. A sagittal plane biomechanical study. Spine 1999; 24:1186–1190; discussion 91.
52. Kotani Y, Cunningham BW, Abumi K, et al. Biomechanical analysis of cervical stabilization systems: An assessment of transpedicular screw fixation in the cervical spine. Spine 1994; 19:2529–2539.
53. Cunningham BW, Sefter JC, Shono Y, et al. Static and cyclical biomechanical analysis of pedicle screw spinal constructs. Spine 1993; 18:1677–1688.
54. Grubb MR, Currier BL, Stone J, et al. Biomechanical evaluation of posterior cervical stabilization after a wide laminectomy. Spine 1997; 22:1948–1954.
55. Baskin DS, Ryan P, Sonntag V, et al. A prospective, randomized, controlled cervical fusion study using recombinant human bone morphogenetic protein-2 with the CORNERSTONE-SR allograft ring and the ATLANTIS anterior cervical plate. Spine 2003; 28:1219–1225; discussion 25.
56. Sidhu KS, Prochnow TD, Schmitt P, et al. Anterior cervical interbody fusion with rhBMP-2 and tantalum in a goat model. Spine J 2001; 1:331–340.
57. Zdeblick TA, Ghanayem AJ, Rapoff AJ, et al. Cervical interbody fusion cages. An animal model with and without bone morphogenetic protein. Spine 1998; 23:758–765; discussion 66.
58. Okada K, Shirasaki N, Hayashi H, et al. Treatment of cervical spondylotic myelopathy by enlargement of the spinal canal anteriorly, followed by arthrodesis. J Bone Joint Surg Am 1991; 73:352–364.
59. Boni M, Cherubino P, Denaro V, et al. Multiple subtotal somatectomy. Technique and evaluation of a series of 39 cases. Spine 1984; 9:358–362.
60. Brown JA, Havel P, Ebraheim N, et al. Cervical stabilization by plate and bone fusion. Spine 1988; 13:236–240.

61. Orr RD, Zdeblick TA. Cervical spondylotic myelopathy: Approaches to surgical treatment. Clin Orthop Relat Res 1999; 359:58–66.
62. Montgomery DM, Brower RS. Cervical spondylotic myelopathy. Clinical syndrome and natural history. Orthop Clin North Am 1992; 23:487–493.
63. Ebersold MJ, Pare MC, Quast LM. Surgical treatment for cervical spondylitic myelopathy. J Neurosurg 1995; 82:745–751.
64. Beutler WJ, Sweeney CA, Connolly PJ. Recurrent laryngeal nerve injury with anterior cervical spine surgery risk with laterality of surgical approach. Spine 2001; 26:1337–1342.
65. Bazaz R, Lee MJ, Yoo JU. Incidence of dysphagia after anterior cervical spine surgery: A prospective study. Spine 2002; 27:2453–2458.
66. An HS, Simpson JM, Glover JM, et al. Comparison between allograft plus demineralized bone matrix versus autograft in anterior cervical fusion. A prospective multicenter study. Spine 1995; 20:2211–2216.
67. Hanai K, Inouye Y, Kawai K, et al. Anterior decompression for myelopathy resulting from ossification of the posterior longitudinal ligament. J Bone Joint Surg Br 1982; 64:561–564.
68. Tippets RH, Apfelbaum RI. Anterior cervical fusion with the Caspar instrumentation system. Neurosurgery 1988; 22:1008–1013.
69. Kojima T, Waga S, Kubo Y, et al. Anterior cervical vertebrectomy and interbody fusion for multi-level spondylosis and ossification of the posterior longitudinal ligament. Neurosurgery 1989; 24:864–872.
70. Ebraheim NA, DeTroye RJ, Rupp RE, et al. Osteosynthesis of the cervical spine with an anterior plate. Orthopedics 1995; 18:141–147.
71. Saunders RL, Pikus HJ, Ball P. Four-level cervical corpectomy. Spine 1998; 23:2455–2461.
72. Schultz KD Jr, McLaughlin MR, Haid RW Jr, et al. Single-stage anterior-posterior decompression and stabilization for complex cervical spine disorders. J Neurosurg Spine 2000; 93:214–221.
73. Mayr MT, Subach BR, Comey CH, et al. Cervical spinal stenosis: outcome after anterior corpectomy, allograft reconstruction, and instrumentation. J Neurosurg Spine 2002; 96:10–16.

39 | Reconstruction of the Cervical Spine Using Artificial Pedicle Screws

Frank L. Acosta, Jr., Henry E. Aryan, and Christopher P. Ames

Department of Neurological Surgery, University of California, San Francisco, California, U.S.A.

INTRODUCTION

Access to the anterior cervical spinal canal is obstructed by the spinal cord and nerve roots posteriorly, the cervical musculature and vessels laterally, and the vertebral bodies anteriorly. Surgical approaches to lesions affecting the ventral compartment of these regions fall into two categories: (*i*) anterior approaches and (*ii*) posterolateral approaches. Anterior approaches across multiple levels, however, provide only a deep and narrow exposure and are of limited use in resecting lesions that extend over more than two levels or that involve significant lateral extension. Cervical posterolateral approaches allow for visualization of the ventral spinal canal across multiple levels, but require extensive resection of the posterior bony elements and pedicles (1,2,3). Reconstruction after posterolateral approaches, therefore, is often problematic in that three-column stabilization has not traditionally been possible across levels at which a pediculectomy has been performed. As such, lesions of the ventral cervical spinal compartment have proven difficult to access from posterior surgical approaches. We describe in detail the anatomic and surgical principles of a lateral cervical paramedian transpedicular approach—a novel technique that provides access to the ventral cervical spinal canal. This technique is a modification of traditional thoracic posterolateral extracavitary approaches. We also describe single-stage posterior column reconstruction of the cervical spine in which traditional cervical lateral mass screws are used to simultaneously reconstruct the cervical pedicle and allow for three-column stabilization in a continuous posterior screw-rod construct after this approach. Thus, cervical spinal stability is enhanced, as all cervical levels are incorporated into the final screw-rod construct.

TECHNIQUE
Patient Positioning

The patient is fiberoptically intubated after induction of general anesthesia. The patient's head is secured in Mayfield pin fixation and the patient positioned prone on uneven chest rolls at 30° and 45° angles, with the surgeon standing on the side with the steeper angle. The patients' head is kept in neutral position and the neck is flexed to allow for a three-finger-breadth space between the chin and manubrium. The posterior neck is prepped and draped in a sterile fashion from approximately three levels above and below the affected area.

Approach

The operating room table is rotated so that the patient's back and neck are level to the floor for the bone removal and instrumentation portion. This maneuver has been described previously for resection of lesions in the thoracolumbar spine (4). As in the lateral extracavitary exposure for the thoracolumabr spine, an elongated midline incision or a shorter hockey stick incision may be used. Authors have favored a midline incision since for the lateral extracavitary exposure of the upper cervicothoracic junction, the scapula must be mobilized from the midline anyway and the upper thoracic spine is usually relatively superficial. A midline incision is made from three levels above and three levels below the affected area. The paraspinous musculature is detached in a subperiosteal fashion from the spinous processes, lamina, and bilateral facet joints of the levels to be instrumented. This dissection is carried to at least

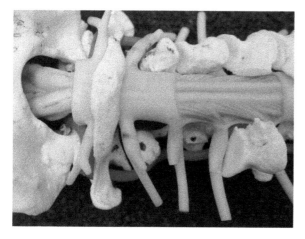

FIGURE 1 Anatomical model of the dorsal cervical spine after unilateral facetectomy and pedicle resection to the floor of the cervical spinal canal have been performed on the side selected for the lateral approach (*left*). The entire nerve root sleeves and dorsal root ganglia of the levels of interest can be clearly seen. Black dots at origins of C2, C3 pedicles at lateral-most aspect of vertebral body indicate planned points of entry for artificial pedicle screws during subsequent cervical spinal reconstruction.

3 cm lateral to the edges of the lateral masses. Contralateral pedicle screws or bicortical lateral mass screws are placed at each level prior to decompression. The screws are then attached to a rod to maintain stability during radical bone removal. This is especially important when there is a destructive lesion of the anterior column, which could cause intraoperative instability, as we will later illustrate. A wide laminectomy over the involved levels is then performed using Kerrison rongeurs. Next, unilateral facetectomies and pedicle resection to the floor of the cervical spinal canal are performed on the side selected for the lateral approach using a high-speed drill and Lempert rongeurs. At this stage of the procedure, the entire nerve root sleeves and dorsal root ganglia of the levels of interest can be clearly seen (Fig. 1).

Vertebral Artery Exposure

Attention is then turned to dissection and mobilization of the vertebral artery. This step is necessary not only to enhance exposure of the ventral cervical spinal cord, but also allows for safe retraction of the vertebral artery during tumor resection or later instrumentation. The nerve root immediately below the level of interest is gently retracted inferiorly (Fig. 2A). A 2 mm Kerrison rongeur is then used to remove the posterior arch of the foramen transversarium (Fig. 2B). Removal of the lateral posterior bony strut of the transverse foramen affords a direct view of the underlying vertebral artery (Fig. 2C). The venous complex surrounding the vertebral artery can be a significant source of blood loss and is therefore coagulated with bipolar cautery. With gentle retraction of the vertebral artery, the Kerrison rongeur is used again to complete the anterior transverse process resection, which forms the anterior margin of the foramen transversarium, providing access to the lateral vertebral body (Fig. 3). With

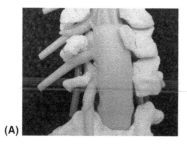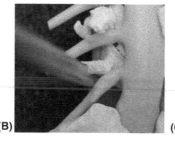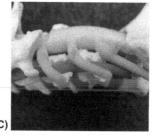

(A)   **(B)**   **(C)**

FIGURE 2 (**A**) Anatomic model of the cervical spine after single-level pediculectomy demonstrating downward retraction of the nerve root below the level of interest to reveal the posterior arch of the foramen transversarium. (**B**) The posterior foramen transversarium is resected using a Kerrison rongeur to provide direct visualization of the underlying vertebral artery. (**C**) Lateral (surgical view) after two-level pediculectomy and resection of the posterior bony border of the foramen transversarium.

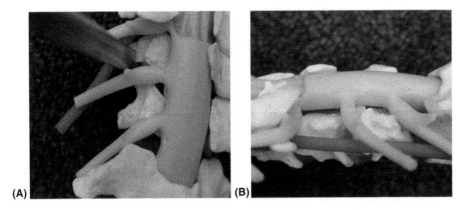

(A) **(B)**

FIGURE 3 (**A**) The anterior bone of the transverse foramen (cervical transverse process) is resected with gentle lateral retraction of the vertebral artery. (**B**) Surgical view after complete vertebral mobilization demonstrating exposure of the vertebral artery and dorsal vertebral body which can be drilled out as needed.

gentle ventral retraction of the vertebral artery and nerve roots, a dorsal corpectomy can be accomplished using a high-speed drill to enhance exposure of the ventral spinal canal, if necessary. Extra large fishhooks are then placed over the lateral soft tissue and secured to a Leyla bar. This tissue is then retracted as ventrally as possible using rubberbands and the retractor arm. This maneuver is critical as it establishes the pure lateral line of sight. After the bone work is complete, the posterior, lateral, and ventral thecal sac are exposed (Fig. 4). Having previously performed a pediculectomy, the nerve roots are no longer tethered in place, and a significant amount of nerve root mobilization can be performed without applying excessive tensile forces to the nerve.

Reconstruction

Following tumor resection, attention is turned to creating a final pedicle/lateral mass screw-rod construct. Bilateral C1 lateral mass screws are placed under fluoroscopic guidance using the technique described by Harms and Melcher (5). "Artificial pedicle screws" are then placed directly into the vertebral body at all levels where a pediculectomy has been performed. The lateral-most aspect of the cervical vertebral body to be instrumented is identified and the corresponding nerve root is gently retracted cephalad (Fig. 5). A starter hole is drilled and tapped under direct visualization. Next, a polyaxial screw is inserted into the vertebral body (Fig. 6A), angled 20° in the sagittal plane, under fluoroscopic guidance to assure bicortical purchase (Fig. 6B). Lateral mass screws are then positioned in the usual fashion in the remaining

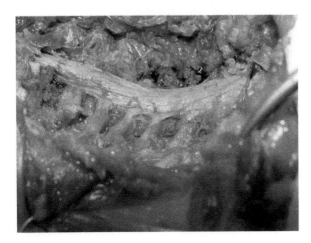

FIGURE 4 Cadaveric specimen demonstrating the wide exposure of the posterior and lateral thecal sac, dorsal vertebral bodies and nerve roots. The ventral dura and epidural space can be fully visualized.

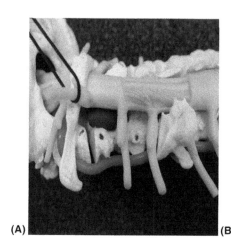
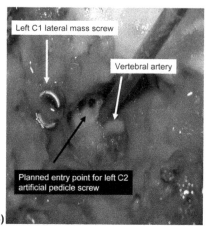

FIGURE 5 (**A**) Spinal model showing insertion point of artifical pedicle screw at C2. (**B**) Intraoperative photograph showing C2 artificial pedicle screw insertion point.

levels down to C6. We typically use pedicle screws beginning at C7. Again, it is important to fixate the contralateral posterior elements with a screw-rod construct prior to bone resection in order to avoid intraoperative instability. Finally, rods are fashioned and secured, followed by thorough decortication of the remaining facet joints and transverse processes and bone graft placement for fusion.

POSTOPERATIVE MANAGEMENT

Anterior-posterior plain radiographs are taken immediately postoperatively. The patient is monitored in the intensive care unit overnight and transferred to the neurosurgical close-observation unit on postoperative day 1. A computed tomography (CT) of the cervical spine, with 2- and 3-D reconstruction, is obtained prior to discharge. The patient is kept in a cervical collar for at least three months postoperatively.

RISKS

The major risks of this technique include injury to the vertebral artery from mobilization and retraction, as well as to the spinal cord and cervical nerve root from extensive dissection,

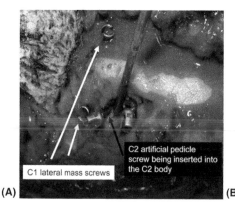
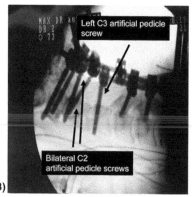

FIGURE 6 (**A**) Intraoperative photo demonstrating initial placement of an artificial pedicle screw in the left C2 vertebral body. (**B**) Lateral intraoperative fluorographic image demonstrating artificial pedicle screws bilaterally at C2 and in the left C3 vertebral bodies. Note that bicortical purchase is achieved.

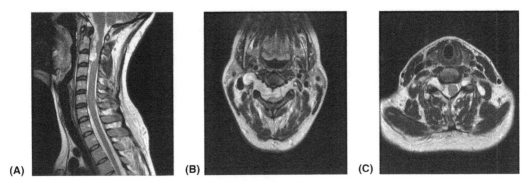

FIGURE 7 (**A**) Sagittal and (**B**, **C**) axial T2-weighted magnetic resonance images of the spine demonstrating large extra and intradural, extramedullary dumbbell-shaped at the C1-2 and C2-3 levels, and on the right at C5-6, causing severe cord compression.

manipulation, and retraction. This is especially problematic in the setting of pre-existing spinal cord dysfunction, in which case a planned retraction of the spinal cord should be avoided. In our experience to date, we have not had difficulty in evaluating the extent of decompression of the ventral canal with the operative microscope. We believe a dental mirror can be used to determine ventral decompression when this is problematic.

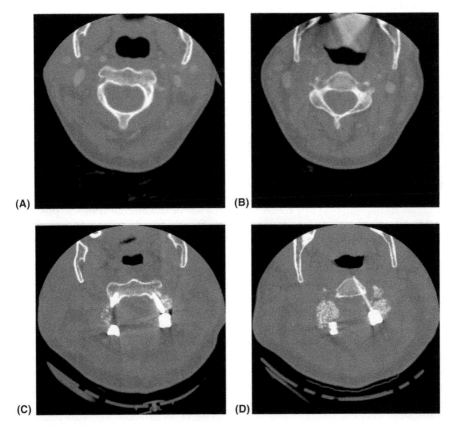

FIGURE 8 Preoperative axial CT scans of the C2 (**A**) and C3 (**B**) vertebral bodies. Postoperative CT scans of the same patient after laminectomy and pediculectomy demonstrating pedicle screws bilaterally at C2 (**C**) and in the left C3 body (**D**).

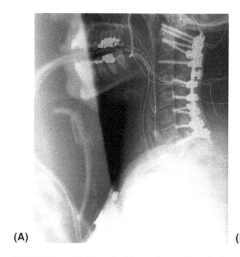
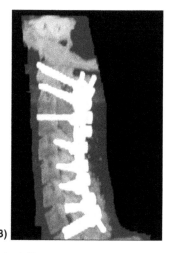

(A)   (B)

FIGURE 9 (**A**) Lateral plain radiograph and (**B**) sagittal CT reconstruction demonstrating the final posterior fusion construct extending from C1 to T1. Note the artificial pedicle screws in the C2 and C3 vertebral bodies.

ILLUSTRATIVE CASE

A 37-year-old woman with a history of neurofibromatosis type 1 (NF1) presented with neck pain and parasthesias involving the legs, arms, and hands. Magnetic resonance imaging of the spine revealed too-numerous-to-count nerve root tumors as well as large dumbbell-shaped extra- and intradural, extramedullary tumors at the C1-2 and C2-3 levels, and on the right at C5-6, causing severe cord compression (Fig. 7).

Using the technique described, one performed a laminectomy from C1-C3 and at C6, bilateral pedicle resection and vertebral artery mobilization at C2 and C3 for removal of all extradural and intradural tumor. Posterior spinal fusion from C1 to T1 was then performed, with "artificial pedicle screws" placed bilaterally at C2 and on the left side at C3 (Fig. 8). The final posterior fusion construct was then created from C1 to T1 (Fig. 9). Pathology revealed these lesions to be neurofibromas. Postoperatively, the patient had mild biceps weakness on the right (4/5), which resolved at two-month follow-up.

CONCLUSIONS

The lateral paramedian transpedicular approach is a variation of traditional thoracic postero-lateral transpedicular extracavitary approaches and offers direct access to intra and extradural lesions of the dorsal, lateral, and ventral cervical and cervicothoracic spinal canal. This approach can be used to treat ventral intra and extradural pathology affecting the cervicothor-acic junction without violating the mediastinum, pleural space, or pharynx. The vertebral artery is mobilized after careful resection of the three boney borders of the foramen transver-sariuim. This approach avoids the morbidity of anterior transcervical, transoral, or transthor-acic procedures, while providing a view of the entire ventral canal. Although, such a radical deconstruction of the posterior cervico-thoracic spine is rarely necessary, one recommend our technique for resecting large ventral intra and extradural masses spanning three or more levels of the anterior cervical spine and/or cervicothoracic junction. It is especially useful in cases where significant pathology of the trachea or esophagus precludes an anterior approach to the cervical spine. We have used this technique in a total of six patients with no compli-cations to date. Single-stage cervical pedicle reconstruction after pediculectomy can be achieved using traditional cervical lateral mass screws to serve as artificial cervical pedicles. This can be incorporated into a posterior screw-rod construct, thus allowing simultaneous three-column stabilization after radical posterior column resection of the cervical spine. More-over, artificial pedicle screws can be used in the instance of a fractured lateral mass at the top of any cervicothoracic construct and prevents having to instrument the adjacent cephalad level while avoiding the risk of vertebral artery injury during pedicle screw insertion.

REFERENCES

1. Bucci MN, McGillicuddy JE, Taren JA, Hoff JT. Management of anteriorly located C1-C2 neurofibromata. Surg Neurol 1990; 33:15–18.
2. Hakuba A, Komiyama M, Tsujimoto T, et al. Transuncodiscal approach to dumbbell tumors of the cervical spinal canal. J Neurosurg 1984; 61:1100–1106.
3. Martin NA, Khanna RK, Batzdorf U. Posterolateral cervical or thoracic approach with spinal cord rotation for vascular malformations or tumors of the ventrolateral spinal cord. J Neurosurg 1995; 83:254–261.
4. Lesoin F, Rousseaux M, Lozes G, et al. Posterolateral approach to tumours of the dorsolumbar spine. Acta Neurochir (Wien) 1986; 81:40–44.
5. Harms J, Melcher RP. Posterior C1-C2 fusion with polyaxial screw and rod fixation. Spine 2001; 26:2467–2471.

40 | Posterior Fixation for Atlantoaxial Instability: Various Surgical Techniques with Wire and Screw Fixation

Naohisa Miyakoshi, Yoichi Shimada, and Michio Hongo
Department of Orthopedic Surgery, Akita University School of Medicine, Akita, Japan

INTRODUCTION

Atlantoaxial instability is caused by rheumatoid arthritis, trauma, tumor, infection, and conge-
nital disorders. Several different techniques have been described for stabilization of the C1–C2
junction. Since the first report of posterior atlantoaxial fusion for the treatment of atlantoaxial
instability by Gallie in 1939 (1), various posterior wiring techniques for atlantoaxial instability
have been developed to provide fixation of C1–C2 segments, including Brooks fusion, modi-
fied-Gallie techniques, and the Halifax interlaminar clamp (1–5). Since 1987 when Magerl
and Seeman (6) introduced the technique of transarticular screw placement, it has become
the standard procedure for posterior fusion of C1–C2. In addition, other methods, such as posterior intraarticular screw fixation (7), posterior screw-rod fixation (8), and anterior transarticular screw fixation (9), have been reported for treatment of atlantoaxial lesion. In this Chapter, the
authors summarize various techniques of posterior atlantoaxial fixation and review clinical and
radiological records of their patient series who have undergone posterior atlantoaxial fixation.

MCGRAW'S POSTERIOR WIRING

Classic instrumentation for the atlantoaxial instability with posterior wiring has been used for
many years in the form of the Brooks or Gallie fusion (1–3). Before the introduction of transarticular screw fixation, posterior wiring was considered the gold standard for treating atlantoaxial instability. There are numerous reports in the literature detailing successful clinical
outcomes using posterior wiring methods (2,3,10,11). However, several biomechanical
studies have shown that this form of instrumentation does a poor job resisting rotational
and lateral bending forces (12,13). This is likely the reason for the high-nonunion rate for
this technique compared to transarticular screw fixation, despite postoperative Halo vest
immobilization (14–16). In 1973, McGraw modified the original Gallie wiring techniques (4).
Between 1979 and 1992, the authors' institution had adopted McGraw's technique for the treatment of atlantoaxial instability.

SURGICAL PROCEDURE OF MCGRAW'S POSTERIOR WIRING

For two or three weeks prior to the procedure, the head is held in traction using Crutchfield's
device or Halo traction to reduce the dislocation of C1–C2. The patient is placed in the spine
frame in the prone position, while the head and neck are maintained in the extended position
with traction. A rectangular cortico-cancellous graft, measuring ~3 cm in length, is cut from the
posterior iliac crest. Notches are fashioned in the graft to accommodate the spinous process of
the C2. A graft is placed between the curettaged laminae of the atlas and axis, and fixed with a
stainless steel wire (i.e., 0.97 mm in diameter) passing around the arch of the atlas and beneath
the spinous process of the axis. Postoperatively, the patient is held in a Halo vest for approximately one month, followed by application of a SOMI or Philadelphia cervical orthosis for
three months. A representative case that underwent McGraw's posterior wiring is presented
in Figure 1.

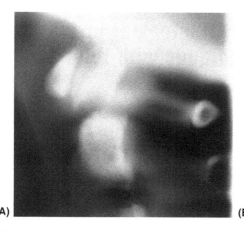 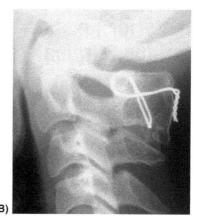

(A)   (B)

FIGURE 1   A 20-year-old male with os odontoideum underwent McGraw posterior wiring. (**A**) Preoperative sagittal tomogram showing subluxation at C1–C2. (**B**) Lateral radiographs obtained 6 years after the surgery demonstrating solid fusion.

SURGICAL RESULTS WITH MCGRAW'S POSTERIOR WIRING (17)

In the authors' institution, 19 consecutive patients (10 males, 9 females) with a mean age of 42.5 years (range, 10–74 years) were treated with McGraw's wiring technique. The cause of atlantoaxial instability included rheumatoid arthritis (nine patients), os odontoideum (six patients), post-traumatic (two patients), and other causes (two patients). Seventeen (89%) of the 19 patients had complained of neck pain as the main symptom. Neurologic abnormalities were found in seven patients (37%).

No cases of severe complications such as vertebral artery injury, iatrogenic neurological deficit, or deep wound infection were observed. Clinical outcomes, assessed according to relief of pain (Table 1), were rated as excellent in 10 patients (53%), good in five patients (26%), fair in 3 patients (16%), and poor in 1 patient (5%). The average follow-up period was 12.2 years (range, 2–22 yrs). Sixteen patients (84%) achieved solid osseous fusion and three patients developed pseudoarthrosis. The fusion rate of the McGraw or modified Gallie procedure has been previously reported to be 50% to 96% (11,18–20), which is comparable to the fusion rate of the authors' series (84%).

TRANSARTICULAR SCREW FIXATION

Magerl and Seeman (6) developed the transarticular screw procedure in an attempt to improve biomechanical stability and fusion rates at the C1–C2 segment (6). Transarticular screw fixation provides immediate rigid fixation of the C1–C2 segment (13,21–23), higher fusion rates (14,24–28), and reduction in the periods of external fixation compared with posterior wiring techniques.

Numerous biomechanical studies have shown that the transarticular screw fixation technique offers increased stability compared with fusion obtained by posterior wiring techniques (13,21,22,25,29–31). In a biomechanical study, Grob et al. (12) found that Magerl's transarticular

TABLE 1   Evaluation of Neck Pain

Rating	Remarks
Excellent	Near complete relief of pain
Good[a]	Occasional discomfort in the neck, necessitating occasional nonnarcotic medication
Fair	Intermittent discomfort in the neck, improvement compared with the preoperative conditions
Poor	Marked discomfort in the neck, necessitating nonnarcotic medication

[a]Patients with a good result had significant improvement, compared with the preoperative condition.

screw fixation technique generally produced significantly less rotation in flexion, extension, axial rotation, and lateral bending compared with the Gallie wiring technique. Henriques et al. (13) also demonstrated that the transarticular screws effectively restrict the motion of the C1–C2 joint in axial rotation and lateral bending, although transarticular screws alone do not increase stiffness compared with either the intact spine or the McGraw technique. The combination of transarticular screws and posterior bone grafting has produced excellent stability in all directions (13). The advantages of the atlantoaxial transarticular screw fixation have been documented in several clinical series (14,15,24,25,32–34). Fusion rates using the transarticular screw are between 92% and 100% (14,24,25, 28,32,33).

Transarticular screw fixation is also believed to produce better postoperative spinal alignment compared to posterior wiring or interlaminar clamps. Since biomechanical stability of posterior wiring or interlaminar clamps depends mainly on the compression force between grafted bone and the C1–C2 laminae, these procedures have a tendency to fix the C1–C2 joint in the hyperlordotic position (35). However, the transarticular screw fixation does not depend on compression forces so that hyperlordotic fixation at C1–C2 can be avoided (35). Between 1992 and 2002, the authors' institution had adopted Magerl's transarticular screw fixation technique for the treatment of atlantoaxial instability.

SURGICAL PROCEDURE OF TRANSARTICULAR SCREW FIXATION

The fusion procedure for Magerl's transarticular screw fixation is performed with the head secured using a Mayfield head fixation set. The atlantoaxial subluxation is reduced using fluoroscopic control. Intraoperatively, a guide wire, which is parallel to the sagittal plane, is inserted into the medial edge of the C2–C3 facet with the tip aimed just at the tubercle of the anterior arch of the atlas. A cannulated drill is passed over the guide wire to prevent the guide wire from penetrating the mucous membrane of the pharynx. After the drill has satisfactorily entered the atlas, a 3.5-mm AO cannulated cancellous screw is inserted. Following bilateral screw fixation, posterior bone grafting is added using either the McGraw procedure or Halifax interlaminar clamps (OSTEONICS, Allendale, New Jersey, U.S.A.) Postoperatively, each patient wears a cervical orthosis for three to four months.

In our retrospective series of 17 patients with 34 bilateral screws there were no vertebral artery injuries (17) and no other major complications, such as neurologic deficits, apoplexy, or infection, were encountered. A representative case that underwent transarticular screw fixation with posterior bone grafting is presented in Figure 2.

POSSIBLE COMPLICATIONS WITH TRANSARTICULAR SCREW FIXATION

The authors believe that atlantoaxial transarticular screw fixation can be performed safely by surgeons who are familiar with both, the procedure and the patient's anatomic situation. However, the technique carries the risk of screw malpositioning and neural and vascular injury (27,36–40). The vertebral artery injury is the most dangerous complication because it can be lethal (27,36,40–42).

The reported rates of vertebral artery injury for this procedure range from 4.1% to 8.2% (14,27,40). Vertebral artery injury can occur not only because the screw is malpositioned, but also because the location of the vertebral artery is anatomically variable and consequently the isthmus of C2, through which the screw is inserted, sometimes is too narrow (27,39,43). In ∼80% of individuals, the vertebral artery makes an acute lateral bend just under the superior articular facet of C2 (44). If this bending point is too medial, too posterior, and/or too high, the height and/or the width of the isthmus of the axis is narrowed, a condition described as a high-riding vertebral artery (Fig. 3) (23,45). Therefore, the risk of vertebral artery injury is much higher for the situation when there is a narrow isthmus with a high-riding vertebral artery.

In studies using computed tomography (CT), 11.9% to 25.9% of the patients had a high-riding vertebral artery on at least one side of the axis that would prohibit the placement of transarticular screws (23,46,39). Therefore, many authors recommend that the anatomical situation of the isthmus of C2 be evaluated preoperatively using CT reconstruction

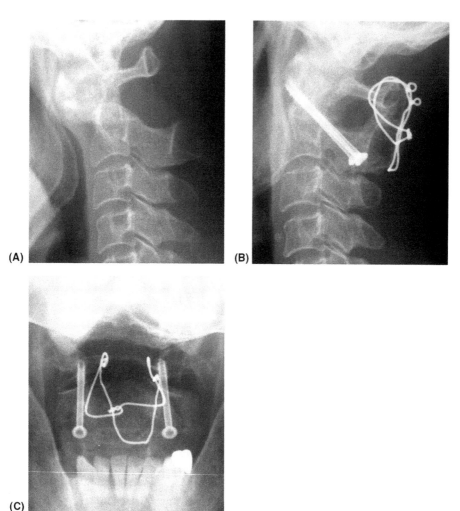

FIGURE 2 A 67-year-old female with rheumatoid arthritis underwent transarticular screw fixation with posterior bone grafting. (**A**) Preoperative lateral flexion radiograph showing subluxation at C1–C2. (**B**) and (**C**) Lateral and anteroposterior radiographs obtained five years after surgery demonstrating good positioning of the transarticular screw and solid fusion.

(6,14,24,27,37,39,47), and advise that insertion of the screw should be abandoned if the isthmus is too narrow (24,39,42,46). Neo et al. (23), however, suggested that even in patients with a high-riding vertebral artery, it is possible to insert a transarticular screw when the surgeon aims for the most posterior and medial part of the isthmus, although precision of the screw placement is essential. According to their procedure, they experienced no major complications such as vertebral artery injury, but they did report that two out of seven screws inserted in patients with a high-riding vertebral artery seemed to breach the cortex of the vertebral artery groove (23).

INTRAARTICULAR SCREW FIXATION

In 1996, Tokuhashi et al. (7) developed a new screw fixation technique for atlantoaxial posterior stabilization, in which the screw is inserted into the atlantoaxial joint along the articular surface under direct view without radiographic control. This screw fixation device was applied in combination with a posterior fixation device such as the Halifax interlaminar clamp (OSTEONICS, Allendale, New Jersey, U.S.A.). Tokuhashi et al. (7) reported the first clinical outcomes of

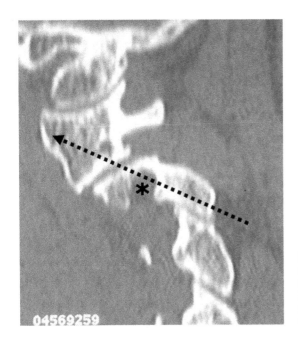

FIGURE 3 A sagittal computed tomography reconstruction of a case with high-riding vertebral artery. This section was obtained 3 mm lateral to the left lateral edge of the spinal canal. Vertebral artery groove (*asterisk*); course of transarticular screw (*dotted arrow*).

11 patients with atlantoaxial instability who had been treated with intraarticular screw fixation in combination with a Halifax interlaminar clamp. In their series, occipital and neck pain, and neural deficit improved. In addition, bony fusion with no correction loss was shown on radiography without any patients experiencing vascular or neural complications (7). Since 2002, the authors' institution has adopted this procedure for the treatment of atlantoaxial lesions.

SURGICAL PROCEDURE OF INTRAARTICULAR SCREW FIXATION (7)

In this procedure, the patient is placed in the prone position while maintaining C1–C2 reduction as much as possible; the reduction is confirmed with C-arm fluoroscopy or radiography. A midline exposure of C1 and C2 posterior elements is then achieved. Careful dissection with a small dissector is performed along the superior laminar ridge of C2 until the atlantoaxial joints are exposed (Fig. 4A). When the dissector reaches the atlantoaxial joints, the surgeon can detect a light sensation of penetration of the capsule because of the loss of resistance. The capsule usually can be dissected free with a small dissector and retracted cranially together with the C2 nerve root. Venous bleeding, if it is encountered, can be controlled by packing with Avitene (Davol Inc., Woburn, Massachusetts, U.S.A.). After exposure of the joint surfaces is achieved, a 1-mm Kirschner wire is inserted into the atlantoaxial joints as a guide for screw insertion (Fig. 4B).

A titanium intraarticular screw (5.0–6.5 mm in diameter, 8.0 to 10.0 mm in length; KISCO-DIR, Co. Ltd., Osaka, Japan) is inserted after interlaminar clamp fixation and hemicortical bone grafting from the posterior iliac crest (Fig. 4C). After the reduced position is confirmed by radiography, fine adjustment of the clamp is performed, the position of the atlantoaxial joints is checked, and tapping and screw insertion are performed using a Kirschner wire as a guide (Figs. 4D and 4E). The intraarticular screws are buried in the atlantoaxial joints, with care taken to avoid the greater occipital nerves located medially and running superficially to the C1–C2 articulation (Fig. 4F). As the final step, the clamp is tightened again to place cephalocaudal pressure on the intraarticular screws. The patients are allowed to sit and walk with a Philadelphia orthosis three days after surgery. The orthosis is applied for three months.

Because this screw can be inserted under a direct view without radiographic control, it potentially decreases the risk of damage to the spinal cord, dura matter, and vertebral

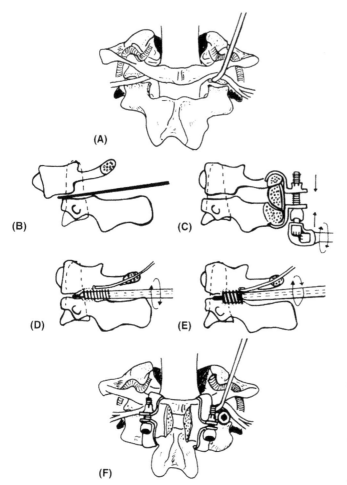

(A)

(B)   (C)

(D)   (E)

(F)

FIGURE 4 Surgical procedure for intraarticular screw placement for atlantoaxial instability. (**A**) Exposure of posterior atlantoaxial joints. (**B**) Insertion of a 1-mm Kirschner wire into the atlantoaxial joints as a guide for screw insertion. (**C**) Interlaminar clamp fixation in the reduced position of atlantoaxial joints and hemicortical bone grafting. (**D**) Tapping using a Kirschner wire as a guide. (**E**) Intra-articular screw insertion using a Kirschner wire as a guide. (**F**) Buried intraarticular screws in the atlantoaxial joints. *Source*: From Ref. 7.

artery (7). To counter the risk of massive bleeding from the periarticular venous plexus during exposure of the atlantoaxial joints, it is important to expose only the joint surface and retract the capsule of the atlantoaxial joints cranially with the C2 nerve root and the periarticular venous plexus (7). A representative case that underwent intraarticular screw fixation with posterior bone grafting is presented in Figure 5.

BIOMECHANICAL STUDY OF INTRAARTICULAR SCREW FIXATION

In a biomechanical study using a bone model of the cervical spine (SAWBONES, Pacific Research Laboratories, Inc., Vashon, Washington, U.S.A.), Tokuhashi et al (7) evaluated atlantoaxial instability after the following three types of instrumentations:

1. Intraarticular screw fixation with Halifax interlaminar clamp
2. Magerl's transarticular screw fixation with Halifax clamp
3. Halifax clamp alone

They measured axial rotation around the base of the dens and flexion around the anterior edge of the base of the dens using an Instron universal testing machine (UTM-10, A & D, Yokohama, Japan). In their study, the Magerl's transarticular screw fixation with the Halifax clamp had significantly greater flexion stiffness than the intraarticular screw fixation with the Halifax clamp

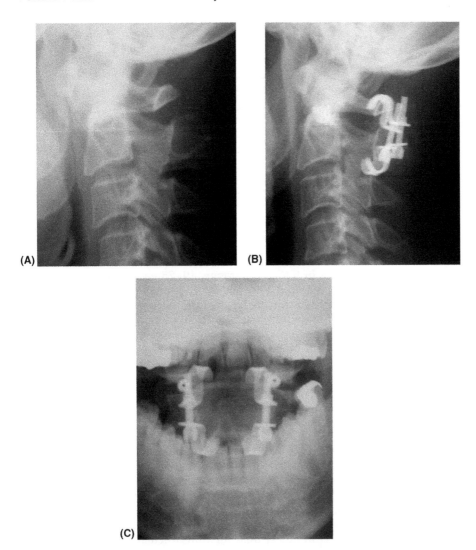

FIGURE 5 A 57-year-old male with posttraumatic atlantoaxial instability underwent intraarticular screw fixation with posterior bone grafting. (**A**) Preoperative lateral flexion radiograph showing subluxation at C1–C2. (**B**) and (**C**) Lateral and anteroposterior radiographs obtained one year after surgery demonstrating good positioning of the intraarticular screws (buried in the atlantoaxial joints) and solid fusion.

or the Halifax clamp alone (Fig. 6), but the torsional resistance of the intraarticular screw fixation with the Halifax clamp was significantly greater than that of the Magerl's transarticular screw fixation with the Halifax clamp or the Halifax clamp alone (Fig. 7). The results of this biomechanical study indicate that intraarticular screw fixation with a posterior interlaminar clamp is effective in strengthening the rotational stability of the atlantoaxial fixation and is considered useful for atlantoaxial posterior stabilization.

COMPARISON BETWEEN INTRAARTICULAR AND TRANSARTICULAR SCREW FIXATION

The authors reviewed clinical and radiological records of 23 consecutive patients with atlantoaxial lesion who underwent either intraarticular screw fixation with bone grafting or transarticular screw fixation with bone grafting at the authors' institution. Seventeen patients

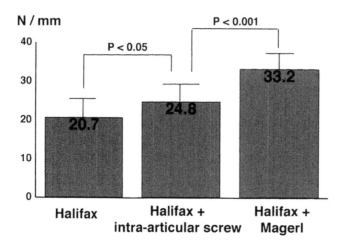

FIGURE 6 Stiffness against flexion in the three fixation techniques. *Source:* From Ref. 7.

(4 males, 13 females) with a mean age of 55.5 years (range, 10–75 years) were treated with Magerl's transarticular screw fixation between 1992 and 2002, and six patients with a mean age of 60.5 years (range, 38–79 years) were treated with intraarticular screw fixation with bone grafting since 2002. The causes of atlantoaxial lesions and symptoms in both groups are shown in Table 2. The data for the patients with transarticular screw fixation was partially obtained from the authors' previous presentation (17). There was no significant difference with regard to the clinical symptoms between the groups. Operation time, blood loss, and complications during and after surgery were compared between the two groups. On plain radiographs, the atlantodental interval (ADI) and fusion rates were evaluated. The criteria for fusion were based on radiographic evidence of trabecular crossings and absence of intersegmental motion at the fusion site in a dynamogram. The evaluations for neck pain were listed previously (Table 1).

During and after surgery, no cases of vertebral artery injury, iatrogenic neurological deficit, infection, or instrumentation failure were observed in either group. No complications were encountered when the intraarticular screw fixation was used. Complications related to the transarticular screw fixation technique included one case of screw penetration of the mucous membrane of the pharynx, but the patient showed no clinical symptoms. The surgeries lasted significantly longer for cases with intraarticular screw fixation with bone grafting (average, 281 minutes; range, 198–353 minutes) than for transarticular screw fixation with bone grafting (average, 203 minutes; range, 170–330 minutes) ($p = 0.002$). However, there was no significant difference in blood loss between the two groups. The mean blood loss

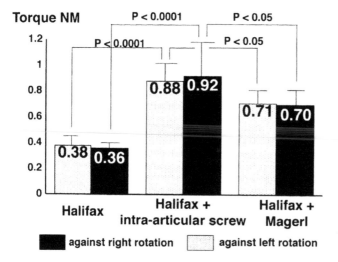

FIGURE 7 Torque against torsion in the three fixation techniques. *Source:* From Ref. 7.

TABLE 2 Background Data of the Patients Who Underwent the Two Surgical Procedures for Atlantoaxial Lesions

	Transarticular screw fixation	Intraarticular screw fixation
Age	55.5 (10–75)	60.5 (38–79)
Gender (M:F)	4:13	2:4
Type of instability		
Rheumatoid arthritis	10	0
Os odontoideum	2	0
Post-traumatic	5	5
Idiopathic	1	1
Symptoms		
Neck pain	14	6
Neurologic deficits	9	2

during surgery was 154 g (range, 31–477 g) for intraarticular screw fixation with bone grafting and 171 g (range, 40–397 g) for transarticular screw fixation with bone grafting.

Table 3 provides a summary of the clinical and radiological outcomes of the patients studied. In both procedures, no patients showed worsening symptoms after surgery. There were no significant differences in reduction of neck pain after surgery, or pre- and postoperative ADIs between the groups. The fusion rate of intraarticular screw fixation with bone grafting (100%) was comparable with that of transarticular screw fixation with bone grafting (94%), although the number of patients was smaller and the mean follow-up period was shorter in the former group. These findings demonstrate that intraarticular screw fixation is a safe and effective technique and its clinical and radiological outcomes are comparable to those with transarticular screw fixation.

OTHER TECHNIQUES FOR ATLANTOAXIAL INSTABILITY

In addition to transarticular screw fixation and intraarticular screw fixation, other techniques have also been developed (8,9,48,49). Among them, an alternative rigid fixation technique for C1–C2 instability is posterior fixation with C1 lateral mass and C2 pedicle screw (8,48). In 1988, Goel et al. (49) developed this technique for C1–C2 fixation, which minimizes the risk of injury to the vertebral artery and allows intraoperative reduction. More recently, the technique proposed by Goel et al. has been modified to the screw and rod fixation system (8,48). Application of this system to the C1–C2 complex does not require the acute angle of approach associated with transarticular screw fixation and has been performed with satisfactory clinical results (48,50). In a cadaveric study comparing screw and rod fixation and transarticular screw fixation, bilateral application in both procedures was similarly effective across the C1–C2 segment (51). However, the screw and rod fixation afforded higher stability than the transarticular screw fixation in flexion and extension modes (51).

TABLE 3 Clinical and Radiological Outcome of the Two Procedures for Atlantoaxial Lesions

	Transarticular screw fixation	Intraarticular screw fixation
Follow-up period (yrs)	6.4 (2–9)	2.8 (2–4)
Pain		
Excellent	9 (53%)	3 (50%)
Good	5 (29%)	2 (33%)
Fair	3 (18%)	1 (17%)
Poor	0	0
Radiographic evaluation		
Atlantodental interval (mm)		
Preoperative	9.0 (2–17)	6.2 (1–11)
Postoperative	2.7 (1–5)	2.3 (1–4)
Follow-up	3.1 (1–5)	2.7 (1–6)
Fusion rate	16/17 (94%)	6/6 (100%)

CONCLUSIONS

Various posterior stabilization techniques with wiring, including McGraw's technique, have been developed to manage atlantoaxial instability. Ever since Magerl and Seeman developed the transarticular screw fixation technique, it has been the standard procedure for posterior atlantoaxial fixation. However, the technique is technically demanding and poses a risk of injury to the nerves and vertebral arteries. Alternatively, the intraarticular screw fixation technique developed by Tokuhashi et al., in which the screw is inserted into the atlantoaxial joint along the articular surface under direct view without radiographic control, is a safe and effective procedure for the treatment of atlantoaxial lesion. In the authors' series, the clinical and radiological results of the intraarticular screw fixation technique were comparable with those of transarticular screw fixation technique, but without any complications.

REFERENCES

1. Gallie WE. Fractures and dislocations of the cervical spine. Am J Surg 1939; 46(3):495–499.
2. Anderson LD, D'Alonzo RT. Fractures of the odontoid process of the axis. J Bone Joint Surg Am 1974: 56(8):1663–1674.
3. Brooks AL, Jenkins EB. Atlanto-axial arthrodesis by the wedge compression method. J Bone Joint Surg Am 1978; 60(3):279–284.
4. McGraw RW, Rusch RM. Atlanto-axial arthrodesis. J Bone Joint Surg Br 1973; 55(3):482–489.
5. Moskovich R, Crockard HA. Atlantoaxial arthrodesis using interlaminar clamps. An improved technique. Spine 1992; 17(3):261–267.
6. Magerl F, Seemann PS. Stable posterior fusion of the atlas and axis by transarticular screw fixation. In: Kehr P, Weidner A, eds. Cervical Spine I. Wien: Springer-Verlag, 1987:322–327.
7. Tokuhashi Y, Matsuzaki H, Shirasaki Y, et al. C1-C2 intra-articular screw fixation for tlantoaxial posterior stabilization. Spine 2000; 25(3):337–341.
8. Harms J, Melcher RP. Posterior C1-C2 fusion with polyaxial screw and rod fixation. Spine 2001; 26(22):2467–2471.
9. Reindl R, Sen M, Aebi M. Anterior instrumentation for traumatic C1-C2 instability. Spine 2003; 28(17):E329–E333.
10. Coyne TJ, Fehlings MG, Wallace MC, et al. C1-C2 posterior cervical fusion: Long-term evaluation of results and efficacy. Neurosurgery 1995; 37(4):688–693.
11. Ranawat CS, O'Leary P, Pellicci P, et al. Cervical spine fusion in rheumatoid arthritis. J Bone Joint Surg Am 1979; 61(7):1003–1010.
12. Grob D, Crisco JJ, Panjabi MM, et al. Biomechanical evaluation of four different posterior atlantoaxial fixation techniques. Spine 1992; 17(5):480–490.
13. Henriques T, Cunningham BW, Olerud C, et al. Biomechanical comparison of five different atlantoaxial posterior fixation techniques. Spine 2000; 25(22):2877–2883.
14. Farey ID, Nadkarni S, Smith N. Modified Gallie technique versus transarticular screw fixation in C1-C2 fusion. Clin Orthop Relat Res 1999; 359: 126–135.
15. Jeanneret B, Magerl F. Primary posterior fusion C1/2 in odontoid fractures: indications, technique, and results of transarticular screw fixation. J Spinal Disord 1992; 5(4):464–475.
16. Govender S, NgCelwane MV. Post-traumatic ligamentous instability of the atlantoaxial joint: a comparison between the Gallie and Brooks fusions. Injury 1993; 24(2):126–128.
17. Hongo M, Shimada Y, Miyakoshi N, et al. Posterior fixation for atlantoaxial instability: a comparison between McGraw's method and Magerl's transarticular screw fixation. 22nd World Congress of SICOT/SIROT, Aug 23–30, 2002. San Diego: Abstract book, 505.
18. Ferlic DC, Clayton ML, Leidholt JD, et al. Surgical treatment of the symptomatic unstable cervical spine in rheumatoid arthritis. J Bone Joint Surg Am 1975; 57(3):349–354.
19. Larsson SE, Toolanen G. Posterior fusion for atlanto-axial subluxation in rheumatoid arthritis. Spine 1986; 11(6):525–530.
20. Thompson RC Jr, Meyer TJ. Posterior surgical stabilization for atlantoaxial subluxation in rheumatoid arthritis. Spine 1985; 10(7):597–601.
21. Naderi S, Crawford NR, Song GS, et al. Biomechanical comparison of C1-C2 posterior fixations. Cable, graft, and screw combinations. Spine 1998; 23(18):1946–1956.
22. Smith MD, Kotzar G, Yoo J, et al. A biomechanical analysis of atlantoaxial stabilization methods using a bovine model. C1/C2 fixation analysis. Clin Orthop Relat Res 1993; 290:285–295.
23. Neo M, Matsushita M, Iwashita Y, et al. Atlantoaxial transarticular screw fixation for a high-riding vertebral artery. Spine 2003; 28(7):666–670.
24. Dickman CA, Sonntag VK. Posterior C1-C2 transarticular screw fixation for atlantoaxial arthrodesis. Neurosurgery 1998; 43(2):275–281.

25. Grob D, Jeanneret B, Aebi M, et al. Atlanto-axial fusion with transarticular screw fixation. J Bone Joint Surg Br 1991; 73(6):972–976.
26. Jeanneret B. Posterior transarticular screw fixation of C1-C2. Tech Orthop 1994; 9:49–59.
27. Madawi AA, Casey AT, Solanki GA, et al. Radiological and anatomical evaluation of the atlantoaxial transarticular screw fixation technique. J Neurosurg 1997; 86(6):961–968.
28. Stillerman CB, Wilson JA. Atlanto-axial stabilization with posterior transarticular screw fixation: Technical description and report of 22 cases. Neurosurgery 1993; 32(6):948–955.
29. Hajek PD, Lipka J, Hartline P, et al. Biomechanical study of C1-C2 posterior arthrodesis techniques. Spine 1993; 18(2):173–177.
30. Hanson PB, Montesano PX, Sharkey NA, et al. Anatomic and biomechanical assessment of transarticular screw fixation for atlantoaxial instability. Spine 1991; 16(10):1141–1145.
31. Mitchell TC, Sadasivan KK, Ogden AL, et al. Biomechanical study of atlantoaxial arthrodesis: Transarticular screw fixation versus modified Brooks posterior wiring. J Orthop Trauma 1999; 13(7):483–489.
32. Eleraky MA, Masferrer R, Sonntag VK. Posterior atlantoaxial facet screw fixation in rheumatoid arthritis. J Neurosurg 1998; 89(1):8–12.
33. Haid RW Jr, Subach BR, McLaughlin MR, et al. C1-C2 transarticular screw fixation for atlantoaxial instability: a 6-year experience. Neurosurgery 2001; 49(1):65–70.
34. Silveri CP, Vaccaro AR. Posterior atlantoaxial fixation: The Magerl screw technique. Orthopedics 1998; 21(4):455–459.
35. Yoshimoto H, Ito M, Abumi K, et al. A retrospective radiographic analysis of subaxial sagittal alignment after posterior C1-C2 fusion. Spine 2004; 29(2):175–181.
36. Coric D, Branch CL Jr., Wilson JA, et al. Arteriovenous fistula as a complication of C1-2 transarticular screw fixation: Case report and review of the literature. J Neurosurg 1996; 85(2):340–343.
37. Gebhard JS, Schimmer RC, Jeanneret B. Safety and accuracy of transarticular screw fixation C1-C2 using an aiming device: An anatomic study. Spine 1998; 23(20):2185–2189.
38. Madawi AA, Solanki G, Casey AT, et al. Variation of the groove in the axis vertebra for the vertebral artery: Implications for instrumentation. J Bone Joint Surg Br 1997; 79(5):820–823.
39. Paramore CG, Dickman CA, Sonntag VK. The anatomical suitability of the C1-2 complex for transarticular screw fixation. J Neurosurg 1996; 85(2):221–224.
40. Wright NM, Lauryssen C. Vertebral artery injury in C1-2 transarticular screw fixation: results of a survey of the AANS/CNS section on disorders of the spine and peripheral nerves. American Association of Neurological Surgeons/Congress of Neurological Surgeons. J Neurosurg 1998; 88(4):634–640.
41. Apfelbaum RI. Screw fixation of the upper cervical spine: Indications and techniques. Contemp Neurosurg 1994; 16(7):1–8.
42. Weidner A, Wahler M, Chiu ST, et al. Modification of C1-C2 transarticular screw fixation by image-guided surgery. Spine 2000; 25(20):2668–2674.
43. Mandel IM, Kambach BJ, Petersilge CA, et al. Morphologic considerations of C2 isthmus dimensions for the placement of transarticular screws. Spine 2000; 25(12):1542–1547.
44. Goel A, Gupta S. Vertebral artery injury with transarticular screws. J Neurosurg 1999; 90(2):376-377.
45. Bloch O, Holly LT, Park J, et al. Effect of frameless stereotaxy on the accuracy of C1-2 transarticular screw placement. J Neurosurg 2001; 95(1 Suppl):74–79.
46. Song GS, Theodore N, Dickman CA, et al. Unilateral posterior atlantoaxial transarticular screw fixation. J Neurosurg 1997; 87(6):851–855.
47. Fuji T, Oda T, Kato Y, Fujita S, Tanaka M. Accuracy of atlantoaxial transarticular screw insertion. Spine 2000; 25(14):1760–1764.
48. Resnick DK, Benzel EC. C1-C2 pedicle screw fixation with rigid cantilever beam construct: case report and technical note. Neurosurgery 2002; 50(2):426–428.
49. Goel A, Laheri V. Plate and screw fixation for atlanto-axial subluxation. Acta Neurochir(Wien) 1994; 129(1-2):47–53.
50. Goel A, Desai KI, Muzumdar DP. Atlantoaxial fixation using plate and screw method: A report of 160 treated patients. Neurosurgery 2002; 51(6):1351–1357.
51. Kuroki H, Rengachary SS, Goel VK, et al. Biomechanical comparison of two stabilization techniques of the atlantoaxial joints: Transarticular screw fixation versus screw and rod fixation. Neurosurgery 2005; 56(1 Suppl):151–159.

Index

9 780367 389499